GESUNDHEITSSYSTEMFORSCHUNG

Herausgegeben von W. van Eimeren und B. Horisberger

F. W. Schwartz B. Badura J. G. Brecht
W. Hofmann K.-H. Jöckel A. Trojan (Hrsg.)

Public health

Texte zu Stand und Perspektiven
der Forschung

Redaktionelle Mitarbeit:
M. Klein-Lange und B. P. Robra

Mit 23 Abbildungen und 61 Tabellen

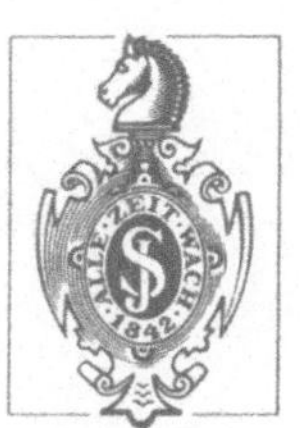

Springer-Verlag

Berlin Heidelberg New York
London Paris Tokyo
Hong Kong Barcelona Budapest

Prof. Dr. Friedrich Wilhelm Schwartz
Dipl. Soz. wiss. Werner Hofmann
Abteilung Epidemiologie und Sozialmedizin, Medizinische
Hochschule Hannover,
Konstanty-Gutschow-Str. 8, 3000 Hannover 61

Prof. Dr. Bernhard Badura
Institut für Soziologie, Technische Universität Berlin,
Dovestr. 1, 1000 Berlin 10

Dr. Josef Georg Brecht
Institut für Gesundheits-System-Forschung,
Weimarer Str. 8, 2300 Kiel-Wik

Priv.-Doz. Dr. Karl-Heinz Jöckel
Bremer Institut für Praventionsforschung und Sozialmedizin,
Abteilung Biometrie und EDV,
St.-Jürgen-Str. 1, 2800 Bremen

Prof. Dr. Dr. Alf Trojan
Institut für Medizin-Soziologie, Universität Hamburg,
Martinistr. 52, 2000 Hamburg 20

ISBN-13: 978-3-540-53185-2   **e-ISBN-13: 978-3-642-84312-9**
DOI: 10.1007/ 978-3-642-84312-9

Satz. Fotosatz-Service Kohler, Wurzburg
19/3140-5 4 3 2 1 0 – Gedruckt auf saurefreiem Papier

Vorwort

Zur Problematik des Begriffs Public health

Der Begriff „Public health", wie er insbesondere durch die
Geschichte, die Arbeitsweisen und die Arbeitsergebnisse der
amerikanischen „Schools of Public Health" geprägt ist, läßt sich
nicht ohne Probleme unmittelbar ins Deutsche übertragen. Die
direkte deutsche Entsprechung, „öffentliche Gesundheit" oder
„öffentliche Gesundheitspflege" muß sich, jedenfalls im bundesdeutschen Sprachraum, mit einer Konnotation des Teilbegriffs
„öffentlich" auseinandersetzen, der in unserem Sprach- und
Politikverständnis immer noch mit hoheitlicher Staatstätigkeit
verbunden ist, geprägt von einem geschichtlichen Vorverständnis,
das in der Medizinalpolizei Preußens (und anderer deutscher
Territorialstaaten) wurzelt und die Geschichtserfahrung des Dritten Reiches zu verarbeiten hat.

Die tatsächlichen, unter Public health zu lösenden Aufgaben
liegen in der Analyse, Bewertung und Organisation von Ursachen,
Entwicklungen und Maßnahmen, die die Gesundheit der Bevölkerung oder zumindest großer Bevölkerungsgruppen betreffen.
Dabei können, aber müssen nicht Staatstätigkeiten berührt werden. Zentral ist vielmehr die Idee des Bevölkerungsbezugs. Die
Deutsche Gesellschaft für Sozialmedizin und Prävention hat daher
als Übersetzung für „Public health" 1987 die Begriffe „Bevölkerungsmedizin und Gesundheitspflege" vorgeschlagen und eine
entsprechende Arbeitsgemeinschaft zur Vorbereitung von deutschen universitären Postgraduiertenstudiengängen nach dem Vorbild der „Schools of Public Health" gebildet.

Multidisziplinarität

Eine weitere, im deutschen Sprachraum bislang allenfalls in ersten
Ansätzen verwirklichte Besonderheit des nordamerikanischen
„Public-health"-Modells liegt in seiner strikten Multidisziplinarität. Während im individual-medizinisch orientierten Gesundheitswesen die biologisch-naturwissenschaftlich geprägte Medizin alleinige Leitwissenschaft ist, treten im sozialen Raum von Gesundheit

und Gesundheitswesen sozial- und verhaltensorientierte, ferner
ökonomische Leitwissenschaften hinzu. Dies hat vielfach, v. a.
wiederum in Nordamerika, zur Bildung eigenständiger „Schools
of Public Health" beigetragen, ein Modell, dessen akademische
Übertragbarkeit auf die Bundesrepublik Deutschland strittig ist,
ohne daß damit zugleich der Grundsatz der Multidisziplinarität in
Frage gestellt wäre.

Akademische Neubelebung von „Public health" in der Bundesrepublik Deutschland

Die gegenwärtig als kritisch erlebten Grenzen einer sich allein auf
das Individuum konzentrierenden Medizin, die relative Hilflosigkeit gegenüber verbreiteten Gesundheitsrisiken in der Bevölkerung
und Finanzierungs- und Organisationskrisen unseres Gesundheitswesens haben zu einem neu belebten Interesse an Public health
in mehreren Industriestaaten, so auch in der Bundesrepublik,
geführt.

Diese öffentlich diskutierten Ideen, unterstützt durch Ver-
öffentlichungen in führenden deutschen Tageszeitungen zu diesem
Problembereich, durch Stellungnahmen aus dem Kreise des
„Sachverständigenrates für die Konzertierte Aktion" beim Bundesministerium für Arbeit und Sozialordnung in seinen Gutachten
(Sachverständigenrat 1987, 1988) zu Bestandsaufnahme und Perspektive des bundesdeutschen Gesundheitswesens, ferner durch
Stellungnahmen des Wissenschaftlichen Beirates der Bundesärztekammer (Vorstand und Wissenschaftlicher Beirat 1989) und des
Bundesgesundheitsrates (Bundesgesundheitsrat 1989), haben zu
einer Reihe sich rasch entwickelnder Aktivitäten in verschiedenen
universitären und nichtuniversitären Einrichtungen in der Bundesrepublik geführt.

Die ohne Hochschulanbindung arbeitenden Akademien für
das öffentliche Gesundheitswesen in München und Düsseldorf
haben Erweiterungen ihrer Ausbildungsprogramme vorgelegt
(1987/1988), teilweise mit dem Ziel (Düsseldorf), einen dem Magi-
sterabschluß (MPH) der amerikanischen „Schools of Public
Health" vergleichbaren Abschluß für deutsche Ärzte zu ermöglichen. Allerdings konzentriert sich diese Ausbildung auf Ärzte
für den öffentlichen Gesundheitsdienst in der Bundesrepublik
Deutschland. Sie beschränken sich damit auf zwar wichtige, aber
nur einen Ausschnitt unseres pluralistischen Gesundheitswesens
berührende Aufgaben.

Getragen durch mehrere Fachbereiche unter Federführung der
soziologischen Fakultät hat die Universität Bielefeld zum
Sommersemester 1989 einen Zusatzstudiengang zum „Diplom-
Gesundheitswissenschaftler" eingerichtet, der Absolventen ver-

schiedener Grundstudiengänge offen steht. In Bochum (seit 1987) und München seit (1988) werden Vorbereitungen zur Etablierung eines Zusatzstudienganges zur Erlangung eines Diploms in „Epidemiologie" getroffen. Epidemiologie bildet eine der wichtigen methodischen Grundlagenwissenschaften im Bereich Public health. Auch die Universität Düsseldorf bereitet einen Studiengang „Gesundheitswissenschaften und Sozialmedizin" vor, der allerdings nur Medizinern zugänglich sein soll. Noch deutlicher auf soziale Leitwissenschaften des Gesundheitswesens und der bevölkerungsbezogenen Gesundheitsförderung hin orientierte Bemühungen werden in Berlin durch die Technische Universität (Institut für Soziologie) verfolgt. Am bestehenden „Zentrum für Öffentliche Gesundheitspflege" in der Medizinischen Hochschule Hannover hat im Herbst 1990 im Ergänzungsstudiengang „Bevölkerungsmedizin und Gesundheitswesen" mit den Wahlschwerpunkten „Management im Gesundheitswesen", „präventive Dienste und Gesundheitsförderung" und „Epidemiologie" (für unterschiedliche Grundstudiengänge) der Studienbetrieb begonnen. Überlegungen zur akademischen Etablierung entsprechender Studiengänge sind ferner aus Hamburg, Marburg und Ulm bekannt. Diese Aufzählung kann bereits bei ihrer Drucklegung überholt sein.

Zur Lage der Forschung

Die Dynamik in der (Re)etablierung einer akademischen Lehre in Public health ist Ausdruck der Überzeugung, daß bevölkerungsmedizinische und auf das Gesundheitswesen als funktionales Ganzes bezogene Fragestellungen bislang in der Bundesrepublik vernachlässigt wurden. Dies gilt gleichsinnig für die Forschung.

Die skizzierten Initiativen greifen jedoch alle nur einen wichtigen Aspekt des in der Bundesrepublik bestehenden Nachholbedarfs auf, den der Lehre. Vernachlässigt sind bislang Bestandsaufnahmen zum Stand und zur Förderung der Forschung in den genannten Aufgabengebieten. Dies ist nicht nur eine unerläßliche Voraussetzung für eine anspruchsvolle akademische Lehre, sondern eine Notwendigkeit aus eigenem Recht. Eine Bestandsaufnahme zur einschlägigen Forschung der Gesellschaft für Strahlen- und Umwelt-Forschung, München (Klein-Lange 1990), zeigt, daß in der Bundesrepublik an vielen, aber nach Zielsetzung, Arbeitsweise und Organisation kaum verbundenen Stellen gesundheitssystembezogene oder bevölkerungsmedizinische Forschungsfelder bearbeitet werden.

Insbesondere durch das Fehlen einer langfristigen, zielorientierten, auf den kontinuierlichen Aufbau einer leistungsfähigen wissenschaftlichen Infrastruktur abzielenden Forschungsförderung sind die Arbeiten in der Regel miteinander wenig verbunden und episodisch angelegt. Die Zuständigkeit nach Fachgesellschaften ist zersplittert; nur teilweise bestehen gemeinsame Arbeitsgruppen (Arbeitsgruppen „Epidemiologie" und „Umweltmedizin" der Deutschen Gesellschaft für Sozialmedizin und Prävention und der Deutschen Gesellschaft für Medizinische Dokumentation, Informatik und Statistik).

In den Bewertungsgremien der öffentlichen Forschungsförderung bestehen vielfach noch Unsicherheiten hinsichtlich der Gegenstände, der Methoden und der qualitativen Standards entsprechender Forschungsarbeiten. Auch die Deutsche Forschungsgemeinschaft befaßt sich inzwischen (1990) mit der Überprüfung dieser Forschungslandschaft mit der Überzeugung, daß es hier forschungspolitischer Impulse bedarf. Bei Redaktionsschluß lag eine Entscheidung über die Etablierung eines entsprechenden Förderbereichs noch nicht vor. Diese Entwicklung unterstreicht die wachsende forschungspolitische Bedeutung der in diesem Reader vorgestellten Thematik.

Aufgabenstellung des Readers

Im Herbst 1988 hat das zuständige Referat im Bundesforschungsministerium an ein Mitglied des Herausgeberkreises die Anregung gegeben, einen Reader zusammenzustellen, der wichtige Forschungsfelder im Bereich von Public health an exemplarischen deutschen Arbeitsbeispielen den an Forschungsfragen und Forschungsförderung in diesen Gebieten grundsätzlich Interessierten vorstellen und einen Einblick in Thematik und Arbeitsweise vermitteln soll. Angesichts des gegenwärtigen Mangels an deutscher Public-health-Literatur in einem größeren thematischen Zusammenhang ist dieser Reader auch geeignet, Studenten und Praktikern dieses Gebietes einen Überblick und zugleich eine für Studium und Unterricht nutzbare, anderweitig nur schwer zugängliche Stoffsammlung zu geben.

Die Herausgeber wollten weder Vollständigkeit in den Gegenständen noch in den Forschungsmethoden anstreben. Die Einführungen zu den einzelnen Forschungsfeldern sind überwiegend knapp gehalten, wenn die ausgewählten Arbeiten für sich selbst sprechen. Die Angabe von weiterführender Literatur zu jedem Forschungsfeld soll zum Selbststudium anregen.

Herrn Dr. Buschbeck und Herrn Hocks vom BMFT gilt für ihre Anregungen und tätige Unterstützung bei diesem Projekt der besondere Dank der Herausgeber.

Literatur

Bundesgesundheitsrat (1989) Votum vom 13. April 1989 zur Verwirklichung
    der Einzelziele der WHO-Strategie „Gesundheit 2000" in der Bundesrepu-
    blik Deutschland. Bundesgesundheitsblatt 7:277–281
Klein-Lange M (1990) Public-Health-Forschung in der Bundesrepublik, hrsgg.
    v. Gesellschaft für Strahlen- und Umweltforschung München, Pro-
    jektträger Gesundheitsforschung, München
Laaser U, Wolters P, Kaufmann FX (Hrsg) (1990) Gesundheitswissenschaften
    und öffentliche Gesundheitsförderung. Aktuelle Modelle für eine Public-
    health-Ausbildung in der Bundesrepublik Deutschland. Springer, Berlin
    Heidelberg New York Tokyo
Sachverständigenrat (1987) für die Konzertierte Aktion im Gesundheitswesen:
    Medizinische und ökonomische Orientierung (Jahresgutachten 1987).
    Nomos, Baden-Baden
Sachverständigenrat (1988) für die Konzertierte Aktion im Gesundheitswesen:
    Medizinische und ökonomische Orientierung (Jahresgutachten 1988).
    Nomos, Baden-Baden
Vorstand und Wissenschaftlicher Beirat der Bundesärztekammer (1989)
    Weiterentwicklung des Gesundheitswesens: Postgraduiertenstudium „Öf-
    fentliche Gesundheit (Public Health)". Dtsch Ärztebl 86/14:39–41 (B-723-
    B-725)

Inhaltsverzeichnis

II Ausgewählte Texte zu speziellen Anwendungsfeldern ... 239

Autorenverzeichnis

Ahrens, Günther, Prof. Dr.
Zahn-, Mund- und Kieferklinik,
Universitätskrankenhaus Eppendorf,
Martinistr. 52, 2000 Hamburg 20

Ahrens, Wolfgang, Dipl.-Biologe
Bremer Institut für Präventionsforschung und Sozialmedizin,
St.-Jürgen-Str. 1, 2800 Bremen

Andersen, Hanfried H., Dr.
FS Marktprozeß und Unternehmensentwicklung,
Wissenschaftszentrum für Sozialforschung,
Reichspietschufer 50, 1000 Berlin 30

Badura, Bernhard, Prof. Dr.
Institut für Soziologie, Technische Universität Berlin,
Dovestr. 1, 1000 Berlin 10

Birkner, Barbara, Dr.
Fachbereich Volkswirtschaftslehre,
Universität der Bundeswehr München,
Werner-Heisenberg-Weg 39, 8014 Neubiberg

Brecht, Josef Georg, Dr.
Institut für Gesundheits-System-Forschung,
Weimarer Str. 8, 2300 Kiel-Wik

Cooper, Brian, Prof. Dr.
Abteilung Epidemiologische Psychiatrie,
Zentralinstitut für Seelische Gesundheit,
Postfach 5970, 6800 Mannheim 1

Deutsche Herz-Kreislauf-Präventionsstudie
c/o Dr. H. Kreuter
Wissenschaftliches Institut der Ärzte Deutschlands,
Godesberger Allee 54, 5300 Bonn 2

Eckart, Wolfgang U., Prof. Dr.
Abteilung Geschichte der Medizin,
Medizinische Hochschule Hannover,
Konstanty-Gutschow-Str. 8, 3000 Hannover 61

Ferber, Christian von, Prof. Dr.
Institut für Medizinische Soziologie, Universität Düsseldorf,
Moorenstr. 5, 4000 Düsseldorf 1

Frentzel-Beyme, Rainer, Dr.
Deutsches Krebsforschungszentrum,
Im Neuenheimer Feld 280, 6900 Heidelberg

Gitter, Wolfgang, Prof. Dr.
Lehrstuhl für Zivilrecht, Arbeits- und Sozialrecht,
Universität Bayreuth,
Universitätsstr. 30, 8580 Bayreuth

Henke, Klaus-Dirk, Prof. Dr.
Abteilung Öffentliche Finanzen, Universität Hannover,
Färberstr. 10, 3000 Hannover 91

Hofmann, Werner, Dipl. Soz. wiss.
Abteilung Epidemiologie und Sozialmedizin,
Medizinische Hochschule Hannover,
Konstanty-Gutschow-Str. 8, 3000 Hannover 61

Huerkamp, Claudia, Dr.
Fakultät für Geschichte und Philosophie, Universität Bielefeld,
Universitätsstr. 25, 4800 Bielefeld

Jöckel, Karl-Heinz, Priv.-Doz. Dr.
Bremer Institut für Präventionsforschung und Sozialmedizin,
Abteilung Biometrie und EDV,
Grünenstr. 120, 2800 Bremen 1

Kaufmann, Franz-Xaver, Prof. Dr.
Institut für Bevölkerungsforschung und Sozialpolitik,
Universität Bielefeld,
Universitätsstr. 25, 4800 Bielefeld

Kirchberger, Stefan, Priv.-Doz. Dr.
Institut für Medizinische Soziologie,
Westfälische Wilhelms-Universität,
Domagkstr. 3, 4400 Münster

Leber, Wulf-D.
Sachverständigenrat für die
Konzertierte Aktion im Gesundheitswesen,
Lengsdorfer Hauptstr. 31, 5300 Bonn 1

Leidl, Reiner, Dr.
Institut für Medizinische Informatik
und Systemforschung (MEDIS),
GSF-Forschungszentrum für Umwelt und Gesundheit, GmbH
Ingolstädter Landstr. 1, 8042 Neuherberg

Müller, Wolfgang, Dr.
Akademie für öffentliches Gesundheitswesen,
Auf'm Hennekamp 70, 4000 Düsseldorf 1

Radebold, Hartmut, Prof. Dr.
Gesamthochschule Kassel,
Postfach 101380, 3500 Kassel

Raspe, Hans-Heinrich, Prof. Dr. Dr.
Institut für Sozialmedizin, Medizinische Universität zu Lübeck,
Sophienstr. 3–5, 2400 Lübeck 1

Redaktionskomitee der
Forschungsgruppe Gesundheitsberichterstattung
c/o Dr. J. G. Brecht
Institut für Gesundheits-System-Forschung
Weimarer Str. 8, 2300 Kiel-Wik

Robra, Bernt-Peter, Dr., MPH
Abteilung Epidemiologie und Sozialmedizin,
Medizinische Hochschule Hannover,
Konstanty-Gutschow-Str. 8, 3000 Hannover 61

Schach, Elisabeth, Dipl.-Volkswirtin, M. Sc.
Rechenzentrum, Universität Dortmund,
Postfach 500500, 4600 Dortmund 50

Schwartz, Friedrich Wilhelm, Prof. Dr.
Abteilung Epidemiologie und Sozialmedizin,
Medizinische Hochschule Hannover,
Konstanty-Gutschow-Str. 8, 3000 Hannover 61

Schwefel, Detlef, Prof. Dr.
Institut für Medizinische Informatik und Systemforschung
(MEDIS),
GSF-Forschungszentrum für Umwelt und Gesundheit, GmbH,
Ingolstädter Landstr. 1, 8042 Neuherberg

Selbmann, Hans-Konrad, Prof. Dr.
Institut für Medizinische Informationsverarbeitung,
Westbahnhofstr. 55, 7400 Tübingen

Trojan, Alf, Prof. Dr. Dr.
Institut für Medizin-Soziologie, Universität Hamburg,
Martinistr. 52, 2000 Hamburg 20

Troschke, Jürgen von, Prof. Dr.
Abteilung für Medizinische Soziologie,
Albert-Ludwigs-Universität,
Stefan-Meier-Str. 17, 7800 Freiburg

Wahrendorf, Jürgen, Prof. Dr.
Deutsches Krebsforschungszentrum,
Institut für Epidemiologie und Biometrie,
Im Neuenheimer Feld 280, 6900 Heidelberg

Waltz, Millard, Lic. oec.
Institut für Soziologie, Technische Universität Berlin,
Dovestr. 1, 1000 Berlin 10

Wichmann, Heinz-Erich, Prof. Dr. Dr.
Arbeitssicherheit und Umweltmedizin, Bergische Universität–
Gesamthochschule Wuppertal,
Gauss-Str. 20, 5600 Wuppertal

I Ausgewählte Texte zu Grundlagendisziplinen

Einleitung

Die *Epidemiologie* beschäftigt sich mit der Verteilung von Krankheiten und deren Determinanten in Gruppen von Menschen. Im Zentrum des Interesses stehen damit im Unterschied zur klinischen Medizin nicht ein oder wenige Individuen, sondern eine oder mehrere Populationen. Neben der Deskription wird und wurde in vielen epidemiologischen Studien ein Beitrag zur Ätiologie von Krankheiten geleistet, indem die Epidemiologie sich nicht nur der Ergebnisse der medizinischen und biologischen Wissenschaften bedient, sondern selber mögliche Zusammenhänge aufzeigt und/oder aufgrund gefundener Auffälligkeiten Hinweise für die weitere Forschung gibt, z. B. Karzinogenität von Tabakrauch oder Asbest oder der Zusammenhang von Ernährung und Krebserkrankung. Dieses Thema spricht der Beitrag von Wahrendorf an. Neben dieser eher „biologisch" orientierten Epidemiologie gewinnen immer mehr Ansätze an Gewicht, die Krankheit und Krankheitsursachen im Zusammenspiel mit sozialen Faktoren verstehen und analysieren. Dieser „Sozialepidemiologie" ist der Beitrag von Waltz et al. zuzuordnen. Er wendet das theoretische und methodische Instrumentarium der modernen Sozialepidemiologie auf die Analyse der Bewältigung eines Herzinfarkts an.

Eine weitere wichtige Entwicklung betrifft die Methodenlehre, die sich in immer stärkerem Maß der Biometrie, und dort v. a. der angewandten Statistik bedient. Obwohl die Epidemiologie nicht als Methodenwissenschaft (miß)verstanden werden darf, spielen methodische, insbesondere biometrische Aspekte eine prominente Rolle: von der adäquaten Planung und der Modellwahl bis zur biometrisch-statistischen Auswertung wird die wissenschaftliche Qualität einer Studie auch und vor allem durch die biometrische Methodik bestimmt. Dabei besteht eine gegenseitige Beeinflussung und Befruchtung von Biometrie und Epidemiologie. Dieser Zusammenhang wird im Beitrag von Wahrendorf deutlich am Beispiel der Weiterentwicklung des Konzepts des zuschreibbaren Risikos („attributable risk").

Die *Medizinsoziologie* ist für Public health insofern von besonderer Bedeutung, als sie Beiträge sowohl zum Thema Gesellschaft und Gesundheit wie auch zur Analyse von Versorgungseinrichtungen liefert. Die Ergebnisse der Medizinsoziologie sind von praktischer Relevanz sowohl für Prävention und Gesundheitsförderung als auch für die Anpassung des Gesundheitswesens an den sozialen Wandel. Der Beitrag von Badura et al. gibt einen Überblick über Forschungsgegenstände und Fragestellung der Medizinsoziologie.

Präventivmedizin befaßt sich mit Ursachen und fördernden bzw. hemmenden Determinanten für Auftreten und Verbreitung von Krankheiten, funktionalen

Behinderungen und vorzeitigem Tode und mit den Bedingungen der erfolgreichen Umsetzung ihrer Ergebnisse in bevölkerungsbezogenen Anwendungen. Der Beitrag der Deutschen Herz-Kreislauf-Präventionsstudie (The German Cardiovascular Prevention Study (GCP)) behandelt primär präventive bevölkerungsweite Ansätze bei der Bekämpfung kardiovaskulärer Erkrankungen. Der Beitrag Schwartz und Robra befaßt sich mit sekundär präventiven (d. h. auf Verhütung klinischer Manifestationen früher Krankheitsstadien zielenden) Maßnahmen und der Beitrag Birkner und Neubauer mit Rahmenbedingungen am Beispiel der Privathaushalte.

Die *Gesundheitsökonomie* untersucht den Einsatz und die Verwendung (knapper) Ressourcen und ihre ökonomischen Wirkungen im Gesundheitswesen. Der Beitrag von Andersen und Schulenburg gibt eine Übersicht zu Forschungsfragen und Gegenständen. Der Beitrag von Henke befaßt sich mit der Finanzierung des Ressourceneinsatzes in der Sozialversicherung aus finanzwissenschaftlicher Sicht. Leidl liefert einen Beitrag zur ökonomischen Bewertung von Produktionsleistungen im Krankenhaus.

Gesundheitspolitik ist in der Bundesrepublik Deutschland in der akademischen Forschung nicht als eigenständige Disziplin etabliert. Sowohl von der Politik und Sozialwissenschaft als auch neuerdings der Sozialmedizin und der Ökonomie sind dazu Beiträge geliefert worden. Der Beitrag von Robra befaßt sich aus sozialmedizinischer Sicht mit Inhalt und Voraussetzungen für Gesundheitsziele als einem Mittel der Gesundheitspolitik. Der Beitrag von Leber stellt aus ökonomischer Sicht ein sozialpolitisches Forschungsthema dar.

Auch *Verwaltung und Recht im Gesundheitswesen* haben trotz ihres hohen empirischen Gewichts bislang keine eigenständige akademische Präsenz. Die Arbeit von Gitter liefert aus sozialrechtlicher Perspektive einen Beitrag zur rechtlichen Bewertung von Finanzierungsalternativen in der Krankenversicherung.

Die *historische Analyse des Gesundheitswesens* ist wesentlicher Teil einer Public-health-Perspektive. Huerkamp befaßt sich mit den historischen Entstehungsbedingungen der Gesetzlichen Krankenversicherung im Deutschen Reich, Eckart mit der Entwicklung der öffentlichen Gesundheitspflege in der Weimarer Zeit und der Frühphase der Bundesrepublik Deutschland.

1 Epidemiologie und Biometrie

An Estimate of the Proportion of Colorectal and Stomach Cancers Which Might Be Prevented by Certain Changes in Dietary Habits*

J. Wahrendorf

Introduction

The role of life-style risk factors in cancer etiology is difficult to quantify, and estimates presented so far differ appreciably (Wynder and Gori 1977; Higginson and Muir 1979; Doll and Peto 1981). The uncertainties behind these estimates expressed by wide ranges of acceptable estimates are substantial. For example, Doll and Peto (1981) give 35% as the best estimate of the proportion of cancer deaths in the United States which could be attributed to diet, with acceptable estimates ranging from 10% to 70%. These figures appear to be derived from comparing cancer mortality figures in different populations, and the role diet may play in cancer etiology is supported by detailed mechanistic considerations. However, concrete reference to figures derived from specific epidemiological studies cannot be found.

Such estimates are generally based on the concept of attributable risk which is defined as the rate of disease in exposed individuals that can be attributed to exposure (MacMahon and Pugh 1970) and can be estimated under certain circumstances both from cohort studies and from case-control studies (Schlesselmann 1982; Breslow and Day 1980). As there has occasionally been confusion about the precise definition, we define below what we shall refer to as "population attributable risk" (AR). Let Π_0 and Π_1 be the overall incidence or mortality rates for the nonexposed and exposed subgroups, respectively, $r = \Pi_1/\Pi_0$ the relative risk, and p the proportion of subjects in the population exposed to the risk factor, then $AR = [p(\Pi_1 - \Pi_0)]/[p\Pi_1 + (1-p)\Pi_0] = p(r-1)/[p(r-1)+1]$.

The concept of attributable risk is a simple and useful one putting epidemiological observations into a public health context. Knowledge is required of p, the proportion of subjects in the population who are exposed to the factor of interest. This points to two limitations. First, in case-control studies, the proportion of exposed persons in the control series is often considered as an estimate of p although this generalization to the underlying population is not always fully justified. Second, and probably most important, the majority of exposures of interest are not simply dichotomous – absent or present – but are assessed on a metric or ordinal scale. Frequently, a continuous exposure measure is categorized into three, four, or more ordered categories. This is, for example, the case for intake of foods or nutrients for which categorization depends on the dietary method used in collecting information and convenience of analysis.

---

* First published in *International Journal of Cancer* (1987) 10:625–628.

In this report we shall outline a method of calculating a parameter similar to the population attributable risk which can be applied when exposure is given in ordered categories and when changes in population exposure are modeled accordingly. This approach will be applied to studies on stomach and colorectal cancer to derive an estimate of what proportion of these cancers might be preventable if populations were to alter their dietary habits.

Material and Methods

Preventable Proportion

Consider that a risk factor is prevalent at $K + 1$ ordered levels, the proportions of the population being exposed to it being $p_0, p_1, \ldots, p_K$ which may be considered as a $(K + 1) -$ vector p. The associated relative risks may be $r_0 = 1.0, r_1, \ldots, r_K$, again denoted as a vector, r.

Consider that an intervention alters the population exposure distribution p into another exposure p^*, say, with proportions $p_0^*, p_1^*, \ldots, p_K^*$. The change from p to p^* may for the moment be completely arbitrary; examples will be discussed later. The proportion of risk removed by this change in exposure distribution is

$$PP = \frac{\sum_{i=0}^{K} p_i r_i - \sum_{i=0}^{K} p_i^* r_i}{\sum_{i=0}^{K} p_i r_i}$$

where PP stands for preventable proportion.

An artificial example may help in understanding this concept. In Table 1 we consider the situation in which the relative risks in the middle and upper thirds of a population are 2.0 and 4.0, respectively. A shift to situation (a) reduces the population risk by 14%, even a change to (b) results in a small gain, but clearer effects are seen with shifts (c) and (d).

Table 1. Preventable proportion of different shifts of an exposure distribution (artificial example)

					PP
	p:	0.33	0 33	0.33	
	r:	1.0	2 0	4.0	
(a)	p^*:	0 5	0.25	0.25	14%
(b)	p^*:	0 6	0	0 4	5 6%
(c)	p^*:	0 6	0 4	0	39.9%
(d)	p^*:	0.5	0.5	0	35.8%
(e)	p^*:	0.666	0.333	0	43%
(f)	p^*:	0.3666	0.333	0.3	4.3%

Shift of Exposure

The change from p to p^* can be modeled completely arbitrarily. However, it is useful to consider simple parametrizations of such a shift which represent reasonable assumptions of how a population might change its exposure distribution. For this purpose we consider that in each exposure category above the baseline category a certain proportion, $s\%$, of individuals might change down into the next exposure category. This is exemplified in (e) and (f) of Table 1. In the situation (e) 100% change downward, whereas in (f) only 10% are considered to change downward. The preventable proportion is in this case a linear function of the shifting proportion s:

$$PP_s = s \frac{\sum_{i=1}^{K} p_i(r_i - r_{i-1})}{\sum_{i=0}^{K} p_i r_i}$$

This shifting model appears to represent a reasonable intermediate description of what may happen in a population when measures of primary prevention are implemented.

Results

We subsequently apply this method to a selected number of case-control studies on diet and colorectal cancer or stomach cancer. The results are summarized in Table 2. For each study we indicate the site examined and whether the data refer to both sexes jointly or one sex only. A brief term for the factor under consideration is given and will be explained in the respective text. The data listed include, for the different ordered factor levels, starting on the left with the baseline category, the proportion (p) of controls exposed to the respective levels of the factor, the relative risks (r) associated with these levels, the estimated proportions (p^*) of the population exposed to the various levels after a shift of $s = 100\%$ or $s = 50\%$ of the population from each above baseline category to the next one down and, finally, the corresponding preventable proportion PP_s. Note that the number of levels considered for a factor can differ from study to study depending on the categorization used.

The first example given in Table 2 is the case-control study on diet and colorectal cancer reported by Jain et al. (1980). The authors consider three categories of consumption of saturated fat and use neighborhood controls to estimate the population prevalence of exposure. Applying the 100% shift model of change in exposure distribution would lead to a 24% reduction in risk in males, whereas in females, for whom the categories are chosen with different cut-off points and the relative risk estimates are larger, the reduction would be 37%. In both cases the reduction would be half as much in the case of 50% of the population in consumption levels above the baseline category shifting to the next category down.

Table 2. Preventable proportion (PP_s) for specific risk factors identified in case-control studies on colorectal cancer and stomach cancer

Study	Site/Sex	Factor	p, r, p^*					s	PP_s
Jain et al. (1980)	Colon and rectum, males	Saturated fat	p: 0.39	0.31	0.3				
			r: 1.0	2.0	2.3				
			p^*: 0 7	0.3	0			100%	24%
			p^*: 0 545	0.305	0.15			50%	12%
	Colon and rectum, females		p: 0.4	0.35	0.25				
			r: 1.0	1.8	3.5				
			p^*: 0 75	0.25	0			100%	37%
			p^*: 0.575	0 3	0.125			50%	18.5%
Graham et al. (1978)	Colon, males	Cabbage	p: 0.197	0.189	0.202	0.241	0 171		
			r: 1.0	1 78	3.04	2 49	2.98		
			p^*: 0 368	0 202	0.241	0.171	0	100%	15.6%
			p^*: 0 292	0.196	0.222	0.206	0.086	50%	7.8%
	Rectum, males		p: 0.211	0.191	0 205	0.220	0 173		
			r: 1.0	1.36	1.44	1.29	1 53		
			p^*: 0.402	0.205	0.220	0.173	0	100%	7.1%
			p^*: 0.307	0.198	0.213	0.197	0.087	50%	3.6%
Dales et al. (1979)	Colon and rectum, males and females	Fat/fiber	p: 0 223	0.649	0.129				
			r: 1.0	1.37	2.68				
			p^*: 0.872	0.129	0			100%	28.1%
			p^*: 0 548	0.390	0.065			50%	14.1%

Table 2. (continued)

Study	Site/Sex	Factor		p, r, p^*					s	PP_s
Manousos et al. (1983)	Colon and rectum, males and females	Risk score	p:	0.27	0.28	0.27	0.12	0.06		
			r:	1.0	0.6	0.8	3.1	8.0		
			p^*:	0.55	0.27	0.12	0.06	0	100%	34%
			p^*:	0.41	0 275	0.195	0.09	0.03	50%	17%
Trichopoulos et al. (1985)	Stomach, males and females	Risk score	p:	0.38	0 27	0.18	0.09	0.07		
			r:	1.0	4.8	9 3	24.5	40.2		
			p^*:	0.66	0.18	0.09	0.07	0	100%	51%
			p^*:	0.515	0.225	0.135	0.08	0.035	50%	25.5%
Jedrychowski et al. (1986)	Stomach, males and females	Protein score	p:	0.24	0.63	0.14				
			r:	1.0	1 30	4.35				
			p^*:	0.86	0.14	0			100%	37.6%
			p^*:	0 55	0.38	0.07			50%	18.8%
		Vegetable score	p:	0.11	0 64	0.25				
			r:	1.0	0 97	4.23				
			p^*:	0.75	0.25	0			100%	44.9%
			p^*:	0.43	0.44	0.13			50%	22 5%

Graham et al. (1978) report in their hospital-based case-control study significantly increasing gradients in risk for colon and rectum cancer with decreasing frequency of consumption of cabbage. In this example there are four categories above the baseline, and shifting to lower categories would imply less pronounced changes in risk; thus for $s = 100\%$ the preventable proportion is only 15.6% for colon cancer and 7.1% for cancer of the rectum.

Only three categories of fat/fiber consumption are considered in the hospital-based case-control study of Dales et al. (1979) in blacks. Low fat/high fiber represents the baseline, high-fat/low-fiber the third category associated with the highest relative risk. In this example the 100% shift model would consider 64.9% of the population to move into the baseline category, resulting in a risk reduction of 28.1%.

In the hospital-based case-control study of Manousos et al. (1983) from Greece, risk scores were computed on the basis of individuals' consumption of two food items increasing risk (beef and lamb) and three vegetables that appeared to be protective (cabbage or lettuce, spinach, beets). This score was distributed into five categories and resulted in a strong increase in relative risk at the upper end of the risk score scale. In this example, the 100% shift model removes 34% of the risk.

A similar concept was used by the same group (Trichopoulos et al. 1985) reporting on a case-control study of stomach cancer in Greece. A risk score based on nine discriminatory food items provides the picture of a very strong gradient in risk, which, as discussed and investigated subsequently (data not shown), may very well be an exaggeration of reality. However, as only a small proportion of the population can be found in the very high risk categories, under the 100%-shift model about half of the excess risk would be removed and, accordingly, one-quarter under the 50% model.

The final example is derived from a hospital-based case-control study on stomach cancer in Cracow, Poland (Jedrychowski et al. 1986). Two particular risk factors were considered. One was derived as a combination of the reported frequency of consumption of protein-containing foods and showed increased risk with increasing consumption, and the other was based on the consumption of vegetables, salads, and fruits and showed an inverse gradient of risk. For the purpose of this presentation both scores were organized in such a way that the associated risks appeared in increasing order. For both scores the proportion of controls exposed to the middle category where the risk was not elevated (1.30 or 0.97), was dominant; thus, the preventable proportion derived under our shift model reflects mainly what could be expected for alteration of the high-risk exposures (very frequent consumption of protein-containing foods or rare consumption of vegetables, salads, and fruits). As the high-risk exposure in relation to vegetable consumption is more prevalent, the preventable proportion under our shift model is slightly larger in this case (22.5% under the 50% model), compared to the protein score (18.8% under the 50% model).

Discussion

The relative importance of different risk factors in the etiology of cancer is the subject of considerable debate. For some well-defined exposures which are associated with a clearly increased risk and whose population prevalence is well estimated or estimatable, population attributable risks are easily calculated and have led, in particular, to estimates of cancers attributable to occupational risk factors.

As stated above, the situation is not as simple for complex exposures such as diet. There are only two epidemiological studies presenting estimates of attributable risk in this framework. Jain et al. (1980) used data from their case-control study on colorectal cancer to calculate population attributable risk for the consumption of saturated fat. For this purpose they dichotomized the exposure categories using the lowest category as reference, and derived 41 % for males and 44 % for females as population attributable risk for saturated fat. Lower figures were derived using for the same data the concept of preventable proportion under a one-parameter shift model (Table 2).

Another report gives figures on attributable risk of dietary relationships with colorectal cancer. It is based on a cohort study among Seventh-Day Adventists (Philips and Snowdon 1985) and identifies three risk factors (high consumption of coffee and eggs, and overweight) for colorectal cancer within their cohort. Applying prevalence figures of these factors to the US population they conclude that these factors may explain a substantial proportion of the colorectal cancer mortality differential between Adventists and US whites (62 % for males and 30 % for females).

The preventable proportion calculated under a shift model yields lower estimates than the classical attributable risk concept. However, we feel very strongly that the general change of an exposure distribution p into another distribution p^* is much closer to reality than considering that everybody moves to the baseline category associated with no increased risk. The one-parameter shift for the change from p to p^*, although very simple, is felt to be not unrealistic and offers useful interpretations. However, the isolated alteration of a single dietary factor may still represent some simplification, or the lowest risk category in each specific population may not represent the theoretical lowest risk category. Thus, a proportion of individuals in these categories may accomplish an additional reduction in risk by appropriate changes.

It is difficult to foresee which dietary changes are likely to take place in practice. Limited data from some investigations (Møller Jensen et al. 1984) and general experience from nutritional research seem to indicate that the magnitude of dietary changes in a population which are likely to materialize should be judged with extreme caution. In terms of our one-parameter shift model, $s = 50\%$ may be used as a yardstick, i.e., 50 % of the population who currently have dietary habits associated with an increased risk of cancer are considered to change their habits into the next category down associated in general with a lower risk. Looking through the results derived in Table 2 from six different studies, it is gratifying to note that the PP_s estimates are all of the same order of magnitude; for $s = 50\%$ one can conclude that the preventable proportion is about 15 % – 20 %.

Doll and Peto (1981) had estimated that 35 % of all US cancer deaths, and even 90 % of stomach and large-bowel cancers, are attributable to diet. Although our figures of preventable proportion derived from studies on colorectal and stomach cancer are considerably lower, they do not necessarily contradict the high values of attributable risks. They seem, however, to reflect much more exactly the reality of possible achievements of intervention measures in a population. The estimates of preventable proportion refer only to single, well-identified risk factors. It may well be that intervention addressing the totality of diet-related risk factors removes a larger proportion of excess risk, although this should be viewed as a complex process to which the individual factors do not contribute independently. Furthermore, it is unlikely that all diet-related aspects of cancer causation will be identified simultaneously.

The exposure distribution p refers to the population prevalence of the different levels of a risk factor. In most of the studies considered, series of hospital controls were used to derive these estimates. It is difficult to judge whether this may have introduced any substantial bias. If one assumes that the prevalence of the high-risk category may be overestimated, one has also to consider that the relative risk derived from the data of a hospital-based study would in this case be an underestimation. These two individual biases are thus likely to be canceled out in the calculation of the preventable proportion.

The preventable proportion (PP) proposed in this report, which takes into account dose-response information on a single risk factor, can easily be generalized to the multivariate exposure situation. In this case p would represent a multivariate exposure distribution with associated relative risks r, and p^* the resulting distribution after some changes. The change from p to p^* would have to be modeled according to the anticipated changes in exposure to single risk factors as well as their interrelationship.

There is a large body of statistical literature concerning the estimation of attributable risk, including approaches in the direction used here (Walter 1980). Attributable risk may also be estimable using the proportion of exposed cases only (Miettinen 1974), and this was recently incorporated into the context of multivariate analysis (Bruzzi et al. 1985). Our study has emphasized application of the concept of preventable proportion in the field of diet-related cancers. A similar application to cardiovascular risk was given by Deubner et al. (1980).

We conclude that the measure of preventable proportion is a useful generalization of the concept of attributable risk. The impact of moderate changes in exposure prevalence can be assessed by this measure. In particular, exposures occurring on a continuous scale and which are unlikely to experience complete removal can be studied in this framework. Using data from several case-control studies on colorectal and stomach cancer, we point out that changes in specific dietary habits may lead to the elimination of about 15 % – 20 % of the excess incidence. This figure was derived consistently from studies with different designs and conducted in different cultural settings.

Acknowledgements. Part of this work was accomplished when working for the International Agency for Research on Cancer, Lyon, France. This paper is dedicated to Professor Gustav Wagner on the occasion of his 70th birthday.

References

Breslow NE, Day NE (1980) Statistical methods in cancer research, Vol 1: The analysis of case-control studies, IARC Sci Publ 32

Bruzzi P, Green SB, Byar DP, Brinton LA, Schairer C (1985) Estimating the population attributable risk for multiple risk factors using case-control data. Am J Epidemiol 122:904–914

Dales LG, Friedman GD, Ury HK, Grossman S, Williams SR (1979) A case-control study of relationships of diet and other traits to colorectal cancer in american blacks. Am J Epidemiol 109:132–144

Deubner DC, Wilkinson WE, Helms MJ, Tyroler HA, Hames CG (1980) Logistic model estimation of death attributable to risk factors for cardiovascular disease in Evans County, Georgia. Am J Epidemiol 112.135–143

Doll R, Peto R (1981) The causes of cancer JNCI 66·1191–1308

Graham S, Dayal H, Swanson M, Mittelman A, Wilkinson G (1978) Diet in the epidemiology of cancer of the colon and rectum. JNCI 61:709–714

Higginson J, Muir CS (1979) Environmental carcinogenesis: misconceptions and limitations to cancer control. JNCI 63:1291–1298

Jain M, Cook GM, Davis FG, Grace MG, Howe GR, Miller AB (1980) A case-control study of diet and colorectal cancer. Int J Cancer 26:757–768

Jedrychowski W, Wahrendorf J, Popiela T, Rachtan J (1986) A case-control study of dietary factors and stomach cancer risk in Poland. Int J Cancer 37:837–842

MacMahon B, Pugh TF (1976) Epidemiology: principles and methods. Little, Brown, Boston

Manousos O, Day NE, Trichopoulos D, Gerovassilis F, Tzonou A, Polychronopoulou A (1983) Diet and colorectal cancer: a case-control study in Greece. Int J Cancer 32:1–5

Miettinen OS (1974) Proportion of disease caused or prevented by a given exposure, trait or intervention. Am J Epidemiol 99.325–332

Møller Jensen O, Wahrendorf J, Rosenqvist A, Geser A (1984) The reliability of questionnaire-derived historical dietary information and temporal stability of food habits in individuals. Am J Epidemiol 120:281–290

Phillips RL, Snowdon D (1985) Dietary relationships with fatal colorectal cancer among Seventh-Day Adventists JNCI 74:307–317

Schlesselman JJ (1982) Case-control studies. Design, conduct, analysis. Oxford University Press, New York

Trichopoulos D, Ouranos G, Day NE, Tzonou A, Manousos O, Papadimitriou CH, Trichopoulos A (1985) Diet and cancer of the stomach: a case-control study in Greece. Int J Cancer 36:291–297

Walter SD (1980) Prevention for multifactorial diseases. Am J Epidemiol 112:409–416

Wynder EL, Gori GB (1977) Contribution of the environment to cancer incidence: an epidemiologic exercise. JNCI 58:825–832

Marriage and the Psychological Consequences of Heart Attack: A Longitudinal Study of Adaptation to Chronic Illness After 3 Years *

M. Waltz, B. Badura, H. Pfaff, and T. Schott

Introduction

An impressive body of theoretical and empirical literature has been evolving in social epidemiology and other fields of behavioural research on the pivotal role of social factors in human well-being. The social environments of people are considered a salient factor not only as a precursor of disease (Joseph and Syme 1982; Syme and Seeman 1983; Groen 1987) but also as a determinant of subsequent coping behaviour and adjustment to physical illness (Di Matteo and Hays 1981; Cohen and McKay 1983; Finlayson 1976; Young 1983; Pearlin et al. 1981; Cohen and Lazarus 1980; Lazarus and Folkman 1983). Like the Roman god Janus, social factors can have two faces, a health-promoting one and a disease-enhancing one. This is particularly true of the marital environment and its impact during the life-span on subjective well-being, as well as on mental and physical health (Finlayson 1976; Thoits 1983; Diener 1984; Headey et al. 1984; Brown and Harris 1978; O'Connor and Brown 1984; Brown 1985; Lowenthal and Haven 1968; Miller and Lefcourt 1983; Maxwell 1985; Norton 1983). One reason for this is differences in the availability and provision of social support in marital contexts with particular characteristics (Brown and Harris 1978; Pearlin and Johnson 1977; Groen 1987). In an early theoretical paper, Kaplan et al. (1977) delineated support mechanisms, such as tangible help, approval, intimacy opportunities, affiliation, and cognitive guidance or the chance to evaluate 'what's going on'. These supports will be provided more so in some marital environments and less so or not at all in others. In the wake of a life event like serious illness, emotionally close and gratifying marriages can be envisaged as providing a strong sense of coherence and security (Antonovsky 1984) which facilitate cognitive processes for evaluating what has happened and its implications (Pearlin et al. 1981; Cohen and Lazarus 1980; Lazarus and Folkman 1983). Social processes in marriage which lead to the knowledge that one is loved and valued may similarly favour the emotional management of the stress syndrome triggered by illness. A lack of coherence and security, social stress in marriage, and the nonprovision of emotional and esteem support may hinder effective coping behaviour at the cognitive and affective levels and, therefore, be predictive of elevated psychological distress. (See also Cohen and Syme 1985; Sarason and Sarason 1985; Caplan 1974; Cobb 1976; Leavey 1983; Lin et al. 1985).

---

* First published in *Social Science and Medicine* (1988) 27(2):149–158.

Krantz (1980) has argued that cognitive processes and subjective health perceptions are particularly important determinants of behaviour and mood state during recovery from myocardial infarction (MI). One major pathway of marital contextual influences on post-MI adjustment may be the area of cognitive coping behaviour associated with the assessment of threat, harm, and loss (Pearlin et al. 1981; Cohen and Lazarus 1980; Lazarus and Folkman 1983; Krantz 1980). Cohen and Lazarus (1980) have termed this aspect of coping "the primary appraisal of the stress of illness". This means the evaluation of what has happened and its implications for the individual's post-MI cognitive mapping of reality. Social environmental influences can be envisaged as having an effect on primary appraisal processes via their impact on 'secondary appraisal' processes. The latter encompass the assessment of what is to be done and the resources available for coming to terms with the sequelae of illness (Cohen and Lazarus 1980; Lazarus and Folkman 1983; Moos 1984). Patients with a supportive marital environment probably view their resources as adequate for meeting the tasks confronting them and, therefore, arrive at an evaluation of the situation which is less negative and more optimistic. In contrast, individuals from social contexts characterised by long-standing marital role strains may feel themselves threatened both by the stress of illness and by the stress originating in their spouse relationships. The patient may, therefore, frequently view himself as confronted by an extremely adverse total life situation and lacking the social support resources that other married patients have available. This double burden may lead to the development of overly negative appraisals of threat, harm, and loss following onset of illness.

As Rook (1984) noted, past research on the stress process has emphasised the provision of social support in adequate interpersonal relationships and neglected negative influences of adverse social environments. A relative stability in the socioenvironmental conditions of many people, e.g. low intimacy and high conflict marriages, has similarly been neglected. In longitudinal investigations of adaptation following serious illness, these aspects of the social environment may be particularly important for several reasons:

- Long-standing social stress and other psycho-social factors have been suggested as possible precursors of pathogenesis in multifactorial, aetiological models of disease (Joseph and Syme 1982; Syme and Seeman 1983; Groen 1978; Baltrusch and Waltz 1986; Jenkins 1976; Appels 1980; Price 1982; Ladwig 1986).
- For this reason, individuals with adverse social environments may be overrepresented in populations of cardiac patients.
- If particular social contexts are 'pathological' due to their negative impact on pre-illness coping behaviour, it seems likely that they will be predictive of problems in post-illness cognitive adjustment, as well as of elevated emotional distress.

Other proposed psychosocial precursors of cardiovascular disease, including the coronary-prone behaviour pattern (Jenkins 1976; Appels 1980; Price 1982; Ladwig 1986) and pre-illness mental health problems termed by Appels (1980; see also Ladwig 1986) as the 'vital exhaustion' syndrome, may similarly be associated with coping styles which define an at-risk group of patients. Hostility or basic mistrust of others has been suggested as a disease-enhancing component of the type A pattern (TABP). This may mean that many type As who develop symptomatic cardiac disease have less adequate marital and other ties. Furthermore, type As with chronic, stressful social environments may be at greater risk for developing the 'vital exhaustion' syndrome or depressive symptomatology as a trigger of MI, as Groen (1987) has proposed.

Hypotheses

Physical health status should be a major determinant of long-term mood state several years after onset of illness, but this influence is primarily mediated by the subjective health perceptions and cognitive adaptation of the patient (Cohen and Lazarus 1980; Lazarus and Folkman 1983; Krantz 1980; Moos 1984). Positive psychosocial factors, in particular social support, facilitate effective coping behaviour and should be inversely associated with the level of dysphoric affect (Cohen and McKay 1983; Brown and Harris 1978). Negative factors, in particular long-standing marital problems but also lower social class status, the TABP and 'vital exhaustion' should have the opposite effect and be associated with overly negative illness-related cognitions and psychological distress.

Figure 1 presents a causal model of variables collected in a longitudinal study on adaptation to MI for testing these three hypotheses. Exogenous or 'background' factors include medical status at the end of the 1st year (T_3), the

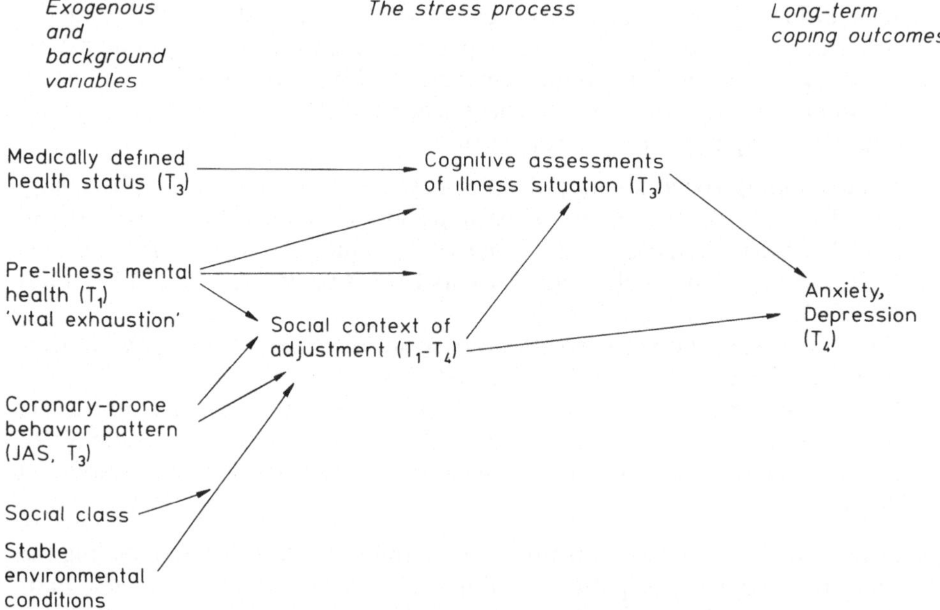

Fig. 1. A causal model of variables in the analyses for predicting long-term distress

TABP, pre-MI depressed mood or mental health problems, social class, as well as relatively stable socioenvironmental conditions based on the reports of both husband and wife over an extended period of time. Medical health status defined as poor by the physician at time three is viewed as the source of a stress syndrome, encompassing cardiac symptoms, disability in everyday activities, and wide-reaching changes in the life situation of physically impaired patients. This post-MI health and life situation should be reflected in the patient's cognitions.

Patients with the same medical diagnosis, however, may experience and evaluate their health situations more positively or more negatively depending on the psychosocial context of adaptation depicted in Fig. 1. The model shows possible moderating influences, which have already been discussed in the preceding remarks. All of these psychosocial factors may have an impact on the patient's cognitive appraisals during the 1st post-MI year as measured at T_3. The buffering hypothesis postulates that social support is inversely related to level of dysphoric affect (Cohen and Syme 1985; Cohen and McKay 1983; Brown and Harris 1978). Subjective health perceptions may or may not be a mediating mechanism. These questions will be explored in two models for predicting psychological distress at 3-4 years after onset of illness. The models are based on previous research of psychological response to MI (Doehrman 1977; Gulledge 1979; Dellipiani et al. 1976; Cay et al. 1982; Mayou 1984; Krantz 1986; Croog and Levine 1977; Wiklund et al. 1984).

Methods

The analyses to be reported on are based on a sample of almost 400 patients for whom we have a complete data set on the subjects and their spouses over a 5-year period. The original sample of approximately 1000 middle-aged, male patients with a medically verified first MI were from a national sample from over 200 participating hospitals. No substantial effects on sample characteristics due to panel and natural mortality were found, except for a small underrepresentation of the self-employed and unskilled workers. Mailed questionnaires were used to collect data at relevant points of time during the 5 years post-MI. Paper and pencil measures of standardised scales, as well as item batteries especially developed for a German-language cardiac population, were included in the questionnaires, as has been described in greater detail elsewhere (Waltz 1986a, b; Badura et al. 1987 a, b; Waltz and Badura 1988). These measures all had adequate psychometric properties. Data was collected from the patient at 2 weeks, 6 and 12 months, 3.5-4 years and 5 years post-MI.

Stable Socioenvironmental Conditions of Adjustment

Retrospective and prospective information related to salient aspects of the marital situation was collected from both husband and wife. The aim of this extensive data collection was to investigate the degree of stability of the socioenvironmental conditions of the patient and to develop empirical measures for tapping these long-term influences. A composite index consisting of 12 items was focused on chronic marital problems and social stress originating in the marriage. This index included reports from both husband and wife on the frequency of marital conflict, on negative changes in the marriage following MI, as well as on the lack of common interests and friends. This marital conflict scale had a Cronbach *alpha* of 0.86 and was found to be moderately correlated with the UCLA loneliness scale, as well as with measures of marital dissatisfaction and long-term role strains. It appeared to have a high degree of construct validity and to be tapping important negative aspects of the marital environment.

A corresponding measure of positive social resources was the intimate attachment scale consisting of 19 items, with a Cronbach *alpha* of 0.92. This composite index included assessments of the emotional quality of the conjugal bond from both spouses. Love and affection, sexual compatability, pleasant socialising, confiding behaviour, and the wife's demonstration of concern and commitment were salient aspects of intimate attachment measured. The index was inversely associated with scores on the UCLA scale ($rho = -0.48$) and a correlate of measures of experienced social support, the adequacy of social support, and marital satisfaction. A focal item in the scale for measuring intimacy, which was repeatedly used retrospectively and prospectively at times one to five was the following: "My spouse and I felt very close to each other (*nah und vertraut*) in the past few weeks" [rated on a scale ranging from 'seldom or never at all' (1) to 'very frequently' (4)]. Similar items were used for tapping everyday patterns of socialising, including "We spent a cosy (*gemütlich*) evening sitting together and talking" and "We laughed together" rated on the same frequency scale. Additional items [rated on a scale ranging from 'very much disagree' (1) to 'agree very much' (4)] were the following: "My spouse is loving and affectionate", "We get along well with each other sexually", "He/she is very warm/cordial towards me", and only applicable for the wife, "I showed my husband that he means very much to me", "I talked with him about my personal problems and worries", and "I let him feel my affection for him".

Medical Status and Subjective Health Perceptions

A number of measures were developed for operationalising the theoretical construct health status, including scales and single-item indicators of physical impairment/disability, health attitudes, and the definition of the situation after MI. These measures were based on reports from the patient and his spouse throughout the study and on time three physician assessments. The general practitioner reported his diagnosis and prognosis of the patient, as well as information with which a three-category index of physical impairment was formed, ranging from low to high cardiac impairment. A single-item measure of subjective health defined on a scale ranging from 'very good' to 'poor' was used at each wave of the study and may be viewed as a fairly broad assessment of a 'sense of being chronically ill' or of recovery and normalisation. Perceived disability in social activities was measured after time two and the scale includes 20 items from both spouses on illness-related problems with a Cronbach *alpha* of 0.88. The various empirical measures of health status and subjective health perceptions, as reported in greater detail elsewhere (Waltz 1986a, b; Badura et al. 1987 a, b; Waltz and Badura 1988) were found to correlate with one another, whereby 'objective' and 'subjective' measures were weakly to moderately correlated. The assessments of the husband and the wife on the experiences of the former, however, appeared to be more strongly associated and to reflect a similar definition of the post-MI life situation of the patient. Several of these measures will be used in the analyses to be discussed.

A major process and outcome variable developed in the study was aimed at measuring the outcome of cognitive appraisal activities of the patient from the time of hospitalisation and has been used thus far in five waves of the study. It is very probable that patient cognitive assessments of the impact of MI may be influenced by the medical diagnosis and physician recommendations, as well as by the observations and attitudes of the spouse. The scale is an attempt at operationalising Lazarus' theoretical construct of primary appraisal processes. In an important article summarizing their approach, Cohen and Lazarus (1980) have emphasised assessments of the stress of illness in the following theoretical dimensions: threats of bodily injury or disability, permanent physical changes, negative symptoms, the endangering of life goals, loss of autonomy, as well as threats to social and occupational functioning. These aspects of the after-effects of illness were operationalised by means of 18 items at T_1 in the hospital respectively 12 items at later measurement points. The Cronbach *alpha* of the 12-item scale was 0.92 with a test-retest coefficient at weeks of 0.77 (see "Appendix").

Data were collected with the primary appraisal scale, as well as with some 20 major process and outcome measures (Waltz 1986a, b; Badura et al. 1987 a, b; Waltz and Badura 1988) at each wave of the study beginning in the hospital (T_1), approximately 6 months afterwards (T_2), at the end of the 1st year (T_3), as well as at approximately 42 months post-MI (time four) and at the end of a 5-year period. Two measures of psychological response to illness were the Hopkins anxiety and depression scales, as adapted from Pearlin et al. (1981) and used at each of the five waves. These two scales in their German-language adaptation had satisfactory psychometric properties. The Cronbach *alpha* values were 0.88 and 0.86 with 6-week test-retest coefficients of 0.81 and 0.77. A short 17-item German version of the Jenkins activity survey (JAS) with an *alpha* of 0.67 was used to operationalise the type A behaviour pattern.

Results

Bivariate Analyses Among Selected Variables of the Model

The matrix of Pearson product-moment coefficients displayed in Table 1 contains two measures of T_4 psychological distress and seven predictor variables. The latter correlated with T_4 anxiety and depression scores as was expected. The largest correlation coefficients were with the cognitive predictor, T_3 scores on the primary appraisal scale. This measure of the patient's illness-related cognitions was more strongly associated with the criterion variables than medical status at

Table 1. Correlation among selected health and psychosocial measures between T_1 and T_4

	1	2	3	4	5	6	7	8	9
1. Intimate attachment scale									
2. Marital conflict	− 0.36								
3. Primary appraisal (T_3)	− 0.21	0.28							
4. Pre-MI mental health	− 0.18	0.18	0.28						
5. TABP (JAS scores)	− 0.07	0.26	0.30	0.22					
6. Social class	0.07	0.00	− 0.14	0.01	0.16				
7. Medical status (T_3)	− 0.04	0.09	0.35	0.15	0.15	−0.08			
8. Hopkins anxiety (T_4)	− 0 18	0.25	0.53	0.35	0.23	−0.19	0.27		
9. Hopkins depression (T_4)	− 0.29	0.30	0.55	0.36	0.24	−0.21	0.22	0.77	
Mean	18.6	8.4	16 3	3.4	185.8	3 0	2.2	10.5	8.3
Standard deviation	9.1	5.3	7.8	0.8	71.0	1.4	0.7	7.0	6.3

the same point of time. These findings are suggestive of the proposition discussed in hypothesis 1, that early patient cognitions are a major mediator of the medically defined and objective consequences of the heart attack. This question will be discussed more completely in the section on two multivariate models of anxiety and depressed mood.

Many of the seven predictors showed low to moderate covariation among themselves. Coronary-prone behaviour, as measured by the JAS, correlated most strongly with the primary appraisal variable and with marital conflict but did not appear to discriminate between high- and low-intimacy marriages. Type A persons assessed their post-MI situation more negatively, had greater marital role strains, reported more frequently pre-MI mental health problems, were in poorer physical health at T_3, and were more distressed at T_4 than other patients. Poor pre-MI mental health, possibly indicating what has been termed 'vital exhaustion' as a precursor of disease, was similarly associated with negative patient cognitions and elevated anxiety and depression several years later. We speculate that these findings are suggestive of an important role of pre-MI aetiological factors on adjustment to the heart attack, i.e. the coronary-prone behaviour pattern, depressed mood and 'vital exhaustion', as well as basic mistrust of others and conflictual interpersonal relationships (Groen 1987; Price 1982; Williams et al. 1985; Henley and Williams 1986).

The social class variable was a correlate of several of the seven predictor variables. Blue-collar workers, in particular the unskilled and semi-skilled, appraised their health situation more negatively and displayed greater long-standing psychological distress than other patients, although social class was not inversely related to JAS scores. The social class measure did not, however, discriminate between different types of marital context nor between patients with high and low physical impairment.

The two indicators of the marital situation correlated only moderately with one another, the Pearson coefficient being -0.36. High-intimacy marriages tended to have relatively low levels of interpersonal problems. Many couples reported low conflict but also low spouse intimacy. The two marital scales also correlated moderately with four psychological variables. Individuals from low-intimacy and high-conflict marriages reported greater pre-MI depression, more negative assessment of their illness situation, and greater dysphoric mood at T_4.

Primary Appraisal Scale Scores

A second group of analyses was focused on the patients' subjective health cognitions over time as monitored by the primary appraisal scale. Scale scores were highest in the hospital several weeks after myocardial infarction (T_1) with a mean for the total sample of 19.9 and gradually decreased over the subsequent period of investigation to 16.1 at T_3 and 14.6 at T_4. Almost all patients appeared to experience a relatively high level of threat, harm, and loss shortly after hospitalisation. During the following 1st year, mean scores were found to decrease most markedly in a small group of patients $(n=64)$ who may be defined as being in fairly good physical health. These individuals came from families in which both

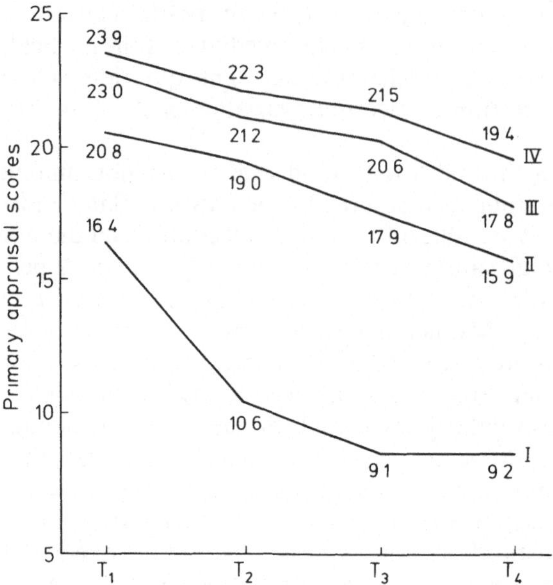

Fig. 2. Time profiles of mean primary appraisal scale scores in four patient groups. Group I, little or no disability ($n=64$). Group II, some to extensive disability ($n=259$). Group III, same as II, extreme type A ($n=75$). Group IV, same as II, extreme type A and high marital conflict ($n=41$)

husband and wife assessed the patient as having 'little' or 'no' cardiac symptoms, physical disability, or other illness-related problems according to a composite index of disability. The majority of patients ($n=259$) were classified as having 'some to extensive' disability according to the reports of both spouses during the 1st year. The dichotomy 'little to no' versus 'some to extensive' experienced disability appeared to be a salient cut-off for understanding subjective health perceptions. In group II the higher the level of disability, the more negative were the patients' primary appraisals.

As displayed in Fig. 2, group means in the low-disability group (I) dropped from 16.4 to 10.6 during the first half year, levelling off at a value close to 9 at T_3 and T_4. The physically more impaired group (II) reported significantly higher scale scores during the first half a year and afterwards ($p \leq 0.001$). Group mean scores were 20.8, 19.0, 17.9 and 15.9 at T_1-T_4. Multivariate analyses, which were performed but cannot be discussed here in greater detail, showed that a number of empirical measures of physical health status and patient experiences with an impaired cardiovascular system were important predictors of primary appraisal scores, as was expected; psychosocial factors were statistically significant but explained a much smaller proportion of variance. Psychosocial influences on cognitive adjustment were found to be most marked in group II, and these included the coronary-prone behaviour pattern and marital conflict.

For this reason, Fig. 2 includes the time profiles of two subgroups of group II. Subgroup III ($n=75$) was defined by characteristics 'some to extensive disability' and 'extreme type A'ness' (i.e. being located in the upper quartile of the JAS score distribution). In addition, 41 of the individuals in group III reported high marital conflict and formed a group IV. These individuals, who were extreme type A and had both health and marital problems, reported the highest group means on the primary appraisal scale from the time of hospitalisation onwards. Average group scores were 23.9, 22.3, 21.5 and 19.4 at T_1-T_4.

Psychosocial factors appeared to have some moderating influence on how patients perceived and evaluated their post-MI situation and health status. Patients with extensive marital problems assessed their situation more negatively than those in low-conflict marriages. The same was true of extreme type A relative to B. Psychological hyperresponsiveness or a tendency of those in type A to appraise environmental demands in an overly negative manner has been suggested by other researchers (Price 1982; Ladwig 1986; Henley and Williams 1986). This tendency was most marked if those in type A also reported spouse conflict and pre-MI mental problems.

Differences in Anxiety Following MI

Elevated anxiety is a frequent psychological response to serious illness and to such after-effects as angina pectoris, experienced disability, and sexual problems. During the first half year following onset of illness and hospitalisation, almost one-half of the patients reported that they were 'frequently' upset and nervous. Scores on a German version of the Zung anxiety scale (T_4) suggested that as many as half of the patients were experiencing elevated levels of anxiety when compared with a male German population in the same age group. According to the reports of the wives at T_3, a larger proportion of the patients were in poor than in good health (215/151). These spouse assessments were probably influenced by their husbands' experiences with different degrees of impairment since hospitalisation [10]. The patient group whose wives judged them to be in 'poor health' displayed as a group rising mean anxiety scores during the 1st year and substantially higher long-term scores than their counterparts assessed as being in 'good health'. Mean scores were 9.3, 12.4 and 11.8 at T_1, T_3 and T_4 respectively. In the healthy group mean scores rose and then decreased to a long-term value of 6.7. The statistically significant differences ($p \leq 0.001$) suggested that chronic health problems post-MI are associated with long-term elevated anxiety.

The time profiles displayed in Table 2 allow a comparison of four patient groups with different configurations of illness-related and marital problems. According to their scores on the marital conflict scale, the sample could be allocated to high-, moderate-, and low-conflict marriages. Approximately 100 subjects each were classified as belonging to a high- and a low-conflict group. Similar numbers of patients in both marital classifications were then found to be in 'good' and 'poor' physical health based on the assessments their wives made at 1-year post-MI. Group I ($n = 43$) may be viewed as a subsample of individuals with relatively low levels of problems in the life domains marriage and health.

They had correspondingly lower mean scores on the anxiety scale throughout the period of investigation than other patients, whereby anxiety appeared to

Table 2. Hopkins anxiety scores in four patient groups from T_1 to T_4

	Group			
	I	*II*	*III*	*IV*
Wave				
T_1 (x = 8.2)	5.8	7.3	9.0	10.0
T_2 (x = 10.4)	4.6	10.2	10.8	14.0
T_3 (x = 10.1)	4.4	8.4	11.7	14.2
T_4 (x = 9.7)	4.9	8.7	10.4	13.5

Selected patient groups
I, Good health/low conflict ($n=43$); II, good health/high conflict ($n=37$); III, poor health/low conflict ($n=66$); IV, poor health/high conflict ($n=77$).

decrease after the initial period of hospitalisation. At T_1 the score of this subsample was 5.8 and 1 year later 4.4. Their counterparts in group III ($n=66$), who were similar regarding marital conflict but who were in poor health status, reported substantially greater anxiety in the hospital (9.0). The group mean scores rose during the first 12 months post-MI and attained a value of 11.7 at T_3, decreasing then during the next 3 years to 10.4. Group IV ($n=77$) displayed a similar pattern of emotional adjustment at a markedly higher level of anxiety scores. These subjects had both substantial illness-related and conjugal problems, whereas group III had only the former. At T_4 both subsamples differed significantly with mean anxiety scores of 10.4 and 13.5 ($p \leq 0.01$), indicating an important role of marital context relative to short- and long-term emotional adjustment after infarction. The same sort of social influence can be assumed when comparing the time profiles of groups I and II. Both sets of subjects were in relatively good health according to their wives but differed in respect to the level of chronic interpersonal problems in the family. As already discussed, anxiety scores showed on average a decreasing tendency in group I, whereas in group II they rose between hospitalisation and T_2 from 7.3 to 10.2, subsequently decreasing in the following 3 years. We interpreted these findings as substantiating our hypothesis that post-MI impairment and disability, when experienced under adverse socioenvironmental conditions, pose a two-fold threat to the individual, which is reflected in elevated anxiety. Group IV would appear to be a high-risk group.

The step-wise regression analyses displayed in Table 3 were performed for investigating a multifactorial model of medical and psychosocial causal influences for predicting anxiety scores on the Hopkins scale at T_4. Model 1 included a medical assessment of health status at T_3 based on data collected from the general practitioner or cardiologist but not the subjective appraisals or health perceptions of the patient. Model 2 contained both types of assessment of physical health in order to explore the relative importance of both 'objective' and 'subjective' indicators of health status on emotional adjustment. Control variables were selected to include sociodemographic characteristics of the patient, his

Table 3. Standardised regression analyses predicting T_4 anxiety ($n = 372$)

Predictor variables	Model 1	Model 2	R^2
Age	n.s.	n.s.	0.000
Social class (low/high)	− 0.18	− 0.11	0.035
Medical status (T_3)	0.17	n.s.	0.103
Pre-MI mental health	0.21	0.15	0.209
TABP (JAS scores)	0.14	n.s.	0.235
Intimate attachment	n.s.	n.s.	0.243
Marital conflict	0.14	n.s.	0.259
Primary appraisal scores (T_3)	–	0.29	0.361
Subjective health (good/poor) (T_3)	–	0.21	0.389
R^2	0.26	0.39	
Adjusted R^2	0.24	0.36	
F	11.1	16.1	

pre-MI mental health situation, as well as a measure of the coronary-prone or type A behaviour pattern. Two empirical measures of what we have termed stable socioenvironmental conditions were focused on negative and positive aspects of the marital context of adaptation.

Of the seven predictor variables in model 1, all except age and marital intimacy were found to be statistically significant. Blue-collar workers, in particular the unskilled and semi-skilled, appeared to have higher long-term anxiety than their professional and white-collar counterparts. As discussed in the previous section, poor health (based here on a medical diagnosis) was associated with high anxiety, explaining approximately 7% of the variance in scale scores. Possible dispositional influences, i.e. mental health problems prior to illness and the TABP, similarly explained about 13% of the variance in the criterion measure. As reported elsewhere (Waltz 1986b; Badura et al. 1987a, b), both variables may be tapping influences related to a 'pathological coping style', since they were found to be predictive of elevated scores on the primary appraisal scale at T_2 and T_3. In a final step of the analysis, the two measures of social explanatory factors were introduced into the predictor equation; only the scores on the marital conflict scale were found to be significantly associated with T_4 anxiety. Differences in this aspect of the spouse relationship appeared to discriminate between subjects reporting high and low levels of anxiety several years following their infarction.

One-quarter of the observed variance in the Hopkins scores could be explained by this first model; the F value was 11.1 ($p \leqq 0.01$). Medical, psychological, and social factors appeared to be related to the success of the patient at attaining his emotional equilibrium at T_4. Substantial health problems and an unfavourable psychosocial context of adaptation, as defined by the following four factors appeared to be linked to long-run emotional distress:

− lower social class status;
− poor pre-MI mental health status;
− being type A rather than B;
− substantial chronic role strains in the marital domain

The analysis in model 1 was expanded to include two additional measures related to the cognitive processing of the illness and its after-effects. The first measure was patient T_3 scores on the primary appraisal scale, which was aimed at operationalising Lazarus' concept of the subjective stress of illness. The second was a single-item measure of subjective health. These two indicators of the patient's definition of the situation were found to be the most important predictors of anxiety scores, explaining an increase of variance of 13%. After their introduction in the analysis, only two of the previous explanatory variables were still included in the predictor equation, social class and pre-MI mental health. We may conclude that 'objective' health, as well as the other predictors in model 1, primarily impact on processes of adjustment related to anxiety as they are mediated by the health-related cognitions of the individual.

Differences in Depressed Mood Following MI

Total sample mean scores on the Hopkins depression scale rose from 7.7 in the hospital to 8.7 1 year later and were significantly higher at T_4 than at T_1. These average scores, however, conceal different patterns of adjustment in various groups of patients. Those in good health appeared to quickly overcome feelings of depressed mood after return home and the gradual 'normalisation' of their lives between T_1 and T_2. Average scale scores in this 'healthy' group of patients dropped from 6.4 in the hospital to 5.6 at T_2 and remained fairly stable in the subsequent period. In the group of patients whose wives described them as being in poor health, depressive affect appeared to increase during the first 12 months and to decrease gradually during the subsequent period of the recovery process studied. The mean scores in this set of subjects at T_3 and T_4 were 10.7 and 10.2 respectively, almost twice as high as in the 'healthy' group of patients. Zung depression scores at T_4 showed that as many as one in three of the patients had substantial depressed mood.

Prior to MI one-fifth of the patients reported frequently being 'sad and in the blues'. This measure is open to possible recall bias because it was collected retrospectively, but we view it as a primitive indicator of pre-illness mental health status and of possible 'vital exhaustion'. At T_2 and third of the patients had similar feelings which appeared to be linked to a personal assessment of 'being sickly' or 'being chronically disabled'. During the following period of recovery, this percentage dropped to under 20% of the sample, whereby only a third of the subjects reported 'never or seldom' feeling depressed. Our sample might, therefore, be considered to contain a sizable number of individuals displaying what could be termed chronic demoralisation (Table 4). Since social support and a confiding relationship have been suggested as possibly playing a major protective role in processes leading to depression following an adverse life event, the sample was divided up into groups characterised by high and low marital intimacy and differences in physical health. Of the total sample of 400 subjects approximately 100 each was assigned to high- and low-intimacy groups based on their scores on the composite index of intimate attachment. In the high-intimacy subset, the subgroups with good and poor health were fairly equal, each containing about 50 in-

Table 4. Hopkins depression scores in four patient groups from
T_1 to T_4

	Group			
	I	*II*	*III*	*IV*
Wave				
T_1 (x = 7.7)	5.9	7.9	8.3	9.5
T_2 (x = 8.3)	4.3	7.9	9.5	11.9
T_3 (x = 8.7)	4.2	7.3	9.8	12.8
T_4 (x = 8.4)	4.5	8.6	9.6	11.6

Selected patient groups:
I, Good health/high intimacy ($n = 45$); II, good health/low intimacy ($n = 29$); III, poor health/high intimacy ($n = 52$); IV, poor
health/low intimacy ($n = 76$).

dividuals. In the low-intimacy subset, one-quarter versus three-quarters were assigned to the good- and poor-health categories.

At T_1, several weeks post-MI, depressive affect appeared to be lower in the
healthy and higher in the unhealthy group. In each, patients with an emotionally
close marital bond reported significantly lower Hopkins scale scores. A linear
gradient between depression scores and group allocation appeared visible with
average scores of 5.9, 7.9, 8.3, and 9.5. The same appeared to be the case at later
points of time. At T_3, 12 months post-MI, group differences were particularly
marked: 4.2, 7.3, 9.8, and 12.8. In group I mean scores decreased after return
home from medical treatment. This subset of subjects with a favourable health
and marital situation appeared to have adjusted rather quickly to their illness. In
groups III and IV, who were assessed by their wives as being in poor physical
health during the 1st year, depressive affect was found to increase and to remain
at a relatively high level. Many of these individuals may be viewed as having
serious psychosocial morbidity as a concomitant of their extensive cardiac impairment and disability. Depression as measured by the Hopkins scores,
however, appeared to be lower in group III than in group IV patients. At T_3, year
post-MI, the high-intimacy subsample differed significantly from the low-
intimacy subsample with mean depression scores of 9.8 and 12.8, respectively
($p \leq 0.01$). At T_4 depressive affect appeared to have decreased somewhat in this
latter group of individuals. Nevertheless, this subsample reported the highest
level of psychological distress in regards to depressed mood. The level of intimate
attachment appeared to discriminate between serious and moderate depression in
the subsample of seriously ill patients with group averages at T_4 of 9.6 and 11.6,
respectively ($p \leq 0.01$), in high-versus low-intimacy marriages. A comparison of
groups I and II showed similar score differentials in high- and low-intimacy marriages. Both groups were reported to be in relatively good health, but depression
was found to rise somewhat in the low intimacy group over the 4 years of the
study reported here. Approximately 6 months post-MI, the respective group
average scores were 4.3 and 7.9; at T_4 they were 4.5 and 8.6 ($p \leq 0.01$).

Stepwise regression analyses for predicting long-term depression scores at 3–4
years after onset of illness, displayed in Table 5, showed all the variables of model

Table 5. Standardised regression analyses predicting T_4 depression ($n = 372$)

Predictor variables	Model 1	Model 2	R^2
Age	n.s.	n.s.	0.006
Social class (low/high)	− 0.20	− 0.14	0.048
Medical status (T_3)	0.13	n.s.	0.095
Pre-MI mental health	0.23	0.17	0.208
TABP (JAS scores)	0.14	n.s.	0.238
Intimate attachment	− 0.15	− 0.11	0.275
Marital conflict	0.15	n.s.	0.292
Primary appraisal scores (T_3)	–	0.36	0.406
Subjective health (good/ppor) (T_3)	–	n.s.	0.411
R^2	0.29	0.41	
Adjusted R^2	0.27	0.39	
F	13.1	17.6	

1 with the exception of age to be statistically significant. In this partial model higher depression scores were found among individuals with lower social status, with extensive cardiac impairment, with poor pre-MI mental health, among type A rather than B individuals, as well as among those patients with low marital intimacy or high spouse conflict. After the introduction of the two measures of illness-related cognitions, three of these predictors were excluded from the equation. Scores on the primary appraisal scale at T_3 were the best predictor variable, explaining 11% of the variance in the criterion variable. In addition, the measure of subjective health was not statistically significant. In model 2 social class, poor mental health prior to MI, and the level of marital intimacy were included as factors associated with differences in long-standing morale. These findings indicated that the objective health situation of the patient, marital stress, and the type A pattern influence depression scores as mediated by cognitive assessment processes. The inverse relation between the scores on the intimate attachment and Hopkins depression scales we interpreted as a possible buffering effect of the social support provisions of an emotionally close spouse tie. Pre-illness mental health problems have been shown in several studies to be predictive of difficulties in adaptation to physical illness and of long-standing psychosocial distress. The Dutch psychologist Appels has argued that a form of depression, characterised by vital exhaustion and sleep problems, which our retrospective measure may be tapping, is especially frequent among type A individuals confronted with excessive environmental demands.

Discussion

Three hypotheses were tested regarding the role of subjective health cognitions and contextual factors in psychological response to a heart attack at approximately 42 months (T_4) after onset of illness and hospitalisation. Health status as defined by the physician and illness-related cognitions of the patient, both measured at the end of the 1st year (T_3), were found to discriminate between individuals with low and high psychological distress. Other measures of health status, such as the wife's assessment or a composite index of experienced disability and symptoms (i.e. reports from both husband and wife from T_2 onwards), were similarly found predictive of different time profiles of anxiety and depression scores. Of all the variables measured in the study, physical health status, assessed as 'poor' by different definers, appeared to be the single most important determinant of high dysphoric affect. In order to test the first hypothesis of a causal path between objective health, patient cognitions, and mood state, stepwise regression models were used. Medically defined health status was entered first in the regression equations and found to explain a relatively large proportion of variance in anxiety and depression scale scores. After the introduction of the cognitive predictors, the former was no longer retained as a statistically significant explanatory factor. We, therefore, concluded that the patients' subjective cognitions were a chief mechanism connecting the objective sequelae of MI and long-term mood state, as Krantz has argued. The upper portion of the model displayed in Fig. 1 appeared to be supported by our longitudinal data set.

Results from a series of analyses investigating the determinants of patient scores on the primary appraisal scale were reported on in a highly abridged manner, but we attempted to show that social and dispositional factors did have some influence on cognitive processes of adaptation. In the regression analyses, several predictor variables were found to be statistically significant in model 1 but not in the full model, which included the subjective health and primary appraisal variables. We, therefore, concluded that poor objective health status, the coronary-prone behaviour pattern, and marital conflict may be causally related to emotional distress primarily as mediated by negative health cognitions. Two other predictors in the full model, i.e. lower social class status and pre-illness mental health problems, may similarly influence cognitive and affective responses to MI, but they also seemed to be directly associated with high levels of anxiety and depressed mood.

The availability and provision of social support, as measured by differences in intimacy attachment in the marital sphere, were not found to be associated with differences in anxiety scores. This social predictor was, however, inversely related to the level of depressed mood, possibly indicating a buffering effect of a confiding relationship, as suggested by the work of Brown, Lowenthal, and others. Patients with little or no post-MI health problems reported low levels of depressive affect if they experienced MI in a high-intimacy marriage. Among the large group of patients with more extensive health problems, who may also have experienced forced retirement and other adverse life changes during the period of investigation, the intimacy variable also appeared to discriminate between individuals with more moderate and more severe depressive mood, group IV subjects having the highest depression scores at each wave of the study. Patients experiencing MI in high-intimacy marriages had significantly lower scores on the Hopkins depression scale than individuals lacking such a supportive marital relationship. This social support, however, did not completely protect all patients, as was the case in a study on life events and depressive caseness reported on by Brown and Harris (1978). One possible explanation for these different findings may be the life situation of the high-disability group. They experienced a serious life event MI, which in many cases triggered a number of other stressors, both problems of a chronic nature and other life events during the subsequent 4 years, e.g. forced retirement or a recurrence of the heart attack. Chronic illness-related problems and concerns despite adequate social support from the spouse may be an important cause of psychological distress in this physically impaired group of individuals.

Based on the assumption that the marital environments of middle-aged cardiac patients may have relatively stable characteristics along the dimensions intimacy and interpersonal conflict, two composite measures of social context were developed and used in the analyses discussed. The intimate attachment scale with 19 items was based on reports of both husband and wife over an extended period of time regarding the feeling of being very close to one another. The high Cronbach *alpha* (0.92) was suggestive of a certain stability in perceptions of high and low intimacy, as had been postulated. The same was true of the 12-item marital conflict scale with an *alpha* of 0.86. Both scales together should be indicative of supportive versus unsupportive contexts of recovery. Over the past 20 years, numerous research groups have conceptualised and measured the provisions of social support systems in various ways. In our study experience of social support in the hospital and similar measures were used, but more comprehensive scales tapping long-term social influences appeared necessary, as has been discussed in the introduction. The high Cronbach *alpha* values are suggestive of a certain stability of long-term perceptions of both spouses concerning the level of intimate attachment and interpersonal problems in their marriages.

The analyses showed that processes associated with elevated anxiety and depressed mood may be influenced by different aspects of the family environment. Psychological adaptation linked to overcoming depressed mood may best be supported in high-intimacy marriages, which provide confiding opportunities and the ability to maintain self-esteem. Anxiety has been less extensively researched in relation to social support, but stressful marriages probably pose a threat to the individual and are, therefore, associated with elevated anxiety. This would mean that the institution of marriage, as long as it is characterised by low chronic role strains, may play a supportive role in recovery. Unsupportive, stressful environments may be an expression of the hostility/mistrust dimension of the TABP linked to a high risk of developing the 'vital exhaustion' syndrome. Further research should explore this possible precursor of disease and cause of adaptational difficulties as has been outlined by Groen (1987), Joseph and Syme (1982), Syme and Seeman (1983), Price (1982), and Williams et al. (1985).

Appendix

Primary Appraisal Scale Items

How strongly do you feel strained/stressed (*belastet*) by the following possible aspects of your infarction?

- the possibility of a second heart attack;
- the possibility of not getting well again;
- the recurrence of pains associated with infarction;
- fear of death;
- not being able to make plans for the future;
- not being able to achieve those things in life I had planned to do;
- not knowing what I am still able of doing;
- the possibility of a worsening of my health;
- no longer being able to cope with physical and mental strain;
- never again becoming what I was before the heart attack;
- a decrease in functional capacity;
- having to give up many things in the future;
- being sometimes helpless and alone;
- being reminded of my illness by fatigue and cardiac symptoms;
- having to cut back what I expected and aimed at in life;
- the possibility of a loss of independence in the future;
- an adverse impact of illness on my relations to other people;
- no longer to look forward to the same joy in life as before the heart attack.

The test-retest coefficient at 6 weeks was 0.77 and the Pearson *rho* between T_3 and T_4 scores was 0.74, between T_4 and T_5 the coefficient was 0.76.

References

Antonovsky A (1984) The sense of coherence as a determinant of health. In: Matarazzo JD, Weiss SM, Herd JA, Miller NE, Weiss SN (eds) Behavioral health: a handbook. Wiley, New York, pp 114–129

Appels A (1980) Psychological prodomata of myocardial infarction and sudden death. Psychother Psychosom 34:187–195

Badura B, Kaufhold G, Lehmann H, Pfaff H, Schott T, Waltz M (1987a) Life after a heart attack. A social epidemiological study. Springer, Berlin Heidelberg New York

Badura B, Kaufhold G, Lehmann H, Pfaff H, Richter R, Schott T, Waltz M (1987b) Life after a heart attack: 4½ years afterwards. Research Report to the Federal Ministry of Research and Technology, University of Oldenburg

Baltrusch HJF, Waltz M (1986) Early family attitudes and the stress process. A life-span and personological model of host-tumor relationships. In: Day S (ed) Cancer, stress, and death, 2nd edn. Plenum, New York, pp 262–282

Brown GW (1985) Early loss and depression. In: Parkes GM, Stevenson-Hinde J (eds) The place of attachment in human behaviour. Tavistock, London, pp 232–268

Brown GW, Harris T (1978) The social origins of depression, Free, New York

Caplan G (1974) Support systems and community mental health. Behavioral, New York

Cay EL, Dugard P, Philip AE (1982) Psychological problems in patients after a myocardial infarction. Adv Cardiol 29:108–112

Cobb S (1976) Social support as a mediator of life stress. Psychosom Med 38:300–314

Cohen F, Lazarus RS (1980) Coping with the stress of illness. In: Stone GC, Cohen F, Adler NE (eds) Health psychology – a handbook. Jossey-Bass, San Francisco, pp 217–254

Cohen S, McKay G (1983) Social support stress and the buffering hypothesis: an empirical review. In: Singer JE, Taylor SE (eds) Handbook of psychology and health. Erlbaum, Hillsdale

Cohen S, Syme SL (eds) (1985) Social support and health. Academic, New York

Croog SH, Levine S (1977) The heart patient recovers. Social and psychological factors. Human Sciences, London
Dellipiani AW, Cay EL, Philip AE, Vetter NJ, Colling WA, Donaldson RJ, McCormack P (1976) Anxiety after a heart attack. Br Heart J 38:752–757
Diener E (1984) Subjective well-being. Psychol Bull 95:542–575
Di Matteo R, Hays R (1981) Social support and serious illness. In: Gottlieb B (ed) Social network and social support. Sage, London
Doehrman SR (1977) Psychosocial aspects of recovery from coronary heart disease: a review. Soc Sci Med 11:119–218
Finlayson A (1976) Social networks as coping resources. Soc Sci Med 10:97–103
Groen JJ (1987) From clinical experience to tested hypothesis: the role of psychosocial factors in coronary heart disease. In: Schmidt T, Dembroski T, Blümchen G (eds) Biological and psychological factors in cardiovascular disease. Springer, Berlin Heidelberg New York
Gulledge AD (1979) Psychological aftermaths of myocardial infarction. In: Gentry WD, Williams RB (eds) Psychological aspects of myocardial infarction and coronary care. Mosby, St Louis, pp 113–130
Headey B, Holmström E, Wearing A (1984) Well-being and ill-being: different dimensions? Soc Ind Res 14:115–139
Henley AC, Williams RL (1986) Type A and B subjects' self-reported cognitive/affective/behavioral responses to descriptions of potentially frustrating situations. J Hum Stress 12:168–174
Jenkins CD (1976) Recent evidence supporting psychological and social risk factors for coronary disease. N Engl J Med 294:987–994
Joseph J, Syme L (1982) Social connection and the etiology of cancer: an epidemiological review and discussion. In: Cohen J, Cullen J, Martin R (eds) Psychosocial aspects of cancer. Raven, New York
Kaplan B, Cassel J, Gore S (1977) Social support and health. Med Care 15:47–58
Krantz D (1980) Cognitive processes and recovery from heart attack: a review and theoretical analysis. J Hum Stress 6:27–38
Krantz DS (ed) (1986) Stress management in health and rehabilitation. J Cardiopulm Rehabil 5
Ladwig KH (1986) Kardiovaskuläre Hyperreaktivität and Depression. Springer, Berlin Heidelberg New York
Lazarus RS, Folkman S (1983) Coping and adaptation. In: Gentry WD (ed) The handbook of behavioral medicine. Guilford, New York
Leavey RL (1983) Social support and psychological disorder: a review. Am J Commun Psychol 11:3–21
Lin N, Dean A, Ensel W (1985) Social support, life events, and depression. Academic, New York
Lowenthal M, Haven C (1968) Interaction and intimacy as a critical variable. Am Soc Rev 33:20–30
Maxwell G (1985) Behavior of lovers: measuring the closeness of relationships. J Soc Pers Relat 2:215–238
Mayou RA (1984) Prediction of emotional and social outcome after a heart attack. J Psychosom Res 28:17–25
Miller R, Lefcourt H (1983) Social intimacy: an important moderator of stressful life events. Am J Community Psychol 11:127–139
Moos RM (ed) (1984) Coping with physical illness: new perspectives. Plenum, New York
Norton R (1983) Measuring marital quality: a critical look at the dependent variable. J Marriage Fam 45:141–151
O'Connor P, Brown GW (1984) Supportive relationships: fact or fancy? J Soc Pers Relat 1:159–175
Pearlin LI, Johnson JS (1977) Marital status, life-strains, and depression. Am Soc Rev 42:704–715
Pearlin L, Lieberman M, Menaghan E, Mullan J (1981) The stress process. J Health Soc Behav 22:337–356
Price VA (1982) Type A behavior pattern. A model for research and practice. Academic, New York

Rook KS (1984) The negative side of social interaction: impact on psychological well-being. J Pers Soc Psychol 46:1097–1108
Sarason IG, Sarason BR (eds) (1985) Social support: theory, research, and application. Nijhoff, Den Haag
Syme L, Seeman T (1983) Sociocultural risk factors in CHD. In: Herd A, Weiss S (eds) Behavior and arteriosclerosis. Plenum, New York, pp 55–71
Thoits P (1982) Conceptual, methodological, and theoretical problems in studying social support as a buffer against stress. J Health Soc Behav 23:145–159
Waltz M (1986a) A longitudinal study on environmental and dispositional determinants of life quality: social support and coping with physical illness. Soc Ind Res 18:71–93
Waltz M (1986b) Marital context and post-infarction quality of life: is it social support or something more? Soc Sci Med 22:791–805
Waltz M, Badura B (1988) Subjective health, intimacy and perceived self-efficacy after a heart attack: predicting life quality five years afterwards. Soc Ind Res 20:87–110
Wiklund I, Sanne H, Vedin A, Wilhelmsson C (1984) Psychosocial outcome one year after a first myocardial infarction. J Psychosom Res 28:309–321
Williams RB, Barefoot JC, Shekelle RB (1985) The health consequences of hostility. In: Chesney MA, Rosenman RH (eds) Anger and hostility in cardiovascular and behavioral disorders. Hemisphere, Washington, pp 173–185
Young R (1983) The family-illness intermesh: theoretical aspects and their application. Soc Sci Med 17:395–398

Weiterführende Literatur zum Thema „Epidemiologie und Biometrie"

Abramson JH (1984) Survey methods in community medicine: an introduction to epidemiological and evaluative studies, 3rd edn. Livingstone, Edinburgh London
Ackermann-Liebrich U, Gutzwiller F, Keil U, Kunze M (1986) Epidemiologie: Lehrbuch für praktizierende Ärzte und Studenten. Meducation Foundation, Wien
Annual Review of Public Health, vol 8/1987
Blohmke M (Hrsg) (1986) Sozialmedizin, 2., neu bearb. Aufl. Enke, Stuttgart
Cohen DR, Henderson JB (1988) Health, prevention and economics. Oxford Univ Press, Oxford
Coleman M, Wahrendorf J (eds) (1989) Directory of on-going research in cancer epidemiology 1989/90. International Agency for Research on Cancer, Lyon (IARC Scientific Publication; 101)
Elwood JM (1988) Causal relationships in medicine: a practical system for critical appraisal. Oxford Univ Press, Oxford
Epidemiologic Reviews, vol 10/1988
Feinstein AR (1985) Clinical epidemiology. Saunders, Philadelphia
Fleiss JL (1981) Statistical methods for rates and proportions, 2nd edn. Wiley, New York
Kleinbaum DG et al. (1982) Epidemiologic research: principles and quantitative methods. Lifetime Learning, New York
Last JM (ed) (1986) Maxcy-Rosenau public health and preventive medicine, 12th edn. Appleton-Century-Crofts, Norwalk/CT
Morrell D (ed) (1988) Epidemiology in general practice. Oxford Univ Press, Oxford (Oxford General Practice Series; 4)
Sackett D, Haynes RB, Tugwell P (1984) Clinical epidemiology: a basic science for clinical medicine. Little, Boston
Waller H (1985) Sozialmedizin. Kohlhammer, Stuttgart

2 Medizinsoziologie

Medizinsoziologie und Public health

B. Badura, T. Schott, A. Trojan

Gegenstand und Fragestellung

Pflanz definiert Medizinsoziologie als „Anwendung soziologischer Theorien und Methoden auf das Gesundheitswesen sowie auf die Phänomene Gesundheit und Krankheit" (Pflanz 1979, S. 238). In den Anfängen der Medizinsoziologie war es üblich, zwischen „Soziologie der Medizin" und „Soziologie innerhalb der Medizin" zu unterscheiden. Soziologie der Medizin beschäftigt sich demnach mit der Analyse von Institutionen wie dem Krankenhaus (z. B. Rohde 1962), ungleichen Zugangschancen zur medizinischen Versorgung und sozialer Ungleichheit und Krankheitsrisiko (z. B. Collatz et al. 1983), Professionsforschung (z. B. Huerkamp 1985), Gesundheitspolitik (z. B. Deppe 1987) oder Bevölkerungspolitik (z. B. Kaupen-Haas 1986), d. h. mit grundlegenden sozialen Bedingungen von Krankheit und Gesundheit, ohne Berücksichtigung der Frage, ob sich dieses Wissen innerhalb der klinischen Praxis der Medizin anwenden läßt oder nicht.

Soziologie innerhalb der Medizin wurde im Unterschied dazu als Teildisziplin begriffen, die nicht zuletzt auch den praktischen Bedürfnissen der medizinischen Versorgung zu dienen habe. Bevorzugte Themen dieses Teilbereichs sind beispielsweise die Arzt-Patienten-Interaktion, die Krankenrolle und medizinsoziologische Probleme bestimmter Kranken- und Bevölkerungsgruppen (vgl. dazu z. B. von Ferber 1975; Pflanz 1979; Gerhardt 1986; Döhner u. Freese 1986; Siegrist 1988).

Obwohl die genannten Themen innerhalb der Medizinsoziologie weiter an Gewicht behalten, zeigen neuere soziologische Beiträge zum Bereich Gesundheit und Krankheit sowohl innerhalb der Krankheitsursachenforschung als auch in der Erforschung von Institutionen und Prozeduren des Gesundheitswesens, daß die Grenzen zwischen Medizinsoziologie und Epidemiologie einerseits und zwischen Medizinsoziologie und Versorgungsforschung andererseits immer mehr verwischen. Die Medizinsoziologie mündet heute in eine interdisziplinäre Bemühung, die in angelsächsischen Ländern mit „Public health" bezeichnet wird, was sich auf Deutsch vielleicht am besten mit Gesundheitswissenschaften übersetzen läßt. Eine für das Fach insgesamt richtungweisende Publikation: *Applications of social science to clinical medicine and health policy"* (Aiken u. Mechanic 1986) spiegelt diese Entwicklung u. E. am deutlichsten wider. Die Kapitelüberschriften dieses Werks lauten:

1) Social contexts of health care and health policy.
2) Major medical problems and monitoring health outcome.

3) Health and illness over the life-cycle.
4) Prevention and caring.
5) Organization and delivery of health services.

Heute geht es zum einen um die systematische Erforschung der Zusammenhänge zwischen sozialen, psychischen und somatischen Prozessen und zum zweiten um Politik, Verwaltung, Planung und Evaluation des vorhandenen Gesundheitsversorgungssystems. In den vergangenen Jahrzehnten haben Soziologen im einzelnen zu folgenden Fragestellungen und Gegenständen beigetragen (nach Aiken u. Mechanic 1986):

- Soziale Voraussetzungen für Wohlbefinden und Gesundheit;
- soziale Rahmenbedingungen und Auslöser von Krankheit;
- soziale und institutionelle Einflüsse auf Genesung und Lebensqualität;
- Sozialversicherung, Gesundheitsdienste und Gesundheitsberufe als Gegenstand sozialhistorischer, ökonomischer, politischer und organisationssoziologischer Forschung;
- Technikeinsatz in der Medizin und ihre Folgen für die Organisation und Qualität der Versorgung;
- ethische Probleme im Spannungsfeld zwischen medizinischer Technik und Patientenbedürfnissen;
- Arzt-Patienten-Interaktion und ihre Konsequenzen für Wohlbefinden und Compliance;
- Gesundheitsselbsthilfe in der Familie und in Selbsthilfegruppen, Nutzung medizinischer Dienste;
- Entwicklung und Evaluation von Präventionsprogrammen und Evaluation einzelner medizinischer Behandlungsformen und Versorgungssektoren (Qualitätssicherung im Gesundheitswesen).

In der Bundesrepublik Deutschland wurde die Medizinsoziologie Anfang der 70er Jahre in das medizinische Curriculum eingeführt und in ca. 10–15 Universitäten in unterschiedlicher Form institutionalisiert. Der geplante Aufbau des Faches Sozialmedizin blieb deutlich dahinter zurück. Auch Epidemiologie hat bis heute kaum eine institutionelle Basis und Infrastruktur an den deutschen Universitäten. Aus dieser Situation erklärt es sich, daß die Medizinsoziologie für „Public health" und Gesundheitswissenschaften einer der wichtigsten Kristallisationskerne geworden ist und dabei eine Rolle übernommen hat, die in anderen Ländern eher mit den Disziplinen Sozialmedizin und Epidemiologie verknüpft ist. Einen guten Überblick über thematische Vielfalt und Ergebnisse medizinsoziologischer Forschung in der Bundesrepublik Deutschland vermittelt der Ergebnisband des Kongresses „Soziologie und Medizin" (Medizinsoziologie 1985).

Für die soziologische Gesundheitsforschung insgesamt von großer Bedeutung waren Fortschritte bei der Identifizierung einzelner Krankheitsursachen, die sich knapp mit den Etiketten „psychosozialer Streß", „soziale Isolation" und „Lebensstil" kennzeichnen lassen. Die medizinsoziologische Gesundheitssystemanalyse hat insbesondere von vergleichenden Forschungsansätzen und von der Anwendung sozialepidemiologischer Methoden und Fragestellungen zur Evaluation einzelner Versorgungsbereiche und Behandlungsprogramme profitiert. Auf diesen auch für „Public health" besonders relevanten Bereich wird daher im

Abschn. „Soziale Einflüsse auf Gesundheit und Krankheit" (S. 42) noch einmal ausführlich eingegangen.

Theoretische und methodische Grundlagen

Die Vermutung, daß soziale Faktoren auf Gesundheit und Krankheit Einfluß nehmen, läßt sich bis weit in die Geschichte verfolgen (vgl. Rosen 1975). Von Virchow stammt der vielzitierte Satz: „Medizin ist eine Sozialwissenschaft und Politik nichts anderes als Medizin im Großen." Diese Äußerung umriß das Programm der Sozialmedizin im 19. Jahrhundert.

Neben der Sozialmedizin wurde die durch Sigmund Freud begründete Psychosomatik zu einem zweiten wichtigen Wegbereiter der modernen Medizinsoziologie. Substantielle Forschungsbeiträge von Soziologen zum Thema Gesundheit und Gesellschaft zeichneten sich jedoch erst nach dem 2. Weltkrieg ab. Als Pionierleistungen dürften hier die theoretischen Arbeiten von Parsons über die kurative Praxis des Arztes (Parsons 1951) und die ersten empirischen Beiträge zur Erforschung des Zusammenhangs zwischen Schicht und psychischer Störung (Hollingshead u. Redlich 1958) gelten. In einschlägigen Dogmengeschichten dieser jungen und aus den USA „importierten" Subdisziplin Medizinsoziologie wird dabei oft übersehen, daß bereits Durkheim mit seinem Werk über den Selbstmord noch vor der Jahrhundertwende nicht nur die empirisch orientierte Soziologie begründete, sondern zugleich auch einen ersten Beitrag zur Sozialepidemiologie psychischer Störungen geliefert hat.

Die theoretischen Grundlagen der Medizinsoziologie im engeren Sinne wurzeln zum einen in der soziologischen Klassik und hier insbesondere in den Arbeiten von Karl Marx (Ideologiebegriff, Entfremdungs- und Ausbeutungstheorem), Emile Durkheim (Epidemiologie des Selbstmords, Arbeitsteilung, soziale Integration) und Max Weber (Herrschaftssoziologie, Bürokratietheorie, Handlungsbegriff) gelegt. Sie wurzeln zum zweiten in aktuellen Ansätzen des Mutterfachs wie der phänomenologischen Soziologie, dem symbolischen Interaktionismus, der Systemtheorie und Ethnomethodologie, wobei sich auf der einen Seite ein verstärktes Interesse an makrosoziologischen Fragestellungen herauskristallisiert und auf der anderen ein verstärktes Interesse an mikrosozialen Zusammenhängen mit entsprechenden Bezügen entweder zur Ökonomie und Sozialpolitik oder zur Sozialpsychologie und Psychophysiologie.

Auch die wichtigsten methodischen Instrumente der Medizinsoziologie entstammen der Mutterdisziplin. Es handelt sich hierbei um Methoden und Techniken der empirisch-quantitativen Sozialforschung und um Vorgehensweisen der empirisch-qualitativen Soziologie. Die vielleicht wichtigste methodische Neuentwicklung auf dem Gebiet sozialwissenschaftlicher Gesundheitsforschung ist die Verknüpfung von Epidemiologie und Soziologie zur Interdisziplin „Sozialepidemiologie".

Soziale Einflüsse auf Gesundheit und Krankheit

In den vergangenen Jahrzehnten hat die sozialwissenschaftliche Krankheitsursachenforschung wesentliche Fortschritte gemacht. Dies gilt insbesondere für die Erforschung krankheitsunspezifischer Sozialfaktoren. Die sozialen Bedingungen von Gesundheit sind demgegenüber noch wenig oder gar nicht erforscht. Im Zentrum der Erforschung sozialer Krankheitsrisiken stehen die folgenden Thesen:

- Armuts- bzw. soziale Ungleichheitsthese,
- Streßthese,
- soziale Unterstützungsthese,
- Lebensstilthese.

Armutsthese

Sie ist die älteste, der traditionellen Sozialmedizin zugrundeliegende Annahme. Sie besagt kurz zusammengefaßt, daß materielles Elend gleichbedeutend sei mit mangelhafter Ernährung, schlechten Wohn- und Arbeitsverhältnissen und wenig gesundheitsbewußtem Verhalten. Die Folge davon sei einerseits eine Schwächung der körpereigenen Widerstandskräfte und andererseits eine erhöhte Exposition gegenüber krankmachenden Umweltfaktoren (z. B. Bakterien, Unfallrisiken, Viren). Diese Forschungstradition behandelt heute mit erweiterter Fragestellung das Thema soziale Ungleichheit und Gesundheit. Soziale Schichtzugehörigkeit ist in der Tat auch heute noch eine der besten Prädiktoren selbstdestruktiver Verhaltensweisen (z. B. Rauchen) und vorzeitigen Todes (Helberger 1977; Neumann u. Liedermann 1981; Black Report 1982; Marmot u. Madges 1987). Woran es bisher fehlt, sind überzeugende Belege dafür, welche Sozialfaktoren zur Erklärung des Schichtgradienten in der Mortalität verschiedener Krankheiten in Frage kommen. Als Hauptkandidaten werden bisher diskutiert: Streßthese, soziale Integrationsthese und Lebensstilthese.

Streßthese

Die Streßforschung hat ihre Wurzeln in der experimentellen Physiologie der 20er und 30er Jahre. Physiologen wie Walter Cannon and Hans Selye beschäftigten sich mit biochemischen Reaktionen des menschlichen Körpers auf physikalische Umwelteinflüsse. Aus diesen Arbeiten entstand ein breites interdisziplinäres Bemühen zur systematischen Rekonstruktion der Zusammenhänge zwischen sozialen, psychischen und physiologischen Vorgängen. International führende Streßforscher teilen heute die Auffassung, daß eine leistungsfähige Psychophysiologie des Stresses von einem hinreichenden Verständnis nicht nur physischer, psychischer, sondern auch sozialer Faktoren abhängt (z. B. Lazarus u. Folkman 1984, S. 12).

Die Streßforschung bearbeitet heute 3 eng zusammenhängende Forschungsgegenstände: 1) die Ursachen von Streß (Stressoren), 2) die Mediatoren von Streß und 3) die Manifestationen von Streß (Streßreaktionen). Intensive Forschungsbemühungen richten sich auf die Identifikation unterschiedlicher Stressoren am Arbeitsplatz (Karmaus et al. 1979; Karmaus 1984; Badura u. Pfaff 1989; Pfaff 1989).

Sehr viel weniger erforscht sind Stressoren in der Freizeit und innerhalb der Familie (Paerlin u. Turner 1987). Auch die Einsicht, daß eine schwere Krankheit zusätzlich zu den direkten krankheitsbezogenen Folgen einen Streßprozeß auslöst, der die Krankheitsbewältigung begleitend beeinflußt und von psychosozialen Faktoren abhängt (Persönlichkeit, soziale Umwelt, Bewältigungsverhalten), die ihrerseits auf den Verlauf der Primärerkrankung zurückwirken können, hat sich noch längst nicht durchgesetzt (vgl. dazu Badura et al. 1987a, b). Bei sozialen Stressoren wird heute zwischen chronischen Belastungen (z. B. Ehestreß), kritischen Lebensereignissen (z. B. Verlust des Arbeitsplatzes) und belastenden Lebenspassagen (z. B. Pubertät, Verrentung) unterschieden.

Mediatoren sind psychosoziale Faktoren, die die Stärke der von den Stressoren ausgehenden Einflüsse auf psychische, physische und soziale Streßreaktionen entweder verstärken oder abschwächen. Der persönliche Bewältigungsstil (z. B. Typ A) scheint ein solcher Mediator zu sein. Aber auch situationsabhängige Formen des Bewältigungshandelns (Coping), soziale Unterstützung aus dem sozialen Umfeld, Qualifikation (Bildungsniveau) und Handlungsspielraum am Arbeitsplatz (z. B. Pfaff 1989).

Bei den Streßreaktionen werden kurzfristige und längerfristige Auswirkungen auf Kognition, Emotion, das Herz-Kreislauf-System, das Immunsystem, das Hormonsystem, auf den Lebensstil (z. B. Rauchen) und das soziale Verhalten (z. B. Reizbarkeit, sozialer Rückzug) untersucht. Der in Tabelle 1 gegebene Überblick von Lazarus u. Folkman verdeutlicht den Grad an Komplexität und Interdisziplinarität, den die moderne Streßforschung mittlerweile erreicht hat (Lazarus u. Folkman 1984, S. 308).

Große Schwierigkeiten bereitet nach wie vor der Nachweis krankheitsspezifischer Streßfolgen. Während bei experimentellen Tierversuchen im Labor der Zusammenhang zwischen spezifischen Stressoren (z. B. Elektroschocks) und spezifischen Krankheitssymptomen (z. B. Magengeschwüren) zweifelsfrei reproduzierbar ist, ist ein solcher krankheitsspezifischer Zusammenhang im Rahmen von sozialepidemiologischen Feldstudien nur noch durch statistische Zusammenhänge belegbar. Der Zusammenhang zwischen Streß und koronarer Herzkrankheit ist epidemiologisch gut belegt (vgl. dazu Siegrist et al. 1980). Ähnliches gilt für den Zusammenhang zwischen Streß und Krankheitsbewältigung (Badura et al. 1987a, b).

Soziale Unterstützungsthese

In der Streßforschung wird heute immer häufiger die Auffassung vertreten, nicht die Belastungen an sich, mit denen Menschen im Laufe ihres Lebens konfrontiert würden, seien das Problem – bilden sie doch einen unaufhebbaren Teil der menschlichen Existenz –, sondern die Art und Weise, wie wir mit ihnen umgehen. Selbst wenn man diese fatalistische Haltung nicht teilt – auf die Bekämpfung vermeidbarer Stressoren zu verzichten, erscheint unsinnig –, bleibt doch festzuhal-

Tabelle 1. Three levels of analysis (3 Stufen der Analyse). (Aus Lazarus u. Folkman 1984)

	Causal Antecedents	Mediating Processes	Immediate Effects	Long-term Effects
Sozial	SES Cultural templates Institutional systems Group structures (e.g., role patterns) Social networks	Social supports as proffered Available social/ institutional means of ameliorating problems	Social disturbances Government responses Sociopolitical pressures Group alienation	Social failure Revolution Social change Structural changes
Psychologisch	Person variables: values-commitments beliefs-assumptions, e g., personal control cognitive-coping styles Environmental (Situational) variables: situational demands imminence timing ambiguity social and material resources	Vulnerabilities Appraisal-Reappraisal Coping: problem-focused emotion-focused cultivating, seeking & using social support Perceived social support: emotional tangible informational	Positive or negative feelings Quality of outcome of stressful encounters	Morale Functioning in the world
Physiologisch	Genetic or constitutional factors Physiological conditioning-individual response stereotype (e.g., Lacey) Illness risk factors- e.g., smoking	Immune resources Species vulnerability Temporary vulnerability Acquired defects	Somatic changes (precursors of illness) Acute illness	Chronic illness Impaired physiological functioning Recovery from illness Longevity

ten, daß selbstverständlich auch das individuelle Bewältigungsverhalten für das persönliche Wohlbefinden bedeutsam ist, daß eben dieses Bewältigungsverhalten jedoch ebenfalls von sozialen Rahmenbedingungen abhängt: z. B. von finanziellen Restriktionen und von den Optionen, die Menschen in einer Situation wahrnehmen, bzw. von den sozialen Unterstützungspotentialen, die ihnen zur Verfügung stehen.

Die herkömmliche Streßforschung konzentriert sich auf die potentiell belastenden Aspekte der sozialen Umwelt. Sie übersieht dabei die potentiell gesundheitsförderliche Kraft sozialer Netzwerke, einzelner sozialer Beziehungen und konkreter zwischenmenschlicher Prozesse. Und sie übersieht die Möglichkeit, daß die soziale Umwelt einen erheblichen positiven Einfluß darauf haben kann, wie der einzelne mit chronischen oder akuten Stressoren umgeht, z. B. durch verstärkte Anerkennung, Ermunterung und Information oder durch kommunikative oder praktische Unterstützung bei der Auswahl und Anwendung konstruktiver Bewältigungsstrategien. Der Begriff „soziale Unterstützung" zielt auf diese positive, gesundheitsförderliche Seite sozialer Beziehungen und zwischenmenschlicher Prozesse. In seiner theoretischen Deutung stützen wir uns insbesondere auf den symbolischen Interaktionismus und die phänomenologische Soziologie. Beide Traditionen betonen seit jeher die große Bedeutung kognitiver Prozesse („Definition der Situation") für die Lebensbewältigung und die Tatsache, daß der Mensch (z. B. bei der Ausbildung eines stabilen und positiven Selbstbildes) ein auf direkte soziale Kommunikation angewiesenes Wesen ist.

Auch die schützende oder stützende Wirkung alltäglicher Signale, Zuwendungen und Selbstbestätigungen aus der sozialen Umwelt, hängt somit stets davon ab, wie sie vom einzelnen wahrgenommen und bewertet werden. Die soziale Umwelt entfaltet, so gesehen, ihre destruktive wie auch gesundheitsfördernde Wirkung über ihren Einfluß auf die kognitive, emotionale und praktische Lebensbewältigung des einzelnen. Unter sozialer Unterstützung verstehen wir in unserer Oldenburger Longitudinalstudie (OLS) Eigenschaften sozialer Netzwerke, einzelner sozialer Beziehungen und konkreter zwischenmenschlicher Prozesse, die als wertvoll, hilfreich oder erfreulich empfunden werden. Auf der Meßebene unterscheiden wir dabei die folgenden empirischen Korrelate sozialer Unterstützung: Netzwerkmerkmale, interpersonelle Prozesse und Netzwerkkognitionen in den verschiedenen Lebensbereichen eines Herzpatienten (Tabelle 2). Die gesundheitsförderliche Wirkung sozialer Unterstützung sehen wir: 1) in der Verhinderung kognitiver Desorientierung bzw. in der Wiedergewinnung einer kohärenten Weltsicht; 2) in der Überwindung negativer Emotionen und der Wiedergewinnung des emotionalen Gleichgewichts; 3) in dem Erhalt oder der Wiedergewinnung eines positiven und stabilen Selbstbildes. Im Falle einer schweren Krankheit erleichtert soziale Unterstützung, z. B. in Form von Gesprächen und Beratung, die Verstehbarkeit dieses Ereignisses und die Vorhersehbarkeit seiner Folgen, reduziert Ängste und Befürchtungen, trägt dadurch und durch Trost und Zuspruch zur Wiedergewinnung des seelischen Gleichgewichts, eines positiven Selbstwertgefühls und zur Wiedergewinnung von Zuversicht und Selbstvertrauen bei. Verbunden mit den kurativen und pflegerischen Bemühungen fördert so verstandene soziale Unterstützung die Krankheitsstreßbewältigung und weckt und bestärkt die Selbstheilungskräfte des Patienten (Badura et al. 1988).

Die direkt gesundheitsförderliche wie auch die streßreduzierende Wirkung sozialer Unterstützung ist mittlerweile in zahlreichen prospektiven Longitudinalstudien nachgewiesen. Auf die Selbstmordstudie von Durkheim wurde bereits

Tabelle 2. Quellen und Meßdimensionen sozialer Unterstützung in der Oldenburger Longitudinalstudie

Meß- Dimensionen \ Quellen	Medizinische Versorgung	Ehe/Familie	Freizeit	Arbeitswelt
Netzwerk- eigenschaften	Mitarbeit in ambulanten Koronargruppen	Familienstand Anzahl der Kinder Anzahl der Vertrauens- personen in der Verwandtschaft Bekannte	Soziale Freizeit- aktivitäten Soziale Kontakte Soziale Eingebundenheit Anzahl der Freunde Soziale Isolation Anzahl der Vertrauens- personen	Anzahl der Bekannten am Arbeitsplatz Anzahl der Ansprechpartner Anzahl der Vertrauens- personen am Arbeitsplatz
Interpersonelle Prozesse	Ärztliche Beratung Psychosoziale Leistungen von ambulanten Koronargruppen	Soziale Unterstützung durch die Partnerin in den Dimensionen: – gefühlsmäßige Nähe – Selbstwertstärkung – konkrete Hilfestellung Soziale Unterstützung durch die Kinder	Psychosoziale Unterstützungsleistungen aus dem Freundeskreis	Unterstützungsleistungen von Vertrauenspersonen Problembezogene Hilfen Informelle Kommunikation
Netzwerk- kognitionen	Zufriedenheit mit ärztlicher Beratung Qualität ärztlicher Beratung Bewertung der Kontakte mit Ärzten, Pflegepersonal etc.	Qualität der Ehebeziehung (Partnerschaft) Angemessenheit der Partnerbeziehung Angemessenheit des Verhältnisses zu den Kindern Allgemeine (Lebens-) Zufriedenheit im Bereich Ehe/Familie	Soziale Integration Angemessenheit sozialer Beziehungen Allgemeine (Lebens-) Zufriedenheit im Bereich Freizeit	Gruppenkohäsion Angemessenheit sozialer Beziehungen Rückhalt am Arbeitsplatz

hingewiesen. Unverheiratete haben, das zeigen die vorhandenen Studien immer wieder, eine deutlich höhere Mortalitätsrate als Verheiratete, und sie sind auch krankheitsanfälliger. Einen guten Überblick über die empirische Evidenz zur sozialen Unterstützungsthese geben House et al. (1988). In eigenen Studien konnten wir selbst zahlreiche sozialepidemiologische Belege für die Gesundheitsrelevanz sozialer Unterstützung in der Familie (Waltz et al. 1988), durch die medizinische Versorgung (Lehmann 1987) und am Arbeitsplatz (Zelder et al. 1985; Richter 1985; Pfaff 1989) finden. Aus unseren eigenen Arbeiten liegen ferner Hinweise auf Zusammenhänge zwischen Typ A und sozialer Unterstützung vor (Kaufhold 1987) sowie ein Versuch zur Exploration der Zusammenhänge zwischen sozialer Unterstützung und Bewältigungsverhalten in einer qualitativen Studie mit Krebspatienten (Schafft 1987).

Lebensstilthese (gesundheitsförderliches bzw. selbstdestruktives Verhalten)

Die Lebensstilthese ist eine der ältesten Gesundheitsthesen. Sie läßt sich bis in die Lehrmeinungen der Antike zurückführen. Ein enges Verständnis von Lebensstil wird in der medizinischen Risikofaktorenforschung verwendet. Hier geht es um den Nachweis, daß z. B. Rauchen, Ernährungsverhalten, Bluthochdruck (kein Verhaltens-, sondern durch Verhalten induzierter physiologischer Parameter), Alkoholkonsum usw. Risikofaktoren für verbreitete Zivilisationskrankheiten, z. B. für Herzinfarkt und Krebs, sind. In neuerer Zeit wird immer wieder betont, daß ein zur „Lebensweisenforschung" erweitertes Risikofaktorenmodell die sozial-kulturelle und sozial-strukturelle Bedingtheit von Risikoverhalten zu berücksichtigen hat (z. B. von Ferber 1980; Europäische Monographien 1983). Ein sehr weites Verständnis von Lebensstil bezieht sich schließlich auf gesundheitsrelevante Laienperspektiven (Laientheorien und Laienaktivitäten), die kulturell vorgeprägt und durch die Sozialisation innerhalb der Familie oder durch andere wichtige Bezugspersonen oder Bezugsgruppen vermittelt sind. Diese gesamte Forschungsrichtung leidet unter 2 gegenwärtig schwer lösbaren Problemen: 1) unter der Tatsache, daß der Begriff „gesundheitsrelevantes Verhalten" unter Experten oft recht umstritten ist, und 2) unter der Tatsache, daß die Komplexität sozialer, kultureller, politischer und ökonomischer Bedingungen, die den Lebensstil einer Population über den gesamten Lebenszyklus ihrer Mitglieder hinweg prägen, die theoretische und empirische Leistungskraft der modernen Sozialwissenschaften auf eine arge Probe stellt. Gleichwohl handelt es sich hier um ein für die Volksgesundheit bedeutsames Forschungsgebiet, in das sehr wohl einzelne wissenschaftliche „Schneisen" geschlagen wurden und auch in Zukunft geschlagen werden können (Badura 1984; Pill, im Druck). Großangelegte „health surveys" sollten sich daher auf die Erfassung von Verhaltensweisen konzentrieren, über deren Gesundheitsrelevanz unter Experten weithin Konsens besteht und für die ein für den Zweck der Intervention theoretisch hinreichendes Verständnis vorliegt. Als höchst plausibel darf die Annahme gelten, daß Alltagstheorien über Gesundheit, Krankheit, über Körper und Seele, über bestimmte Stressoren und über soziale Beziehungen eine hohe Gesundheits- weil Verhaltensrelevanz haben,

z. B. das Nutzungsverhalten gegenüber Gesundheitsdiensten und Professionellen jeder Art beeinflussen. Die konkreten Inhalte dieser Theorien, ihre soziokulturellen Ursachen, ihre Verbreitung und tatsächliche Handlungsrelevanz bedürfen aber noch sehr intensiver Forschung.

Zur sozialen Dimension der gesundheitlichen Versorgung

Es ist kein Zufall, daß in der eingangs zitierten Definition der Medizinsoziologie von Pflanz die „Anwendung soziologischer Theorie und Methoden auf das Gesundheitswesen" als erstes genannt wird. Eine (oft kritische) Betrachtung ärztlichen Handelns und der medizinischen Versorgung kennzeichnet historisch die Anfangsphase medizinsoziologischer Untersuchungen. Insofern kann Medizinsoziologie als Mitbegründerin einer breiter angelegten Forschungsrichtung „Systemanalyse des Gesundheitswesens" gelten. Hier eröffnen sich, neben der Erforschung des Zusammenhangs zwischen Gesellschaft (Arbeitswelt, Familie, Freizeit), Gesundheit und Lebensqualität, zukünftig eine Vielzahl von Problemstellungen, zu denen die Medizinsoziologie wesentliche Beiträge liefern kann und in der Vergangenheit auch geliefert hat.

Professionalisierung und Medikalisierung

Von einer Professionalisierung der westlichen Medizin kann erst seit weniger als 200 Jahren gesprochen werden (Freidson 1970; Huerkamp 1985). Ärztliche Professionalisierung muß in Zusammenhang mit der Ausbildung der modernen Industriegesellschaft und ihrer zunehmenden Medikalisierung gesehen werden, d. h. mit der Ausweitung eines Marktes für medizinische Dienstleistungen bei gleichzeitigem Ausbau sozialstaatlicher, auf Gesundheit ausgerichteter Sicherheiten (Siegrist 1988). Gleichzeitig bewirkte der wissenschaftliche Fortschritt der Naturwissenschaften im 19. Jh. auch eine Verwissenschaftlichung der Medizin, was eine Rollendifferenzierung in medizinisch-naturwissenschaftliche Forscher und behandelnde Ärzte sowie eine Institutionalisierung der unterschiedlichen Fachdisziplinen der Medizin zur Folge hatte. Hinzu kamen erhöhte Anforderungen an die ärztliche Ausbildung bei gleichzeitiger staatlicher Kontrolle von Qualität, Dauer, Prüfungsanforderungen des Medizinstudiums sowie der Zulassung zur professionellen Berufsgruppe (Approbation) und schließlich – gegen Ende des 19. Jahrhunderts – die Gründung ärztlicher Standesorganisationen (Siegrist 1988). In weniger als 100 Jahren waren die Professionalisierung einer Berufsgruppe gesellschaftlich durchgesetzt, staatlich legitimiert und Strukturen ausgebildet, die heute unser Gesundheitssystem ausmachen.

Siegrist (1988) nennt folgende Kriterien einer Profession: spezialisiertes, auf einer Hochschule erworbenes und danach weiterentwickeltes Expertenwissen; staatlich legitimierte Monopolisierung von Leistung; kollegiale Eigenkontrolle bzw. teilweiser Entzug sozialer Kontrolle durch „Nichtexperten"; hohes Maß an beruflicher Autonomie; in der Regel hohes Sozialprestige. Die These der Professionalisierung und Medikalisierung (Foucault 1976, Zola 1972) stützt sich in erster Linie auf die Merkmale Monopolisierung, Kontrolle und berufliche Autonomie, wobei der Grad der beruflichen Autonomie durch die Ausprägungen von Monopolisierung und den Möglichkeiten der Kontrolle gekennzeichnet ist. Eine soziologisch reflektierte Analyse professionellen Handelns differenziert zwischen verschiedenen Ebenen: der gesellschaftlichen Reichweite professionellen Handelns, der Ebene der Kooperation und der Arbeitsteilung innerhalb des Gesundheitssystems sowie der alltäglichen Arzt-Patient-Beziehung.

Mythos und Wirklichkeit professionellen Handelns und die darin enthaltenen Widersprüche und Konflikte können an mehreren Beispielen deutlich gemacht werden. Schon zu Beginn der Professionalisierung der Medizin vor dem Hintergrund der französischen Revolution war der Grundwiderspruch von Professionalisierung und Medikalisierung erkennbar.

> Die Jahre ... haben zwei große Mythen auftauchen sehen, die einander polar entgegengesetzt sind: den Mythos eines nationalisierten ärztlichen Berufsstandes, der in der Art des Klerus organisiert ist und auf der Ebene der Gesundheit und des Körpers mit ähnlichen Vollmachten ausgestattet ist wie jener im Hinblick auf die Seelen; und dann den Mythos eines vollständigen Verschwindens der Krankheit in einer Gesellschaft, die zu ihrem heilen Ursprung zurückgefunden hat und ohne Wirren und Leidenschaften lebt. ... Die beiden Träume sind isomorph: der eine schildert die rigorose, militante und dogmatische Medizinierung der Gesellschaft durch eine quasi religiöse Bekehrung und die Einsetzung eines Klerus der Heilkunst; der andere Traum erzählt von derselben Medizinierung, aber in einer triumphierenden und negierenden Tonart, nämlich von der Verflüchtigung der Krankheit in einem korrigierten, organisierten und überwachten Milieu, in dem schließlich mit ihrem Gegenstand und mit ihrer Existenzberechtigung die Medizin selber verschwindet (Foucault 1976, S. 48/49).

Senkung der Mortalitätsraten und Verbesserung der Lebenschancen im 19. Jahrhundert konnten lange als Ergebnisse des medizinischen Fortschritts ausgegeben und zur Mehrung des Prestiges der Medizin verwendet werden. Heute wissen wir, daß dies in weitaus stärkerem Maße das Ergebnis sozial-staatlicher und sozialhygienischer und nicht kurativer Leistungen war (McKeown 1982; Szreter 1988).

Sicherlich erklären Professionalisierungs- und Medikalisierungsthese nicht die gesamte Wirklichkeit der gegenwärtigen Situation des Gesundheitswesens in der Bundesrepublik Deutschland. Akzeptiert man sie jedoch bis zu einem gewissen Grad, so erschließt sich hieraus ein Grundverständnis, weshalb im Vergleich zur kurativen Individualmedizin der Bereich „öffentliche Gesundheit" nur ein Mauerblümchendasein fristet.

Der erste, von Foucault beschriebene Traum, konnte in Erfüllung gehen. Wie sieht es mit dem zweiten aus? Die Grenzen medizinisch-professionellen Handelns sind mittlerweile zu offensichtlich, und selbst innerhalb der Medizin setzt ein Umdenken ein:

> Die Erfolge der kurativen Medizin im Laufe der letzten Jahrzehnte hatten weit verbreitet zu der Überzeugung geführt, daß es möglich sein werde, mit weiteren Fortschritten alle gesundheitlichen Probleme in der Bevölkerung individualmedizinisch zu lösen. Diese Überzeugung ist ins Wanken geraten ... (*Deutsches Ärzteblatt* 1989).

Kooperation und Arbeitsteilung im Gesundheitswesen

Kooperationsbeziehungen und Arbeitsteilung im Gesundheitswesen waren bisher eher am Rande Gegenstände medizinsoziologischen Interesses. Grundlage der Betrachtung ist nach wie vor die These von Freidson (1970), daß Kooperation und Arbeitsteilung innerhalb der Gesundheitsberufe im wesentlichen durch die auf Kontrolle basierende Vormachtstellung der Medizin geprägt sind. Diese Vormachtstellung ist gesellschaftlich legitimiert, sie beruht auf dem Recht und der Befähigung zur Erstellung der Diagnose, zu operativen Eingriffen sowie zur Verordnung von Heilmaßnahmen und Medikamenten. Aus soziologischer Perspektive interessant sind auch Monopolisierungschancen und Besetzungspolitik an medizinischen Fakultäten sowie Leitungsstellen in Wissenschaft, Gesundheitsverwaltung und Gesundheitspolitik (Siegrist 1988). Trotz einiger Sammelbände, die Kooperation und Arbeitsteilung im Gesundheitswesen als forschungs- und praxisrelevantes Themenfeld aufgreifen, ist dieser Bereich insgesamt betrachtet ein empirisch weitgehend „unbeackertes Feld" geblieben (z. B. Kaupen-Haas 1968; Trojan u. Waller 1980 a, b; Waller 1982).

Arzt-Patient-Interaktion

Die Arzt-Patient-Beziehung ist innerhalb der Medizinsoziologie ein wohlbeforschtes Gebiet. Aus soziologischer Sicht ist die Interaktion zwischen Arzt und Patient eine strukturell asymmetrische Beziehung, was in der Regel beinhaltet, daß der Patient Laie und der Arzt Experte ist und nur ihm Handlungs- und Informationsmöglichkeiten gegeben sind (Expertenmacht); ferner über eine gesellschaftlich legitimierte Definitionsmacht des Arztes (d. h. Diagnoseerstellung; Krankschreibung etc.) unterschiedliche soziale Rollen zugewiesen werden; und drittens in der Situation der Interaktion die Steuerungsmacht ebenfalls beim Arzt liegt, d. h., daß er über Zeitpunkt und Dauer des Kontaktes, über die Wahl der Therapie bis hin zum Verhängen von Sanktionen Möglichkeiten der Einflußnahme hat (Siegrist 1988). Während in der ambulanten Versorgung Wahl- und Einflußmöglichkeiten des Patienten größer erscheinen und die Chance eines eher symmetrischen Interaktions- und Kommunikationsprozesses bzw. eines „therapeutischen Arbeitsbündnisses" gegeben ist, besitzt das normale Krankenhaus noch immer wesentliche Merkmale einer „totalen Institution" (Goffman 1972; Huppmann u. Fischl 1988).

Neuere Ergebnisse medizinsoziologischer Forschung weisen noch immer auf Defizite bei den interaktiven Handlungskomponenten hin, was – jedoch nicht ausschließlich – mit der während des Studiums und der Weiterbildung des Arztes schwerpunktmäßig erworbenen instrumentellen Kompetenz und der Vernachlässigung der Schulung interaktiver Kompetenzen erklärt werden kann. Weitere Begründungen sind z. B. die Organisationsstruktur im Krankenhaus sowie die Reduktion von Krankheit auf ihre biomedizinischen Aspekte. Das Verhältnis der Arzt-Patient-Beziehung im Krankenhaus schwankt z. B. in Abhängigkeit von der Schwere der Erkrankung (je leichter eine Erkrankung ist, um so einfacher scheint es für den Arzt zu sein, eine stärker symmetrische Beziehung herzustellen), von dem sozioökonomischen Status des Patienten sowie von der Art der Einrichtung (Allgemeines Kreiskrankenhaus vs Krankenhaus mit psychosomatischer Abteilung) (Rohde 1962; Hollingshead u. Redlich 1958; Siegrist et al. 1985; Ridder 1988; Siegrist 1988; Huppmann u. Wilker 1988).

Ein weiteres Merkmal der Arzt-Patient-Beziehung im Krankenhaus ist die relative soziale Distanz, zumindest in zweierlei Hinsicht: Zum einen nimmt die Zeit für Visite und Patientengespräch nur einen geringen Anteil am beruflichen Alltag des Krankenhausarztes ein, die psychosoziale Betreuung der Patienten bleibt in der Regel dem Pflegepersonal überlassen. Zum anderen ist die ärztliche Beratung in vielen Fällen nicht am Beratungsinteresse des Patienten, sondern überwiegend an medizinischen Problemstellungen orientiert. Lehmann (1987) konnte nachweisen, daß Herzinfarktpatienten im Akutkrankenhaus zwar zu 92 % über Krankheit und Medikamenteneinnahme ausführlich beraten wurden, zur nervlichen Belastung in Familie und Beruf (59 %), zur Sexualität (19 %), zur Wiederaufnahme der Arbeit (63 %) und zu Fragen der Berentung (23 %), also zum Leben mit einer chronischen Krankheit, jedoch deutlich seltener ausführlich beraten wurden, obwohl der Wunsch der Patienten nach Beratung zu diesen Themen nahezu gleichbleibend groß war.

> Sie [die Ärzte] beschränken ihre Beratungstätigkeit auf das biomedizinisch Notwendige, und dies zudem oft nur – wie in Patienteninterviews zu erfahren war – in der Form von Geboten oder Verboten. Nur ein geringer Teil der Ärzte im Akutkrankenhaus ist bereit, die medizinisch relevanten Informationen auch im psychosozialen Kontext des Patienten zu interpretieren und zu besprechen (Lehmann 1987, S. 67).

Obwohl die Voraussetzungen in der ambulanten Versorgung zu einer besseren und lebensnäheren Beratung der Patienten günstiger sind, ergibt sich hier ein ähnliches Bild mit einer zusätzlichen und riskanten Variante: Viele Hausärzte tendieren zu einer Medikalisierung psychosozialer Probleme und der Verordnung von Psychopharmaka (Lehmann 1987; Badura 1989). Als Folgen des Aufklärungsdefizits können genannt werden: Hilflosigkeit des Patienten im Umgang mit seiner Krankheit; signifikant schlechtere subjektive Befindlichkeit und höhere Angst bei schlechter Beratung; hohe Komplikationsrate, erhöhter Schmerzmittel- und Psychopharmakaverbrauch; geringe Bereitschaft, ärztliche Ratschläge und medizinisch-therapeutische Verordnungen zu befolgen (Non-Compliance) (Haynes et al. 1982; Raspe 1983; Badura et al. 1987a, b).
Ein weiteres Ergebnis der Oldenburger Longitudinalstudie über das Leben mit einem Herzinfarkt war, daß in die Beratung zur Krankheit Angehörige und insbesondere der Lebenspartner des Patienten nur völlig unzureichend einbezogen sind, obwohl gerade ihre Bedeutung für die Bewältigung einer schweren Krankheit als sehr hoch einzuschätzen ist (Schott 1987b; Schott u. Badura 1988).

Familie, Laiensystem und Selbsthilfegruppen

Medizinsoziologische Untersuchungen zum Zusammenhang zwischen Gesundheit und Krankheit einerseits und den Leistungen von Familie und Laiensystem andererseits berücksichtigen zumindest 2 Gesichtspunkte: die Frage nach den sozialen Ursachen von Krankheit (Soziogenese) und die Frage nach den Gesundheitsleistungen von Familie und Laiensystem sowie den gesundheitsrelevanten Ressourcen sozialer Netzwerke. Über Jahrzehnte hinweg wurde die Rolle der Familie aus einer psychoanalytischen und psychosomatischen Tradition heraus eher unter dem Gesichtspunkt der Verursachung von Krankheit betrachtet. Die Bedeutung der „Laien" für Krankheitsbewältigung und Gesundheitsförderung wird von Forschung und Praxis noch weniger wahrgenommen als Arbeitsteilung und nichtärztliche Berufsgruppen im Gesundheitswesen. Die Medizinsoziologie war ebenso „arztfixiert" wie die Gesundheitspolitik. Erst in den 70er Jahren fanden die Gesundheitsleistungen von Familie und Laiensystem wieder das Interesse der Forscher. Als Ursache dieser Wiederentdeckung können genannt werden:

1) ein gewandeltes Krankheitspanorama, d. h. Abnahme der Infektionskrankheiten und Zunahme chronischer Krankheiten in ihrer Bedeutung für Morbidität und Mortalität;
2) ein gewandelter altersdemographischer Aufbau der Bevölkerung, d. h. Zuwachs des Anteils der über 60jährigen an der Gesamtbevölkerung und eine damit verbundene Zunahme altersbedingter Erkrankungen;
3) eine Medizinkritik, die die „Enteignung der Gesundheit durch Experten" beklagt und in deren Folge es verstärkt zur Bildung von Selbsthilfegruppen kam.

Zur Erforschung der alltäglichen Bedeutung und Leistung des Laiensystems für die Gesundheitsvorsorge und Krankheitsbewältigung wurde 1979, gefördert vom Bundesministerium für Forschung und Technologie, der Forschungsverbund „Laienpotential, Patientenaktivierung und Gesundheitsselbsthilfe" gegründet. In ihm waren 6 sozialwissenschaftliche Forschungsprojekte eingebunden, die zu den Themen „Selbsthilfe im Gesundheitswesen", „Gesundheitsselbsthilfegruppen", „gemeindebezogene Gesundheitsvorsorge", „Gesundheitsvorsorge am Arbeitsplatz", „soziale, psychische und somatische Faktoren bei der Bewältigung einer chronischen Krankheit", „patientenorientierte Intensivmedizin" arbeiteten. Die im Verbund gewonnenen Ergebnisse sollten den Wandel von einer anbieter- zu einer stärker am Konsumenten gesundheitlicher Leistung orientierten Gesundheits- und Sozialpolitik unterstützen, indem sie Fragen zu Art und Umfang von Laienhandeln, seiner Qualität, der Verzahnung von Laien- und professionellem Handeln sowie den gesellschaftlichen Voraussetzungen und Rahmenbedingungen beantworten halfen (v. Ferber u. Badura 1983; v. Ferber 1987; Grunow et al. 1983; Trojan 1986; Abt 1986; Badura et al. 1987a, 1987b; Grote et al. 1983; v. Ferber u. Schroer 1984).

Umfang und Bedeutung familiärer Hilfeleistung im Falle von Krankheit werden an folgenden Zahlen deutlich: organmedizinische Krankheitsepisoden werden – sofern sie keinen schwereren Grad erreichen – in mehr als 90 % der Fälle in familiärer Selbsthilfe bewältigt (Grunow et al. 1983). Über 80 % der Fälle von Pflegebedürftigkeit werden zu Hause gepflegt (Socialdata 1980). Angesichts gesellschaftlicher Entwicklungen wie Zunahme des Anteils alter Menschen, häufigere soziale Isolation, Zerstörung gewachsener Gemeinschaften durch stärkere soziale Mobilität etc. müßte medizinsoziologische Forschung die Gefährdung der uns zu Unrecht selbstverständlich erscheinenden „Gesundheitsselbsthilfe im Alltag" jedoch erheblich stärker analysieren als dies bisher geschieht.

Doch nicht nur der quantitative Aspekt, noch stärker der qualitative Aspekt heben die Gesundheitsleistungen von Familie und sozialem Netzwerk hervor. In einer mittlerweile umfangreichen nationalen und internationalen Forschung ist die Bedeutung sozialer Integration und sozialer Unterstützung für Gesundheitsförderung und erfolgreiche Rehabilitation nach einer chronischen Krankheit nachdrücklich dokumentiert (als Überblick: Badura 1981; House et al. 1988). Soziale Isolation als Risikofaktor bezüglich Morbidität und Mortalität kann als die eine Seite eines Kontinuums angesehen werden, das nach der anderen, positiven Seite eine erhebliche Ausdifferenzierung erfährt. So sind z. B. bezüglich Bewältigungsmuster und Chancen erfolgreicher Krankheitsbewältigung Unterschiede zwischen verschiedenen Familientypen festzustellen, wobei Schicht, die Qualität der Partnerbeziehung, Rigidität und Verteilung sozialer Rollen zwischen den Ehepartnern von Bedeutung sein können (Finlayson u. McEwan 1977; Gerhardt 1986; Gerhardt u. Friedrich 1982; Ruberman et al. 1984; Schott u. Waltz 1985; Waltz 1981, 1986; Waltz et al. 1988). Wenn als Fazit sozialwissenschaftlicher Gesundheitsforschung die herausragende Bedeutung der Familie bei der Überwindung von Lebenskrisen steht, so muß gleichzeitig auch auf das Defizit in der Praxis bezüglich der „Unterstützung der Unterstützer" hingewiesen werden (Schott 1987 b; Schott u. Badura 1988). Bessere Beratung und intensiveres Miteinbeziehen der wichtigsten Angehörigen im Falle einer chronischen Krankheit und weiterreichende Hilfe im Falle häuslicher Pflege sind hierfür nur 2 Beispiele, die genannt werden sollen.

Für Selbsthilfegruppen läßt sich feststellen, daß sie eine erhebliche soziale Ressource für die bessere Bewältigung von Krisen und Krankheiten darstellen, daß sie eine emanzipative Bedeutung für die „Laien" gegenüber der erwähnten „Dominanz der Experten" haben, daß sie jedoch professionelle Dienste in der Regel nicht ersetzen können (vgl. z. B. Kickbusch u. Trojan 1981; Trojan 1986). Im Bereich der Gesundheitsförderung und Prävention ist der Beitrag von „Laien", Bürgerinitiativen und ähnlichen Zusammenschlüssen unmittelbar plausibel und auch empirisch belegt (vgl. z. B. Enkertz u. Schweigert 1987; Trojan 1989). Die kooperative Verknüpfung mit anderen Trägern der Prävention und die praktische Umsetzung von Bürgerbeteiligung bzw. „community participation" werfen jedoch erhebliche Probleme auf und erfordern weitere anwendungsorientierte Grundlagenforschung in diesem Bereich (vgl. z. B. Trojan u. Faltis 1987).

Ein weiteres wichtiges Gebiet für Prävention und Gesundheitsförderung aus sozialwissenschaftlicher und medizinsoziologischer Sicht ist die Arbeitswelt (von Ferber u. Schroer 1984; Slesina 1987). Neben dem klassischen Arbeitsschutz (Reduktion der Unfallgefahr und gesundheitsschädigenden Umweltbedingungen am Arbeitsplatz) und der Reduktion von körperlicher Arbeitsbelastung sowie von Arbeitsstreß, wird es Zukunftsaufgabe sein, bei der Arbeitsgestaltung – insbesondere bei der Einführung neuer Techniken – soziale gesundheits- und wohlbefindssteigernde Faktoren zu berücksichtigen. Wie durch die Forschung gut belegt ist, sind hier als mögliche Ansatzpunkte zu nennen: Verbesserung von Kooperation, Kommunikation und Kohäsion durch Netzwerkförderung, Einrichtung von Gesundheitszirkeln als Möglichkeit der gesundheitsgerechten Arbeitsgestaltung unter Mitarbeit der Beschäftigten (Friczewski 1988; Hauß u. Laußer 1987; Karmaus 1984; Marstedt u. Mergner 1986; Pfaff 1989; Renner 1988).

Entwicklungsperspektiven

Die Medizinsoziologie in der Bundesrepublik Deutschland sollte weiter ausgebaut werden. Bisher haben noch längst nicht alle medizinischen Fakultäten entsprechende Institute oder Lehrstühle. Zugleich sollte durch „joint appointments" die Zusammenarbeit mit der Mutterdisziplin erleichtert werden. Anzustreben ist ferner eine engere Kollaboration mit den übrigen nichtkurativ orientierten Gesundheitswissenschaften („public health"), insbesondere mit Gesundheitspsychologie, Politikwissenschaft und mit der Epidemiologie, die selbst jedoch erst einmal zu entwickeln wäre. Welche Erwartungen hat der Medizinsoziologe z. B. gegenüber der Epidemiologie? Und was soll in Zukunft der originär medizinsoziologische Beitrag zur (Sozial)epidemiologie sein? In der Bundesrepublik Deutschland stellt sich zudem die Frage, in welchem Umfang und in welcher Weise das im Medizinercurriculum verankerte Fach Sozialmedizin zu Epidemiologie speziell und Gesundheitswissenschaften allgemein beitragen könnte und sollte.

Der enge Zusammenhang zwischen Epidemiologie und Medizinsoziologie zeigt sich schon im ersten deutschsprachigen Sammelband von König u. Tönnesmann (1958), in dem Pflanz in seinem Beitrag eingangs feststellt, daß seinerzeit etwa die Hälfte aller Forschungsarbeiten in der empirischen medizinischen Soziologie auf der epidemiologischen Methode beruhte.

Vor dem Hintergrund dieses engen Zusammenhangs ist auch eine neuere Veröffentlichung des Medizinsoziologen Levine und des Epidemiologen Lilienfeld aufschlußreich. In der Einleitung zu ihrem 1987 erschienen Band *Epidemiology and Health Policy* beschäftigen sie sich u. a. mit der Frage, warum die Epidemiologie als eine der wichtigsten Grunddisziplinen der Gesundheitsforschung keine größere Anerkennung, Förderung und praktische Verwertung erfährt. Sie kommen dabei zu folgenden Ergebnissen:

1) Die moderne Epidemiologie orientiert sich an einem Klassifikationssystem von Krankheiten, das aus der klinischen Medizin stammt und soziale und Umweltfaktoren unberücksichtigt lasse. Vorgeschlagen wird ein Klassifikationssystem, in dem verschiedene Krankheiten nach gemeinsamen Merkmalen zusammengefaßt werden, wie z. B. Krankheiten des Industriesystems, Begleiterkrankungen bestimmter psychischer und physischer Erkrankungen oder Krankheiten, die durch Streß verursacht werden. Eine derartige Klassifikation würde eine wirksamere Prävention selbst dort erlauben, wo wir noch wenig über die spezifischen Krankheitsursachen und Krankheitsverläufe wissen.
2) Epidemiologen seien in der Regel zu selbstkritisch hinsichtlich der Validität und Reliabilität ihrer Erkenntnisse. Zu häufig würden sie selbst methodenkritische Argumente liefern, die einer praktisch-politischen Nutzung ihrer Erkenntnisse im Wege stehen.
3) Das Ansehen der Epidemiologie innerhalb des Medizinsystems sei gering, und das sei im übrigen eine Folge des geringen Ansehens auch aller sonstigen public-health-orientierten (nichtkurativen) Forschungsaktivitäten.
4) Es fehle an einer aktiven Förderung und Unterstützung innerhalb einzelner Bevölkerungsgruppen und innerhalb der wissenschaftlichen Gemeinschaft,

u. a. weil es zu wenig Adressaten und Umsetzer epidemiologischer Erkenntnisse gebe.

5) Epidemiologische Erkenntnisse stoßen oft auf Widerstände aus der Industrie, da sie deren Bedingungen und Entscheidungen kritisch gegenüberstehen. Nicht das gesundheitsschädigende Verhalten einzelner Konsumenten (z. B. von Tabakwaren, Alkohol, Medikamenten usw.) allein gelte es zu verändern, sondern auch die Produktpalette und das agressive Marketingverhalten auf seiten der Produzenten gesundheitsschädigender Güter.

Trotz aller Breite der Erkenntnisse weist der internationale Forschungsstand erhebliche Lücken auf. Die größte liegt in unserem (mangelhaften) Wissen über die *Möglichkeiten zur Gesundheitsförderung und Krankheitsverhütung*. Was wir wissen, wird viel zu unzulänglich und zu selten in die Praxis umgesetzt. Die Versorgung chronisch Kranker bereitet auch international erhebliche Probleme. Das gilt in besonderem Maße für die Versorgung psychisch Kranker. Aiken u. Mechanic unterscheiden hier sehr zu recht zwischen primären, d. h. unmittelbar durch eine Krankheit bewirkten Behinderungen, und sekundären Behinderungen, die durch den Umgang mit der Krankheit und ihrer primären Folgen durch die Betroffenen selbst und durch ihre soziale Umwelt (inklusive medizinischer Versorgung und Sozialversicherung) ausgelöst werden und möglicherweise verschärfend auf die primären Behinderungen zurückwirken (Aiken u. Mechanic 1986).

Die organisatorischen Folgen und psychischen Kosten zunehmender Technisierung in der Medizin sowie technikbedingte Änderungen im ärztlichen Handeln (Diagnose, Therapie) bedürfen zukünftig ebenfalls erheblich vermehrter Aufmerksamkeit. Das gilt auch für die Versorgung Pflegebedürftiger. Verstärkte Aufmerksamkeit verdient schließlich die Gesundheitsverträglichkeit einzelner Techniken und politischer Entscheidungen, der Transport-, Technologie- und Preispolitik zum Beispiel.

Die Modernisierung des Versorgungssystem steht in allen hochindustrialisierten Gesellschaften auf der politischen Tagesordnung. Hier geht es um grundlegende Fragen der Ausbildung, Finanzierung und Organisation medizinischer und sonstiger gesundheits- und krankheitsrelevanter Dienste und um die Frage, wer wo am besten durch wen mit welcher Methode zu versorgen ist. Nicht nur das gewandelte Krankheitspanorama und die sich wandelnde Altersstruktur der Bevölkerung, sondern auch der ebenfalls in zahlreichen hochindustrialisierten Ländern beobachtbare grundlegende Wandel elementarer Formen sozialen Zusammenlebens erfordert dies. Immer mehr Menschen leben allein, erziehen allein oder lassen sich scheiden, ohne wieder zu heiraten. Dies hat vermutlich erhebliche Folgen für die Krankheitsentstehung. Es hat mit Sicherheit Folgen für die Arbeitsteilung zwischen bezahlten Dienstleistungen und informeller Selbsthilfe im Falle von Krankheit, Behinderung und Pflegebedürftigkeit.

Eine systematische Erforschung des angesprochenen Zusammenhangs zwischen sozialen Faktoren, psychischen und physischen Prozessen sowie gesundheitsrelevanten Verhaltensweisen ist in der Bundesrepublik Deutschland nur in Ansätzen gegeben und hat nur in ganz wenigen Fällen internationale Anerkennung erfahren. Es gibt keine eigenen Publikationsorgane, und die Projektförmigkeit der Forschung erschwert deren Kontinuität und die systematische Entwicklung qualifizierten Personals.

Die Methoden und Instrumente der empirischen Sozialforschung sind für die hier angesprochenen Fragestellungen überall dort zentral, wo die Gesundheitsforschung nicht unter kontrollierten Laborbedingungen stattfindet, sondern unter natürlichen Feldbedingungen. Dies gilt nahezu für das gesamte Gebiet sozialwissenschaftlicher Gesundheitsforschung mit Ausnahme der Psychophysiologie. Dringend geboten scheint zugleich eine stärkere Theorieorientierung. Denn, wie sagt der Philosoph Whitehead zu Recht: „There is nothing more practical than a good theory."

Die Medizinsoziologie ist ein *inter*disziplinäres Fach, d. h. Fach *zwischen* anderen Fächern. Sie hat in der Vergangenheit methodisch und inhaltlich aus vielen Bereichen der Gesundheitswissenschaften geschöpft und in vielfältiger Weise zum Wissensbestand des Gebiets Public health beigetragen. Gerade ihr Charakter als verbindendes und vermittelndes Fach zwischen anderen Spezialdisziplinen wird von großem Wert für die Integration von Forschung und Ausbildung in „Schools of Public Health" sein.

Literatur

Abt HG (1986) Förderung des Gesundheitsverhaltens in der Gemeinde. In: Silomon H et al. (Hrsg) Sozialmedizin, Sozialrecht und Gesundheitsökonomie Springer, Berlin Heidelberg New York Tokyo, S 144–151

Aiken LH, Mechanic D (eds) (1986) Applications of social science to clinical medicine. Rutgers Univ Press, New Brunswick

Angermeyer MC, Freyberger H (Hrsg) (1982) Chronisch kranke Erwachsene in der Familie Enke, Stuttgart

Badura B (Hrsg) (1981) Soziale Unterstützung und chronische Krankheit. Zum Stand sozialepidemiologischer Forschung. Suhrkamp, Frankfurt am Main

Badura B (1984) Life-style and health: some remarks on different viewpoints. Soc Sci Med 19:341–347

Badura B (1989) Interaktionsstress. Zum Problem der Gefühlsregulierung in der modernen Gesellschaft. Zeitschrift für Soziologie 19/5:317–328

Badura B, Pfaff H (1989) Stress, ein Modernisierungsrisiko? Mikro- und Makroaspekte soziologischer Belastungsforschung im Übergang zur postindustriellen Zivilisation. Kölner Z Soziologie und Sozialpsychologie 41:654–668

Badura B, Kaufhold G, Lehmann H, Pfaff H, Schott T, Waltz M (1987a) Leben mit dem Herzinfarkt. Eine sozialepidemiologische Studie. Springer, Berlin Heidelberg New York Tokyo

Badura B, Kaufhold G, Lehmann H, Pfaff H, Richter R, Schott T, Waltz M (1987b) Leben mit dem Herzinfarkt: 4½ Jahre nach dem Erstinfarkt. Eine sozialepidemiologische Langzeitstudie über einen Zeitraum von 4½ Jahren nach dem Infarkt. Selbstverlag, Oldenburg

Badura B, Kaufhold G, Lehmann H, Pfaff H, Richter R, Schott T, Waltz M (1988) Soziale Unterstützung und Krankheitsbewältigung – Neue Ergebnisse aus der Oldenburger Longitudinalstudie 4½ Jahre nach Erstinfarkt. Psychother Psychosom Med Psychol 38:48–58

Black Report (1982) Inequalities in health. Penguin, London

Collatz J et al. (1983) Perinatalstudie Niedersachsen und Bremen. Urban & Schwarzenberg, München

Deppe H-U (1987) Krankheit ist ohne Politik nicht heilbar. Suhrkamp, Frankfurt am Main

Deutsches Ärzteblatt (1989) 86/14:B-723

Döhner H, Freese H (Hrsg) (1986) Alternsforschung 1985. Deutsches Zentrum für Alternsfragen, Beiträge zur Gerontologie und Altenarbeit. Bd 63. Deutsches Zentrum für Altersfragen, Berlin

Enkerts V, Schweigert I (Hrsg) (1988) Gesundheit ist mehr. Soziale Netzwerke für eine lebenswerte Zukunft. Ergebnisse-Verlag, Hamburg

Europäische Monographien zur Forschung in Gesundheitserziehung (1983) 5. Lebensweisen und Gesundheit. Bundeszentrale für gesundheitliche Aufklärung, Köln

Ferber C von (1975) Soziologie für Mediziner. Springer, Berlin Heidelberg New York

Ferber C von (1985) Selbsthilfe im Sozialstaat. Selbsthilfe 5:4–8

Ferber C von (Hrsg) (1987) Gesundheitsselbsthilfe und professionelle Dienstleistungen. Springer, Berlin Heidelberg New York Tokyo

Ferber C von (1989) Strukturreform oder Weiterentwicklung des gegliederten Sozialleistungssystems der Bundesrepublik. In: Lüschen G, Cockerham WC, Kunz G (Hrsg) Gesundheit und Krankheit in der BRD und den USA. Oldenbourg, München

Ferber C von, Badura B (Hrsg) (1983) Laienpotential, Patientenaktivierung und Gesundheitsselbsthilfe. Oldenbourg, München

Ferber L von, Schroer A (1984) Arbeitsunfähigkeitsdaten als Grundlage der Verlaufsbeobachtung chronischer Krankheiten. Öff Gesundheitsw 46:71–79

Finlayson A, McEwen J (1977) Coronary heart disease and patterns of living. Croom Helm, London New York

Foucault M (1976) Die Geburt der Klinik. Ullstein, Frankfurt am Main

Freidson E (1970) Profession of medicine. A study of the sociology of applied knowledge. New York (dt. 1979: Der Ärztestand; dt Übersetzung von Hannelore Nuffer; herausgegeben von J. J. Rohde u. U. W. Schöne, Enke, Stuttgart)

Friczewski F (1988) Sozialökonomie des Herzinfarkts. Untersuchung zur Pathologie industrieller Arbeit. Berlin

Gerhardt U (1986) Patientenkarrieren. Eine medizinsoziologische Studie. Suhrkamp, Frankfurt am Main

Gerhardt U, Friedrich H (1982) Familie und chronische Krankheit – Versuch einer soziologischen Standortbestimmung. In: Angermeyer MC, Freyberger H (Hrsg) Chronisch kranke Erwachsene in der Familie. Enke, Stuttgart, S 1–25

Goffman E (1973) Asyle. Suhrkamp, Frankfurt am Main

Grote C von, Sprenger A, Weingarten E, Schuster H-P (1983) Patientenorientierte Intensivmedizin – Einige strukturelle und interaktionelle Bestimmungselemente für die Realisierung. In: Ferber C von, Badura B (Hrsg) Laienpotential, Patientenaktivierung und Gesundheitsselbsthilfe. Oldenbourg, München, S 141–189

Grunow D, Breitkopf H, Dahme H-J, Engfer R, Grunow-Lutter V, Paulus W (1983) Gesundheitsselbsthilfe im Alltag. Ergebnisse einer repräsentativen Haushaltsbefragung über gesundheitsbezogene Selbsthilfeerfahrung und -potentiale. Enke, Stuttgart

Hauß F, Laußer A (1987) Überlegungen zu Konzeption und Realisierungsbedingungen der betrieblichen Gesundheitsförderung, IGES-Papier. Berlin

Haynes RB, Taylor DW, Sackett DL (1982) Compliance-Handbuch. Oldenbourg, München Wien

Helberger C (1977) Ziele und Ergebnisse der Gesundheitspolitik. In: Zapf W (Hrsg) Lebensbedingungen in der Bundesrepublik. Campus, Frankfurt am Main, S 677–742

Hollingshead AB, Redlich FC (1964) Social class and mental illness. Wiley, New York

House J, Landis KR, Umberson D (1988) Social relationships and health. Science 241:540–545

Huerkamp C (1985) Der Aufstieg der Ärzte im 19. Jahrhundert. Vandenhoeck and Ruprecht, Göttingen

Huppmann G, Fischl B (1988) Arzt-Patient-Beziehung: Einfluß institutioneller Rahmenbedingungen. In: Huppmann G, Wilker F-W (Hrsg) Medizinische Psychologie, Medizinische Soziologie. Urban & Schwarzenberg, München Wien Baltimore

Huppmann G, Wilker F-W (Hrsg) (1988) Medizinische Psychologie, Medizinische Soziologie. Urban & Schwarzenberg, München Wien Baltimore

Karmaus W (1984) Bewältigung von arbeitsbezogenen Belastungen und Beschwerden. Campus, Frankfurt New York

Karmaus W, Müller V, Schienstock G (1979) Stress in der Arbeitswelt. Bund, Köln

Kaufhold G (1987) Zur Bedeutung des Type-A-Verhaltensmusters für die Herzinfarktrehabilitation. In: Badura et al. (Hrsg) Leben mit dem Herzinfarkt. Springer, Berlin Heidelberg New York Tokyo, S 286–320

Kaupen-Haas H (1968) Soziologische Probleme medizinischer Berufe. Westdeutscher Verlag, Köln Opladen

Kaupen-Haas H (Hrsg) (1986) Der Griff nach der Bevölkerung. Aktualität und Kontinuität nazistischer Bevölkerungspolitik. Greno, Nördlingen

Kickbusch I, Trojan A (Hrsg) (1981) Gemeinsam sind wir stärker! Selbsthilfegruppen und Gesundheit. Selbstdarstellungen, Analysen, Forschungsergebnisse. Fischer, Frankfurt am Main

König R, Tönnesmann M (Hrsg) (1958) Probleme der Medizinsoziologie. Westdeutscher Verlag, Köln

Lazarus RS, Folkman S (1984) Stress, appraisal, and coping. Springer, New York

Lehmann H (1987) Die psychosoziale Dimension im Rehabilitationsverfahren. In: Badura B et al. (Hrsg) Leben mit dem Herzinfarkt. Eine sozialepidemiologische Studie. Springer, Berlin Heidelberg New York Tokyo, S 65–86

Levine S, Lilienfeld G (1987) Epidemiology and health policy. Tavistock, New York

Marmot MG, Madges N (1987) An epidemiological perspective on stress and health. In: Kasl SV, Cooper CL (eds) Stress and health: issues in research methodology. Wiley, Chichester, pp 3–26

Marstedt G, Mergner U (1986) Psychische Belastung in der Arbeitswelt. Westdeutscher Verlag, Opladen

McKeown T (1982) Die Bedeutung der Medizin. Suhrkamp, Frankfurt am Main

Medizinsoziologie (1985) Sammelband der auf dem Kongreß „Soziologie und Medizin – Bilanz und Perspektiven medizinsoziologischer Forschung" ausgestellten Poster; Infratest Gesundheitsforschung. München

Neumann G, Liedermann A (1981) Mortalität und Sozialschicht. Bundesgesundheitsblatt 24/11:173–181

Parsons T (1951) Illness and the role of the physician. Am J Orthopsychiatry 21:452–460

Pearlin L, Turner HA (1987) The family as a context of the stress process. In: Kasl SV, Cooper CL (eds) Stress and health: issues in research methodology. Wiley, Chichester, pp 143–165

Pfaff H (1989) Streßbewältigung und soziale Unterstützung. Zur sozialen Regulierung individuellen Wohlbefindens. Deutscher Studienverlag, Weinheim

Pflanz M (1958) Die epidemiologische Methode in der medizinischen Soziologie. In: König R, Tönnesmann M (Hrsg) Probleme der Medizin-Soziologie. Kölner Z für Soziol Sozialpsychol (Sonderheft 3)

Pflanz M (1979) Medizinsoziologie. In: König R (Hrsg) Handbuch der empirischen Sozialforschung. Enke, Stuttgart, S 238–244

Pill R (im Druck) Issues in lifestyles and health: lay meanings of health and health behaviour. In: Badura B, Kickbusch I (eds) Issues in health promotion

Raspe H (1983) Aufklärung und Information im Krankenhaus. Vandenhoeck u. Ruprecht, Göttingen

Renner A (1988) Konzepte und Modelle zum Zusammenhang von Arbeit und Gesundheit. Ein Überblick. In: Peter G (Hrsg) Arbeitsschutz, Gesundheit und neue Technologien. Westdeutscher Verlag, Opladen, S 65–97

Richter R (1985) Arbeitsstreß und soziale Unterstützung bei Lokführern der Deutschen Bundesbahn. Diplomarbeit, Universität Oldenburg

Ridder P (1988) Einführung in die Medizinische Soziologie. Teubner, Stuttgart

Rohde JJ (1962) Soziologie des Krankenhauses. Enke, Stuttgart

Rosen G (1975) Die Entwicklung der sozialen Medizin. In: Deppe H-U, Legus M (Hrsg) Seminar: Medizin, Gesellschaft, Geschichte. Suhrkamp, Frankfurt am Main, S 74–134

Ruberman W, Weinblatt AB, Goldberg JD, Chandhary B (1984) Psychosocial influences on mortality after myocardial infarction. N Engl J Med 311:552–559

Schafft S (1987) Psychische und soziale Probleme krebserkrankter Frauen. Über die Bewältigung einer Krebserkrankung im sozialen Umfeld, in der medizinischen Versorgung und in Selbsthilfegruppen. Minerva, München

Schott T (1987a) Die Rückkehr zur Arbeit. In: Badura B et al. (Hrsg) Leben mit dem Herzinfarkt. Springer, Berlin Heidelberg New York Tokyo, S 179–203

Schott T (1987b) Ehepartnerinnen von Herzinfarktpatienten: Ein Exkurs. In: Badura B et al. (Hrsg) Leben mit dem Herzinfarkt. Springer, Berlin Heidelberg New York Tokyo

Schott T, Badura B (1988) Wives of heart attack patients: the stress of caring. In: Anderson R, Bury M (eds) Living with chronic illness. The experience of patients and their families. Unwin and Hyman, London, pp 117–136

Schott T, Waltz M (1985) Soziale Unterstützung und Genesungsverlauf nach Herzinfarkt. In: Langosch W (Hrsg) Psychische Bewältigung der chronischen Herzerkrankung. Springer, Berlin Heidelberg New York Tokyo, S 193–203

Siegrist J (1988) Medizinische Soziologie, 4. völlig neu bearbeitete Aufl. Urban & Schwarzenberg, München

Siegrist J (1978) Arbeit und Interaktion im Krankenhaus. Enke, Stuttgart

Siegrist J et al. (1980) Soziale Belastung und Herzinfarkt: Eine medizinsoziologische Fall-Kontroll-Studie. Enke, Stuttgart

Slesina W (1987) Arbeitsbedingte Erkrankungen und Arbeitsanalyse. Enke, Stuttgart

Socialdata (1980) Anzahl und Situation zu Hause lebender Pflegebedürftiger, Bd. 80. Schriftenreihe des Bundesministers für Jugend, Familie und Gesundheit. Kohlhammer, Stuttgart

Szreter S (1988) The importance of social intervention in Britain's mortality decline c. 1850–1914: A re-interpretation of the role of public health. Soc Hist Med 1:1–37

Trojan A (Hrsg) (1986) Wissen ist Macht. Fischer, Frankfurt am Main

Trojan A (im Druck) Community groups and voluntary organizations as a setting for health promotion. In: Badura B, Kickbusch I (eds) Issues in health promotion.

Trojan A, Faltis M (1987) Re-Animation des „Sozialen" und Demokratisierung des „Systems". Zwei Schwerpunkte für die Zukunft der Gesundheitssicherung. In: Hildebrandt H, Trojan A (Hrsg) Gesündere Städte – kommunale Gesundheitsförderung. Sozialwissenschaft u. Gesundheit e. V., Hamburg

Trojan A, Waller H (Hrsg) (1980a) Gemeindebezogene Gesundheitssicherung. Einführung in neue Versorgungsmodelle für medizinische und psychosoziale Berufe. Urban & Schwarzenberg, München

Trojan A, Waller H (Hrsg) (1980b) Sozialpsychiatrische Praxis. Akademische Verlagsgesellschaft, Wiesbaden

Waller H (1982) Sozialarbeit im Gesundheitswesen. Ausbildungskonzepte, Praxisberichte, Forschungsergebnisse. Bosch/Beltz, Weinheim

Waltz M (1981) Soziale Faktoren bei der Entstehung und Bewältigung von Krankheit – ein Überblick über die empirische Literatur. In: Badura B (Hrsg) Soziale Unterstützung und chronische Krankheit. Suhrkamp, Frankfurt am Main

Waltz M (1986) Marital context and post-infarction quality of life: Is it social support or something else? Soc Sci Med 22:791–805

Waltz M, Badura B, Pfaff H, Schott T (1988) Marriage and the psychological consequences of a heart attack: a longitudinal study of adaptation to chronic illness after 3 years. Soc Sci Med 27:149–158

Zelder K, Windler A, Roth F et al. (1985) Arbeit und Gesundheit des Lokführers der deutschen Bundesbahn, eine sozialepidemiologische Studie. Oldenburg

Zola IK (1972) Medicine as an institution of social control. Soc Rev 20:487–504

Weiterführende Literatur zum Thema „Medizinsoziologie"

Aiken LH, Mechanic D (eds) (1986) Applications of social science to clinical medicine and social policy. Rutgers Univ Press, New Brunswick
Morgan M, Calnan M, Manning N (1985) Sociological approaches to health and medicine. Croom Helm, London
Siegrist J (1988) Medizinische Soziologie, 4., völlig neu bearb. Aufl. Urban & Schwarzenberg, München

3 Präventivmedizin

The German Cardiovascular Prevention Study: Design and Methods *

GCP Study Group

Introduction

The German Cardiovascular Prevention Study (GCP) is a multicentre community-oriented investigation for the primary prevention of ischaemic heart disease (IHD) and stroke. The concepts and methods for this programme were developed during a pilot phase from 1979 to 1983, using experience obtained in completed, as well as ongoing, community-intervention studies in North Karelia, Finland (Puska et al. 1983), German- and French-speaking towns in Switzerland (Gutzwiller et al. 1985), Eberbach and Wiesloch, FRG (Nüssel 1985), and Pawtucket (Elder 1986), Minnesota (Blackburn et al. 1984) and cities in the Stanford area in the United States (Farquhar et al. 1985).

There is sufficient evidence from various longitudinal epidemiological studies linking the risk for cardiovascular diseases to certain individual characteristics. These risk factors include elevated arterial blood pressure and total serum cholesterol, cigarette smoking, overweight, physical inactivity, type A, behaviour, and deficient psychosocial support (Paffenbarger et al. 1986; Pooling Project Research Group 1978; Cooper et al. 1981).

Controlled clinical trials have further demonstrated the effectiveness of treating severe as well as moderately elevated arterial blood pressure to reduce cardiovascular risk (Veterans Administration Cooperative Study Group 1967, 1970; Hypertension Detection and Follow-Up Program Cooperative Group 1979; Management Committee 1980; Medical Research Council Working Party 1985) and the possibility of decreasing the incidence of coronary heart disease by pharmacologically controlling hypercholesterolaemia (Lipid Research Clinics Program 1984). These studies strengthen the causal relationship between these risk factors and cardiovascular disease.

For the prevention of cardiovascular diseases, however, the logical progression from controlled clinical trials is the implementation of community intervention studies. Many of the latter have already demonstrated or suggested that a broad multifactorial and multidisciplinary community-oriented prevention programme directed towards the main cardiovascular risk factor is feasible, effective and results in a reduced incidence of disease.

---

* First published in *European Heart Journal* (1988) 9:1058–1066. This study is funded by the Federal Ministry for Research and Technology and the Federal Ministry for Youth, Family, Women's Affairs and Health (Federal Republic of Germany).

Aims

The aims of the GCP for an intervention period of 8 years (1984–1991) are as follows:

1. The development and implementation of a feasible community-oriented prevention programme, which at the end of the intervention period would be further carried out by the study communities themselves. The programme should also be transferable to other communities in the FRG having characteristics similar to those in the present study. A provisional judgement regarding feasibility of the intervention programme in the study communities should be available after 2 years of intervention.
2. A reduction in the prevelance of cardiovascular risk factors as compared to the FRG as a whole, as a result of the interventive process, among target populations of German males and females, aged 25–59 years at the beginning of the study. A trend towards risk-factor reduction should be measurable after 4 years of intervention.
3. A decrease in cardiovascular morbidity and mortality (ICD-9 410–414, 430–438) in males and females aged 25–69 years, as compared to rates of the rest of the FRG population. A similar trend in total mortality should be observed, assuming no compensatory increases in other causes of death.

Required Population Size

In order to determine the necessary population size required to detect a reduction in cardiovascular mortality, several considerations have been made in the statistical planning stage. The problem is complex since: individuals may not be considered statistically independent (clustering effect); the mechanisms by which intervention affects mortality are not yet completely understood; and secular trends and variability in the reference may distort the effects.

Therefore, the statistical methods normally adopted for clinical trials cannot be used (Campbell and Stanley 1963). However, the methods may be considered as an approximate solution to the problem. Based upon results of interventions in other studies, a relative reduction of cardiovascular mortality of between 5% and 10% should be expected within a decade. An 8% reduction of age-specific cardiovascular mortality is to be detected (with a probability of at least 90% at a significance level of 5%) by the GCP for the ICD-9 categories 410–414 and 430–438 at the end of the 8-year intervention period. It is further assumed that this reduction is achieved nonlinearly over a period of 8 years (no effect before the 3rd year and a linear increase in effect of up to 8% between the 3rd and 8th year). Cumulative cardiovascular mortality over the 8-year period would then be reduced by 5.6% (based on the assumption of a decreasing secular trend of 2% over the 8 years). With this in mind and given the German age and gender distribution for 1984, the necessary sample size for a one-sided test would be 282 000 at the beginning of the study.

Reference Concept

A true experimental design is difficult to achieve when conducting community-based intervention studies for the following reasons. Total populations and not individuals are the basic units. Furthermore, the randomization process to intervention and reference units is not easy because of the difficulties in finding adequate numbers of communities where such studies can be conducted and that are sufficiently comparable at the start or remain comparable over the study period. Regarding the latter, local crises, such an unemployment, are not easily controlled by research methods. Lastly, the decision by control communities to remain as such may be altered when knowing that intervention seems to be successful.

Because of the above considerations, only quasiexperimental study designs are at our disposal. The GCP study group decided to use a national reference frame, instead of single communities, for study control. This allows a reduction of the required sample size for the intervention regions (one sample situation). It permits specific comparisons by using particular subsets of the reference population. A reduction in 'contamination' of the reference by the regional prevention programme is likewise achieved. (Single control communities are not found far from intervention communities, so as to maintain comparability.) Selective secular trends in both intervention and single community reference areas could easily impair one-to-one community comparisons.

Reference data are being obtained via a national health examination and interview survey programme which utilizes the same study procedures and documentation as those of the intervention communities.

Selection of Communities

The study population comprises the resident population of selected communities in five study regions spread over the FRG (Table 1). The effect of intervention is

Table 1. Regional structure of the study population

Study region	Total population 1984	Evaluation population[a]
Berlin-Spandau	208 600	67 300
Bremen North and West	190 100	53 600
Stuttgart West and Vaihingen	338 900	94 700
Karlsruhe with Bruchsal and Mosbach[b]	348 200	99 100
County of Traunstein, Bavaria	142 600	41 100
Total	1 228 400	355 800
FRG	61 175 000	24 970 000[c]

[a] Based upon a yearly migration rate of 4.5% (out of the intervention regions) accumulating over 8 years to 30% males and females aged 25–59 years at the start of the stuy.

[b] Mortality figures are available only for Karsruhe, with a subpopulation of 64 860.

[c] Migration neglected.

Table 2. Selected regional characteristics, 1984

Items	Pool of intervention regions	FRG
Persons aged 25–59 years (%)	44.6	44.5
Foreigners (%)	11.5	7.1
Marriages per 1000 inhabitants	6.0	6.0
Unemployed persons (%)	9.3	9.5
Females (%)	52.6	52.2
Gross domestic product per capita (1000 DM, adjusted), 1980	26.4	24.2
Occupation (%)		
Agriculture	0.8	5.4
Production	41.6	41.6
Trade, transport	21.3	18.3
Other services	36.3	34.7
Inhabitants/physician	1377	1690

Table 3. Age-specific cardiovascular mortality rates per 100000 inhabitants (ICD-9 410–414; 430–438), 1981–1982 (mean)

	Age-specific rate			
	30–39	40–49	50–59	60–69
Men				
Berlin-Spandau	14	101	290	921
Bremen	16	82	349	901
Stuttgart	16	64	255	822
Traunstein	–[a]	35	196	925
Four regions[b]	15	72	274	879
FRG	17	82	327	1007
Women				
Berlin	11	46	119	376
Bremen	4	33	68	368
Stuttgart	2	18	46	275
Traunstein	–[a]	5	69	376
Four regions	5	23	71	337
FRG	7	21	81	363

[a] No information available due to privacy law restrictions.
[b] Data for Karlsruhe, Bruchsal, Mosbach not yet obtained.

to be measured more specifically in the resident German population aged 25–59 years at the beginning of the study. The five regions selected comprise a population of 1 228 400 persons of all ages which gives – after consideration of a migration rate of 30% (out of the study regions) over 8 years or 4.5% per year – a mid-study German population for the age group of interest of 355 800 (Table 1).

The GCP study regions are communities of different sizes of urban or rural structure and of divergent degrees of industrialization. They have been selected in order to fulfil the following requirements. The combined population of the study communities should not differ substantially regarding sociodemographic characteristics from the population of the FRG. The anticipated success of the intervention efforts should, therefore, allow conclusions to be drawn about the potential results of a global intervention in the FRG (Table 2).

A comparison of cardiovascular mortality, the final outcome within both the intervention region and the FRG as a whole, is presented in Table 3.

Intervention Concept

The intervention strategies of the GCP are based upon the social learning theory of Bandura (1977) and the theory of diffusion of innovations of Rogers (1983). Many of the intervention procedures have been adopted from ongoing or completed community studies, especially those in Minnesota (Blackburn et al. 1984), Stanford (Farquhar et al. 1985), and Pawtucket (Elder et al. 1986); see Fig. 1.

Prevention here aims at the modification in the total population of faulty health behaviours (among others, smoking, poor nutritional habits and physical inactivity) directly associated with a greater cardiovascular disease risk. Because healthy behaviour is, in general, incorporated within the pattern of a person's daily life, effective prevention must involve the development of favourable conditions for healthy life styles (in the terminology of the World Health Organization: 'making the healthier choice the easier choice'). The GCP programme is attempting to achieve the latter by means of involvement within the living spheres: family, neighbourhood, education and training, work place and leisure time. Specific methods have been developed to promote public information, train professional and lay individuals and support, self-help activities. Health education at these levels centres around the following issues: elevated blood pressure, healthy nutrition, especially with regard to fat, cholesterol and salt intake, improved physical activity and the promotion of non-smoking.

The achievement of the desired effect within the relatively short study period relies significantly not only upon the intense involvement of all important public persons, groups and organizations in the community, but the appropriate use of mass media and professional multipliers and support of lay activities, as well. Health committees are formed to provide community-wide coordination in the production and distribution of health goods and services. Special efforts are made to involve the physicians and medical associations, as they are important for the effective promotion of the preventive activities.

The individual programme elements must be adapted to the specific needs of the cooperating partners in the community, while considering that proposals and support must be offered in a way that facilitates the final administration of the programme by the community itself. Coordination of study activities is provided by the Study Secretariat and by the local health task forces working under the principle of equal partnership (interventive strategy type A, known as *kooperative Prävention*).

In order to gain the maximum support from the medical profession, the study group responsible for Karlsruhe, Bruchsal and Mosbach decided to make all in-

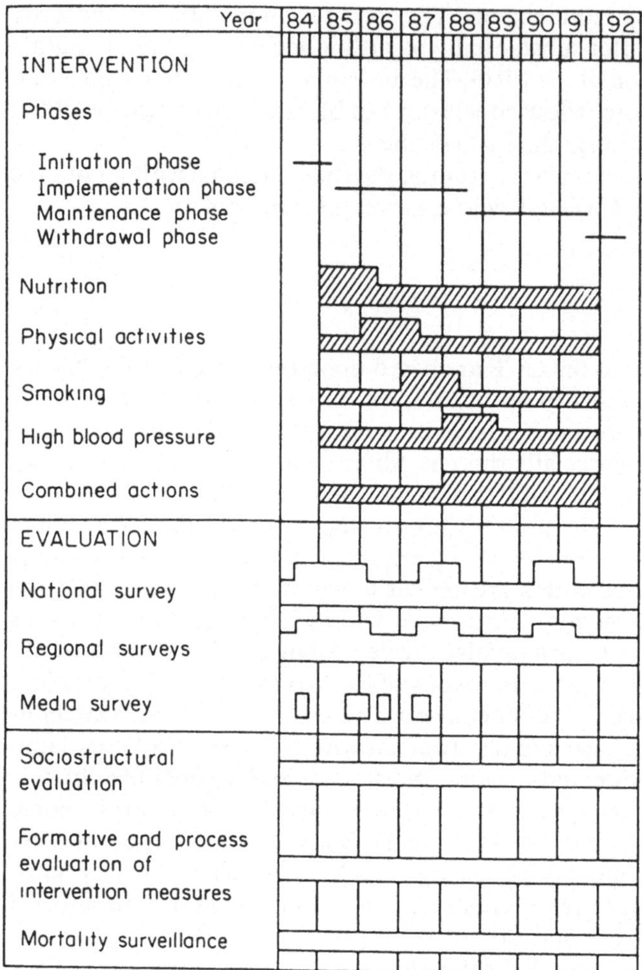

Fig. 1. GCP study: time schedule, 1984–1992

tervention activities dependent on the positive vote of the regional medical association (interventive strategy type B, known as *kommunale Prävention*). It remains to be seen whether the differences between A and B type strategies lead to differences in field work, participation of physicians, or risk-factor reduction throughout the course of the study.

Process Evaluation

As in recent community-oriented intervention studies (Farquhar et al. 1985), special emphasis is put on process evaluation to document the intervention measures carried out as well as the reactions to such processes within target persons and in the social field of the community over time.

The immediate outcome of such interventions are analysed in terms of (a) the number of persons and types of groups in the population having changes regarding health knowledge related values, and (b), changes at the community level in particular in preventive services and provision of goods. Such outcomes will be related to both specific intervention programmes of the study centres and to other preventive activities in the community.

For the purpose of general presentation and an integration of the vast amount of data, the GCP is developing a 'baseline-indicator-system'. This involves: (a) Bi-annual reports and qualitative description of the intervention measures and strategies carried out; (b) qualitative and quantitative procedures, including annual survey to evaluate immediate and long-term health-related changes at both the personal and sociostructural level; and (c) documentation of both the organizational processes within the study centres themselves and description of their effects on intervention.

Survey Design

Health examination and interview surveys have been conducted in all intervention regions before the start of the preventive measures in order to acquire baseline data on initial health attitudes, health behaviour and cardiovascular risk-factor prevalence. This information will serve as a basis for intermediate analyses of interventive efforts in the regions. Subsequent cross-sectional surveys using identical methods will be carried out at the midpoint and at the end of the intervention period. The pooled data of regional surveys will be compared to the parallel conducted National Health Examination and Interview Survey results. The regional samples are randomly drawn for German males and females from the compulsory residency registries in the study areas: (a) follow-up examination of the baseline sample will allow for a longitudinal comparison within the sample over the whole period of 8 years; and (b) the specific intervention approach B in Karlsruhe, Bruchsal and Mosbach will be compared at study years 4 and 8 with the other study regions (approach A) in terms of risk-factor reduction.

The baseline samples per study region will comprise a total of 1800 examinees. Given an approximate participation rate of 70% of all those invited, the gross sample amounts to about 2500 per region.

The National Health Examination and Interview Survey utilizes 200 sample points representative of the FRG primary units to give a net sample of 36 participants in each cluster and thus a total of 7200 participants. This provides, at a presumed participation rate of 70%, approximately 5000 examinees.

Furthermore, 15840 randomly drawn persons from an additional 880 sampling points spread all over the FRG are contributing about 11000 interviews (National Health Interview Survey; see Table 4).

The National Health Examination Survey comprises the following anthropometric and medical measurements: height, weight, resting blood pressure (taken twice in the sitting position), resting pulse rate, serum HDL cholesterol, serum total cholesterol ad thiocyanate.

Table 4. Sample sizes and response rates of baseline surveys, 1984–1985

Type of survey	Total sample	Returns	Response rate (%)
Regional Surveys			
Berlin-Spandau	2637	1857	70.4
Bremen North and West	2542	1807	71.1
Stuttgart West including Vaihingen	2524	1802	71.4
County of Traunstein, Bavaria	2604	1958	75.2
Karlsruhe	2583	2002	77.5
Bruchsal and Mosbach	2604	2168	83.3
National Health Survey	7252	4836	66.7
National Health Interview Survey	15713	10949	69.7

The questionnaire used in the National Health Examination Survey the National Interview Survey and the regional surveys comprises among other topics: sociodemographic variables, food frequency list, smoking history, work activity (including work satisfaction), leisure time activity, the Bortner scale, the OECD symptom list, the Rose angina questionnaire, a medical history covering major groups of disease, a history of drug therapy and items covering usage of the health care system. The questionnaire has been developed as a self-administered instrument, but it has been decided that in the Health Examination Survey the physician drawing blood should ask the questions regarding the medical history.

Data Sources for Mortality and Approach to Validation

Data from official statistics serve as the basis for the assessment of cardiovascular and total mortality in both the regional and national studies. Analyses of official mortality statistics from previous years for the study regions as well as for selected countries of the FRG show yearly changes in both total and cardiovascular mortality that could not be explained by chance alone. For several time periods such fluctuations are far greater than the reduction of cardiovascular mortality aimed at through intervention in the GCP (Table 5). To control these disparate trends, a validation of mortality data is planned. The validation will be done in several ways: (a) determination of coding practices of death certificates in the statistical offices (intra- versus inter-observer variation); (b) determination of validity of diagnoses on death certificates; and (c) further investigations of statistical peculiarities. The main objective of these studies is to determine whether a systematic error exists and, if so, whether it remains constant over the 8-year study period.

Substantial changes in case fatality would also effect the interpretation of study results, i.e. the reduction of cardiovascular mortality, especially when these differ between the study regions and the FRG as a whole. Such changes are most likely due to improvements in curative medicine, e.g. treatment of hypertension

Table 5. Relative age-adjusted mortality: males (25–64 years) City of Bremen versus the FRG, 1970–1984[a]

Year	Cause of death			Total mortality
	410–414	430–438	410–414 430–438	
1970	107　(227)	84　(57)	101　(284)	103　(1136)
1971	107　(230)	71[b]　(47)	98　(227)	104　(1108)
1972	109　(229)	97　(61)	106　(290)	106　(1103)
1973	99　(203)	86　(51)	96　(254)	109[b]　(1095)
1974	97　(190)	92　(48)	96　(238)	101　(975)
1975	102　(195)	77　(41)	96　(236)	103　(982)
1976	115[b]　(216)	117　(55)	115[b]　(271)	107[b]　(966)
1977	119[b]　(209)	85　(38)	112　(247)	108[b]　(913)
1978	119[b]　(210)	62[b]　(26)	108　(236)	105　(870)
1979	135[c]　(222)	81　(32)	124[c]　(254)	108[b]　(860)
1980	97　(160)	137[b]　(55)	105　(215)	116[c]　(892)
1981	106　(186)	127　(51)	110　(237)	119[c]　(931)
1982	91　(151)	101　(42)	93　(193)	108[b]　(853)
1983	92　(149)	124　(48)	98　(197)	109[b]　(833)
1984	111　(182)	101　(38)	109　(220)	120[c]　(909)

[a] Standard population for the city of Bremen in 1970 of males aged 25–64 years. Absolute numbers in parentheses.
[b] Beyond the 95% confidence limit (Poisson).
[c] Beyond the 99% confidence limit (Poisson).

and coronary bypass surgery. As a complete registration of all relevant events in the intervention regions as well as in the rest of the country is not feasible, the incidence of coronary heart disease and stroke could be estimated by use of individual cases. The latter becomes more likely as a recent administrative decree obliges hospitals in the FRG to provide one discharge diagnosis for each patient. The validity of these statistics can be investigated in collaboration with the ongoing WHO MONICA studies in Germany (Keil 1985).

Statistical Analysis

Intermediate and final-phase analysis of changes in risk-factor prevalence between pooled intervention regions and the reference sample will involve standard statistical methods and examination of prevalence rates, means and medians (Kish 1965; Goodman 1978; Huntsberger and Leaverton 1970).

Table 6 shows the detectable differences for some risk factors, if both one intervention region versus another and all intervention regions versus the National Health Survey are compared. The samples are large enough to allow for a detailed analysis of specific age and gender groups as well as social strata.

Besides basic analyses described above, methods which consider the study regions and clusters in the reference as experimental units will be applied. This

Table 6. Detectable differential changes of risk factors based on preliminary data ($\alpha = 0.05$, $\beta = 0.10$)[a]: one-tailed test

Risk factors and indicators	Differential change in one intervention region versus another[b]		Differential change in all intervention regions versus reference	
	Absolute change	Relative change (%)	Absolute change	Relative change (%)
BMI (kg/m)	0.58	2.28	0.30	1.17
Cholesterol (mmol/l)	0.17	2.89	0.09	1.48
Smoking (% smokers)	6.65	18.18	3.41	9.33
Systolic blood pressure (mmHg)	3.71	2.82	1.90	1.44
Diastolic blood pressure (mmHg)	2.26	2.77	1.16	1.42

[a] Smoking is shown as age- and sex-standardized prevalence. For blood pressure, second measurement values have been used; for diastolic blood pressure, phase V Korotkoff sound.
[b] Assuming a sample of 1800 in each centre and 5000 individuals in the reference.

will result in a drastic reduction of degrees of freedom and may be regarded as a conservative way of testing the intervention effects.

In order to assess the effect of the prevention programme on cardiovascular and total mortality, these rates for the pooled study regions will be compared with those of the national reference (Elandt-Johnson and Johnson 1980). The test procedure will be based on $\Sigma(T_i - ET_i)$, where T_i denotes the cumulative number of relevant deaths (ICD-9 410–414, 430–438, and 000–999) in the appropriate age and gender groups for the pool of intervention regions, and ET_i represents the cumulative expected number of respective deaths calculated from the mortality in the reference population. The summation is over all relevant age and gender groups. Because incidence information will not be available and the validity of the available mortality data is questionable, the following additional analyses will be carried out in order to arrive at quantitative estimates of the study-effects on mortality: (a) the secular trends of unverified heart disease death rates will be compared between study regions and the reference via regression models; and (b) the mortality figures in the study regions will be further compared with those of selected regions in the reference.

Discussion

The study design of the GCP is the result of several years of pretesting with regard to the definition and development of feasible prevention programmes and available data sources (Greiser et al. 1978; Laaser 1986).

The GCP displays several features common to other completed and ongoing community intervention studies (Puska et al. 1983; Gutzwiller et al. 1985; Nüssel 1985; Elder et al. 1986; Blackburn et al. 1984; Farquhar et al. 1985). Among these are: (a) the quasi-experimental design; (b) the use of process evaluation to assist in the adaptation and monitoring of preventive activities; (c) the use of health examination surveys and mortality surveillance to evaluate the effect of primary prevention measures on both the risk-factor levels and disease endpoints; and (d) the application of community-oriented interventive strategies based upon the principles of community organization, social marketing und self-help.

As the USA community intervention study groups had to face nation-wide prevention programmes such as the National High Blood Pressure Education Programme, a National High Blood Pressure Programme (Projektgruppe Nationales Blutdruck-Programm 1985) in the FRG is emerging that will most probably have lasting effects on the detection and control of hypertensive patients throughout the country. Other regional or country-wide preventive activities – for example the country-wide prevention programme of the Medical Association of the state of Baden-Württemberg or numerous self-help initiatives – might well influence trends in life style and risk behaviour, thus shaping secular trends of risk factors and cardiovascular mortality.

On the other hand, there are striking discrepancies to be noted when comparing the GCP with other ongoing community intervention studies.

1. All the USA studies have, or had to, confront a steep downward trend in cardiovascular and total mortality which has developed since 1968 and which, at least in part, was a consequence of rapidly changing nutrition and consumption habits, life-style patterns and factors concerning the medical care system. In contrast, the FRG mortality figures over the last few years do not show such a decrease. A massive positive change of nutrition and smoking habits in the German population is not indicated by available data. Recent blood pressure surveys show a comparatively low rate of efficient blood pressure control, comparable to the situation in the U.S.A. at the start of the 1970s. However, the level of cardiovascular mortality is considerably lower in the FRG than in the USA.

2. Unlike the USA studies, the selection of the communities for the GCP was done with the intention of allowing generalizability of the study results, thus enabling a transfer of methods and procedures of prevention into national health policies.

3. The use of the nation as a reference for the intervention regions seems a feature unique to the German study.

4. As a by-product of the decision to fund the GCP, the National Health Examination Survey emerged, which will provide not only reference data for the GCP but also valuable data on the state of health, health attitudes and health behaviour of the nation as a whole for the development of future health strategies. In the USA and many other countries, National Health Surveys existed prior to the start of community-based intervention studies.

An important difficulty for the evaluation of the GCP is the limited availability of disaggregated and valid mortality data. In addition, the present population denominators have to be based upon year-to-year estimations using the 1970 census data, the last exact information on the German resident population.

Appendix

Principal Investigators

E. Greiser, Bremen Institute for Prevention Research and Social Medicine (BIPS), Bremen.

J. Hoeltz, Infratest Health Research Inc., Munich.

H. Hoffmeister, Institute for Social Medicine and Epidemiology, Federal Health Office, Berlin (West).

K.-D. Hüllemann, Clinical Institute for Physiology and Sports Medicine, (KIPSI), Hospital St. Irmingard, Prien.

H. Kreuter, Scientific Institute of the German Medical Association (WIAD), Bonn.

U. Laaser, German Institute for High Blood Pressure Research (DIBHB), Heidelberg.

E. Nüssel, Division of Clinical Social Medicine, Department of Internal Medicine, University of Heidelberg, Heidelberg.

J. v. Troschke, Division of Medical Sociology, University of Freiburg, Freiburg.

This manuscript has been prepared by E. Greiser and K.-H. Jöckel (BIPS), U. Laaser (DIBHB), M. Zachcial (WIAD).

References

Bandura A (1977) Social learning theory. Prentice Hall, Englewood Cliffs

Blackburn H, Luepker RV, Kline FG, et al. (1984) The Minnesota Heart Health Program: a research and demonstration project in cardiovascular disease prevention In: Matarazzo JD, Miller NE, Weiss SM, et al. (eds) Behavioural health: a handbook of health enhancement and disease prevention. Wiley, Silver Spring, pp 1171–1178

Campbell DT, Stanley JC (1963) Experimental and quasi-experimental design for research. Rand McNally, Chicago

Cooper T, Petre T, Weiss SM, et al. (1981) Coronary prone behaviour in coronary heart disease: a critical review. Circulation 63:1200–1215

Elandt-Johnson RC, Johnson NL (1980) Survival models and data analysis. Wiley, New York

Elder JP, McGraw SA, Abrams D, et al. (1986) Organizational and community approaches to community-wide prevention of heart disease: the first two years of the Pawtucket Heart Health Program. Prev Med 15:107–117

Farquhar JW, Fortmann SP, Maccoby N, et al. (1985) The Stanford Five-City-Project: design and methods. Am J Epidemiol 122:323–334 .

Goodman LA (1978) Analyzing qualitative/categorical data. Addison-Wesley, London

Greiser E, Hoffmeister H, Klesse R, et al. (1978) Preliminary study-design of a German multifactorial intervention trial on diabetes and cardio-vascular diseases. Trans Eur Soc Cardiol 1:86

Gutzwiller F, Junod B, Schweizer W (eds) (1985) Wirksamkeit der gemeindeorientierten Prävention kardiovaskulärer Krankheiten: Ergebnisse des Nationalen Forschungsprogramms 1 A. Prävention von Herz-Kreislauf-Krankheiten in der Schweiz. Huber, Bern

Huntsberger DV, Leaverton PE (1970) Statistical inference in the biomedical sciences. Allyn and Bacon, Boston

Hypertension detection and follow-up program cooperative group (1979) Five-year findings of the hypertension detection and follow-up program. I Reduction in mortality of persons with high blood pressure, including mild hypertension. JAMA 242:2562–2571

Keil U (1985) MONICA Project: Herz-Kreislauf-Studie der Weltgesundheitsorganisation. Herz 2:99

Kish L (1965) Survey sampling. Wiley, New York

Laaser U (1986) Die Deutsche Herz-Kreislauf-Präventionsstudie (DHP): Das Modell einer kooperativen Prävention. In: Halhuber C, Traenckner K (eds) Die koronare Herzkrankheit – eine Herausforderung an Gesellschaft und Politik. perimed, Erlangen

Lipid Research Clinics Program (1984) The lipid research clinics' coronary primary prevention trial results. I. Reduction in incidence of coronary disease. JAMA 251:351–364

Management Committee (1980) The Australian therapeutic trial in mild hypertension. Lancet 1:1260–1267

Medical Research Council Working Party (1985) MRC trial of treatment of mild hypertension: principal results. Br Med J 291:97–104

Nüssel E (1985) Community-based prevention: the Eberbach-Wiesloch Study. In: Hofmann H (ed) Primary and secondary prevention of coronary heart disease. Springer, Berlin Heidelberg New York, pp 50–59

Paffenbarger RS, Hyde RT, Wing AL, et al. (1986) Physical activity, all-cause mortality and longevity of college alumni. N Engl J Med 314:605–613

Pooling Project Research Group (1978) Relationship of blood pressure, serum cholesterol, smoking habit, relative weight and ECG abnormalities to incidence of major coronary event: final report. J Chronic Dis 31:201–206

Projektgruppe Nationales Blutdruck-Programm (NBP) (1985) Projektbeschreibung. pmi, Frankfurt

Puska P, Tuomilehtto J, Salonen JT, et al. (1983) Ten years of the North Karelia Project: results with community-based prevention of coronary heart disease in Finland. Scand J Soc Med 11:65–68

Rogers EM (1983) Diffusion of innovations, 3rd edn. Free, New York

Veterans Administration Cooperative Study Group (1967) Effects of treatment on morbidity in hypertension. I. Results in patients with diastolic blood pressure averaging 115 through 129 mm Hg. JAMA 202:1028–1034

Veterans Administration Cooperative Study Group (1970) Effects of treatment on morbidity in hypertension. II. Results in patients with diastolic blood pressure averaging 90 through 114 mm Hg. JAMA 213:1143–1152

Stand und Perspektiven der Forschung zur Krebsfrüherkennung *

F. W. Schwartz, B.-P. Robra

Krebsfrüherkennung als Bevölkerungsscreening

Im Rahmen dieses Beitrags sind Krebsfrüherkennungsmaßnahmen als Bestandteil von Screeningprogrammen an großen asymptomatischen Bevölkerungsgruppen („Massenscreening") zu diskutieren.

Screeninguntersuchungen (Filteruntersuchungen) sind definitionsgemäß nicht geeignet, eine endgültige Diagnose zu etablieren. Vielmehr ist es ihre Aufgabe, anscheinend gesunde Teilnehmer am Untersuchungsprogramm möglichst zuverlässig und zutreffend in Gruppen mit hohem und niedrigem Risiko für das Vorhandensein der vorgegebenen Zielkrankheit einzuteilen. Die Einladung zu einem solchen Programm setzt voraus, daß die Entdeckung der Zielkrankheit mit den eingesetzten Methoden früher möglich ist als die durchschnittliche Entdeckung an Patienten, die wegen Symptomen das Versorgungssystem gezielt aufsuchen. Es muß ferner vorausgesetzt werden, daß die damit ermöglichte Behandlung effektiver oder für den Betroffenen weniger belastend ist als die Behandlung zu einem späteren Zeitpunkt.

Forderungen an Programmstruktur und Untersuchungstests

Die Durchführung eines Screenings verlangt eine klare Programmstruktur. Dies setzt die Beschreibung und erfolgreiche Rekrutierung der gewünschten Teilnehmer voraus, die Festlegung zweckmäßiger Untersuchungsintervalle und die Stabilisierung und Qualitätsüberwachung der eingesetzten Untersuchungsmethoden. Die unmittelbare Abklärungsdiagnostik gefundener positiver Fälle ist zu definieren, ebenso die Maßnahmen der Frühtherapie bei gesicherten Frühfällen. Die Einführung eines Früherkennungsprogramms bedingt nach heutiger Auffassung zugleich die Einführung eines begleitenden Evaluationsprogramms einschließlich der Kontrolle der Kosten.

Screening ist zu unterscheiden von Diagnostik. Jede Diagnostik geht von bestimmten, möglicherweise spezifischen Beschwerden von Patienten aus. Die angewandten Untersuchungstests können, müssen aber nicht standardisiert sein.

* Erstmals veröffentlicht in: Projektträgerschaft „Forschung im Dienste der Gesundheit" in der Deutschen Forschungsanstalt für Luft- und Raumfahrt e. V. (1989) Krebsforschung in der Bundesrepublik Deutschland. Kohlhammer, Stuttgart, S. 75–84.

Diagnostik ist mithin jeder Prozeß der Abklärung vorliegender Beschwerden oder Befunde mit variablen (hierarchischen oder parallel aufeinander bezogenen) Untersuchungen mit dem Ziel, in einem individuellen Fall eine endgültige Diagnose zu etablieren. Im pathogenetischen Krankheitsprozeß setzt Screening (die Abklärung seltener früher Zufallsbefunde ausgenommen) deutlich früher ein als jede symptomgeleitete Diagnostik. Viele frühe Krankheitsmerkmale stellen sich weniger distinkt und damit zugleich mehrdeutiger dar als späte. Ähnliche Schwierigkeiten stellen sich vielfach auch für die Abklärungsdiagnostik der durch Screening aufgefundenen frühen Verdachtsfälle. Früherkennung an asymptomatischen Patienten stellt daher hohe Anforderungen an den Screeningtest. Der Test soll sicher, schnell, kostengünstig, einfach durchführbar und für die Teilnehmer akzeptabel sein, zugleich möglichst hohe Sensitivität und Spezifität aufweisen. Je seltener eine Zielkrankheit ist, um so höhere Anforderungen werden insbesondere an die Spezifität gestellt, damit die Zahl der falsch positiven Testergebnisse mit den daraus resultierenden Kosten an Ressourcen, Patientenzeit und Beängstigung möglichst klein, der positive prädiktive Wert möglichst hoch gehalten wird. Unzureichende Spezifität mit falsch positiven Fällen bedeutet bei einer wiederum nicht vollkommen spezifischen Abklärungsdiagnostik die Gefahr definitiv gestellter, falsch positiver Diagnosen und damit, insbesondere im Bereich der Krebsfrüherkennung, nicht notwendiger Behandlung mit erheblichen physischen und psychischen Konsequenzen für die Betroffenen. Die Testeigenschaften müssen vor Beginn eines Programms unter praxisnahen Bedingungen sorgfältig untersucht und die Einhaltung festgelegter Bedingungen im Rahmen der begleitenden Evaluation ständig überwacht werden.

Daß Screeningprogramme nicht für extrem seltene Erkrankungen eingeführt werden sollen, ergibt sich nicht nur aus den zunehmend als notwendig erkannten Grundsätzen einer sparsamen, möglichst effektiven Mittelverwendung, sondern auch aus der mathematischen Abhängigkeit der positiven prädiktiven Werte vom Krankheitsvorkommen. Diese und andere bedenkenswerten Eigenschaften eines Screeningprogramms lassen sich in einer Checkliste zusammenstellen (s. Übersicht).

Kriterien für Zielkrankheiten

- Krankheitslast
  Individuelle Krankheitslast
  (Verlust an Lebensjahren, vermeidbare Behinderung, Schmerz)
  Kollektive Krankheitslast
  (u. a. Prävalenz, bei periodischem Screening auch Inzidenz, Produktionsverlust, Kosten)

- Ätiologie, Pathogenese
  Ausreichend bekannt
  Frühstadien mit ausreichender Latenzzeit, „Sojourn Time"
  Signalstärke, Progressionswahrscheinlichkeit

- Nutzen, Risiken, Kosten
  Akzeptable Frühbehandlung verfügbar, die die Krankheitslast wirksam zu senken verspricht gegenüber der üblichen Versorgung
  Risiken und Kosten stehen in angemessenem Verhältnis zum gesundheitlichen Gewinn (auch im Vergleich zu anderen Gesundheitsaufgaben).

Kriterien für Zielpopulation

- Epidemiologisch
  (alters- bzw. gruppenspezifische Prävalenz, Inzidenz, Signalstärke, „Sojourn Time",
  Progressionswahrscheinlichkeit)

- Sozialpolitisch
  (Krankheitslast, Kosten, Risiken, Nutzen)

- Organisatorisch
  (Bereitschaft zur Beteiligung und Folgecompliance, örtliche und zeitliche Verfügbarkeit
  von Einrichtungen, Integration in kurative Versorgung).

Kriterien für Screeningtests

- Validität
  Sensitivität, Spezifität
  Reliabilität, Beobachterunabhängigkeit
  Analytische Varianz
  Intra- und interindividuelle Merkmalsvarianz
  Validität der Referenztests
  Periodik des Screenings
  Offengelegte Standards für Messung und Ergebniswertung.

- Akzeptabilität, Praktikabilität, Kosten
  für Probanden,
  für Untersucher.

- Diagnostischer Ertrag
  (aus Validität, Akzeptanz, Prävalenz bei periodischem Screening auch Inzidenz).

- Analoge Kriterien
  auch für die verfügbare Abklärungsdiagnostik.

Es sollte beachtet werden, daß die Akzeptanz im Früherkennungsprogramm keineswegs nur von den primär eingesetzten Untersuchungstests abhängt, sondern eine ganze Reihe komplexer Eigenschaften anspricht. Dazu gehören die laienhafte Einschätzung der Therapierbarkeit in bezug auf bleibende Überlebenschancen und verbleibende Lebensqualität, die psychologische und soziale Akzeptanz einer Entdeckung der Krankheit, von deren Existenz die Umgebung Kenntnis nimmt, sowie objektive und subjektive Belastungen durch Abklärungsdiagnostik und Therapie. Unter diesem Gesichtspunkt scheint es plausibel, daß unter den in der Bundesrepublik Deutschland derzeit angebotenen Früherkennungsmaßnahmen (auf Krebserkrankung der Zervix, der Brust, der Haut, des Kolonrektums, der Prostata) die Früherkennung auf Zervixkrebs die größte Akzeptanz findet. Diese Erkrankung ist oberflächennah, hinreichend gut diagnostisch zu erkennen und in der Frühphase mit einem relativ kleinen Eingriff ausreichend sicher beherrschbar. Die Skepsis des Publikums, die sich in seit Jahren unbefriedigenden Teilnahmeraten zeigt, wird – wie wir aus entsprechenden sozialwissenschaftlichen Untersuchungen wissen – nicht zuletzt über die behandelnden (Haus)ärzte vermittelt. Alle werbenden Bemühungen um verbesserte Teilnahmeraten dürfen die Ärzte nicht außer acht lassen. Die beste Werbung liegt zweifellos in einer substantiellen Verbesserung der Programmteile selbst.

Grundlagenwissen zum „naturgesetzlichen" Verlauf der Zielerkrankungen

Zum vertieften Verständnis der Schwierigkeiten eines Früherkennungsprogramms, speziell eines Programms der Krebsfrüherkennung, ist es notwendig, den naturgesetzlichen Ablauf einer unbeeinflußten Zielerkrankung ("natural history") sorgfältig zu analysieren. Folgende Fragen sind in diesem Zusammenhang zu klären: Führen onkologisch faßbare präneoplastische Entwicklungsstufen in allen Fällen zu einem invasiven Karzinom oder gibt es eine nennenswerte spontane Regression (wie für Dysplasien an der Zervix nachgewiesen) bzw. lassen sich die Rückbildungen und das Verschwinden präneoplastischer Veränderungen durch bestimmte nichttherapeutische Maßnahmen (z. B. Verzicht auf Rauchen, auf Alkohol oder Änderungen in Ernährungsgewohnheiten, etwa hinsichtlich der Vitamin-A-Aufnahme) beschleunigen, wie dies etwa für dysplastische Veränderungen des Rachen-Kehlkopf-Raums oder der Speiseröhre diskutiert wird? Wenn Progression stattfindet – welche durchschnittlichen Zeiträume sind maßgeblich, und von welcher Variabilität müssen wir ausgehen? Dies ist wichtig zur Festlegung zweckmäßiger Screeningintervalle und erlaubt auch, die Anforderungen an eine ausreichende Sensitivität der eingesetzten Untersuchungsmethoden zu präzisieren. Wenn Wiederholungsuntersuchungen nach falsch-negativen Voruntersuchungen eine befriedigend hohe Chance haben, noch in eine präneoplastische Latenzzeit zu fallen, ist offensichtlich eine andere Lage gegeben, als wenn unmittelbar die Gefahr übersehener, klinisch manifest werdender Krebsfälle besteht (sog. „Intervallfälle").

"Lead time"-Fehler

Eine weitere Schwierigkeit besteht darin, daß gerade bei langen Latenzzeiten die Früherkennung einer Krebsvorstufe naturgemäß zu sehr viel längeren Überlebenszeiten ab Diagnosezeitpunkt gegenüber fortgeschrittenen Stadien führt, und zwar mit wie ohne Therapie, weil die Beobachtungszeit der Erkrankung dadurch viel länger geworden ist. Man nennt diesen häufigen Fehler, der auch bei einem Vergleich der Überlebenszeiten klinischer Stadien zu beachten ist, nach dem reichhaltigen Schrifttum den "lead time bias". "Lead time" ist die Zeit, die der im Screening entdeckte Krebs durchschnittlich früher entdeckt wird, als seine Entdeckung bei Abwesenheit von Screening wahrscheinlich gewesen wäre.

Verweildauerfehler

Die Wahrscheinlichkeit der Entdeckung von Krebsvorstufen (durch einen in der Regel unvollkommenen Test) ist nicht zuletzt von der Dauer des präklinischen Latenzstadiums einer prämalignen Veränderung abhängig. Es haben langsam verlaufende, lange persistierende Veränderungen bei einem gegebenen periodischen Screening eine höhere Entdeckungschance als schnelle Verläufe. Das

Screening selektiert also günstige Verläufe. Dieser systematische Fehler bei der Bewertung von Screeningprogrammen im Vergleich zu nicht gescreenten Gruppen wird als „length biased sampling" oder „Verweildauerfehler" bezeichnet. Er wird nur wenig durch den Effekt modifiziert, daß die Sensitivität und Spezifität vieler Tests von der Größe der gesuchten Läsion abhängig ist, schnelle Verläufe bei fixem Intervall aber eine größere Chance haben, eine entdeckbare größere Läsion darzustellen, als sehr langsame.

Selbstselektion

Eine weitere Fehlerquelle besteht in der nicht seltenen Selbstselektion der Teilnehmer an einem Früherkennungsprogramm. Gemeint ist, daß einerseits frühe, u. U. äußerst diskrete subjektive oder objektive Warnzeichen Patienten zu einem Screening führen oder andererseits bei stark angstbesetzten Krankheitsbildern wie Krebs ihre Teilnahme verhindern. Es kann die paradoxe Situation eintreten, daß die häufigsten Teilnehmer am Screening diejenigen Personen sind, die es am wenigsten nötig haben. Dies ist beispielsweise beim Zervixscreening bei Frauen aus mittleren Altersgruppen aus der Mittelschicht heute der Fall, während Bevölkerungsgruppen mit objektiv erhöhtem Erkrankungsrisiko aus sozialen oder psychischen Gründen (Distanz zum Untersucher, Zeitmangel, Desinteresse, negatives Selbstbild etc.) die Untersuchungen am geringsten in Anspruch nehmen. Eine ungünstige, risikoinverse Selektion wäre auch bei einem Screening auf neoplastische Veränderungen des oberen aerodigestiven Trakts in bezug auf starke Alkohol- und Tabakkonsumenten zu erwarten.

Risikogruppen

Die Frage einer angemessenen Abgrenzung von Risikogruppen stellt eine wichtige Herausforderung an moderne Früherkennungsprogramme dar. Unser empirisches Wissen zur Risikoverteilung der für ein systematisches Früherkennungsprogramm relevanten Krebslokalisationen ist in den letzten Jahren stark gewachsen. Es lassen sich in vielen Fällen recht exakte relative Risiken für ausreichend gut abgrenzbare Teilgruppen angeben. Bei zweckentsprechender organisatorischer Gestaltung von Früherkennungsprogrammen können damit Prävalenzanreicherungen der Zielerkrankungen im untersuchten Bevölkerungssegment um das 2- bis 70fache erreicht werden (das erste Beispiel trifft für Verwandte ersten Grades von Lungenkrebskranken zu und das zweite Beispiel auf das Lungenkrebsvorkommen bei rauchenden Asbestarbeitern). Die Prävalenzanreicherung durch Bildung von Risikogruppen ist u. U. ein wirksamer Weg, um sowohl die Effektivität wie die Wirtschaftlichkeit von Screeningprogrammen bedeutend zu erhöhen. Für diesen Weg ist es nicht notwendig, den kausalen Zusammenhang zwischen Risikofaktor (oder Risikoindikator) und Zielkrankheit bereits im Detail zu kennen (vgl. zur Hausen 1989). Der Grundgedanke wird etwa in den arbeitsmedizinischen Vorsorgeuntersuchungen zur Überwachung besonders gefährdeter Personenkreise angewandt. Er hat bislang aber nicht in deutschen Programmen der gesetzlichen Krankenversicherung Eingang gefunden, wenn wir von der Festlegung einer unteren Altersgrenze absehen.

Methodik der Programmbewertung

Die geschilderten Schwierigkeiten und „Fallen" bei der Bewertung von Screeningprogrammen haben dazu geführt, daß in den letzten Jahren eine gemeinsam durch Epidemiologie, Klinik und Versorgungsforschung ("health care research") entwickelte Methodik für die Evaluation von Screeningprogrammen bereitgestellt wurde. Die angemessenste Methode zur Klärung der Effektivität eines Screenings unter sonst unsicheren bzw. nur teilweise erklärten Voraussetzungen ist die Durchführung einer randomisierten kontrollierten Studie. Derartige Studien sind beispielsweise erfolgreich durchgeführt worden, um die Frage zu klären, ob das mammographische Screening bei Frauen zu einer Überlebensverbesserung führt (HIP-Studie in New York, Kopparberg-Östergötland-Studie und Malmö-Studie in Schweden). Randomisierte kontrollierte Studien lassen sich sogar noch dann durchführen, wenn in einer Bevölkerung ein Screeningprogramm bereits grundsätzlich eingeführt ist. Es kann dann die Intensität der Einladungsbemühungen (wie in der Kaiser-Permanente-Studie) oder das vorgeschriebene Screeningintervall (wie in der Minnesota-Studie zum kolorektalen Screening) variiert werden. Das völlige Fehlen derartiger randomisierter Studien in der Bundesrepublik Deutschland ist daher keine unabweisbare Konsequenz aus unserer frühen Entscheidung für ein strukturiertes Früherkennungsprogramm, sondern Ausdruck bislang fehlender interdisziplinärer Forschungs- und Förderungsstrukturen in diesem Bereich.

Es haben darüber hinaus eine Reihe von Beobachtungsstudien zu einer verbesserten Evidenz zugunsten der Früherkennung beigetragen. Dazu gehören zeitliche Vergleiche der Krebsinzidenz (Rate neu erkannter Fälle) und der Mortalität in definierten Populationen vor und nach Einführung eines Screeningprogramms. Diese haben allerdings säkulare zeitliche Schwankungen in dem natürlichen Vorkommen und der Mortalität der Erkrankung zu beachten. Räumliche Vergleiche mit Regionen unterschiedlich intensiver Screeningaktivität können die Frage von „Dosis-Wirkungs-Beziehungen" klären helfen. Alle derartigen Studien setzen das Vorhandensein einer funktionierenden Krebsregistrierung für Inzidenz- und Mortalitätsdaten in definierten Regionen voraus. Dies ist für die Bundesrepublik Deutschland nur im Saarland und in Hamburg gegeben (im Saarland ist zudem das Krebsregister aus Datenschutzgründen gefährdet). Die Rahmenbedingungen für wissenschaftliche Arbeiten sind damit in der Bundesrepublik Deutschland an wichtiger Stelle gestört. Für Teilaspekte liefern klinische Tumorregister, die sich sowohl auf Diagnostik, Behandlung wie Nachsorge nichtselektierter Behandlungsverläufe beziehen, wichtige Informationen (vgl. Nagel 1989; v. Kleist 1989). Hier haben Fördermaßnahmen sowohl von privater (Deutsche Krebshilfe) wie staatlicher Seite (BMA, BMJFFG) in den letzten Jahren wichtige Voraussetzungen in der Bundesrepublik Deutschland geschaffen. Während die Nutzung dieser Instrumente für klinische Zwecke [z. B. prognostischer Variablen bei Lungenkrebs (Höpker u. Lüllig 1987)] auf zunehmendes Interesse stößt, sind Ansätze zur Bewertung der Früherkennungsprogramme noch nicht entwickelt.

Ein neueres – inzwischen recht erfolgreich eingesetztes – Instrument zur Screeningevaluation sind Fallkontrollstudien, die nicht nur geeignet sind, alters- und intervallspezifische „Effektschätzer" für definierte Resultatgrößen (v. a. die Mortalität) des Programms zu liefern, sondern man kann mit ihrer Hilfe auch die Wirtschaftlichkeit (im Sinne einer Kosten-Effektivitäts-Analyse) von Screening-varianten untersuchen, sofern unter sonst vergleichbaren Rahmenbedingungen unterschiedliche Varianten im Feld eingeführt worden sind. Fallkontrollstudien lassen sich in sehr viel kürzeren Zeiträumen durchführen als prospektive Studien, zu denen auch die erwähnten „randomisierten" kontrollierten Studien gehören, aber sie setzen die mehrjährige Durchführung von Screeningprogrammen bereits voraus (retrospektiver Ansatz). Sie liegen daher für die Situation, die wir in der Bundesrepublik Deutschland erreicht haben, besonders nahe. Die oben geschilderten Selektionseinflüsse machen nichtrandomisierte Studien allerdings anfällig gegen systematische Fehler. Bisher ist in der Bundesrepublik Deutschland erst eine Studie dieser Art durch Kooperation zwischen Heidelberg (DKFZ), Saarland (Tumorzentrum, Ärzteschaft) und Hannover (Abteilung Epidemiologie und Sozialmedizin der MHH) zur Wirkung des kolorektalen Krebsscreenings in Gang gekommen.

Die dargestellten Schwierigkeiten bei Planung, Organisation und wissenschaftlicher Bewertung von Massenscreeningprogrammen erklären, warum Screeningprogramme im internationalen Vergleich bislang nicht die Verbreitung gefunden haben, die man aufgrund der Erwartungen in den 60er Jahren an derartige Maßnahmen vorhersagte.

Für das entwickelte deutsche Früherkennungsprogramm steht in den nächsten Jahren die Einführung der Mammographie als (unselektive) Maßnahme für alle Frauen ab einer noch zu definierenden Altersgrenze an. Ein Qualitätssicherungsprogramm wird derzeit unter Förderung des BMFT definiert und flächendeckend erprobt.

Die Häufigkeit zytologischer Abstriche vom Gebärmutterhals kann – wie internationale Daten zeigen – ohne wesentlichen Effektivitätsverlust statt des bisher noch empfohlenen jährlichen auf ein 2–3jähriges Intervall zurückgenommen werden, wenn bereits negative Vorbefunde guter Qualität vorliegen. Es fehlt ein Einladungsmodell, mit dessen Hilfe Frauen gezielt an die Früherkennungstermine erinnert werden, und zwar je nach Vorbefund und Alter mit unterschiedlichem Intervall.

Notwendigkeit interdisziplinärer Forschungsgruppen

Früherkennung von Krebsen ist also – trotz oft gegenteiliger Propagierung – nur nach Maßgabe gesicherter frühdiagnostischer und frühtherapeutischer Möglichkeiten und unter Berücksichtigung alternativer Strategien gerechtfertigt. Der Stellenwert eines Früherkennungstests kann daher nur im Kontext des naturgesetzlichen Verlaufs der Zielkrankheit, der Struktur und der Funktion des Programms, in dem er eingesetzt wird, und der Leistungsfähigkeit der diagnostischen und therapeutischen Versorgungskette beurteilt werden. Eine gemeinsame Evaluation solcher aufeinander bezogenen Teilkomponenten von Früherkennungsprogrammen stellt besondere Anforderungen an die Interdisziplinarität und die Integration der Forschung. Dies verlangt den Aufbau interdisziplinärer Arbeitsgruppen zwischen Klinik, Epidemiologie und Gesundheitssystemforschung nach dem Vorbild der klinisch-onkologischen Arbeitsgruppen (vgl. Seeber 1989). Ein solcher Förderungsansatz fehlt bisher. Ohne ihn sind substantielle Fortschritte in der Technik, dem Niveau und der Programmstruktur von Früherkennungsmaßnahmen nicht zu erwarten. Die hohen Kosten für Screeningprogramme lassen die interdisziplinäre Anbindung der Gesundheitsökonomie wünschenswert erscheinen. Die in der Vergangenheit durch das BMFT geförderten „Bestandsaufnahmen" zum Stand der Möglichkeiten einer systematischen Krebsfrüherkennung (insbesondere IABG 1979–1983) haben die hier gestellten Aufgaben nicht lösen können. Dies gilt auch für die isolierte Förderung einzelner frühdiagnostischer Untersuchungstechniken (etwa im Bereich der automatisierten Zytologie). Nagel (1989) weist in seinem Beitrag zu Recht darauf hin, daß viele aus klinischer Sicht entwickelte Untersuchungsansätze an in der Regel kleinen Stichproben in der flächendeckenden Anwendung des Massenscreenings mit Effizienzproblemen zu kämpfen haben, ohne deren vorherige Analyse solche Ansätze oft zum Scheitern verurteilt sind. Ein systematisierter, interdisziplinär angelegter Förderbereich Früherkennung ist demnach ein dringliches Desiderat.

Eine besondere Förderung verdienen in Zukunft Programme an abgrenzbaren Risikogruppen in der allgemeinen Bevölkerung. Die auch von zur Hausen (1989) angesprochene Identifizierung genetischer Risiken als eine Möglichkeit der Risikogruppenidentifizierung wirft im Rahmen einer laufenden prospektiven Überwachung durch Früherkennungsmaßnahmen auch ernstzunehmende verhaltens- und sozialwissenschaftliche Probleme auf. Wir haben bereits darauf hingewiesen, daß die Erfahrungen mit laufenden Früherkennungsprogrammen gezeigt haben, daß die objektiv und subjektiv am stärksten gefährdeten Personengruppen oft ein deutlich angstbesetztes Vermeidungsverhalten zeigen. Trotz beachtenswerter Forschungsbeiträge (z. B. Verres 1986) sind wir weit entfernt davon, die damit verbundenen psychodynamischen und sozialen Mechanismen zu verstehen und in einer Programmstruktur erfolgreich zu berücksichtigen. Organisierte Fortbildungsmaßnahmen der involvierten Ärzteschaft und andere Qualitätssicherungsmaßnahmen müssen einen qualitativen Mindeststandard etablieren und aufrecht erhalten. Solche Standards lassen sich nicht aus klinischer Sicht allein entwickeln, sondern setzen Interdisziplinarität voraus.

In der Förderung interdisziplinärer Arbeitsgruppen sowohl im Bereich der Forschung wie der praktischen Umsetzung liegen die wesentlichen Chancen einer Verbesserung der Früherkennungsprogramme in den nächsten Jahren.

Literatur

Hausen H zur (1989) Wo steht die Krebsforschung? In. Projektträgerschaft „Forschung im Dienste der Gesundheit" (Hrsg), S 33–39

Höpker W-W, Lüllig H (1987) Lungenkarzinom: Resektion, Morphologie und Prognose. Springer, Berlin Heidelberg New York Tokyo

Kleist S von (1989) Krebsbekämpfung durch Privatinitiative. In: Projektträgerschaft „Forschung im Dienste der Gesundheit" (Hrsg), S 45–54
Nagel GA (1989) Forschungsbedarf aus der Sicht der Deutschen Krebsgesellschaft. In: Projektträgerschaft „Forschung im Dienste der Gesundheit" (Hrsg), S 55–67
Projektträgerschaft „Forschung im Dienste der Gesundheit" in der Deutschen Forschungsanstalt für Luft- und Raumfahrt e. V. (1989) Krebsforschung in der Bundesrepublik Deutschland. Kohlhammer, Stuttgart
Seeber S (1989) Perspektiven der Krebstherapieforschung. In: „Projektträgerschaft Forschung im Dienste der Gesundheit" (Hrsg), S 85–91
Verres R (1986) Krebs und Angst: subjektive Theorien von Laien uber Ursachen, Verhütung, Früherkennung, Behandlung und die psychosozialen Folgen von Krebserkrankungen. Springer, Berlin Heidelberg New York Tokyo

Prävention aus der Sicht sozialversicherter Privathaushalte: Erklärungsansätze und Versuch der empirischen Überprüfung*

B. Birkner, G. Neubauer

Problemstellung

Das präventive Gesundheitsverhalten von Privathaushalten kann für sich nicht in Anspruch nehmen, Gegenstand besonderen Interesses der Gesundheitsökonomen zu sein. (Eher schon ist es Forschungsgegenstand der Medizinsoziologie.) Beschäftigen sich Ökonomen mit der Krankheitsprävention, so geschieht dies häufig unter dem Aspekt der Kosten-Nutzen-Gegenüberstellung zur Effizienzbeurteilung von Vorsorgeprogrammen. Fast regelmäßig findet sich bei Befürwortern einer Selbstbeteiligung der Hinweis auf deren „erzieherische" Wirkung auf die Krankheitsvorbeugung durch die Versicherten. Von gesundheitspolitischer Seite wird die Krankheitsprävention mitunter in den Dienst der Kostendämpfung gestellt – ein Weg, der im übrigen in die Irre führt.[1]

Ansatzpunkt der folgenden Überlegungen ist allein der sozialversicherte Privathaushalt, der nicht nur in seiner Rolle als Finanzier und Leistungsempfänger der sozialen Krankenversicherung gesehen wird, sondern als Wirtschaftseinheit, die selbst Gesundheitsleistungen bereitstellt.

Ziel ist es – unabhängig von Kosten-Nutzen-Erwägungen, unabhängig von einer wie auch immer gearteten Indienstnahme der Prävention für sozialpolitische Intentionen – zu fragen, warum und wie Privathaushalte präventiv tätig werden. Daran anschließend ist die Frage zu erörtern, wie die Haushalte bei ihren Bemühungen um Krankheitsvorbeugung durch die Gesundheitspolitik wirksam untertstützt werden können.

Wirkungen von Krankheit auf den sozialversicherten Privathaushalt

Krankheit verursacht eine Reihe von Risiken, die für den Versicherten nur zu jenen Teilen abgedeckt sind, als sie den krankheitsbedingten Konsum von Gesundheitsgütern und -leistungen betreffen sowie denjenigen Einkommensausfall wegen Arbeitsunfähigkeit, der direkt der Krankheitsdauer zuzuordnen ist.[2]

Grundsätzlich beim Haushalt selbst verbleiben die Risiken, durch Krankheit frühzeitig zu sterben, Schmerzen zu erleiden, sozial isoliert zu werden usw., sowie

---

* Erstmals veröffentlicht in: Oberender P (Hrsg) (1988) Neuorientierung im Gesundheitswesen. PCO, Bayreuth (Schriften zur Gesundheitsökonomie, Bd. 2, S. 143–164).

[1] Vgl. unten, Fußnote 18.

[2] Vgl. Müller-Groeling H (1968) Zur ökonomischen Problematik der Gesetzlichen Krankenversicherung. ORDO 19:489.

das Risiko einer krankheitsbedingten Einschränkung der Dispositionsfreiheit bei Einkommenserzielung und -verwendung. So kann eine längerfristige gesundheitliche Beeinträchtigung den Verlauf der Lebenseinkommenskurve ungünstig beeinflussen, sei es durch frühzeitige Verrentung, durch eine im Durchschnitt längere Arbeitslosigkeit,[3] durch einen im Durchschnitt niedrigeren Lohnsatz oder, im ungünstigsten Fall, durch eine kumulierte Wirkung der genannten Faktoren.

Einschränkungen der Wahlmöglichkeiten bei der Einkommensverwendung resultieren dann, wenn krankheitsbedingt der konsumierbare Güterraum schrumpft. Zahlreiche Güter, sei es aus dem Bereich der Ernährung, der Freizeitgestaltung etc., setzen eine ausreichende Gesundheit des Konsumenten voraus. Je nach Art und Schwere vermögen Erkrankungen zu einer Revision des bisher realisierten und für die Zukunft projizierten Lebensstandards zu zwingen. Krankheit kann also auch bei Krankheitsvollkostenversicherung zur Restriktion für das Wirtschaften des Haushalts werden; sie gewinnt damit eine ökonomische Eigenschaft, die jener des Einkommens ähnlich ist, indem auch sie das Niveau des Lebensstandards limitiert.

Die einzige Möglichkeit des Haushalts, sich vor den skizzierten nichtversicherbaren Risiken zu schützen, besteht darin, der Krankheitsentstehung vorzubeugen. Prävention wäre mithin als eine Art „Zusatzversicherung" aufzufassen.

Prävention und Krankenversicherung

Tatsächlich lassen sich Analogien zwischen Prävention und regulärer Versicherungsnahme feststellen: Ein unsicherer aber großer Verlust, die Erkrankung, wird in seiner Eintrittswahrscheinlichkeit herabgesenkt durch einen kleinen, sicheren Verlust. Als Prämiensurrogat ist sowohl der monetäre Preis etwaiger Präventionsgüter denkbar als auch, im Falle der Krankheitsvorbeugung durch Konsumverzicht, der Nutzenentgang beim Verzicht auf gesundheitsriskante Güter. Allerdings – und hierin liegt ein gewichtiger Unterschied zur regulären Versicherung, die ja mit Sicherheit die finanziellen Lasten im Schadensfalle übernimmt – werden lediglich Eintrittswahrscheinlichkeiten bestimmter präventiv beeinflußbarer Krankheiten gesenkt. Mit Sicherheit kann nicht ausgeschlossen werden, dennoch daran zu erkranken; erst recht nicht kann ausgeschlossen werden, an Krankheiten (oder Unfallfolgen) frühzeitig zu sterben, deren Auftreten nicht vom eigenen Verhalten abhängt.

In der Versicherungsökonomie wird üblicherweise von einem konkurrierenden Verhältnis zwischen einer Verminderung der Schadenswahrscheinlichkeit durch den Versicherten (Prävention) und Versicherungsnahme ausgegangen.[4] Dies mag für bestimmte Versicherungszweige, z. B. Diebstahlversicherungen, zutreffen, ebenso für Teile des präventiv beeinflußbaren Krankheitsspektrums, also

---

[3] Vgl. Brinkmann C (1983) Verbleib und Vermittlungsprobleme von Arbeitslosen, Material Arbeitsmarkt Berufsforsch 5:7f.

[4] Vgl. Ehrlich SJ, Becker GS (1972) Market insurance, self-insurance and self-protection, J Pol Economy 80:641ff. Für die Krankenversicherung vgl. Nordquist G, Wu S (1976) Joint demand for health insurance and preventive medicine. In: Rosett RN (ed) The role of health insurance in the health service sector. New York, pp 35ff.

teilweise auch für die Krankenversicherung. Von einer Konkurrenzbeziehung beider Strategien ist jedoch dann nicht mehr a priori auszugehen, wenn 2 Bedingungen erfüllt sind: 1) der Erfolg der Prävention ist ungewiß, und 2) der Verlust im Schadensfall läßt sich nicht allein durch den Ersatz des Einkommens- und Vermögensschadens durch die Versicherung vollständig „heilen". Je gravierender der Versicherte die nichtversicherbaren Krankheitsfolgen einschätzt, je höher das bei ihm verbleibende Risiko ist, desto eher ist Prävention trotz Vollversicherung zu erwarten. Umgekehrt muß, wenn gesundheitsgefährdendes Verhalten vorliegt, auch nach Gründen hierfür gesucht werden, die außerhalb des Versichertenstatus liegen.

Überlegungen zum Entscheidungshintergrund

Wovon hängt es ab, ob sich jemand präventiv verhält oder es unterläßt? Die Entscheidung dürfte von folgenden Faktoren beeinflußt sein:

- von der Risikoaversion,
- vom Preis der Prävention, also vom Geldpreis oder von nichtmonetären Preisbestandteilen wie z. B. dem Nutzenentgang beim Konsumverzicht,
- von den Informationen über Eintrittswahrscheinlichkeiten präventiv beeinflußbarer Krankheiten sowie von Krankheiten und Unfällen, die nicht vom eigenen Verhalten abhängen,
- vom Zeithorizont, sofern es sich um die Vorbeugung von Krankheiten des höheren Lebensalters handelt.

Es lassen sich nun, ausgehend von diesem Entscheidungskatalog, Hypothesen bilden, die hier allerdings nur kurz angesprochen werden können.[5]

So ist von einer mit dem Alter steigenden Risikoaversion auszugehen. Höheres Alter dürfte auch den Zukunftsbezug des Handelns begünstigen, da die Zeit, in der die „Erträge" der präventiven Lebensweise anfallen, näher liegt als bei jungen Menschen.

Eine stärkere Risikoaversion und eine Einbeziehung künftiger Belange in die gegenwärtigen Dispositionen ist wohl auch eher zu erwarten von Personen, die sich für ihnen nahestehende Menschen verantwortlich fühlen, mithin von Verheirateten und von Eltern. Geht man von altruistisch verbundenen Nutzenfunktionen in der Familie aus, so mag dies die Verzichtsleistung, die eine präventive Lebensweise erfordern kann, erleichtern. Überdies kann in der Familie das Gesundheitsverhalten der Mitglieder einer gegenseitigen Kontrolle unterzogen werden. Generell dürfte ferner gelten, daß der Preis, sofern als gegenwärtiger Verzicht für künftige „Erträge" zu erbringen, dann als hoch empfunden wird, wenn die Gegenwart von Sorgen belastet ist.[6]

---

[5] Vgl. hierzu Birkner B (1986) Privathaushalt und Gesundheit – Erklärungsansätze für das präventive Gesundheitsverhalten von Privathaushalten und Versuch der empirischen Überprüfung anhand ausgewählter Beispiele. Dissertation, Universität der Bw München, S 110ff.

[6] Siehe ergänzend hierzu den Erklärungsansatz von V. R. Fuchs für die niedrigere durchschnittliche Lebenserwartung verwitweter und geschiedener amerikanischer Männer. Fuchs VR (1974) Some economic aspects of mortality in developed countries. In: Perlman M (ed) The economics of health and medical care. London, pp 189f.

Besondere Beachtung in der Gesundheitsökonomik und der Medizinsoziologie findet der Konnex zwischen Ausbildung und Gesundheitsverhalten. Eine höhere Ausbildung begünstigt ein adäquates Gesundheitsverhalten. Als Begründung hierfür lassen sich keine naheliegenden Erklärungen finden wie für die Variablen Alter und Familienstand, entsprechend zahlreich sind die Interpretationsansätze. Es muß, der gebotenen Kürze halber, auf die dazu vorliegende Literatur verwiesen werden.[7]

Ergebnisse der empirischen Analyse

Da es unmöglich ist, das präventive Gesundheitsverhalten von Privathaushalten, das sich z. T. aus vielen alltäglichen Verhaltensweisen zusammensetzt, im Rahmen dieses Beitrags darzustellen, muß eine Auswahl getroffen werden.

Es wurden 3 Beispiele präventiver Maßnahmen herausgegriffen, 2 davon sind der Konsumsphäre des Haushalts entnommen: der Verzicht auf Zigarettenrauchen und die Ernährung mit Bio- bzw. Naturkost. Als drittes Beispiel wurde die Nutzung eines Präventionsangebots der Gesetzlichen Krankenversicherung, der Krebsfrüherkennungsuntersuchungen (KFU), gewählt.[8]

Alle 3 Maßnahmen lassen sich für den Ökonomen durch eine Nachfrage- bzw. Inanspruchnahmeanalyse sinnvoll darstellen. Es wurde dabei jeweils eine Querschnitt- und eine Längsschnittbetrachtung vorgenommen, deren Ergebnisse im folgenden kurz wiedergegeben werden.[9]

Zigarettenkonsum

Im Querschnittvergleich zeigte sich eine Abhängigkeit des Zigarettenkonsums sowohl hinsichtlich des Anteils von regelmäßigen Rauchern je Gruppe als auch der Konsumintensität je Raucher von Alter und Geschlecht. Mehr Männer (ca. 30 % der männlichen Bevölkerung ab 14 Jahre) als Frauen (ca. 20 %), mehr junge Menschen als ältere rauchen Zigaretten. Die höchsten Raucherquoten finden sich bei jungen Männern. In der Gruppe der jungen Menschen sind die Raucherquoten von Männern und Frauen am ehesten angeglichen. Die Konsumintensität liegt bei männlichen wie weiblichen Rauchern in mittleren Lebensjahren am höchsten. Unter allen demographisch abgrenzbaren Bevölkerungsgruppen war und ist das Rauchen in der heute älteren Frauengeneration am wenigsten verbreitet; dies zeigt sich an den jeweils niedrigsten Raucher- wie Exraucheranteilen. Bei Männern steigt der Anteil der ehemaligen Zigarettenraucher mit dem Alter tendenziell an.

---

[7] Vgl. die Zusammenstellung in Birkner B (1986) S 120ff., vgl. Fußnote 5.

[8] Die Auswahl der Beispiele erfolgte nicht nach deren präventiver Effizienz. Für den Verzicht auf Zigaretten, auch für die Inanspruchnahme der KFU wird diese wohl von keinem medizinischen Experten bestritten. Nicht unumstritten ist die krankheitsvorbeugende Wirkung von Biokosternährung. Von den Haushalten selbst – dies läßt sich mit Umfrageergebnissen belegen – wird auch letztere als präventiv wirksam eingeschätzt.

[9] Zur ausführlichen Darstellung sowie den verwendeten Quellen vgl. Birkner B (1986) S 135ff., s. Fußnote 5.

Die Raucherquote ist bei Männern wie Frauen vom Familienstand abhängig. Verheiratete weisen bei beiden Geschlechtern die niedrigsten Raucherquoten auf, ledige Männer sowie geschiedene und getrennt lebende Frauen die jeweils höchsten. Relativ hoch ist der durchschnittliche monatliche Zigarettenverbrauch (nach der Einkommens- und Verbrauchsstichprobe des Statistischen Bundesamtes) im Haushaltstyp „Elternteil mit einem Kind", in dem zu über 80 % eine Frau Haushaltsvorstand ist.

Für Männer läßt sich eine Sozialschichtabhängigkeit der Rauchgewohnheiten nachweisen. Mit der Anzahl der Ausbildungsjahre sinkt die Raucherquote. In Arbeiterberufen liegt der Anteil der regelmäßigen Zigarettenraucher am höchsten, bei Selbständigen am niedrigsten. Für den Zigarettenkonsum der Frauen zeigt sich keine eindeutige Abhängigkeit von der Sozialschicht. Einer nicht nach Geschlecht getrennten Erhebung zufolge steigt der Anteil der Exraucher mit der Sozialschicht an.

Zigaretten sind ein inferiores Gut. Der durchschnittliche monatliche Verbrauch steigt bis zu einer mittleren Einkommensgruppe an und sinkt danach ab. In den unteren Einkommensklassen besitzen sie mit einer Mengenelastizität von 1,75 dagegen den Charakter eines Luxusgutes. Während die Inferiorität eines Gutes eher auf einen Verbrauchsrückgang in der Zukunft schließen läßt, deutet die hohe Mengenelastizität im unteren Einkommensbereich auf einen bei steigendem Realeinkommen zunehmenden Verbrauch hin. Aus den Querschnittsanalysen läßt sich somit nicht eindeutig auf die künftige Verbrauchsentwicklung schließen.

Im Längsschnitt (Zeitraum ca. 20 Jahre) zeigt sich ein leichter Rückgang der Raucherquote insgesamt, der aber bedingt wird durch ein deutliches Sinken der Raucherquote bei Männern (um ca. 17%), das nicht ganz kompensiert wird durch ein Ansteigen der Raucherquote der Frauen (um ca. 10%). Im gleichen Zeitraum stieg die durchschnittliche tägliche Konsummenge je Raucher um 10 Zigaretten an.

Als schlecht prognostizierbar gilt die weitere Entwicklung der Rauchgewohnheiten der Frauen. Es spricht jedoch einiges dafür, daß sich der Rückgang des Rauchens bei Frauen nach der Aufbauphase (die stärksten Zuwächse der weiblichen Raucherquoten lagen zwischen 1965 und 1975!) in ähnlicher Weise sozialschichtabhängig einstellt, wie dies für Männer bereits heute nachzuweisen ist.[10]

Wie sich die Verbrauchsentwicklung in den sozialen Schichten vollzog, kann zumindest näherungsweise anhand des durchschnittlichen monatlichen Konsums in den Haushaltstypen des Statistischen Bundesamtes dargestellt werden. In den 60er Jahren glichen sich die Verbrauchsmengen in den Haushaltstypen 2 (4 Personen, mittleres Einkommen, Haushaltsvorstand Arbeiter oder Angestellter) und 3 (4 Personen, höheres Einkommen, Haushaltsvorstand Angestellter oder Beamter) noch weitgehend, waren sogar in einigen Jahren in Typ 3 höher. Danach sank der Verbrauch bis in die 80er Jahre im Typ 2 geringfügig, im Typ 3 deutlich ab. Dem steht eine beträchtliche Verbrauchszunahme im Haushaltstyp 1 (2 Personen, niedriges Einkommen, Renten- oder Sozialhilfeempfänger) gegenüber.

---

[10] Vgl Birkner B (1986) S 53, s. Fußnote 5.

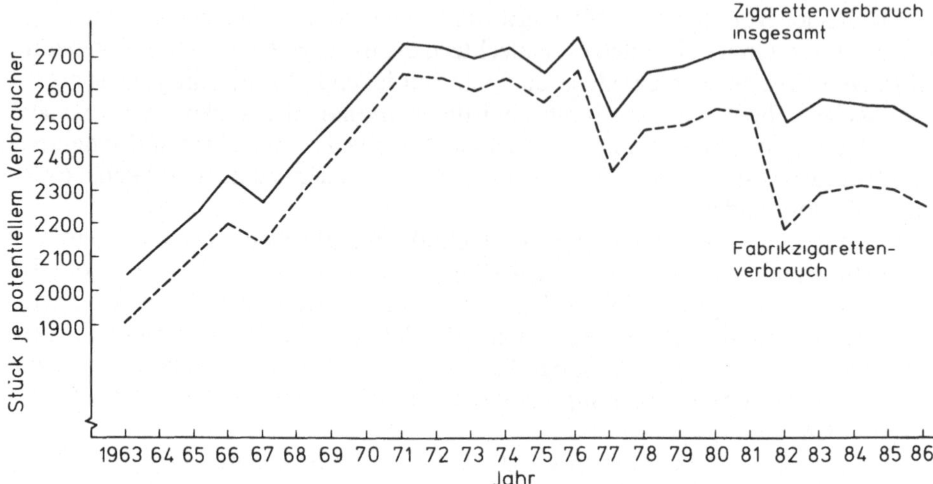

Abb. 1. Entwicklung des Zigarettenverbrauchs in der Bundesrepublik Deutschland von 1963 bis 1986 – Bevölkerung ab 15 Jahren. Verbrauch von Fabrikzigaretten und Zigarettenverbrauch insgesamt. Fabrikzigaretten und „Selbstgedrehte" je potentiellem Verbraucher; (Statistische Jahrbücher der Bundesrepublik Deutschland, Stuttgart und Mainz, verschiedene Jahrgänge; eigene Berechnungen)

Darin manifestiert sich die aus dem Einkommensquerschnitt abgeleitete hohe Einkommenselastizität im Bereich unterer Einkommen.

Um die Entwicklung des gesamten Zigarettenverbrauchs in der Bundesrepublik Deutschland (wiederum ca. 20 Jahre) möglichst genau erheben zu können, wurde der jährliche Verbrauch als Summe von Fabrikzigaretten und von aus Feinschnitt selbstgedrehten Zigaretten zugrunde gelegt (Abb. 1).

Der Verbrauch stieg von den beginnenden 60er bis zu den beginnenden 70er Jahren mit nur einem leichten, durch eine Tabaksteuererhöhung bedingten Rückgang auf 1967 kontinuierlich an. Zu Beginn der 70er Jahre stagnierte der Verbrauch, seit Anfang der 80er Jahre entwickelt er sich zurück.

Deutliche Einbrüche verursachten die steuerbedingten Preiserhöhungen von 1977 um ca. 17 % und 1982 um ca. 22 %;[11] im Jahr nach der Preiserhöhung stiegen die Verbrauchsmengen jedoch jeweils wieder an. Eine näherungsweise Berechnung der Preiselastizität der Nachfrage durch Fabrikzigaretten auf der Grundlage der Durchschnittspreise und Durchschnittsmengen je 2 Jahre vor und nach der Preiserhöhung ergab für 1975/76 auf 1977/78 einen Wert von ca. −0,4 für 1980/81 auf 1982/83 von ca. −0.6.[12] Dieser, trotz einer Steigerung in den 80er

---

[11] Berechnet für eine Schachtel Zigaretten gängiger Preislage, vgl. Statistisches Bundesamt (Hrsg) Preise und Preisindizes für die Lebenshaltung. Stuttgart Mainz.

[12] Die Durchschnittsbildung wurde vorgenommen, um die Schwankungen des Kurvenverlaufs, die durch Vorratskäufe verursacht sind, zu glätten (deutlich für 1976). 1982 wurde die Steuererhöhung zur Jahresmitte wirksam, die Bevorratung fand also in der ersten Jahreshälfte statt. Strenggenommen müßten also zur Elastizitätsberechnung die Durchschnittswerte jeweils zum Halbjahr zugrundegelegt werden. Dies ist jedoch mit den vorliegenden Daten nicht möglich. Die angegebenen Elastizitäten sollen auch lediglich einen groben Hinweis auf die Mengenreaktion liefern.

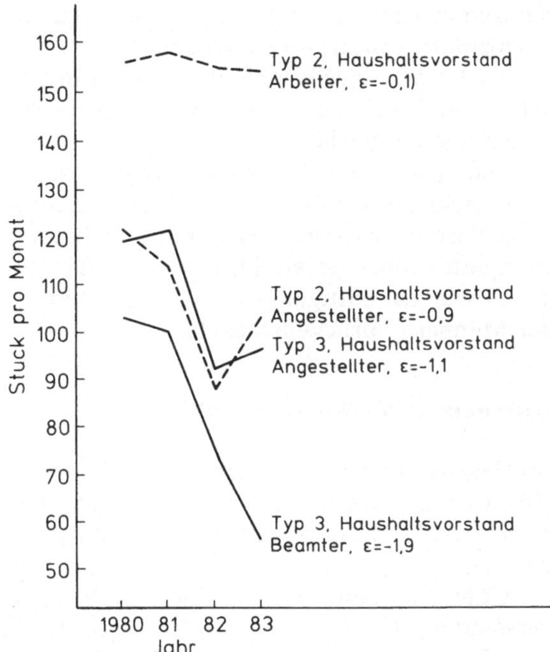

Abb. 2. Verbrauchsreaktion bei Fabrikzigaretten auf die steuerbedingte Preiserhöhung von 1982 in den Haushaltstypen 2 und 3 nach der Stellung im Erwerbsleben des Haushaltsvorstandes [Statistisches Bundesamt (Hrsg.), Einnahmen und Ausgaben ausgewählter privater Haushalte, Stuttgart und Mainz, verschiedene Jahrgänge; eigene Berechnungen]

Jahren, eher unelastischen Nachfrage nach Fabrikzigaretten steht eine hohe Kreuzpreiselastizität von Feinschnittmenge und Fabrikzigarettenpreis gegenüber (1975/76 auf 1977/78: 3,3; 1980/81 auf 1982/83: 2,3).[13]

Als Folge der Substitutionsvorgänge verdoppelt sich der Anteil der „Selbstgedrehten" am Gesamtverbrauch nach dem Preisschub von 1977, bleibt auf dem Niveau und steigt nach 1982 nochmals um fast 100 %. Auch wenn er danach wieder leicht sinkt, war 1986 jede zehnte Zigarette selbstgedreht. Selbstgedrehte Zigaretten gelten als weit gesundheitsschädlicher als Fabrikzigaretten!

Aussagen zu Preiselastizitäten in einzelnen Bevölkerungsgruppen können mit dem vorliegenden Datenmaterial für die Bundesrepublik Deutschland nur begrenzt vorgenommen werden. Da seit 1977 das Statistische Bundesamt in den Haushaltstypen 2 und 3 (vgl. oben) die Verbrauchsmengen je getrennt für Arbeiter-, Angestellten- und Beamtenhaushalte ausweist, war es möglich, für den Preisschub Anfang der 80er Jahre die Mengenreaktion in den 4 Haushaltsgruppen zu berechnen (Abb. 2).[14] Am schwächsten fiel die Mengenreaktion in den Haushalten mit der höchsten durchschnittlichen Verbrauchsmenge, den Arbeiterhaushalten aus, am stärksten in den Beamtenhaushalten mit dem niedrigsten

---

[13] Die Berechnung erfolgte nach dem gleichen Modus wie die Preiselastizität der Nachfrage.
[14] Der Berechnung wurden, wie oben, je Zweijahresdurchschnitte zugrunde gelegt.

Konsumniveau. Die beiden Typen der erfaßten Angestelltenhaushalte liegen mit Elastizitäten von ca. −1 dazwischen.

Nach einer amerikanischen und einer britischen Untersuchung ist für Jugendliche[15] und Frauen[16] von einer überdurchschnittlichen Preisreagibilität der Nachfrage auszugehen.

Eine abschließende Beurteilung der künftigen Verbrauchsentwicklung fällt nicht leicht. Jedoch dürften jene Einflüsse, die auf eine weitere Senkung des künftigen Verbrauchs schließen lassen – insbesondere die insgesamt sinkende Raucherquote – überwiegen. Dies gilt v. a. dann, wenn auch der Zigarettenkonsum der Frauen ein Sättigungsniveau erreicht und sich anschließend, ähnlich wie bei den Männern, zurückentwickelt.

Bio- bzw. Naturkostkonsum

Im Gegensatz zum Zigarettenverbrauch, der v. a. mit Hilfe der Tabaksteuerstatistiken exakt zu erheben ist, ist die Datenbasis für diese Produktgruppe eher schmal. Auf Ergebnisse der amtlichen Statistik konnte nicht zurückgegriffen werden.

Unter Bio- bzw. Naturkost werden Produkte des sog. alternativen Landbaus verstanden; sie werden überwiegend von Reformhäusern und Bioläden vertrieben. Die Gruppe regelmäßiger Konsumenten von Biokost ist relativ klein, sie dürfte ca. 7 % aller Konsumenten umfassen.

Die demographische Struktur der Käufer entspricht in etwa dem Bevölkerungsdurchschnitt, lediglich die durchschnittliche Haushaltsgröße und Kinderzahl liegt über dem Durchschnitt. Eine gesunde Ernährung der Kinder wird entsprechend häufig als Konsummotiv genannt. Deutliche Abweichungen vom Bevölkerungsdurchschnitt zeigt das sozioökonomische Profil der Käufer. Es überwiegen Personen mit gehobenem Bildungsabschluß, Käufer aus Angestellten-, Beamten- und Selbständigenhaushalten. Käufer aus Arbeiterhaushalten stellen die kleinste Gruppe. Relativ stark vertreten sind Nichterwerbstätige, Studenten und Schüler sowie Rentner.

Die Mehrheit (ca. 90 %) der Gesamtbevölkerung hält offenbar Bio- und Naturkost für gesünder als herkömmlich erzeugte Lebensmittel. Daß dennoch die Gruppe der Konsumenten so klein ist, liegt an den hohen Preisforderungen der Bioanbieter. Das hohe Preisniveau wird als das wesentliche Kennzeichen dieses Marktes genannt. Die Preisabstände zu vergleichbaren Waren des konventionellen Lebensmittelhandels dürften etwa zwischen 50 und 100 %, z. T. sogar darüber liegen. Schätzungen, die Aussagen über die Höhe der Mehrausgaben für Ernährungszwecke bei Biokonsumenten erlauben, waren mit dem vorliegenden Datenmaterial nicht möglich.

---

[15] Vgl. Lewitt EM, Coate D, Grossman M (1981) The effects of government regulation on teenage smoking. J Law Economics 24:568.

[16] Vgl. Atkinson AB (1974) Smoking and the economics of government intervention. In: Perlman M (ed) The economics of medical care. London, p 436. Daß dies auch für die Bundesrepublik Deutschland gilt, ist anzunehmen; so nannten mehr weibliche Exraucher aller Altersgruppen als männliche finanzielle Gründe für das Aufhören. Vgl. Birkner B (1986) S 141, s. Fußnote 5.

In den 70er bis in die 80er Jahre expandierte das Produktionsvolumen des alternativen Landbaus kräftig, ausgehend allerdings von einem niedrigen Niveau. Nach allen einschlägigen Quellen wird eine weitere Expansion des Biokostmarktes auch in der Zukunft erwartet. Die günstigen Prognosen veranlassen zunehmend mehr Lebensmitteleinzelhändler, Biokostprodukte in ihr Sortiment aufzunehmen und somit als Konkurrenten der Reformhäuser und Bioläden aufzutreten. Falls dies, wie zu erwarten, auf das Preisniveau drückt, dürften in Zukunft auch Nachfrager zum Zuge kommen, die bisher von den hohen Preisforderungen abgehalten wurden.

Inanspruchnahme der Krebsfrüherkennungsuntersuchungen (KFU)

Der Querschnittsvergleich zeigt eine mehr als doppelt so hohe Beteiligung der berechtigten Frauen (ca. 30 %) als der Männer (ca. 13 %) am Vorsorgeprogramm. Ab dem mittleren Lebensalter nimmt die Teilnahmequote bei beiden Geschlechtern kontinuierlich ab, sie ist bei Frauen ab 70 Jahren sogar niedriger als in den Vergleichsgruppen der Männer.

Analog dem Verzicht auf Zigarettenrauchen nehmen prozentual mehr verheiratete Männer und Frauen die KFU regelmäßig in Anspruch.

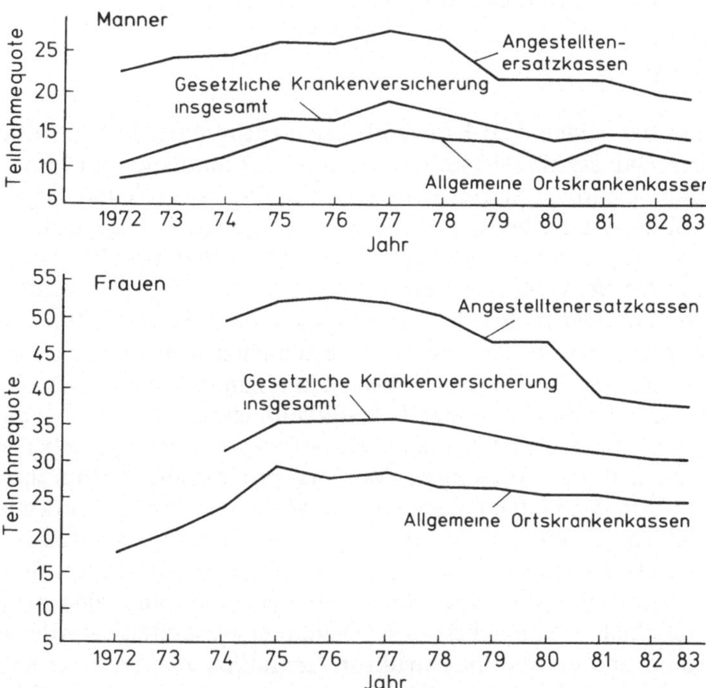

Abb. 3. Teilnahme an der Krebsfrüherkennungsuntersuchung in Prozent der Berechtigten. Bundesrepublik Deutschland 1972–1983 [Statistisches Bundesamt (Hrsg.), ausgewählte Zahlen für das Gesundheitswesen, Stuttgart und Mainz; verschiedene Jahrgänge]

Nicht eindeutig läßt sich eine Abhängigkeit von Sozialfaktoren nachweisen. Die Kassenzugehörigkeit kann als (allerdings grober) Indikator für die Zugehörigkeit zu einer sozialen Gruppe angesetzt werden. Die höchste Teilnahmequote bei Männern findet sich bei den Versicherten der Angestelltenersatzkassen, überdurchschnittlich hoch ist auch die Beteiligung der weiblichen Ersatzkassenversicherten.

Die höchsten Teilnahmequoten jedoch weisen die weiblichen Mitglieder der Arbeiterersatzkassen auf. Jeweils unterdurchschnittlich hoch ist die Beteiligung der AOK-Versicherten am Vorsorgeprogramm.

Während für die beiden anderen Beispiele präventiven Verhaltens, den Zigarettenverzicht und die gesundheitsbewußte Ernährung, auf eine Ausbreitung in der Bevölkerung (insbesondere in höheren sozialen Schichten) zu schließen ist, nimmt die Inanspruchnahme der KFU seit 1977, dem Jahr der bei beiden Geschlechtern höchsten Beteiligung, ab. Anders, eigentlich konträr zu den beiden anderen Beispielen, vollzieht sich die Entwicklung in den sozialen Gruppen (wenn wiederum die Kassenzugehörigkeit als Indikator verwendet wird): Der Rückgang der Inanspruchnahme seit 1977 ist bei den Versicherten der Angestelltenersatzkassen stärker ausgeprägt als bei den Versicherten der Ortskrankenkassen (insbesondere beim Frauenprogramm), so daß sich die Teilnahmequoten in beiden Kassenarten angleichen. Über den gesamten Zeitraum seit Einführung der gesetzlichen KFU betrachtet, stieg die Beteiligung der AOK-Versicherten, sank die Beteiligung in den Ersatzkassen der Angestellten. Dies gilt jeweils für Männer wie Frauen (Abb. 3).

Fazit

Für die beiden dem Konsumbereich entnommenen Präventionsarten gilt sicherlich, daß sie als Bestandteil der sog. „Gesundheits- und Fitneßwelle" anzusehen sind. Deutlich ist (insbesondere für die gewandelten Rauchgewohnheiten der Männer) das Meinungsführerprofil derjenigen Gruppe, von der der Trend zum Nichtrauchen bzw. zur gesundheitsbewußten Ernährung ausgeht. Es läßt sich aus den Beispielen die Vermutung ableiten, daß jene Präventionsmaßnahmen, die von den Haushalten in eigener Regie, ohne Hinzuziehung von Ärzten, erbracht werden, sich in der Bevölkerung tendenziell ausbreiten. Die Inanspruchnahme von Ärzten zu Präventionszwecken – zumindest gilt dies für die KFU – ist von diesem Trend abgekoppelt. Auffallend ist dabei v. a., daß die Inanspruchnahme gerade bei jenem Personenkreis zurückgeht, den Versicherten der Angestelltenkassen, dessen Nutzung des Vorsorgeprogramms überdurchschnittlich hoch ist.

Von den in den Querschnittsanalysen erhobenen Merkmalen zeigten jene Variablen, die die soziale Stellung beschreiben – Ausbildung, Berufsgruppenzugehörigkeit – für die beiden Konsumbeispiele einen Einfluß in der erwarteten Richtung auf präventive Verhaltensweisen. Im Vergleich zur stark beachteten Sozialschichtabhängigkeit des Gesundheitsverhaltens wurde bisher der Familienstand und die Familienstruktur vermutlich zu wenig berücksichtigt. Soweit das vorliegende Datenmaterial eine Auswertung nach diesen Merkmalen überhaupt zuließ, waren die Ergebnisse jeweils eindeutig: Verheiratete verhalten sich gesundheitsbewußter als Nichtverheiratete.

Gesundheitspolitische Überlegungen

Im folgenden sei jenes Teilgebiet der Gesundheitspolitik, dessen Anliegen die Krankheitsprävention ist, als Gesundheitsschutz bezeichnet.[17]

Bevor – bezogen auf die ausgewählten Beispiele – Instrumente des Gesundheitsschutzes diskutiert werden, sind vorab 3 Bedingungen zu stellen:

1) Der Gesundheitsschutz der Bevölkerung ist ein eigenständiges, unabhängiges Ziel der Gesundheitspolitik. Konkret bedeutet dies, Gesundheitsschutz ist als ein von aktuellen Bemühungen um Kostendämpfung unabhängiges Ziel zu behandeln.[18]

2) Bei der Zielvorgabe ist von Utopien abzusehen, wie z. B. der Abschaffung des Rauchens etc. Zum anderen hat sich der Gesundheitsschutz, wie jeder andere Bereich staatlichen Handelns, ordnungspolitischen Normvorgaben zu fügen. So muß es, dem Prinzip der Konsumfreiheit zufolge, jedem gestattet sein, sich beim Konsum Gesundheitsrisiken auszusetzen. Politischer Handlungsbedarf entsteht, wenn
   - der Verbraucher die Risiken nicht kennt,
   - Dritte geschädigt werden,
   - er den Risiken aus eigener Kraft nicht aus dem Wege gehen kann, also zu riskantem Konsum gezwungen ist.[19]

3) Bevor gesundheitspolitische Maßnahmen ergriffen werden, ist die Diagnose zu beachten. Sollte die Beobachtung zutreffen, daß sich präventive Eigenaktivitäten in der Bevölkerung tendenziell ausbreiten, so wäre daraus als allgemeine Politikempfehlung eine moderate Unterstützung der Präventionsbemühungen der Versicherten abzuleiten. Moderat deshalb, weil sich – zum einen – die Rechtfertigung meritorischer Eingriffe abschwächt, wenn sich die Präferenzen von selbst in die gewünschte Richtung einstellen; zum anderen deshalb, weil im Vordringen krankheitspräventiver Eigenaktivitäten der Subsidiaritätsgedanke zum Tragen kommt, der durch ein übermäßiges Angebot an Fremdhilfe durchbrochen werden könnte. Dem Subsidiaritätsgedanken zufolge sind jedoch die privaten Haushalte durch staatliche Vorleistungen in die Lage zu setzen, sich selbst helfen zu können.[20]

Eine Gesundheitsschutzpolitik, die möglichst alle Bevölkerungsgruppen erreichen will, die die unterschiedlichen Motivationen zu gesundheitsschädlichem

---

[17] Vgl. Helberger Chr (1977) Ziele und Ergebnisse der Gesundheitspolitik. In: Zapf W (Hrsg) Lebensbedingungen in der Bundesrepublik. Sozialer Wandel und Wohlfahrtsentwicklung. Frankfurt New York, S 718.

[18] Andernfalls wären Zielkonflikte unvermeidbar, wenn sich nachweisen ließe, daß eine Verlängerung der Lebenserwartung der Bevölkerung die gesamten Kosten der medizinischen Versorgung erhöhen würde, wie dies Leu und Doppmann im Falle einer Beseitigung des Rauchens prognostizieren. Vgl. Leu RE, Doppmann RJ (1984) Gesundheitsverhalten, Gesundheitsstatus und Kosten der medizinischen Versorgung. Vortrag gehalten im Nov. 1984 im 13. Colloquium der Robert Bosch Stiftung, unveröffentlichtes Manuskript.

[19] Wenn z. B. eine Sucht vorliegt, z. B. wenn nur gesundheitsriskante Güter, sofern diese zur Deckung des Subsistenzmittelbedarfs gehören, am Markt angeboten werden, z. B. wenn nichtriskante Güter zu soviel höheren Preisen angeboten werden als riskante, so daß Bezieher niedriger Einkommen vom Konsum ausgeschlossen werden.

[20] Vgl. Nell-Breuning O von (1957) Solidarität und Subsidiarität im Raume von Sozialpolitik und Sozialreform. In: Boettcher E (Hrsg) Sozialpolitik und Sozialreform. Tübingen, S 221.

Verhalten berücksichtigen will, erfordert die Zusammenstellung eines Maßnahmenbündels. Ansatzpunkte können dabei sein:

- die Präferenzen der Haushalte: durch Aufklärung wird versucht, die Bedarfsentscheidungen der Haushalte zu beeinflussen;
- die Budgetrestriktionen der Haushalte: durch pekuniäre Anreize wird der Konsum in die gewünschte Richtung gelenkt;
- die Anbieterseite: z. B. durch Auflagen bei der Produktion und Distribution der Güter.

Gemäß dem Postulat der Konsumfreiheit ergibt sich eine Rangordnung der Maßnahmen in der Reihenfolge, wie sie aufgeführt wurde.

Aufklärung

Der Aufklärung über Risiken des Rauchens wird ein hoher Wirkungsgrad zugeschrieben. Die in den 70er Jahren einsetzenden Aufklärungskampagnen dürften für viele Raucher den Anstoß zum Aufhören gegeben haben. Heute gibt es kaum mehr Raucher aus Unkenntnis. Als ergänzende Maßnahme zur Aufklärung sind die gesetzlichen Werbebeschränkungen der Tabakindustrie zu sehen. Auch wenn deren Wirkung im Vergleich zur Informationspolitik über Gesundheitsgefahren gering ist, sind sie doch unverzichtbar, wenn bei sinkenden Raucherquoten der Zigarettenmarkt an seine Grenzen stößt und der sich verschärfende Wettbewerb zunehmend auch mit Mitteln der Werbung ausgetragen wird.

An eine künftige Aufklärungspolitik sind folgende Forderungen zu stellen: Sie sollte an Zielgruppen orientiert sein; zu nennen sind Jugendliche, Frauen, starke Raucher. Je mehr sich die Raucherquote auf den „harten Kern", also auch auf mutmaßlich starke Raucher reduziert, desto mehr sollte diese Gruppe angesprochen werden. Das Ziel einer realistischen Aufklärungspolitik könnte es dann auch sein, diesen Rauchern Kenntnisse über weniger riskante Arten des Rauchens zu vermitteln.[21] Aufklärung sollte ferner auch Gesundheitsrisiken betonen, die nicht erst im höheren Alter auftreten und zwar insbesondere dann, wenn sie sich an Jugendliche und junge Erwachsene wendet.[22]

Ähnlich wie für die Raucheraufklärung wäre u. U. auch für die Aufklärung zur KFU eine Orientierung an Zielgruppen sinnvoll. Die vom Gesetzgeber intendierte Beteiligung möglichst aller Anspruchsberechtigten wurde seit Einführung der KFU nie erreicht. Bei rückläufiger Inanspruchnahme erscheint sie weniger denn je realisierbar. Es wäre deshalb zu überprüfen, ob nicht eine gezielte Aufklärung von epidemiologisch abgrenzbaren Risikogruppen allgemeinen Appellen vorzuziehen ist. Zweck dieser Maßnahme wäre es, zumindest die Risikogruppe möglichst vollständig der Untersuchung zuzuführen.

Zusätzlich erfolgversprechend könnte eine stärkere Einbeziehung der Ärzte in die Aufklärung über den Nutzen der KFU sein, insbesondere bei jenem Perso-

---

[21] Verzicht auf Rauchen z. B während körperlicher Arbeit, kein Aufrauchen bis zum Filter etc.

[22] Gegenwärtige Risiken sind z. B. eine Leistungsminderung beim Sport, für Frauen im gebärfähigen Alter eine mögliche Schädigung der Frucht, eine geringere Konzeptionswahrscheinlichkeit.

nenkreis (ältere Frauen) deren Arztkontakthäufigkeit überdurchschnittlich, deren Teilnahme am Vorsorgeprogramm aber unterdurchschnittlich ist.

Von der Natur der Sache her ist Aufklärung über gesunde Ernährung schwieriger zu gestalten als etwa Aufklärung über Tabakabusus. Gesunde Ernährung erfordert nicht nur die Berücksichtigung von Gesundheitsbelangen beim Konsum einzelner Güter, sondern die Zusammenstellung eines Güterbündels. Das Lebensmittelrecht der Bundesrepublik Deutschland, dessen primäres Ziel der Gesundheitsschutz ist, kennt zahlreiche Vorschriften zur Erhöhung der Markttransparenz; Verbraucheraufklärung wird insbesondere auch von den Verbraucherzentralen auf Länderebene betrieben. Dennoch liegt das Schwergewicht des Gesundheitsschutzes nach dem Lebensmittelrecht auf Ge- und Verboten für Produzenten und Händler.

Aufklärungspolitik stößt eben dort an ihre Grenzen, wo es um den Konsum lebensnotwendiger Güter geht und wenn es gilt, Marktentnahmen besonders schutzwürdiger Verbrauchergruppen zu steuern.

Pekuniäre Anreize

Der zweite Ansatzpunkt, pekuniäre Anreize zu gesundheitsgerechtem Verhalten, sei an 2 möglichen Instrumenten hierfür expliziert, der Selbstbeteiligung an den Krankheitsfolgen und der Besteuerung von gesundheitsschädlichem Konsum, hier der Tabaksteuer.

Ob die Androhung finanzieller Sanktionen im Krankheitsfall durch eine Selbstbehaltsregelung geeignet ist, ein Verhalten zu ändern, durch das eine erhöhte Wahrscheinlichkeit eines frühzeitigen Todes in Kauf genommen wird, erscheint zweifelhaft. Damit Selbstbehalte verhaltenssteuernd im Hinblick auf Prävention wirken, müssen 3 Bedingungen erfüllt sein: Es muß sich 1) um leichtere Erkrankungen handeln, die im Vergleich zu ihrer geringen Bedrohung für Leib und Leben 2) einen unverhältnismäßig hohen finanziellen Behandlungsaufwand erfordern und deren Entstehung 3) präventiv leicht zu beeinflussen ist. Alle Bedingungen sind erfüllt für die Prophylaxe einiger Zahnerkrankungen. Für Zahnersatz existiert bereits eine Zuzahlungspflicht für die Versicherten der Gesetzlichen Krankenversicherung.

Gegen darüber hinausgehende Selbstbehalte spricht auch die Vermutung einer Ausbreitung von präventiven Eigenleistungen der Versicherten. Setzt sich der Subsidiaritätsgedanke durch, so weist dies auf eine funktionierende Solidargemeinschaft hin. Risikoüberwälzung auf die Versicherten ist aber als Instrument für das Gegenteil, eine nichtfunktionierende, von den Versicherten „ausgebeutete" Solidargemeinschaft konzipiert.

Zur Beeinflussung von riskantem Konsum erscheint es erfolgversprechender, direkt am Preis der riskanten Güter durch Verbrauchssteuern anzusetzen. Auch wenn einerseits die Zigarettennachfrage insgesamt eher schwach preiselastisch ist, andererseits aus ordnungspolitischen Gründen (Konsumfreiheit) prohibitive Steuern ausscheiden, kann die Tabaksteuer bei geeigneter Handhabung ein Instrument der Gesundheitsschutzpolitik sein.

Als Hauptgrund hierfür ist die überdurchschnittliche Preisreagibilität Jugendlicher, also einer besonders schutzbedürftigen Verbrauchergruppe, anzusehen.

Das gilt v. a. dann, wenn es zutrifft, daß Aufklärung über die später im Leben auftretenden Gesundheitsrisiken des Rauchens bei Jugendlichen sogar zu Konsumerhöhungen führen kann, als Kompensation für einen vermeintlich erst später nötigen Verzicht.[23]

Für die Tabaksteuer spricht weiterhin, daß sich die Preiselastizität der Nachfrage erhöhen dürfte, je mehr sich die Rauchgewohnheiten von Männern und Frauen angleichen, da die Preisreagibilität der Frauen ebenfalls als überdurchschnittlich hoch eingeschätzt wird. Schließlich ist, zumindest für erwachsene Raucher, von einer kombinierten Wirkung von Aufklärungskampagnen und nachfolgender Tabaksteuererhöhung auszugehen, da letztere dann häufig den endgültigen Anstoß zum Aufhören gebe.[24] Allerdings wirkt dieser Anstoß in den sozialen Gruppen unterschiedlich stark (vgl. Abb. 3).

Der Einsatz der Tabaksteuer als gesundheitspolitisches Instrument verlangt aber einige Modifikationen, die sowohl die Ausgestaltung als auch die Höhe der Steuer betreffen.

Für Zigaretten und Feinschnitt gilt ein gemischter Steuersatz, mit einem preis- und einem mengenabhängigen Teil. Die Wertsteuer hat einen Anteil von 60 %, die Mengensteuer von 40 % an der Gesamtsteuer. Relativ teuere Tabaksorten werden folglich benachteiligt, jedoch gelten diese als weniger schadstoffbelastet als billigere Sorten. Zu fordern ist also eine Änderung des Verhältnisses beider Steuerbestandteile zugunsten des Mengensteueranteils.[25]

Zu fordern ist weiterhin, den Steuervorteil selbstgedrehter Zigaretten aufzuheben, zumindest aber zu senken. Dies könnte durch eine isolierte, die übrigen Tabakerzeugnisse nicht berührende Anhebung der Feinschnittsteuer geschehen. Beides, der hohe Wertsteueranteil und der Steuervorteil „Selbstgedrehter", lenken die Nachfrage wirtschaftlich schwächerer Raucher, damit auch Jugendlicher, auf schädlichere Zigaretten.

Zu prüfen wäre auch die Möglichkeit, den Schadstoffgehalt (Nikotin, Kondensat, Teer) als Besteuerungsgrundlage heranzuziehen und dadurch die Nachfrage auf sog. Leichtmarken zu lenken. Der größte Teil der regelmäßig Zigaretten konsumierenden Raucher, der Gewohnheitsraucher, würde darauf mit einer Ausweitung der Konsummenge reagieren. Die Erhöhung der Konsumintensität in den vergangenen 20 Jahren war v. a. eine Folge des Übergangs auf leichtere Zigaretten.[26]

Die Veränderung der Steuerhöhe sollte flexibler gehandhabt werden, sich an der Entwicklung der Verbraucherpreise insgesamt orientieren. In den zurückliegenden 20 Jahren wurden alle 5 Jahre die Steuersätze erhöht, was zu sprunghaften Preiserhöhungen führte. Der Steuererhöhung folgten dann Jahre mit stabilen Zigarettenpreisen sowie Jahre, in denen der Preisindex für Tabakwaren zwar stieg, jedoch geringfügiger als der Preisindex der Lebenshaltung.[27] In dieser Zeit stiegen die Verbrauchsmengen jeweils wieder an.

---

[23] Vgl. Atkinson AB (1974) S 436, s. Fußnote 16.
[24] Vgl. Leu RE (1984) Anti-smoking publicity and the demand for cigarettes. J Health Economics 3:111.
[25] Dem stehen aber die Bemühungen um Steuerharmonisierung in der EG entgegen, die eine weitere Erhöhung des Wertanteils vorsehen.
[26] Vgl. Leu RE (1984) S 104, s. Fußnote 24.
[27] Vgl. Birkner B (1986) S 239f., s. Fußnote 5.

Steuererhöhungen in kürzeren Zeitabständen könnten aufgrund der oben angesprochenen kombinierten Wirkung mit Aufklärungskampagnen womöglich einen größeren Nachfragerückgang induzieren. Darüber hinaus provozieren seltene, jedoch sprunghafte Preiserhöhungen gesundheitspolitisch unerwünschte Ausweichreaktionen;[28] sie lassen die Tatsache unberücksichtigt, daß sich Konsumgewohnheiten langsam verändern, gerade im Genußmittelbereich.

Eingriffe auf Anbieterseite

Staatliche Eingriffe auf das Angebot zum Zweck des Gesundheitsschutzes werden in der Bundesrepublik Deutschland seit langem praktiziert. Die Produktion und Distribution von Lebensmitteln unterliegt einer Fülle gesetzlicher Auflagen, ebenso gelten gesetzliche Regelungen für die Zigarettenproduktion, z. B. Zusatzstoffe betreffend.

Als vorrangig ist es gegenwärtig anzusehen, das Vertrauen der Verbraucher in die amtliche Lebensmittelkontrolle wiederherzustellen. Tatsächlich hatten die Verbraucher in den vergangenen Jahren Grund, an der Qualität der angebotenen Lebensmittel zu zweifeln.[29]

Unter dem Aspekt des Jugendschutzes wäre ein Verbot der Zigarettendistribution über Automaten zu erwägen, auch wenn dadurch lediglich Spontan- und Gelegenheitskäufe gesenkt werden könnten, der Konsum von Gewohnheitsrauchern davon jedoch unberührt bliebe.

Als eine am Angebot ansetzende Maßnahme zur Erhöhung der Inanspruchnahme der KFU wäre an eine verstärkte Einbindung von Betriebsärzten in das Vorsorgeprogramm zu denken, um dadurch eine höhere Teilnahmequote männlicher Anspruchsberechtigter zu erreichen.[30]

Schlußbemerkung

Der Gesundheitsschutz umfaßt Politikbereiche, die über die hier beschriebenen hinausgehen. Zu nennen sind die Vorbeugung von Krankheit und Unfall am Arbeitsplatz, im Straßenverkehr, die Umweltschutzpolitik. Appelle oder Verhaltensanreize an die Adresse der Verbraucher büßen an Glaubwürdigkeit und Wirksamkeit ein, wenn sie nicht begleitet werden von Maßnahmen, die auf die Beseitigung von Gesundheitsrisiken zielen, die nicht vom Verhalten des einzelnen zu beeinflussen sind. Wer z. B. seine Gesundheit bedroht sieht durch Schadstoffe in der Luft, der mag zu Vergeblichkeitsreaktionen neigen („ ... was nützt es da noch, das Rauchen aufzugeben ...") und mithin den Beitrag seiner eigenen Aktivitäten zur Gesunderhaltung zu gering einschätzen.

---

[28] Wie z. B. Aufrauchen bis zum Filter, mehr Züge pro Zigarette.

[29] Dafür seien 4 Stichworte genannt, der sog. Weinskandal, angebrütete Eier in der Nudelproduktion, radioaktive Belastung von Grundnahrungsmitteln, Nematoden im Seefisch. Die Reihe ließe sich erweitern.

[30] Vgl. Kirschner W (1984) Krebsfrüherkennungsuntersuchungen in der Bundesrepublik Deutschland. Gründe der Nichtinanspruchnahme und Möglichkeiten zur Erhöhung der Beteiligung. München, S 76.

Weiterführende Literatur zum Thema „Präventivmedizin"

Basler HD (Hrsg) (1989) Gruppenarbeit in der Allgemeinpraxis. Springer, Berlin Heidelberg New York Tokyo (Neue Allgemeinmedizin: Angewandte Heilkunde Praxisforschung)
Berkmann LF, Breslow L (1983) Health and ways of living: the Alameda County Study. Oxford University Press, New York
Gray JAM (ed) (1985) Prevention of disease in the elderly. Churchill Livingstone, London
Horn K, Beier C, Kraft-Krumm D (1984) Gesundheitsverhalten und Krankheitsgewinn: zur Logik von Widerständen gegen gesundheitliche Aufklärung. Westdeutscher Verlag, Wiesbaden
Hudson WT, Reinhart MA, Rose SD et al. (eds) (1988) Clinical preventive medicine: health promotion and disease prevention. Little Brown, Boston/Toronto
Social Science and Medicine (1988) vol 26/5. Special Issue: Worksite Health Promotion

4 Gesundheitsökonomie

Forschungsfragen und Gegenstände der Gesundheitsökonomie

H. H. Andersen, J.-M. Graf v. d. Schulenburg

Frage- und Problemstellung der Gesundheitsökonomie

Die Jahrestagung des Vereins für Socialpolitik 1985 mit dem Thema „Ökonomie des Gesundheitswesens" markiert eine Standortbestimmung in der Entwicklung der Gesundheitsökonomie zu einer anerkannten Subdisziplin der Wirtschaftswissenschaften in der Bundesrepublik Deutschland. Einen ersten Meilenstein für den Beginn einer ökonomisch orientierten Analyse der Sicherung im Krankheitsfall setzte die Sozialenquete von 1966. Schon damals wurde die Frage gestellt, ob die Gesetzliche Krankenversicherung nicht zu teuer sei und ob für die Gesundheit nicht mehr ausgegeben werde als im Sinne eines objektivierten Grenznutzenausgleichs gerechtfertigt sei.

Die „Kostenexplosionsdebatte" – Anfang der 70er Jahre beginnend – erwies sich dann im weiteren Verlauf als treibender Motor. „Kostenexplosion" und „Kostendämpfung" als Begründung ökonomischer Analysen des Gesundheitswesens haben deshalb für die Disziplinentwicklung eine entscheidende Bedeutung gehabt. Aber so bedeutsam dieser Ansatzpunkt für die Ableitung unmittelbarer Handlungsvorschläge auch sein mag und so forschungsbegründend er sich auch auswirkte, so hat die Jahrestagung auch gezeigt, daß das Bemühen um Kostendämpfung nicht die einzige Rechtfertigung einer ökonomischen Analyse darstellt und daß es nicht Aufgabe der Gesundheitsökonomie ist, ein wissenschaftlich begründbares Kostenminimum zu bestimmen. Die Gesundheitsökonomie als Hilfswissenschaft der Kostendämpfungspolitik zu identifizieren verstellt eher den Blick dafür, was ihr die Zukunft als wissenschaftliche Disziplin sichert, nämlich eine besondere Theoriebildung.

Was unter Gesundheitsökonomie zu verstehen sei, wäre am besten mit dem Hinweis auf eine umfassende, eindeutige und möglichst konsensfähige Definition zu beantworten. Eine solche Definition liegt nicht vor. Deshalb gilt zunächst der allgemeine Hinweis, daß Gesundheitsökonomie die Übertragung wirtschaftswissenschaftlicher Frage- und Problemstellungen und die Anwendung des wirtschaftswissenschaftlichen Instrumentariums auf das Gesundheitswesen bedeutet. Was nun mit ökonomischen Frage- bzw. Problemstellungen gemeint ist, sei an Definitionsversuchen amerikanischer Gesundheitsökonomie demonstriert, von denen auch die bundesrepublikanische Gesundheitsökonomie wesentliche Impulse empfangen hat.

> In a formal sense the economics of health may be defined as the economic aspects of health services – those aspects of the health problem that deal with the determination of quantity and prices of scarce resources devoted to this and related purposes and with the combinations in which these resources are employed (Klarman 1965, S. 2).

Ähnlich, aber den ökonomischen Gesichtspunkt alternativer Verwendungszwekke hervorhebend, die folgende Perspektive:

> The economic perspective assumes that resources are scarce relativ to human wants, that these resources have alternative uses, and that people have diverse wants, not all of which can be satisfied (Fuchs 1983, S. 7).

Im Umkehrschluß auf das Gesundheitswesen angewendet hieße dieses, daß die ökonomische Perspektive dann unbegründet wäre, wenn es hinreichende Mittel zur allseitigen Befriedigung der Bedürfnisse nach Gesundheitssicherung und Krankheitsbewältigung gäbe und gesellschaftlicher Konsens darüber besteht, über alternative Verwendungszwecke nicht weiter nachzudenken. Unabhängig davon, wie das Gesundheitswesen organisiert ist und wie über seine Finanzierung entschieden wird: diese Ausgangsbedingungen sind in keiner Gesellschaftsordnung und in keinem Land (außer dem Schlaraffenland) gegeben.

Die Anwendung der ökonomischen Perspektive auf das Gesundheitswesen war immer von teils heftiger Kritik begleitet. Dabei lassen sich eine normative und eine eher methodisch-methodologische Ebene unterscheiden. Der normative Vorwurf gipfelt in Behauptungen wie jener, der Gesundheitsökonomie sei eine letztlich inhumane Tendenz eigen und sie liefe auf eine subtilere Form der Euthanasie hinaus. Dieser Kritik liegt ein Mißverständnis zugrunde. Denn es ist eben nicht Ziel oder Aufgabe der Gesundheitsökonomie zu bestimmen, wieviel ein Individuum oder eine Gesellschaft insgesamt für die Gesundheitssicherung und Krankheitsbewältigung ausgeben soll, sondern Hilfestellung dafür zu geben, daß die Verwendung und Verteilung vorhandener oder erforderlicher Mittel in effektiver und effizienter Weise erfolgen. Es ist natürlich ganz legitim, daß der einzelne Mediziner und der einzelne Krankenhaus- und Heimleiter es für seine ethische Pflicht hält, alles zu versuchen und vom Gesundheitssystem zu verlangen, um seinen Patienten bestmöglichst zu helfen. Dennoch ist jede Mark, die für eine bestimmte Behandlung oder ein bestimmtes Gesundheitsversorgungsprogramm ausgegeben wird, für alternative Verwendungen verloren. Die volkswirtschaftlichen – d. h. gesellschaftlichen – Kosten einer Gesundheitsmaßnahme sind somit gleich dem Nutzen, die alternative Verwendungen, für die die von der Gesundheitsmaßnahme beanspruchten Ressourcen (Arbeit, Boden, Kapital und Energie) auch hätten eingesetzt werden können, gebracht hätten. Dieses Denken in Opportunitäts- oder Alternativkosten, das die Ökonomie lehrt, ist eine gesellschaftliche Pflicht aller derjenigen, die Ressourcenentscheidungen treffen. Es ist somit auch eine ethische Aufgabe, der sich der im Gesundheitswesen Beschäftigte und der Gesundheitspolitiker nicht entziehen kann.

Die methodisch-methodologische Kritik richtet sich dagegen auf die Anwendung bzw. Angemessenheit bestimmter Ansätze, Theorien, Modelle oder Hypothesen auf das Gesundheitswesen. So bedarf es v. a. in der deutschen Tradition immer noch besonderer salvatorischer Klauseln, um Gesundheit als (wenn auch besonderes) Gut, Versorgung als Knappheitsproblem, Therapieformen als Effizienzkalküle oder gewonnene Lebensjahre als Kapital zu betrachten. Nicht die Kritik an der ökonomischen Perspektive an sich, sondern die Kritik an der Anwendung bestimmter Ansätze durch den Hinweis auf die Besonderheiten des empirischen Gegenstandes steht zur Diskussion. Deshalb gilt für die Gesundheitsökonomie allgemein, daß aufgrund der Bedeutung des empirischen Gegenstandes die Anwendung des jeweils gewählten Instrumentariums unter einen besonderen Rechtfertigungsdruck gerät.

Notwendig vereinfachend läßt sich der Stand der gesundheitsökonomischen Forschung in der Bundesrepublik Deutschland folgendermaßen skizzieren. Der gesellschaftliche Bereich Gesundheitswesen ist auf die Fruchtbarkeit und Notwendigkeit einer – wie auch immer definierten – ökonomischen Interpretation abgeprüft. Wenn auch in Einzelfragen aufgrund des sensiblen Gegenstandsbereichs kontrovers, werden im grundsätzlichen kaum mehr Zweifel geäußert, daß ökonomische Ansätze einen sinnvollen Beitrag zur Aufklärung sozialer Realität leisten können. Das Problembewußtsein für die ökonomische Seite des Gesundheitswesens und damit auch für eine Disziplin Gesundheitsökonomie wächst eher noch. Eine kaum mehr überschaubare Zahl unterschiedlicher ökonomischer Ansätze, Theorien und Theoreme, Hypothesen und Modelle sind auf Problemstellungen im Gesundheitswesen angewandt und auf ihre Interpretationskraft getestet worden. Diese Entwicklung hat allerdings auch schon in der Gesundheitsökonomie selbst Zweifel aufkommen lassen, ob diese Phase nicht zu einer Applikationseuphorie geführt hat, die gelegentlich in das „l'art pour l'art" akademischer Glasperlenspiele einmündet. Auch aus diesen Gründen ist eine deutliche Tendenz erkennbar, die auf eine interdisziplinär orientierte und empirisch gestützte Forschung setzt. Das Problem der gesundheitsökonomischen Fragestellung lautet – wiederum vereinfacht – nicht mehr primär, welche Ansätze, Theorien oder Hypothesen vorliegender Denktraditionen auf das Gesundheitswesen anwendbar sind, sondern wie sie modifiziert werden müssen, um für die Spezialität des Gesundheitsbereichs eine spezifische Erklärungs- und Prognosefähigkeit gewinnen zu können. Damit ist letztlich das Ziel gemeint, v. a. durch die Berücksichtigung der Besonderheiten des Gutes Gesundheit und des Marktes für Gesundheitsleistungen oder der Produktionsbedingungen für Gesundheitsleistungen eine gesundheitsökonomisch spezifische Theoriebildung zu entwickeln. Beispiele wären etwa eine Verhaltenstheorie für Nachfrager und Anbieter von Gesundheitsleistungen, die Entwicklung eines gegenstandsspezifischen Steuerungsinstrumentariums oder von Methoden der ökonomischen Evaluierung von Gesundheitsleistungen.

Ökonomische Grundlagendisziplinen

Obwohl – vielfach zu Recht – behauptet wird, daß es nur eine ökonomische Theorie gibt, auf der alles aufbaut, haben sich mit der Zeit doch verschiedene ökonomische Grundlagendisziplinen herausgebildet, die die wirtschaftlichen Vorgänge – und auch das Gesundheitswesen – unter verschiedenen Aspekten betrachten. In diesem Abschnitt sollen deshalb diejenigen ökonomischen Grunddisziplinen kurz vorgestellt werden, die in der Gesundheitsökonomie eine herausragende und eigenständige Bedeutung haben. Es sind dies insbesondere die mikroökonomische Verhaltenstheorie, die Finanzwissenschaft, die Wirtschaftsordnungspolitik, die Versicherungswissenschaft und die Betriebslehre.

Mikroökonomische Verhaltenstheorie

Die mikroökonomische Verhaltenstheorie versucht das ökonomische Verhalten von Individuen zu beschreiben und Hypothesen über Verhaltensänderungen aufgrund von Datenänderungen abzuleiten. Dabei erfolgt diese Analyse in folgenden Schritten. Zunächst wird das Problem genau beschrieben, um dessen Klärung es geht. Beispielsweise die Frage, ob eine bestimmte Selbstbeteiligung zu einer Reduktion der Inanspruchnahme von Gesundheitsleistungen führt oder welche Wirkungen eine bestimmte Umstrukturierung der Gebührenordnungen niedergelassener Ärzte hat. Im zweiten Schritt wird dann anhand eines ökonomischen Individualmodells diese Frage untersucht, wobei ein Modell ein abstraktes Bild der Realität ist, das nur die wesentlichen Beziehungen und Tatbestände wiedergibt.

Es wird beispielsweise ein Modell für einen repräsentativen Versicherten oder Arzt aufgestellt. Typisch für die mikroökonomische Verhaltenstheorie ist es, daß zunächst anhand eines Individuums – des repräsentativen Individuums – argumentiert wird. Die Grundthese der mikroökonomischen Verhaltenstheorie ist es, daß jedes Individuum eine Zielfunktion zu maximieren versucht und dabei bestimmte Nebenbedingungen zu beachten hat. In die Zielfunktion gehen alle wichtigen Ziele ein, wie z. B. das Einkommen, die Lebensqualität, die Arbeitszufriedenheit, die Freizeit usw. Die Nebenbedingungen sind Restriktionen, die das Individuum zu beachten hat: So sind für einen bestimmten Versicherten seine Erwerbsmöglichkeiten und das Gesundheitsversorgungssystem gegeben. Ein Arzt hat die rechtlichen Vorschriften, ethische Normen und die derzeitigen Möglichkeiten der ärztlichen Kunst sowie seine eigenen Möglichkeiten zu beachten.

Im dritten Schritt werden aus dem Modellrahmen im Wege der Deduktion Hypothesen über Verhalten und Verhaltensänderungen abgeleitet. Im vierten Schritt erfolgt dann die Überprüfung der Hypothesen anhand empirischer Daten und mit Hilfe ökonometrischer Verfahren.

Oft reicht es nicht aus, nur ein Individuum zu betrachten, da dessen Verhalten in einem hohen Maße vom Verhalten anderer abhängt. So wird das Verhalten des Versicherten in nicht unwesentlichem Maße vom Verhalten des jeweils behandelnden Arztes beeinflußt. Sein Rat, seine Behandlungsmöglichkeiten und seine ökonomischen und medizinischen Zielsetzungen bestimmen ebenso das Inanspruchnahmeverhalten des Versicherten, wie dessen Verhalten selbst. Die mikroökonomische Verhaltenstheorie fügt deshalb auch in einem nächsten Schritt Individualmodelle zu einem Marktmodell zusammen, um Hypothesen über die Interdependenzen der einzelnen Individuen abzuleiten.

Insbesondere die Anwendung der mikroökonomischen Verhaltenstheorie auf gesundheitsökonomische Fragestellungen hat zu sehr fruchtbaren Ergebnissen geführt. Sie hat zudem die ökonomische Theorie befruchtet, da im Gesundheitswesen die Zielsetzungen und die Beschränkungen sich wesentlich von den sonstigen Märkten unterscheiden, da z. B. Ziele wie Ethik oder Beschränkungen durch staatliche Regulierungen eine übergeordnete Rolle spielen.

Die empirischen Verfahren zur Überprüfung der Aussagen der Gesundheitsökonomie können in deskriptive Verfahren (Clusteranalyse, Faktorenanalyse, Methoden der Indexbildung) und induktive Verfahren unterschieden werden.

Letztere wiederum umfassen die Varianzanalyse und die multiple Regressionsanalyse (Eingleichungsmodelle, Mehrgleichungsmodelle, Logit- und Probitmodelle, Modelle mit latenten Verfahren). So wie die jeweilige theoretische Modellstruktur von der jeweiligen Fragestellung, den Interdependenzen, den individuellen Zielsetzungen und den Handlungsbeschränkungen abhängt, so ist auch die Auswahl empirischer Methoden von verschiedenen Faktoren abhängig. Insbesondere sind hier die zu testende Hypothese, die Art des Datensatzes und das Ziel der empirischen Untersuchung zu nennen.

Finanzwissenschaft

Die Finanzwissenschaft beschäftigt sich traditionell mit der Tätigkeit des Staates. Ihre Methoden finden aber auch Anwendung für die Tätigkeit von Parafisci – wie die Gesetzlichen Krankenkassen – und für die Analyse von Finanzströmen zwischen den Wirtschaftssektoren. So beschäftigt sich die Gesundheitsökonomie u. a. mit den Ausgabe- und Einnahmeströmen zwischen den einzelnen Elementen des Gesundheitsversorgungssystems. Diese Ströme kann man in der Form einer Input-Output-Tabelle oder in Form einer Kreislaufgrafik (vergleichbar dem Blutkreislauf) darstellen. Diese Darstellungen machen dann deutlich, wieviel Mittel von einem Element (z. B. den Krankenkassen) zu einem anderen Element (z. B. den Hilfsmittelherstellern) geflossen sind. Derartige deskriptive Darstellungen sind sehr hilfreich, um die Struktur des Gesundheitswesens zu erkennen und im Zeitvergleich auf Veränderungen aufmerksam zu machen. Sie sind von einigen Gesundheitsökonomen – insbesondere Philipp Herder-Dorneich – auch auf nichtmonetäre Größen erweitert worden, indem er z. B. die Ströme der Scheine im Gesundheitswesen (Krankenscheine und Rezepte) analog dargestellt und interpretiert hat.

Aufbauend auf der Kreislaufdarstellung können die Inzidenzwirkungen – d. h. Verteilungswirkungen von Finanzierungsregelungen – analysiert werden. Diese Aufgabe der Gesundheitsökonomie ist deshalb besonders hervorzuheben, da das Gesundheitswesen einer der größten Umverteiler in der Gesellschaft ist. Es führt nicht nur – z. B. aufgrund der einkommensbezogenen Beiträge – zu einer Querschnittumverteilung, sondern auch zu einer intergenerativen Verteilung, d. h. zu einer Umverteilung der Finanzierungslasten über die Generationen hinweg.

Aufgabe der Finanzwissenschaft ist es auch, den Output öffentlicher Institutionen zu bewerten. Hierzu wurden besondere Verfahren – insbesondere die Nutzen-Kosten-Analyse, die Kostenwirksamkeitsanalyse und die Nutzwertanalyse – entwickelt. Das grundlegende Prinzip ist die Erfassung und Quantifizierung aller Nutzen und Kosten eines Gesundheitsversorgungsprogramms (z. B. eines neuen Präparats, eines Großgeräts, einer präventiven Maßnahme). Die Bewertung und Aggregation der einzelnen Nutzen- und Kostengrößen erfolgt dann durch Verrechnungspreise (Schattenpreise) oder Präferenzskalen.

Nicht zuletzt ist es Aufgabe der Finanzwissenschaft, überhaupt zu klären, welchen Aufgaben sich der Staat annehmen soll und inwieweit er das Geschehen in einzelnen Wirtschaftssektoren reglementieren soll. So wurde im Rahmen der finanzwissenschaftlichen Disziplin eine intensive Diskussion über die Besonderheiten des Gutes Gesundheitsleistungen geführt, welche besondere staatliche Regelungen notwendig machen. Denn es stellt sich natürlich die Frage, durch welche staatlichen Maßnahmen und durch welche Marktorganisation eine den Präferenzen der Bevölkerung am besten genügende Gesundheitsversorgung ermöglicht wird. Damit gehen die Fragen der Finanzwissenschaft über in die Wirtschaftsordnungspolitik.

Wirtschaftsordnungspolitik

Die gesundheitsökonomische Diskussion ist stark geprägt durch ordnungspolitische Fragestellungen, die in die Disziplin der Wirtschaftsordnungspolitik fallen. Als Entscheidungsmechanismus für die Verteilung von Ressourcen oder Rechten bieten sich mehrere Alternativen an: der Markt, eine hierarchische Befehlsstruktur, Wahlen, Verhandlungen usw. Welche Alternative am geeignetsten ist, um die Probleme im jeweiligen Wirtschaftssektor zu lösen, hängt entscheidend von der Ausgangsverteilung und der Informationsstruktur ab. Empfindet man die Ausgangsverteilung in der Bevölkerung als gerecht und haben alle den gleichen Informationsstand, so führt der Markt zu den geringsten Organisationskosten und zum optimalen Ergebnis. Im Gesundheitswesen wurde die ordnungspolitische Diskussion stark beherrscht durch die Positionen der Befürworter von mehr Markt und denjenigen, die das bisherige Modell der Gesetzlichen Krankenversicherung befürworten: den Neokorporatismus.

Ordnungspolitische Fragen sind auch die Abgrenzung zwischen privater Krankenversicherung und Gesetzlicher Krankenversicherung, der Umfang von Selbstbeteiligungen, die Struktur der Krankenkassen und der Umfang des Wettbewerbs zwischen Krankenkassen, die Zulassungspraxis beim Kassenarzt, die Krankenhausfinanzierung usw. Es sollte aber beachtet werden, daß ohne eine ökonomische Fundierung ordnungspolitischer Positionen diese zu reinen Werturteilen degenerieren, über die man zwar vortrefflich streiten kann, die aber in der Diskussion nicht weiterführen.

Eine nichtnormative, sondern positive Frage ist, wie sich die Ordnungsstrukturen des Gesundheitswesens angesichts der demographischen Entwicklungen und der Inzidenzwirkungen des Finanzierungssystems weiterentwickeln werden. Mit Hilfe von Public-choice-Modellen ist diese Frage untersucht worden. Ursprünglich wird die Modellierung von kollektiven Entscheidungsprozessen der finanzwissenschaftlichen Disziplin zugeordnet. Doch angesichts des Umfangs der Literatur und der Eigenständigkeit der entwickelten Methoden kann sie auch als eine eigenständige Disziplin aufgefaßt werden.

Versicherungswissenschaft

Das Herzstück des Gesundheitsversorgungssystems sind die Krankenkassen und Krankenversicherungen. Ihre ökonomische Analyse fällt in den Bereich der Versicherungswissenschaft, die zu einer eigenständigen wirtschaftswissenschaftlichen Disziplin geworden ist. Ihre Aufgabe ist die Beschreibung und die Bewertung des versicherten Risikos und die versicherungstechnische Handhabung des Risikos. Mit Hilfe der Entscheidungstheorie unter Unsicherheit werden Aussagen zum Verhalten der Versicherten und zum Risk-Management der Versicherer gewonnen.

Die Versicherungswissenschaft hat Methoden der Prämienkalkulation und der Bildung von Tarif- und Risikoklassenstrukturen entwickelt, die von Krankenversicherern angewendet werden. Die Versicherungswissenschaft behandelt auch die Frage, inwieweit eine Pflichtversicherung und ein eingeschränkter Wettbewerb zwischen Versicherern nötig ist, da Moral hazard und Adverse selection sonst zu negativen Effekten führen. Unter Moral hazard versteht man eine übermäßige Ausdehnung des Inanspruchnahmeverhaltens bei Bestehen von Krankenversicherungsschutz. Adverse selection liegt vor, wenn sich bei einem Versicherer besonders viele schlechte Risiken sammeln und er hierdurch einen Wettbewerbsnachteil hat.

Betriebslehre

Im Gesundheitswesen werden Leistungen produziert. Im ökonomischen Sinne sind Arztpraxen, Krankenhäuser, Pflegeheime, Apotheken usw. Unternehmen. Aufgabe der Betriebs(wirtschafts)lehre ist es, die internen Strukturen von Unternehmen zu analysieren und Hinweise für eine effiziente marktorientierte Organisation von Betrieben zu liefern. Die Instrumente der Betriebslehre sind auch fruchtbringend auf Gesundheitsbetriebe angewendet worden. Dabei geht es beispielsweise um die Finanzierung und das Controlling im Krankenhaus, die Gestaltung von Managementstrukturen und das Marketing von Gesundheitsleistungen. Als ein besonderer Zweig der Betriebslehre hat sich die Krankenhausbetriebslehre etabliert. Mittlerweile ist aber auch für niedergelassene Ärzte eine betriebswirtschaftliche Ausbildung von großem Nutzen.

Themenschwerpunkte und Forschungsfelder der Gesundheitsökonomie

Da die Gesundheitsökonomie ihre Themen und Fragestellungen einerseits aus der Anwendung des ökonomischen Instrumentariums auf das Gesundheitswesen gewinnt, andererseits die Problemstrukturierung durch die Besonderheiten der verschiedenen Gesundheitsbereiche geprägt ist, lassen sich Themenschwerpunkte und Forschungsfelder der Gesundheitsökonomie nach allgemeinen Dimensionen ökonomischer Analyse oder nach den einzelnen Sektoren bzw. Bereichen des Gesundheitswesens gliedern. Unter dem Gesichtspunkt einer disziplinären Orientierung bieten sich folgende Schwerpunkte an: Bedarf, Nachfrage und Inanspruchnahme; Angebot und Produktion; Finanzierung; Ordnungspolitik und Steuerung; ökonomische Evaluierung von Gesundheitsleistungen.

Bedarf, Nachfrage und Inanspruchnahme

Die gesundheitsökonomische Analyse der Nachfrageseite zeichnet sich immer noch durch terminologische Unklarheiten aus. Dies gilt auch für die zentralen Begriffe Bedarf, Nachfrage und Inanspruchnahme. Trotz der theoretischen, empirischen und politischen Implikationen wird nicht immer eindeutig unterschieden.

Die grundlegenden Differenzen gesundheitsökonomischer Ansätze werden besonders deutlich bei der Frage, ob das neoklassische Instrumentarium eine angemessene Methode zur Analyse der Nachfrage nach Gesundheitsleistungen ist. Einerseits wird die Anwendungsfähigkeit der mikroökonomischen Nachfragetheorie auf das Gesundheitswesen grundsätzlich bestritten und deshalb das Bedarfskonzept für das einzig angemessene gehalten, andererseits wird gerade die Orientierung am Bedarfskonzept für ökonomisch verhängnisvoll gehalten und als gesundheitspolitische Fehlorientierung diagnostiziert.

Die Diskussion Bedarf versus Nachfrage wird auf einer primär politischen, einer primär theoretisch-normativen und einer primär methodisch-methodologischen Ebene geführt. Die politische Diskussion spielt dabei für die hochindustrialisierten Länder keine entscheidende Rolle mehr. Aber unmittelbar einsichtig ist, daß für jene Länder, die nicht über ein ausreichendes Gesundheitsversorgungssystem verfügen, die Planung von Versorgungseinrichtungen unter Zugrundelegung von Bedarfsüberlegungen eine vordringliche Aufgabe ist. Die unter theoretischen und normativen Gesichtspunkten formulierten Positionen unterscheiden sich prinzipiell zunächst in der Einschätzung der individuellen Fähigkeit, autonom nach eigenen Wertvorstellungen und Nützlichkeitserwägungen über die angemessene Inanspruchnahme medizinischer Leistungen entscheiden zu können. Da in der Nachfragetheorie immer auch das Einkommen eine konstitutive Größe darstellt, kann in den beiden Grundpositionen letztlich auch eine normative Grundentscheidung für das „Freiheitspostulat" einerseits und das „Gleichheitspostulat" andererseits gesehen werden. Die methodisch-methodologische Kritik richtet sich v. a. auf die normativen Implikationen, die dem Bedarfskonzept inhärent sind. Denn die externe Festlegung von wünschbaren Zuständen erfordert immer eine hinreichend begründbare Legitimation. Bezweifelt wird, daß durch Expertenurteil, empirische Erhebungen oder politische Richtlinien die entsprechenden Legitimationsgrundlagen zur Steuerung der Gesundheitsversorgung erreicht werden können. Hinzu kommt das Argument, daß der Bedarf letztlich beliebig ausgedehnt werden kann und somit konsensfähige objektive Festlegungen weder für medizinische noch für politische Entscheidungskalküle möglich sind.

Da insbesondere die Begriffe Nachfrage und Inanspruchnahme häufig synonym verwendet werden, sollen die wesentlichen Unterschiede, aber auch Gemeinsamkeiten skizziert werden. Nachfrage im strengen Sinne bezieht sich auf Zahlungsbereitschaft und Zahlungsfähigkeit. Inanspruchnahme unterscheidet sich von Nachfrage zuerst und grundsätzlich dadurch, daß immer der Handlungsvollzug vorausgesetzt ist: also die erfolgte Konsultation des Arztes, die Konsumption des Medikaments oder der Krankenhausaufenthalt.

Ein Grund für die häufige synonyme Verwendung dürfte nun darin zu sehen sein, daß empirische Untersuchungen zu einer „Theorie der Nachfrage nach Gesundheitsleistungen" oder – etwas weniger anspruchsvoll – eines Schätzmodells der Nachfrage auf vergleichbare oder identische Daten zurückgreifen wie die Analysen der Inanspruchnahme. Die Determinanten der Nachfrage sind fast immer auch die Determinanten der Inanspruchnahme; oder: Inanspruchnahme ist die gemessene Nachfrage.

Gerade die empirischen Gemeinsamkeiten bei der Bestimmung der Nachfrage bzw. der Inanspruchnahme von Gesundheitsleistungen verweisen auf Konvergenzen im Hinblick auf eine verhaltenswissenschaftliche Begründung der gesundheitsökonomischen Analyse der Nachfrageseite. Während sich dabei die Inanspruchnahmeanalysen primär auf Verhaltensdimensionen in Form von „Lebensstilvarianten" (z. B. Eß-, Rauch- oder Trinkgewohnheiten; Berufs- und Arbeitsplatzsituationen; Risikoverhalten etc.) beziehen, zielt die nachfragetheoretische Analyse auf grundsätzliche Annahmen. Dies sei an einem Beispiel demonstriert.

Auf dem Schlußplenum der erwähnten Jahrestagung des Vereins für Socialpolitik kam es zu einer kurzen Kontroverse über die mutmaßlichen Konsequenzen einer Steigerung der Kostentransparenz bei den Versicherten. Der eine Diskutant befürwortete solche Maßnahmen, weil er vermutete, daß das Wissen um die Kosten der Inanspruchnahme die Nachfrage eher dämme. Der andere dagegen erwartete genau das Gegenteil. Der Versicherte werde danach trachten, möglichst viel an Leistungen herauszuholen, zumindest soviel, wie er an Beiträgen eingezahlt habe. Es ist offensichtlich, daß beide von sehr verschiedenen Annahmen hinsichtlich des erwarteten Verhaltens der Versicherten ausgehen. Dominiert auf der einen Seite die Annahme eines Solidaritätsgefühls mit der Versichertengemeinschaft, wird auf der anderen Seite das rationale Kalkül eines vermuteten relativen Vorteils unterstellt.

Der Ökonomie – insbesondere in ihrer heute dominierenden neoklassischen Form – ist zum Vorwurf gemacht worden, sie vernachlässige die „menschliche Komponente" und adaptiere eine „mechanistische Sicht der Gesellschaft"; es gelte deshalb, die Ökonomie als verhaltenswissenschaftliche Disziplin zu beleben. Es muß daher gefragt werden, ob eine ökonomische Theorie menschlichen Verhaltens auf das Entscheidungsverhalten im Gesundheitswesen anwendbar ist. Dann ist weiter zu fragen, wie das ökonomische Verhaltensmodell spezifiziert werden muß, um durch die Berücksichtigung der Besonderheiten des Gutes Gesundheit und der Gesundheitsmärkte eine empirisch überprüfbare Erklärungs- und Prognosebasis abgeben zu können. Dies wäre die Formulierung eines Verhaltensmodells, in dem Präferenzen und Restriktionen klar unterschieden werden, die Individuen die Entscheidungsalternativen kennen und entsprechend den relativen Vorteilen handeln. Es bedarf deshalb weiterer empirischer und theoretischer Bemühungen, um über eine Deskription von Lebensstilvarianten und empirischökonometrischen Modellanalysen die Formulierung einer erklärungs- und prognoserelevanten gesundheitsökonomischen Verhaltenstheorie der Nachfrage nach Gesundheitsleistungen zu erreichen.

Angebot und Produktion

Das Angebot an Gütern und Dienstleistungen wird traditionell in folgende Sektoren gegliedert: ambulanter Sektor, stationärer Sektor, Arzneimittel, Heil- und Hilfsmittel. Es sind Sektoren mit jeweils spezifischen „Produktionsbedingungen" und eigenen Entwicklungstendenzen. Nun ist gerade auch das Verhältnis der einzelnen Sektoren zueinander von Interesse sowie die sich ändernden Ausgabenanteile der Gesetzlichen Krankenversicherung. Es wird z. B. die Frage gestellt, warum der Sektor „Heil- und Hilfsmittel" um so viel stärker steigt als alle anderen Sektoren; oder warum die Ausgaben für den stationären Sektor stärker steigen als für den ambulanten Sektor. Es ist deshalb v. a. auch unter Allokationsgesichtspunkten ein Problem der ökonomischen Analyse, nach einer effizienten sektoralen Struktur zu suchen. Es bestehen zwischen allen der hier aufgeführten Sektoren Substitutionsmöglichkeiten.

Der ambulante Sektor

Der Untersuchungsgegenstand des ambulanten Sektors ist durch die Praxis des niedergelassenen Arztes definiert. Untersucht wird, warum der Arzt, unter welchen Produktionsbedingungen, in welcher Form, welche Leistungen erbringt und wie das Entgelt dafür aussieht. So wie es auf der Nachfrageseite ein Ziel gesundheitsökonomischer Analyse ist, ein Verhaltensmodell der Nachfrage nach medizinischen Leistungen zu formulieren, so ist es auf der Angebotseite ein Ziel, ein ökonomisches Entscheidungsmodell für das ärztliche Verhalten zu entwickeln. Dabei ist es v. a. die durch steigende Ärztezahlen veränderte Entscheidungssituation, in der die ökonomische Perspektive zunehmend an Bedeutung gewinnt. Denn aufgrund des steigenden Wettbewerbsdrucks wird ein „trade-off" zwischen Ethik, Freizeit, Attraktivität des Standorts und Einkommen deutlich.

Von der Motivstruktur ärztlichen Entscheidungsverhaltens (partiell) abgekoppelt ist die Analyse der Praxis als organisatorischer Einheit. Dieser Untersuchungsansatz läßt sich näherungsweise mit der „Arztpraxis als betriebswirtschaftlichem Problemfeld" umschreiben. In diesen Problemkreis gehören z. B. Analysen des Produktivitätsfortschritts ärztlicher Leistungen etwa durch Rationalisierung mittels EDV-Anlagen. Vor allem aber sind die ständig an Bedeutung gewinnenden technischen Einrichtungen Gegenstand der Analyse. Die zunehmende Technisierung der Medizin hat nun auch erhebliche Auswirkungen auf das Entscheidungsverhalten des Arztes selbst, überhaupt eine Praxis zu eröffnen. Darüber hinaus werden auch die Formen ärztlicher Leistungen selbst beeinflußt. Die These, daß Apparate einen immanenten Anwendungszwang (Amortisationszwang) induzieren, und die daraus folgenden Konsequenzen für das ärztliche Leistungsgeschehen sind zunehmend Gegenstand nicht nur medizinimmanenter, sondern auch ökonomischer Kritik.

Die in letzter Zeit am häufigsten zu beobachtende Formveränderung des ambulanten ärztlichen Angebots sind die erkennbaren Trends zu Gruppen- bzw. Gemeinschaftspraxen. In einer Reihe auch empirischer Untersuchungen werden mit unterschiedlichen Ansätzen und Fragestellungen das Entstehen, die Motive der Beteiligten, die Arbeitsweisen oder Vor- und Nachteile untersucht. Neben Wünschen im Hinblick auf die Arbeitsplatzgestaltung sind es Gründe der medizinischen Spezialisierung, der gemeinsamen Ausnutzung technischer Geräte und Tendenzen zu ganzheitlicher Medizin, die angeführt werden. Im Vordergrund des ökonomischen Interesses steht v. a., ob sich die Vorteile der „economics of scale" durch die verschiedenen Formen der Gruppen- bzw. Gemeinschaftspraxen ausmachen lassen; eine bisher durchaus kontrovers geführte und keineswegs abgeschlossene Diskussion. Bewegen sich derartige Analysen im Rahmen der Praxis als Betriebseinheit, so gelten andere Fragen den möglichen Einflüssen veränderter Angebotsformen z. B. auf die Wettbewerbssituation, ob also möglicherweise in den Präferenzen bestimmter Patientengruppen die althergebrachte Form der Einzelpraxis immer weniger Zuspruch hat.

Kaum ein Thema hat neben der allgemeinen „Kostenexplosionsdebatte" die Öffentlichkeit zeitweise mehr beschäftigt als die Entwicklung der Ärzteeinkommen. Ihre Höhe hat neben der Beitragssatzentwicklung das Bewußtsein für die hohen Ausgaben im Gesundheitswesen geschärft. Dabei mögen die als zu hoch empfundenen Einkommen und die Einkommensdivergenzen zwischen verschiedenen Facharztgruppen durchaus ein Motiv für den Ökonomen sein, sich diesem Problemkreis zuzuwenden. Die Höhe selbst wird jedoch kaum Maßnahmen zur Dämpfung aus ökonomischer Sicht rechtfertigen können. Es werden vielmehr die Mechanismen der Preisbildung analysiert, nach Defiziten in den Allokationswirkungen gesucht, Strategien der Optimierung entworfen und v. a. alternative Maßnahmen der Steuerung diskutiert. Zwar wird es immer wieder Versuche geben, die seit dem Mittelalter gestellte Frage nach dem „gerechten Preis" auch für medizinische Leistungen in der heutigen Zeit zu beantworten; sei es, daß die Entwicklung des Bruttosozialprodukts eine „Meßlatte" abgeben soll, sei es, daß die Einkommensentwicklung nach bestimmten Kriterien (z. B. Ausbildung) vergleichbarer Berufsgruppen herangezogen wird.

Drei Schwerpunkte der ökonomischen Analyse des Honorierungssystems haben sich herausgebildet: 1) Die Darstellung und die Auswirkungen der verschiedenen Formen und Verfahren, besonders im Hinblick auf deren allokative Wirkungen. Im Mittelpunkt steht dabei v. a. die Analyse von Einzelleistungshonoraren im Vergleich zu den verschiedenen Formen der Pauschalierung. 2) Das geltende System der Einzelleistungshonorierung ist selbst ein Schwerpunkt. Dabei werden Fragen des geltenden Bewertungsmaßstabs diskutiert (z. B. ob die Bewertung technischer Leistungen nicht zu hoch angesetzt ist im Vergleich zur Beratung) oder deren Bedeutung für Höhe und Divergenz der Einkommen untersucht. 3) Ein weiterer Schwerpunkt, der implizit oder explizit in die meisten Analysen der Formen und Verfahren des Honorierungssystems mit eingeht, betrifft die möglichen oder tatsächlichen Steuerungswirkungen des Honorierungssystems. Es sind also Fragen danach, welche Konsequenzen sich z. B. für die Einkommensentwicklung der Ärzte, für die Verteilung der ambulanten Leistungen auf die Versorgung der Bevölkerung und für die Ausgaben der Krankenversicherung ergeben, wenn bestimmte Änderungen im System (z. B. ein Wechsel von der Einzelleistungshonorierung zu Formen der Pauschalierung) vorgenommen würden.

Der stationäre Sektor

Krankenhäuser sind Wirtschaftseinheiten mit einer differenzierten organisatorischen Struktur, mit einem hohen Etat und mit einer großen Zahl von Beschäftigten. Insbesondere der naheliegende und immer wieder aufgenommene Vergleich

mit Industriebetrieben oder bürokratischen Organisationen hat schon vergleichsweise früh eine eigene Disziplin „Krankenhausbetriebslehre" entstehen lassen.
Gesundheitsökonomische Problemstellungen, die sich nicht ausschließlich bzw.
primär den Themen der Krankenhausbetriebslehre zurechnen lassen (Themen
wie etwa Zielanalyse, Zielbestimmung und Zielplanung im Krankenhaus; Organisationsstruktur, Management, Steuerungs- und Kontrollsysteme; Informa-
tions- und Datenverarbeitung; Personalwesen) beziehen sich v. a. auf Planung
und Versorgung, Krankenhausfinanzierung und Wirtschaftlichkeit im Krankenhaus.

Unter Versorgungsgesichtspunkten werden Alternativformen des Angebots
an stationären Leistungen oder Möglichkeiten der Substitution stationärer Leistungen diskutiert. Da von Unterversorgung nicht mehr die Rede sein kann, sondern der „Bettenberg" zum Schlagwort geworden ist, haben sich auch hier die
Problemstellungen verschoben. So sind beispielsweise Ansätze zur Neuordnung
des Krankenhauswesens, die auf einer Wettbewerbskonzeption beruhen, vor dem
Hintergrund tendenzieller Überversorgung diskussionsfähiger als in Zeiten, in
denen eine akzeptable Vorhaltung vordringliche Planungsaufgabe war.

Deshalb wird auch die neuere Planungs- und Versorgungsdiskussion von
Problemen bestimmt, wie eine Begrenzung des überproportionalen Wachstums
der Ausgaben für den stationären Sektor erreicht werden kann. Dazu gehören sowohl die Forderung nach verfeinerten Methoden der Bettenbedarfsplanung wie
die Erörterung von Möglichkeiten, stationäre Leistungen durch Verzahnung mit
dem ambulanten Sektor zu substituieren. Planungsziele sind eher Reduktion und
Differenzierung des Bettenangebots, die Diskussion unter Gesichtspunkten der
Versorgung gerät zunehmend unter den Druck von Substitutionsüberlegungen.

Die Krankenhausfinanzierung ist ein differenziertes System institutioneller
Regelungen, das in verschiedenen Gesetzesvorhaben geregelt wurde. Die wichtigsten Etappen dabei sind das Krankenhausfinanzierungsgesetz (KHG) vom
29.6.1972, das Krankenhauskostendämpfungsgesetz (KHKG) vom 22.12.1981
und das Krankenhausneuordnungsgesetz (KHNG) vom 20.12.1984. Zwei Themen stehen dabei im Vordergrund der ökonomischen Diskussion: Einmal die
Auseinandersetzung um ein duales oder monistisches Prinzip der Finanzierung.
Das duale Prinzip bedeutet, daß der Staat die Investitionskosten übernimmt und
die Betriebskosten über den Pflegesatz abgerechnet werden; das monistische
Prinzip bedeutet, daß alle Kosten über den Pflegesatz kalkuliert werden. Vorschläge, das monistische Prinzip in die Krankenhausfinanzierung einzuführen,
haben sich im Krankenhausneuordnungsgesetz nicht durchgesetzt. Es gilt also
weiter das duale Finanzierungsprinzip.

Das zweite hier im Vordergrund stehende Thema betrifft die Entgeltverfahren. Mehr noch wohl als die Grundprinzipien war das in der Bundespflegesatzverordnung geltende Selbstkostendeckungsprinzip Anlaß ökonomischer Kritik.
Bemängelt wurde v. a., daß die Erstattung von Selbstkosten den Krankenhäusern keine Anreize zu wirtschaftlichem Handeln bieten konnte. Das seit dem
1.1.1986 geltende Pflegesatzrecht hat insofern zu einer gewissen Auflockerung
des Prinzips der Selbstkostendeckung geführt, als die Pflegesätze auf der Grundlage der vorauskalkulierten Selbstkosten mit den Krankenkassen ausgehandelt
werden und deshalb Überschüsse, die bei wirtschaftlicher Betriebsführung entste-

hen, dem Krankenhaus verbleiben und Verluste entsprechend vom Krankenhaus zu tragen sind. Die im neuen Pflegesatzrecht ausgewiesenen Tendenzen zu prospektiven Entgeltverfahren sind v. a. Gegenstand von Überlegungen zur ökonomischen Analyse der Preisgestaltung im Krankenhaus, und die aktuelle Forschung läßt erkennen, daß dieses Thema auch weiterhin Gegenstand theoretischer und empirischer Analysen sein wird.

Da die krankenhausökonomische Diskussion letztlich zum Ziel hat, die stationäre Versorgung auch unter dem Gesichtspunkt der ökonomischen Effizienz zu analysieren, ist die Frage nach der Wirtschaftlichkeit im Krankenhaus als Frage nach dem Stellenwert des ökonomischen Prinzips überhaupt bezeichnet worden. Die Diskussion um die Wirtschaftlichkeit im Krankenhaus setzt deshalb auf einer grundsätzlichen Ebene an, wie sie etwa im (scheinbaren) Gegensatzpaar von „Ökonomie und Humanität" deutlich wird. Da bei allen unterschiedlichen Ansätzen, Methoden oder Indikatoren die Wirtschaftlichkeit immer Ausdruck der Mitteladäquanz der Leistungserstellung ist, sind Grad der Zielerreichung und Leistungsadäquanz des Behandlungsprozesses notwendige Orientierungsmaßstäbe zur Beurteilung der Wirtschaftlichkeit. Dies wiederum ist der gesundheitsökonomische Kern des Themas: zur Beurteilung der Leistungsfähigkeit reichen die ökonomischen Instrumente nicht aus, Ansätze zur Formulierung und Operationalisierung eines krankenhausspezifischen Wirtschaftlichkeitsbegriffs sind deshalb notwendig.

Arzneimittelsektor

Überhöhte Arzneimittelpreise im Vergleich zum Ausland, vergleichsweise hoher Medikamentenverbrauch in der Bundesrepublik Deutschland, hohe Gewinne der pharmazeutischen Industrie oder die wachsende Sensibilität für mögliche negative Auswirkungen von Medikamenten sind öffentlichkeitswirksame Themen des Arzneimittelsektors. Dabei wäre zunächst zu fragen, ob die „pharmazeutische Industrie" überhaupt Gegenstand einer spezifisch gesundheitsökonomischen Analyse ist. Wer nun die gesundheitsökonomische Diskussion in der Bundesrepublik Deutschland verfolgt, wird feststellen, daß seit ihrer Etablierung auch die Ökonomie der pharmazeutischen Industrie als deren integraler Bestandteil gilt. Dies beruht einmal darauf, daß diese Industrie unmittelbar in die hohe Systeminterdependenz des Gesundheitsbereichs eingebunden ist. Ein Hinweis darauf ist etwa die in der RVO vorgesehene Teilnahme an der konzertierten Aktion im Gesundheitswesen.

Auch hat die pharmazeutische Industrie selbst ein besonderes Selbstverständnis, welches aus den Besonderheiten des Markts für Gesundheitsleistungen hergeleitet wird. Die daraus abgeleiteten Besonderheiten der pharmazeutischen Produkte oder die spezifischen strukturellen Ausprägungen dieses Markts sind das gesundheitsökonomisch Spezifische, das immer wieder herausgestellt wird. Hingewiesen wird etwa darauf, daß der Preis als Wettbewerbsparameter eine nur untergeordnete Rolle spielt; eine Tatsache, die sich allerdings durch erhöhte Selbstbeteiligungen und das Vordringen der Generika auf manchen Märkten ändern könnte. Es werden v. a. die im Gesundheitsreformgesetz vorgesehenen Festbetragsregelungen und deren Auswirkungen auf Produktion und Preisgestaltung zu untersuchen sein.

Eine weitere Besonderheit sind die arzneimittelspezifischen Reglementierungen und deren internationale Unterschiede. Hier wird der gemeinsame Binnenmarkt der EG noch zu erheblichen Veränderungen führen. Hervorgehoben werden auch die Konsequenzen aus dem hohen Forschungs- und Entwicklungsaufwand, der sich auch aus dem therapeutischen Auftrag an die pharmazeutische Industrie herleiten läßt. Diese knappen und skizzenhaften Hinweise auf beispielhafte Problemstellungen sollten verdeutlichen, daß jene Argumente, die für eine Begründung einer gesundheitsökonomischen Disziplin herangezogen werden, auch für den Bereich der pharmazeutischen Industrie gelten können.

Die Analysen der Nachfrageseite des Arzneimittelsektors entsprechen einem Schema, wie die Aufspaltung der Nachfrage nach Arzneimitteln generell geschrieben wird: auf den Patienten, der nachfragt und verbraucht, aber nicht entscheidet; auf den Arzt, der entscheidet aber nicht verbraucht und nicht bezahlt; auf die Kasse, die nicht verbraucht oder entscheidet, aber bezahlt. Eindeutig im Vordergrund des Interesses steht dabei die Stellung der Gesetzlichen Krankenversicherung im System der Arzneimittelnachfrage. Da die Kassen – abgesehen von Appellen im Rahmen der Konzertierten Aktion – auf die Preisgestaltung der Pharmahersteller unmittelbar keinen nennenswerten Einfluß ausüben können, werden Maßnahmen v. a. in der Überwindung der Aufspaltung der Nachfrage durch Kooperation der verschiedenen Partner möglich. Deshalb kann als ein Hauptproblem der Untersuchungen zusammenfassend die Frage gelten: Wie können Ärzte, Patienten und Kassen kooperieren, um von der Nachfrageseite her Druck auf Angebots- und Preisstruktur der Pharmahersteller auszuüben, und wie können sie zusammenarbeiten, um die Ausgaben der Kassen für die Arzneimittel auf das geringstmögliche Maß zu senken.

Diskutiert werden Auswirkungen und Möglichkeiten von Positivlisten (Empfehlungen an die Ärzte, bestimmte kostengünstige Präparate zu verordnen) oder von Negativlisten (Ausschluß bestimmter Präparate aus der Erstattungspflicht); analysiert werden Auswirkungen von Reimporten, um die internationalen Preisunterschiede ausnützen zu können. Von zunehmendem Gewicht ist dabei der Einfluß von Generika auf dem Arzneimittelmarkt, d. h. von Präparaten, die dieselbe chemische Zusammensetzung haben wie die am Markt angebotenen Markenpräparate, deren Patentschutz abgelaufen ist.

Wichtigste Voraussetzung für die Wirksamkeit der angesprochenen Maßnahmen ist die Kooperation mit den Ärzten. Deshalb ist die Analyse des Verschreibungsverhaltens und die Diskussion rationeller, d. h. kostengünstiger Arzneimitteltherapien von Interesse. Analysen des Verschreibungsverhaltens von Ärzten setzen nicht nur bei den Ärzten selbst an, sondern lassen sich auch durch die Analyse des Konsums an Medikamenten gewinnen. Ein vieldiskutiertes Thema ist hier der Versuch, die Ausgabensteigerungen für Arzneimittel in eine Mengen-, Preis- und Strukturkomponente aufzuschlüsseln. Wie problematisch trotz der Ärztedominanz das Patientenverhalten in bezug auf den Arzneimittelverbrauch ist, wird an Untersuchungen zur Non-Compliance deutlich. Dabei wird mit Non-Compliance die Nichtbefolgung der Anordnungen und Verschreibungen des Arztes durch den Patienten bezeichnet. Dieses Phänomen deutet darauf hin, daß die Nachfrage nach Arzneimitteln nicht nur aus den Entscheidungen des Arztes allein ableitbar ist. Denn die Non-Compliance-Problematik zeigt, wie die eingangs skizzierte Aufspaltung der Nachfrageseite in Verschreibung, Verbrauch und Finanzierung einerseits durch das konzertierte Vorgehen der beteiligten Parteien überwunden werden kann, daß aber andererseits auch Strategien notwendig sind, die bei den jeweiligen Gruppen selbst ansetzen.

Heil- und Hilfsmittel

Der Markt für Heil- und Hilfsmittel ist hochgradig differenziert und in zahlreiche Marktsegmente aufgegliedert. Auf der Nachfrageseite dominiert die typische Aufspaltung in Arzt, Patient und Krankenversicherung, wie sie auch für Arzneimittel skizziert wurde. Daraus folgt, daß im wesentlichen kollektive Preisvereinbarungen vorherrschen und freie Marktpreisbildung nur im Bereich der „Selbstzahler" existiert (z. B. höherwertige Brillengestelle). Auf der Angebotseite dominieren freiberufliche bzw. selbständige handwerkliche Strukturen mit vorgelagerten industriellen Unternehmenseinheiten.

Die expansive Entwicklung dieses Sektors ist in erster Linie auf den medizinisch-technischen Fortschritt und noch z. T. wenig ausgebildete Steuerungsinstrumente – wie z. B. Verhandlungspreise – zurückzuführen; eine Rolle spielt auch das Vordringen chronisch-degenerativer Krankheiten. Die Steigerungsraten in der Ausgabenentwicklung und das erreichte Ausgabenvolumen dürften auch zu einer erhöhten Aufmerksamkeit für gesundheitsökonomische Analysen dieses Sektors führen.

Finanzierung

Alle hochentwickelten Industrieländer haben im Laufe der Zeit ein umfassendes System der Sicherung im Krankheitsfall ausgebaut. Grundprinzip aller Sicherungssysteme im Gesundheitswesen ist dabei die kollektive Finanzierung. Die Verabschiedung des Krankenversicherungsgesetzes am 15. 6. 1883 im deutschen Reichstag gilt als Beginn moderner sozialer Krankenversicherung.

Ganz generell haben sich 3 grundsätzliche Alternativen der kollektiven Finanzierung herausgebildet: die Finanzierung über den Staat, über beitragsfinanzierte Selbstverwaltungskörperschaften und über nach aktuarischen Grundsätzen arbeitende Privatversicherungen. Die Bundesrepublik Deutschland ist dabei der einzige Staat, in dem die soziale Krankenversicherung von relativ autonomen Selbstverwaltungskörperschaften in staatlichem Auftrag betrieben wird. Da ca. 90 % aller Bundesbürger durch die Gesetzliche Krankenversicherung geschützt sind, kann von einem GKV-zentrierten System der sozialen Sicherung im Krankheitsfall gesprochen werden.

Es ist nun v. a. diese GKV-Zentriertheit, die die außerordentlich hohe Interdependenz des Gesundheitssystems bedingt; und diese Systeminterdependenz hat Konsequenzen für nahezu alle Ansätze zur gesundheitsökonomischen Analyse des Gesundheitsbereichs. Weder die Genese des Anspruchsverhaltens, noch die

Bestimmung der Nachfrage oder die Analyse der Angebotstrukturen sind ohne den Rückgriff auf Formen, Finanzierung oder Leistungen des GKV-Systems zu beschreiben, zu erklären oder zu prognostizieren. Nicht ohne Berechtigung ist deshalb auch die Problemgeschichte der Gesundheitsökonomie in der Bundesrepublik Deutschland als die Problemgeschichte der GKV beschrieben worden. Dabei lassen sich die Schwerpunkte der gesundheitsökonomischen Analyse des GKV-Systems nach den Themen Gestaltungsprinzipien, Beitragsgestaltung und Mitgliederstruktur sowie Leistungsgeschehen näherungsweise gliedern.

Den Kern der Diskussion um die Gestaltungsprinzipien der GKV bildet die Analyse des Solidaritätsprinzips, des tragenden Pfeilers der sozialen Krankenversicherung. Solidargemeinschaft heißt lohnabhängige Beitragsgestaltung und eine durch die Beitragsbemessungsgrenze definierte Zwangsmitgliedschaft. Das Prinzip des Zwanges folgt unmittelbar aus dem Solidaritätsprinzip, denn ohne Elemente der Pflicht zur Versicherung ist eine Solidargemeinschaft nicht zu begründen. An dieses konstitutive Prinzip knüpfen Untersuchungen an, etwa an seine Zeitgemäßheit, an unerwünschte Folgewirkungen, mögliche Alternativen wie dem Einbau äquivalenzprinzipieller Elemente oder der Forderung nach mehr Eigenverantwortung. Zudem stehen die Kassen der GKV in vielfältigen Wettbewerbsbeziehungen zueinander. Dieser Wettbewerb innerhalb der GKV, seine Möglichkeiten und Grenzen, seine erwünschten oder unerwünschten Folgen sind erst in den letzten Jahren verstärkt Gegenstand gesundheitsökonomischer Analysen geworden. Die dabei geäußerten total entgegengesetzten möglichen Wirkungen (Wettbewerb zwischen GKV-Kassen führt über Leistungswettbewerb zur Beitragserhöhung; er führt über Beitragswettbewerb zu einer Beitragssenkung) zeigen beispielhaft auf eine Reihe noch ungeklärter Fragen.

Die Tatsache, daß in einer Zwangsversicherung die Höhe der Beiträge erheblich schwankt, war immer schon ein Ärgernis und wurde als eine Gefährdung des Solidarausgleichs gesehen. Diese Entwicklung verschärft sich z. Z. noch. Da die GKV nahezu ausschließlich über die lohnabhängigen Beiträge finanziert wird, kann nur eine differenzierte Analyse der Mitgliederstruktur Erklärungen zu den Differenzen oder zu den möglichen Entwicklungen liefern und Ansätze zu notwendigen Maßnahmen der finanziellen Absicherung einzelner Kassen wie der GKV insgesamt abgeben (Finanzausgleichsverfahren).

Im Zusammenhang mit der ausdifferenzierten empirischen Analyse der Beitragssatzentwicklung, seiner Unterschiede und den bestimmenden Faktoren zeichnet sich ein gesundheitsökonomischer Forschungszusammenhang ab, der über unmittelbare Finanzierungskonsequenzen hinausgeht. Denn je differenzierter die empirischen Wirkungsanalysen die Erklärungszusammenhänge aufdecken, um so sicherer ist die Indikatoreneigenschaft von Beitragssatzunterschieden etwa für regionale Bezüge, die Morbiditätsentwicklung und das Krankheitspanorama, für das Inanspruchnahmeverhalten oder Angebotsüberhänge.

Im Zusammenhang des Leistungsgeschehens wird grundsätzlich die Kompetenzverteilung zwischen Mittelaufbringung und Mittelverwendung kritisiert. Während die Kassen für die Mittelaufbringung selbst zuständig sind, wird ihnen die Verwendungsseite im wesentlichen vom Staat vorgeschrieben. Dadurch aber sind auch nur begrenzte Steuerungsmöglichkeiten für die GKV auf der Leistungsseite gegeben. Vor allem wird die Ausweitung des Leistungskatalogs der GKV kritisiert und die Durchforstung v. a. im Hinblick auf sog. versicherungsfremde Leistungen gefordert.

Ein gesundheitsökonomisches Dauerthema ist die Auseinandersetzung um die Form der Leistungsgewährung, um das Kostenerstattungs- bzw. das Sachleistungsprinzip. Es geht hierbei um die Frage, ob die Versicherten die Inanspruchnahme von Gesundheitsleistungen zunächst selbst bezahlen, um sie dann von den Krankenkassen ersetzt zu bekommen (wie bei der privaten Krankenversicherung) oder ob die Sachleistungen in Anspruch genommen und die Kosten dann von den Krankenkassen jeweils mit Ärzten, Apotheken, Krankenhäusern abgerechnet werden. Wie die Sozialenquete zeigt, ist die Auseinandersetzung um die möglichen Konsequenzen insbesondere für die Inanspruchnahme schon früh – insbesondere von ökonomischer Seite – geführt worden. Es wurde v. a. argumentiert, daß dieses Prinzip eine Nullpreismentalität fördere und bei den Versicherten kein Bewußtsein für die Kosten medizinischer Behandlungen aufkommen lassen könne. Nun hat allerdings die generelle Einführung des Kostenerstattungsprinzips in der zahnärztlichen Versorgung durch das Gesundheitsreformgesetz zu einer Veränderung geführt, deren Konsequenzen insbesondere für das Inanspruchnahmeverhalten z. Z. noch nicht abgeschätzt werden können. Zu erwarten aber ist, daß die empirischen Analysen der Konsequenzen dieser Strukturveränderung auch ein Test für die Gültigkeit mancher Hypothesen im Hinblick auf den Einfluß der Kostenkenntnis auf das Inanspruchnahmeverhalten sein werden.

Die Finanzierungsmodalitäten der GKV werden darüber hinaus im Hinblick auf die durch sie bewirkten Umverteilungen analysiert. Umverteilungswirkungen heißt, daß bestimmte Individuen bzw. Gruppen relativ mehr an Leistungen aus der GKV erwarten können, als sie Beiträge entrichten. Nicht gemeint sind dabei jene Umverteilungswirkungen von Nichtgeschädigten auf Geschädigte, die das Prinzip jeder Art von Versicherung sind und deshalb auch für das versicherungstechnische Äquivalenzprinzip der privaten Versicherung gelten. Umverteilungswirkungen resultieren v. a. aus der Anwendung des Solidaritätsprinzip (Lohnabhängigkeit der Beiträge; Familienlastenausgleich; Krankenversicherung der Rentner). Diese Umverteilungswirkungen werden ökonomisch kontrovers beurteilt. Vor allem werden die Redistributionswirkungen als versicherungsfremd bezeichnet. Als systemkonformerer Ausgleich wird meist auf entsprechende redistributive steuerpolitische Instrumente verwiesen.

Die steigende Bedeutung der privaten Krankenversicherung – das Gesundheitsreformgesetz hat zu einem Eintrittsschub geführt – in der gesundheitsökonomischen Diskussion liegt nicht nur in ihrem Beitrag zur Finanzierung des Gesundheitswesens, sondern auch in der Rolle des Konkurrenten zur GKV und zur Demonstration der Wirkungsweise anderer, marktkonformerer Finanzierungssysteme. Der fundamentale Unterschied zur GKV liegt zunächst in der Beitragsgestaltung. Während die GKV einen lohnabhängigen Beitrag erhebt, richten sich die Beiträge der PKV nach Eintrittsalter und Geschlecht. Kalkuliert wird nach dem Äquivalenzprinzip, so daß der abgezinste Wert der zu erwartenden Versicherungsleistungen und der abgezinste Wert der zu erwartenden Beiträge einer Risikoklasse in etwa gleich sind. Untersucht wird, ob sich dieses Kalkulationsprinzip nicht auch partiell in der GKV praktizieren läßt, indem z. B. eine Differenzierung zwischen Grund- und Zusatzleistungen vorgenommen wird, wobei letztere durch aktuarisch kalkulierte Prämien finanziert werden.

Aus diesen fundamental anderen Gestaltungsprinzipien, den in der PKV dominierenden differenzierten Formen der Selbstbeteiligung und dem für die PKV geltenden Kostenerstattungsprinzip lassen sich nun Erfahrungswerte ableiten, die in der gesundheitsökonomischen Analyse und in der Begründung möglicher Reformalternativen auch für das GKV-System von erheblicher Bedeutung sind. So greifen Untersuchungen über die mutmaßlichen Auswirkungen von Wahltarifen auch auf PKV-Daten zurück. Da Experimenten im Bereich der sozialen Sicherung enge Grenzen gesetzt sind, kann das System der PKV für die empirische gesundheitsökonomische Analyse partiell als funktionales Äquivalent dienen.

Ordnungspolitik und Steuerung

Die Begriffe Ordnungspolitik und Steuerung haben keine einheitliche Bedeutung; es gibt nur (relativ) übereinstimmende Konventionen. Die ordnungspolitische Diskussion bezieht sich dabei primär auf die Auseinandersetzung um die grundsätzlich möglichen Alternativen, um die „staatliche Planung der Formen", um das Setzen institutioneller Rahmenbedingungen. Steuerung bezieht sich dagegen primär auf die Ausgestaltung der Formen, die konkreten Instrumente und Mechanismen und deren Wirkungsweisen.

Bei allen theoretischen und politischen, d. h. auch wertgebundenen Differenzen über die Angemessenheit der alternativ möglichen ordnungspolitischen Prinzipien und den daraus folgenden Differenzen über die Angemessenheit einzelner Steuerungsinstrumente, gibt es doch weitgehend Grundkonsens bei Wissenschaftlern, Politikern und anderen Beteiligten im Gesundheitswesen über folgendes: Aus den Besonderheiten des Gutes Gesundheit und dem historisch gewachsenen System der sozialen Sicherung folgt, daß für kein einzelnes ordnungspolitisches Prinzip und den daraus abgeleiteten jeweiligen systemkonformen Steuerungsinstrumenten exklusive Geltung beansprucht werden kann. Auch der konsequente Anhänger marktökonomischer Prinzipien erkennt für bestimmte Bereiche die Notwendigkeit von Gruppenverhandlungen oder regulierenden Eingriffen an; und auch dezidierte Verfechter eines staatlichen Gesundheitsdienstes leugnen die partiellen Vorteile wettbewerblicher Steuerung nicht. Neben aller Konkurrenz der Systeme gibt es deshalb einen Grundkonsens bezüglich Komplementarität. Wer z. B. die Selbstbeteiligung für ein wirksames Instrument marktökonomischer Nachfragesteuerung hält, wird – abgeleitet aus dem Solidarprinzip oder allgemeinen politischen Wertvorstellungen – immer auch auf die Notwendigkeit flankierender (regulativer) Eingriffe zugunsten chronisch kranker und älterer Menschen hinweisen; wer die Koordination von Leistungs- und Geldströmen im Gesundheitswesen v. a. durch Gruppenverhandlungen auf Verbandsebene steuern will, muß Mechanismen einbauen, die sichern, daß die errichten Ergebnisse nicht zu Lasten der einzelnen Versicherten ausfallen.

Unter ordnungs- und steuerungspolitischen Gesichtspunkten deutlich Priorität haben in den letzten Jahren jene Überlegungen, die auf die Vorteile eines marktökonomischen Konzepts setzen. Analysiert werden die möglichen Vorteile der Organisationsformen des Wettbewerbs und des Preismechanismus; als normative Grundorientierung werden die Eigenverantwortung betont und als primäres Steuerungsziel die Effizienzsteigerung unter allokativen Gesichtspunkten herausgestellt. „Mehr Markt" und „mehr Wettbewerb" heißen die zu Schlagwörtern geronnenen Forderungen. Daß sich die Bemühungen der Ökonomen insbesondere auf diese Alternative konzentrieren, dürfte v. a. auf folgende Gründe zurückzuführen sein: Auf die empirische Beweiskraft hinsichtlich der Leistungsfähigkeit in anderen Wirtschaftsbereichen; auf das vermeintliche oder tatsächliche Versagen der bisher vorherrschenden regulativen Muster; und auf das Motiv, Innovationen in einen Sektor einzubringen, für den die Wirkungsfähigkeit dieses Instrumentariums noch nicht bestätigt oder verworfen werden kann.

Im Rahmen dieser Diskussion von besonderer Bedeutung ist die Frage der Selbstbeteiligung. Mehr als nur ein Instrument marktökonomischer oder versicherungstechnischer Steuerung ist die Selbstbeteiligung zum Symbol in der Auseinandersetzung um Steuerungsprinzipien überhaupt geworden. Wer marktökonomische Instrumente favorisiert, nimmt auch an dieser Diskussion teil, wer die Marktökonomie ablehnt, wird immer auch auf die Problematik der Selbstbeteiligung verweisen. Die insbesondere unter Wirtschaftswissenschaftlern überaus populäre Forderung nach mehr Marktsteuerung hat nun dazu geführt, gesundheitsökonomie mit Marktökonomie gleichzusetzen. Dieser Eindruck ist unrichtig. Denn grundsätzlich gilt, daß auch weiterhin das Gesundheitswesen in der Bundesrepublik Deutschland weitgehend als ein regulierter Markt zu bezeichnen ist, in dem wettbewerbsorientierte Steuerungsinstrumente keine Priorität haben. Dies zeigen auch die bundesrepublikanischen Besonderheiten in der ordnungs- und steuerungspolitischen Diskussion, nämlich die Funktionen der „Konzertierten Aktion im Gesundheitswesen" und die Selbstverwaltung als politisch-organisatorisches Prinzip.

Die gemeinsame Selbstverwaltung zwischen der Gesetzlichen Krankenversicherung und den Kassen(zahn)ärztlichen Vereinigungen ist ein institutionell verankerter Koordinationsmechanismus, der sich v. a. auf die ambulante Versorgung bezieht, mit großen Einschränkungen auf den stationären Sektor und kaum auf die Arzneimittelversorgung. Die Steuerungswirkungen dieses ordnungspolitischen Prinzips werden insbesondere vor dem Hintergrund der vermuteten bzw. behaupteten Defizite regulativer Steuerungsmodelle einerseits („Staatsversagen") und wettbewerblicher Steuerungsmodelle andererseits („Marktversagen") diskutiert.

Ökonomische Evaluierung von Gesundheitsleistungen

Die Evaluierung von Gesundheitsleistungen zielt zunächst ganz allgemein darauf ab zu bestimmen, daß irgendwer (oder irgendwas) in einem bestimmten Maß durch eine bestimmte Leistung „verbessert" wird. Die ökonomische Evaluierung von Gesundheitsleistungen versucht darüber hinaus, das Verhältnis von Maßnahmen zu Zustandsveränderungen in berechenbaren Einheiten abzubilden. Das Ideal bestände in einer in Geldeinheiten erfaßten und dadurch objektivierbaren Ergebnisbeurteilung.

Das erste Problem besteht nun darin, die Voraussetzungen zu schaffen, um die gemeinten Relationen evaluieren zu können. Trotz der inhärenten Wertproblematik gibt es eine Reihe von theoretischen, methodischen und empirischen Ansätzen, die die unterschiedlich möglichen Ergebnisdimensionen in intersubjektiv einsetzbare Meßeinheiten umsetzen (z. B. Gesundheitszustand, Gesundheitsindikatoren). Die verschiedenen Ansätze bzw. Versuche, Gesundheit zu messen, Indikatoren zu bilden oder hochaggregierte Versorgungsniveaus zu ermitteln, unterscheiden sich v. a. hinsichtlich der Komplexität der zu ermittelnden Meßeinheiten. Sie reichen von der einfachen, binären Schematisierung (Fühlen Sie sich gesund? Ja oder nein?) bis zu hochkomplexen gruppenspezifischen Versorgungsniveaus.

Im Vordergrund der ökonomischen Evaluierung von Gesundheitsleistungen stehen die Kosten-Nutzen- bzw. Kosten-Wirksamkeits-Analysen. Mit diesem Instrumentarium wurde ein früher Zugang gesucht, die ökonomische Dimension in die Analyse des Gesundheitswesens einzubringen. Die Grundidee dieser Ansätze beruht auf der Annahme, daß Indikatoren für Nutzen und Kosten die Zahlungsbereitschaft der Konsumenten bei vollständigen Märkten darstellen. Da in vielen Bereichen das Marktgeschehen eingeschränkt ist, bedarf es einer Simulation zur Ermittlung der Nutzen und Kosten, um den gesellschaftlichen Wert öffentlicher Investitionen zu ermitteln und hierdurch zu einer Rationalisierung der administrierten Allokation beizutragen.

Die theoretische und methodische Ausdifferenzierung und die immer breitere Anwendungspalette mit je spezifischen Anforderungen hat auch zu einer terminologischen Differenzierung geführt. Allen verschiedenen Varianten gemeinsam ist letztlich nur die Evaluierung einer Input-Output-Relation. Dennoch lassen sich 2 Grundmuster unterscheiden, auf die sich die meisten Variationen zurückführen lassen: Kosten-Nutzen-Analysen (KNA) und Kosten-Wirksamkeits-Analysen (KWA). Beide unterscheiden sich grundsätzlich in der Erfassung des Outputs. Während in der KNA versucht wird, alle Maßnahmenkonsequenzen zu monetarisieren (d. h. in Geldeinheiten auszudrücken), werden in der KWA nur die unmittelbar in Geldeinheiten erfaßbaren Größen monetär ausgewiesen und andere Auswirkungen im Hinblick auf definierte Ziele bestimmten Bewertungsverfahren unterzogen.

Unmittelbar einsichtig ist, daß sich nicht nur theoretische und methodische Probleme, sondern v. a. die Wertediskussion auf die Frage konzentriert, ob und in welcher Form oder in welchem Ausmaß sich die Wirkungen gesundheitsbezogener Maßnahmen überhaupt in Geldeinheiten erfassen lassen. Nun kann zwar auch die Fundamentalkritik („das Leben ist unbezahlbar") nicht die grundlegende Tatsache ignorieren, daß jede Verwendungsentscheidung bei knappen Mitteln immer den Ausschluß alternativer Zwecke zur Folge hat und sich deshalb auch immer einer vergleichenden Evaluierung stellen muß. Allerdings stehen den Versuchen, die Wirkungen von Gesundheitsleistungen zu monetarisieren, nicht nur ethisch-moralische Grenzen, sondern v. a. methodische Probleme entgegen. Zwar besteht relativ breiter Konsens darüber, die durch Gesundheitsleistungen erzielte Verlängerung der Lebenszeit mit Hilfe der Human-Kapital-Methode auch in monetären Größen auszuweisen; problematisch bleibt jedoch v. a. der Komplex der „intangiblen Erträge", für die sich zunehmend der Begriff Lebensqualität durchsetzt.

Wenn man nun davon ausgeht, daß die (ökonomische) Evaluierung vom singulären und begrenzten Gesundheitsprojekt bis zur gesamtstaatlichen Gesundheitspolitik, vom einzelnen Medikament bis zur pharmazeutischen Industrie insgesamt, vom einzelnen medizinisch-technischen Gerät bis zum medizinisch-technischen Fortschritt überhaupt, von der therapeutischen Einzelmaßnahme bis zum gesamten Gesundheitswesen reicht, dann wird das potentielle Anwendungsgebiet deutlich. Berücksichtigt man zudem die Spannbreiten monetarisierbarer und nichtmonetarisierbarer Wirkungen, dann zeigt sich die mögliche Komplexität.

Wenngleich es breiten Konsens über die Notwendigkeit des Kosten-Nutzen-Denkens im Entscheidungshandeln in bezug auf die Mittelverwendung im Gesundheitswesen gibt, so zeigt sich doch auch erhebliche Skepsis im Hinblick auf die Bedeutung entsprechender Untersuchungen als wirklich relevanter Entscheidungshilfen. Sie reicht von der Feststellung, daß die Anwendung dieses Instrumentariums auf das Gesundheitswesen noch in den Anfängen stecke und es deshalb verfeinerter Methoden insbesondere auch durch Fortschritte in der medizinischen Evaluierung bedürfe, bis zur Vermutung, daß mehr und verfeinerte Kosten-Nutzen-Analysen nur der Arbeitsbeschaffung für Ökonomen dienten. Es bleibt deshalb eine gewisse Spannung zwischen der Beschwörung von Effektivitäts- und Effizienzdenken einerseits und dem praktikablen Einsatz entsprechender Instrumente andererseits. Schwer abschätzbar bleibt deshalb auch, welcher Stellenwert in Zukunft diesen Ansätzen zukommen wird.

Perspektiven der Gesundheitsökonomie

Da sich die Gesundheitsökonomie als Subdisziplin der Wirtschaftswissenschaften etabliert hat, wird im Hinblick auf die Theoriebildung zu prüfen sein, wieweit diese neue sektoral angewandte Ökonomie zur Verfeinerung und Weiterentwicklung der allgemeinen ökonomischen Methoden beiträgt. Die empirische Ausrichtung wird wesentlich dadurch bestimmt werden, welche Konsequenzen oder Defizite nach Verabschiedung des Gesundheitsreformgesetzes zu erwarten sind bzw. noch bestehen, welche Entwicklungen erkennbar sind, die weiteren Kostendruck auf das Gesundheitswesen ausüben werden und welchen Beitrag gesundheitsökonomische Analysen für die politisch-praktische Umsetzung leisten können.

Unabhängig davon, wie man im einzelnen die Maßnahmen des Gesetzes zur Strukturreform im Gesundheitswesen (Gesundheitsreformgesetz – GRG – vom 20.12.1988) auch beurteilen mag, es muß bezweifelt werden, daß nach diesem Vorhaben kein Handlungsbedarf mehr für weitere Reformmaßnahmen besteht. Trotz oder gerade wegen der gesetzlichen Verankerung des Bemühens um Beitragssatzstabilität wird der Problemdruck bleiben. Verschärft hat sich die Aufmerksamkeit für die weiterhin steigenden Beitragsunterschiede. Und es gehört wohl zu den latenten Folgen des GRG, daß beispielsweise durch Neugründungen von Betriebskrankenkassen – die traditionell vergleichsweise gute Risiken bündeln – nicht nur Arbeitnehmer, sondern auch Arbeitgeber die Vorteile niedriger Beitragssätze nutzen wollen. Das zunehmende Auseinanderdriften der Beitragssätze verschärft die bereits bestehenden Verteilungsprobleme, untergräbt die mit dem Solidaritätsprinzip verbundenen distributiven Absichten und gefährdet somit die Akzeptanz der Grundlagen der sozialen Krankenversicherung. Die geplante Neuorganisation der GKV wird deshalb zu erheblichen Veränderungen im Finanzierungssystem führen müssen.

Auch sind Entwicklungen absehbar, von denen weiterhin ein Druck auf die Kosten im Gesundheitswesen ausgehen werden. Relativ breiter Konsens besteht darüber, daß v. a. 3 Gründe maßgebend sind: Die soziodemographischen Veränderungen der Bevölkerungsstruktur, insbesondere der Anstieg der Rentnerquote; der medizinisch-technische Fortschritt, der im Gesundheitswesen eher kostensteigernd als kostensenkend wirkt; und das Überangebot an Leistungserbringern, das sich in Schlagworten wie Bettenberg und Ärzteschwemme manifestiert. Die möglichen Konsequenzen dieser Entwicklungen und deren effiziente Steuerung sind empirische Herausforderungen an die gesundheitsökonomische Forschung.

Welchen Beitrag nun die Gesundheitsökonomie für die Gestaltung des Gesundheitswesens geleistet hat, leisten kann oder leisten muß, bedürfte selbst einer eingehenden Prüfung. Wer etwa die zahlreichen Entwürfe etablierter Gesundheitsökonomen im Verlauf der Diskussion um die Strukturreform des Gesundheitswesens mit dem Gesundheitsreformgesetz selbst vergleicht, mag bezweifeln, daß entscheidende Impulse aufgenommen wurden. Wer andererseits die Argumentationsstruktur dieser Debatte analysiert, wird feststellen können, daß ökonomische Begründungen im Zentrum auch dieser Reform standen, und es wird die Kritik verständlich, daß ökonomischen Überlegungen ein unzulässiger Primat in Fragen der Gestaltung des Gesundheitswesens eingeräumt werde. Solange jedoch die Ressourcen auch für das System der Gesundheitssicherung und Krankheitsbewältigung knapp sind, alternative Verwendungen ein politisches Entscheidungsproblem bleiben und die individuellen Bedürfnisse und Ansprüche unterschiedlich sind, wird das Gesundheitswesen ein Thema auch der ökonomischen Analyse bleiben. Deren Beitrag aber wird aufgrund der Besonderheiten dieses Bereichs weniger in der Anweisung normativer Handlungsentwürfe als in der Beschreibung, Erklärung und Prognose liegen, im Hinweis auf Ineffizienzen und dem Aufzeigen alternativer Entscheidungsmöglichkeiten.

Literatur

Andersen HH, Schulenburg J-M Graf von der (1987) Kommentierte Bibliographie zur Gesundheitsökonomie. Deutschsprachige Publikationen. edition sigma, Berlin
Bundesverband der Pharmazeutischen Industrie e V.: Basisdaten des Gesundheitswesens, BPI, Frankfurt (erscheint jährlich)
Fuchs VR (1983) How we live. An Economic Perspective on Americans from Birth to Death. Cambridge u. London: Harvard University Press
Gäfgen G (Hrsg) (1986) Ökonomie des Gesundheitswesens. Duncker & Humblot, Berlin
Klarman HE (1965) The Economics of Health. Columbia University Press, New York u. London
Robert-Bosch-Stiftung (Hrsg) (1982ff.) Beiträge zur Gesundheitsökonomie Bleicher, Gerlingen
Sachverständigenrat für die Konzertierte Aktion im Gesundheitswesen (1987, 1988, 1989) Jahresgutachten. Nomos, Baden-Baden

Langfristige Finanzierbarkeit
der Gesetzlichen Krankenversicherung *

K.-D. Henke

Zum zukünftigen Finanzbedarf

Es ist unstrittig, daß es Finanzierungsprobleme in der Gesetzlichen Krankenvercherung (GKV) gibt. Angesichts der zunehmenden Versorgungsdichte (Betten,
Ärzte, Arzneimittel, Heil- und Hilfsmittel), der prognostizierten demographischen Entwicklung der Bevölkerung und der medizinisch-technischen Entwicklung erscheint die Finanzierbarkeit der Gesundheitsversorgung als gefährdet. Allerdings ergibt sich die Gefährdung der Finanzierbarkeit der GKV nicht allein
durch die genannten 3 Faktoren. Vielmehr treten die insbesondere vom Sachleistungsprinzip ausgehenden Anreize für Anbieter und Nachfrager von Gesundheitsleistungen hinzu, die ihrerseits wiederum nicht ohne Verbindung zur Einzelleistungshonorierung, zur derzeitigen Krankenhausfinanzierung und der gewachsenen Kassenartenstruktur gesehen werden können. Alle diese Einflüsse stehen schließlich im Zusammenhang mit dem in der Reichsversicherungsordnung
abgesicherten Anspruch auf eine Gesundheitsversorgung nach den Regeln der
ärztlichen Kunst. Die Interpretation dieser Regeln angesichts der zunehmenden
Ärztezahl kann zu weiteren angebotsseitig induzierten Effekten kommen, die in
der Epidemiologie und Sozialmedizin mit dem Begriff der Arztzahlmorbidität
bezeichnet werden. Die Verwobenheit der aufgezeigten Wirkungen macht es sehr
schwer, einzelne Bestimmungsfaktoren der Ausgabenentwicklung in ihrer quantitativen Bedeutung zu isolieren.[1]

Aus Status-quo-Prognosen geht hervor, daß es zu erheblichen Beitragssatzsteigerungen kommt bzw. bei gewünschter Beitragssatzstabilität erhebliche Leistungseinschränkungen erforderlich sind, wenn nicht eine Reform der GKV zu
einer Situation führt, die allen Beteiligten akzeptabel erscheint.

Bei einer Diskussion des zukünftigen Finanzbedarfs sollte auch Klarheit über
den Finanzierungsgegenstand bestehen, d. h., es muß gefragt werden, was mit
den Ausgaben im Gesundheitswesen „gekauft" werden soll. Handelt es sich um
einen höheren Gesundheitsstand der Bevölkerung, aufgeschlüsselt nach Bevölkerungsgruppen, Krankheitsarten oder Regionen? Geht es um eine noch bessere Infrastrukturqualität im Bereich der ambulanten oder stationären Versorgung?
Soll eine höhere Versorgungsdichte bei gleich hohen Einkommen der Leistungs-

---

* Erstmals veröffentlicht in: Zimmermann H (Hrsg) (1988) Die Zukunft der Staatsfinanzierung.
Marburger Forum Philippinum. Wissenschaftliche Verlagsgesellschaft, Stuttgart, S. 143–159.
[1] Siehe zu den Bestimmungsgründen der zukünftigen Risikovorsorge Henke u. Adam 1987.

anbieter fixiert werden, z. B. deshalb, weil von interessierter Seite die Auffassung vertreten wird, der Staat habe eine Fürsorgepflicht für die ausgebildeten bzw. in Ausbildung befindlichen Ärzte? Wird eine höhere Inanspruchnahme der Gesundheitsleistungen gewünscht in genereller Form oder bezogen auf den präventiven Bereich, auf Notfälle, am Wochenende? Oder soll die „Wachstumsbranche" Gesundheitswesen weiter finanziell unterstützt werden, weil – wie gezeigt werden kann – die neuen Arbeitsplätze, die in der Vergangenheit geschaffen worden sind, in erster Linie dem Gesundheitswesen zuzuordnen sind? Schließlich kann man fragen, ob mit den Ausgaben der GKV ein höheres Humankapital bezahlt wird, das im Rahmen einer längerfristigen Betrachtung durchaus wachstumspolitische Bedeutung haben kann. Diese Auflistung macht deutlich, daß Klarheit über den Finanzierungsgegenstand in der Diskussion über die Finanzierbarkeit der GKV erforderlich ist. Aus gesundheitsökonomischer Sicht läßt sich die Forderung erheben, daß die Qualität und Wirtschaftlichkeit der Gesundheitsversorgung im Vordergrund stehen sollte. Abzulehnen sind sicherlich Umsatzgarantien für bestimmte Anbietergruppen; aus der Fürsorgepflicht des Staates läßt sich keine finanzielle Alimentation bestimmter Berufsgruppen ableiten.

Schließlich gehört zu einer Diskussion über den zukünftigen Finanzbedarf auch ein Blick auf die derzeitige Finanzlage der GKV. Aus Tabelle 1 läßt sich die aktuelle Finanzentwicklung in der GKV, gemessen an den Veränderungen je Mitglied einschließlich Rentner gegenüber dem entsprechenden Vorjahreszeitraum, für die Leistungsausgaben insgesamt und für die verschiedenen Bereiche der Leistungsausgaben entnehmen. Dort ist zu ersehen, daß insbesondere Anfang der 70er Jahre eine „Kostenexplosion" im Gesundheitswesen vorlag, während in den darauffolgenden Jahren die Zuwachsraten deutlich niedriger ausgefallen sind. Finanziert werden diese Ausgaben durch die Sozialabgaben, wobei der Grundlohn als Beitragsbemessungsgrundlage dient. In diesem Zusammenhang läßt sich der Tabelle entnehmen, daß die Zuwachsraten der Grundlohnsumme je Mitglied ohne Rentner im Vergleich zur Bruttolohn- und -gehaltssumme je beschäftigtem Arbeitnehmer im Zeitablauf Schwankungen unterliegen. Für die Finanzierbarkeit der GKV ist es von besonderem Interesse, daß in den Jahren 1986 und 1987 die Zuwachsraten der Bruttolohn- und -gehaltssumme höher ausfallen als die der Grundlohnsumme, aus der die GKV finanziert wird. Ob diese Entwicklung zu einer „Erosion der Bemessungsgrundlage" führen wird, bedarf einer sorgfältigen Beobachtung.

Der Beitragssatz ergibt sich als Quotient zwischen Leistungsausgaben und Grundlohnsumme; wie Tabelle 1 zu entnehmen ist, liegt er seit 1986 über 12%, wobei es sich in der Tabelle um den durchschnittlichen Beitragssatz handelt, der nicht nur zwischen den verschiedenen Krankenkassenarten, sondern auch innerhalb einzelner Krankenkassen schwankt.[2]

Auf die Frage, ob der durchschnittliche Beitragssatz in der GKV zu hoch oder zu niedrig ist, läßt sich aus ökonomischer Sicht keine Antwort geben. So ist es vorstellbar, daß die Bevölkerung einen sehr viel höheren Prozentsatz zu zahlen bereit wäre, andererseits ist denkbar, daß mit einem niedrigeren Beitragssatz nicht zwangsläufig eine schlechtere Gesundheitsversorgung einhergehen muß. In-

---

[2] Siehe hierzu im einzelnen Henke K-D 1983 sowie die dort genannte Literatur.

Tabelle 1. Aktuelle Finanzentwicklung in der Gesetzlichen Krankenversicherung, Veränderungen je Mitglied einschließlich Rentner gegenüber dem entsprechenden Vorjahreszeitraum in %. (Arbeits- und Sozialstatistik BMA, bis 1986 Vordruck KJ 1/ab 1987 Schnellmeldung nach KV 45 – vorläufige Werte)

	1970–1975[a]	1975–1980[b]	1980	1981	1982	1983	1984	1985	1986	1987
1) Leistungsausgaben insgesamt	17,4	6,9 (6,6)[c]	9,3 (8,5)[c]	6,2	0,2	3,5	7,3	4,3	4,2	2,9
davon										
– ärztliche Behandlung	13,5	5,2	7,0	6,3	2,3	5,1	5,9	3,3	2,6	3,2
– zahnärztliche Behandlung	17,2	4,8	4,0	6,5	2,0	3,5	3,9	0,8	6,9	7,1
– Zahnersatz	35,8	10,7	11,8	9,2	−14,1	− 4,6	9,5	3,9	−10,6	−17,7
– Arzneien aus Apotheken	14,0	6,0	8,8	7,3	0,7	4,9	7,0	6,2	5,5	4,5
– Heil- und Hilfsmittel	28,5	12,3	10,3	6,9	− 4,6	3,8	15,2	6,8	10,2	7,5
– stationäre Behandlung	21,7	6,6	7,8	6,2	8,0	4,7	6,6	4,9	6,3	4,5
– Krankengeld (ohne Rentner)	12,4	6,3	9,8	− 4,3	− 8,6	1,8	7,4	0,6	7,0	7,0
2) Grundlohn je Mitglied ohne Rentner[b]	10,9	6,2[d]	5,4	5,0	4,4	3,8	4,5	3,0	3,1	2,0
Bruttolohn- und Gehaltssumme je beschäftigten Arbeitnehmer	10,2	6,2	6,6	4,9	4,1	3,9[e]	3,0[e]	2,8[e]	3,8[e]	3,3[e]
3) Allgemeiner Beitragssatz in % des Grundlohns	1970: 8,2 1975: 10,43	1975: 10,43 1980: 11,38	11,38	11,79	12,00	11,83	11,44	11,80	12,20	12,53

[a] Durchschnittliche jährliche Veränderung.

[b] In den Jahren 1976–1978 errechnet nach der Formel *Beitragseinnahmen in der allgemeinen Krankenversicherung allgemeiner Beitragssatz · 100*, im Jahre 1979 ist erstmals ein Vergleich mit der seit 1978 ermittelten Grundlohnsumme möglich [§ 2 Abs. 1 der Verordnung über das Verfahren zum Ausgleich der Leistungsaufwendung in der Krankenversicherung der Rentner (KVdR-Ausgleichsverordnung) vom 20. 12. 1978].

[c] Werte in Klammern ohne Mutterschaftsurlaubsgeld.

[d] Wegen der Umstellung in der Ermittlung der Grundlöhne ab 1978 kann ein Durchschnittswert für den 5-Jahres-Zeitraum 1975–1980 nicht angegeben werden. Untersuchungen haben jedoch ergeben, daß im Durchschnitt mehrerer Jahre von einer im Trend übereinstimmenden Entwicklung sowohl des Grundlohns als auch der Bruttolohn- und Gehaltssumme (BLGS) ausgegangen werden kann. Die Steigerungsrate der BLGS für die Jahre 1975–1980 betrug durchschnittlich 6,2% pro Jahr.

[e] Statistisches Bundesamt: Stand Januar 1987.

soweit führt die politische Forderung nach Beitragssatzstabilität zu einer Festschreibung der Ausgaben auf einem historisch zufälligen Niveau.

Die Finanzierungsformen

Grundsätzliche Formen der finanziellen Absicherung des Krankheitsrisikos

Bevor die einzelnen Finanzierungsalternativen der GKV untersucht werden sollen, ist es zweckmäßig, sich Klarheit über die grundsätzliche Form der finanziellen Absicherung des Krankheitsrisikos zu verschaffen. Diese Formen lassen sich anhand der Gestaltungsprinzipien und Finanzierungsformen der Daseinsvorsorge in allgemeiner Form entnehmen (Abb. 1). Aus Abb. 1 werden die ordnungspolitischen Alternativen deutlich, von denen – je nach Ausgestaltung – unterschiedliche allokative und distributive Wirkungen ausgehen. In der GKV hat man sich vor über hundert Jahren gegen den reinen versicherungstechnischen Risikoausgleich ausgesprochen, hat also nicht das versicherungstechnische Äquivalenzprinzip zugrunde gelegt, sondern hat es von Anfang an um Solidar- und Sozialziele ergänzt. Die GKV ist – folgt man dem Schema – einerseits durch das Versi-

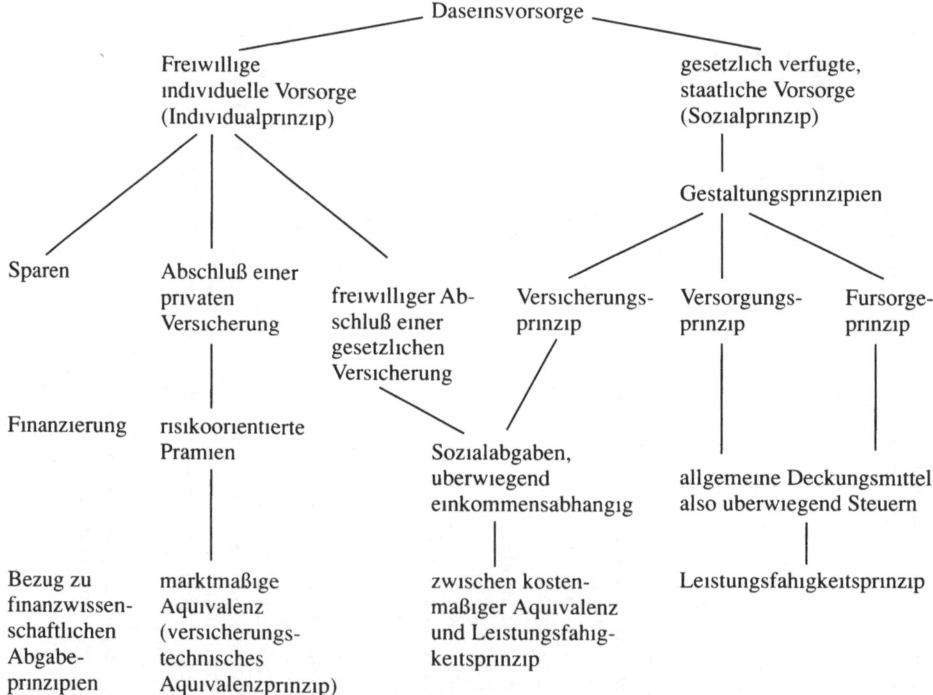

Abb. 1. Gestaltungsprinzipien und Finanzierungsformen der Daseinsvorsorge. [Mod. nach Kath D (1981)]

cherungsprinzip im Rahmen der gesetzlich verfügten staatlichen Vorsorge, zum anderen aber auch durch den freiwilligen Abschluß und damit durch die individuelle Vorsorge gekennzeichnet. Unabhängig davon, ob eine gesetzliche oder freiwillige Mitgliedschaft in der GKV zugrunde liegt, kommt es durch die Konstruktionsprinzipien zu einem Solidarausgleich, der sich aus folgenden Elementen ergibt: partieller Kassenzwang für einen großen Teil der Versicherten, beitragsfreie Mitversicherung der Familienangehörigen, beitragsunabhängiger Anspruch auf Gesundheitsleistungen, einkommensunabhängige proportionale Beiträge bis zur Beitragsbemessungsgrenze mit Arbeitgeberanteil für die Arbeitnehmer. Diese Elemente sind es, die den Solidarausgleich im Vergleich zum versicherungstechnischen Äquivalenzprinzip ausmachen. Aus diesem Solidarausgleich ergeben sich die vielfältigen Verteilungswirkungen in der GKV.[3]

Hinsichtlich einer Reform der GKV bzw. einer Weiterentwicklung des Solidarausgleichs ist der Bezug zu den anderen Formen der Daseinsvorsorge (s. Abb. 1) erforderlich. So ist zu fragen, in welche Richtung das System entwickelt werden soll: stärker zu einer am Risiko orientierten Prämienfinanzierung oder mehr in Richtung einer Finanzierung über Steuern bzw. allgemeine Deckungsmittel. Es geht also um ein Austarieren zwischen der Anwendung des Sozialprinzips und des Individualprinzips. In jedem Fall ist es wichtig, daß man den Solidarausgleich in qualitativer und quantitativer Hinsicht überdenkt, wenn anschließend über Finanzierungsmöglichkeiten gesprochen wird und darüber, welche alternativen Finanzierungsformen zur Verfügung stehen. Jede Veränderung in der Finanzierung hat Konsequenzen für den Solidarausgleich und damit für einen politisch äußerst sensiblen Bereich der Daseinsvorsorge.

Finanzierungsformen der GKV auf lange Sicht

Bei der Finanzierung der gesetzlichen Krankenversicherung handelt es sich um einen vielschichtigen Vorgang. Im folgenden steht die Mittelaufbringung durch die Gesetzlichen Krankenkassen im Vordergrund, d. h., die spezifischen Formen der Finanzierung der Leistungserbringer durch die Kassenarzthonorierung und im Rahmen der Krankenhausfinanzierung werden nicht untersucht. Diese Einschränkung ist im Hinblick auf die von der Finanzierung der Leistungserbringer ausgehenden Anreize nicht unbedeutend. Insbesondere die derzeitige Einzelleistungshonorierung und die duale Finanzierung der Krankenhausleistungen bringen unerwünschte Wirkungen mit sich.[4] Insoweit ist die Finanzierung der GKV im Rahmen der primären Mittelaufbringung nur die erste Stufe einer vielschichtigen Finanzierungsverflechtung.[5]

Ausgeklammert wird mit der Betrachtung der Mittelaufbringung durch die Krankenkassen weiterhin die politisch derzeit im Vordergrund stehende Mobili-

---

[3] Siehe hierzu im einzelnen Sachverständigenrat für die Konzertierte Aktion im Gesundheitswesen 1987, S. 73ff., sowie Behrens 1987

[4] Siehe zu den Honorierungsformen Schulenburg 1981, und zur Krankenhausfinanzierung: Bundesminister für Arbeit und Sozialordnung 1983.

[5] Siehe zur Ausgaben- und Einnahmenverflechtung Statistisches Bundesamt 1987.

sierung von Wirtschaftlichkeitsreserven im Gesundheitswesen. Viele Fachleute sehen in dieser Finanzierungsvariante kurz- und mittelfristig den erfolgversprechendsten Weg. Diese ausgabenseitige Finanzierungsstrategie führt einerseits zur Leistungsausgrenzung, andererseits u. U. aber auch zu einer wirtschaftlicheren Erstellung und veränderten Preisbildung von Gesundheitsleistungen. In diesem Bereich fehlt es an geeigneten Mechanismen und Anreizen, die quasi automatisch zu einer Umstrukturierung der Gesundheitsausgaben im Sinne einer bedarfsgerechten und kostengünstigen Versorgung führen. In dem Maß, wie die Beitragssatzstabilität als politisches Ziel vorgegeben wird, gewinnt die Mobilisierung von Wirtschaftlichkeitsreserven in den verschiedenen Leistungsbereichen der GKV eine besondere Bedeutung.[6]

Nach diesen Vorbemerkungen ist es möglich, die verschiedenen langfristigen und einnahmeseitigen Finanzierungsformen der GKV zu erläutern. Anhand der folgenden Übersicht über die langfristigen Finanzierungsformen der GKV lassen sich Finanzierungsformen danach trennen, ob die derzeitige lohnbezogene Beitragsfinanzierung beibehalten werden soll oder nicht. Im einzelnen lassen sich Sozialabgaben, Erstattungen und Zuweisungen, etwaige Einnahmen aus einer verhaltenslenkenden Beitrags- und Steuerpolitik sowie die verschiedenen Varianten der Selbstbeteiligung als Finanzierungsinstrumente ansehen. Ohne Anspruch auf die Vollständigkeit bei der Zusammenstellung der Finanzierungsformen und ohne eine gleichgewichtige Behandlung aller in der Abb. 2 genannten Finanzierungsformen zu beanspruchen, sei im folgenden auf einige Finanzierungsmöglichkeiten eingegangen.

Bei der Erhöhung der Versicherungspflichtgrenze und der Beitragsbemessungsgrenze handelt es sich um die sensible Frage einer zweckmäßigen Abgrenzung zwischen gesetzlicher und privater Krankenversicherung (PKV). Es geht auch um die Neubestimmung des versicherungspflichtigen und versicherungsberechtigten Personenkreises. Diese Fragen kann man nicht diskutieren, ohne sie in den Zusammenhang mit der Kassenartenstruktur der GKV zu bringen. Hier fehlt es m. E. an klaren, ordnungspolitischen Zielvorstellungen. Im gegenwärtigen System können angemessene Beitragssätze nur garantiert werden, wenn die Abwanderung der guten Risiken zur PKV bei gleichzeitiger freiwilliger Versicherung der schlechten Risiken in der GKV in Grenzen gehalten wird. Hinzu kommt das Problem der Alterslast, das sich in der PKV und in der GKV schon deswegen ganz unterschiedlich stellt, weil die Systeme unterschiedliche Finanzierungsformen aufweisen. Wenn ich einmal vom Rentnerfinanzausgleich absehe, dann schlägt die Alterslast im Rahmen der Umlagefinanzierung in der GKV voll auf die beitragszahlenden Versicherten durch, während sie im Finanzierungsverfahren der PKV durch die Alterungsrückstellungen über den Lebenszyklus partiell geglättet wird.

Zu den Weiterentwicklungsmöglichkeiten in diesem Zusammenhang zählt auch der Vorschlag einer Stärkung der solidarischen Finanzierung der GKV.

---

[6] Siehe hierzu im einzelnen die Jahresgutachten 1987 und 1988 des Sachverständigenrates für die Konzertierte Aktion im Gesundheitswesen. Dort werden detailliert die Leistungsbereiche ambulant-ärztliche und zahnärztliche Versorgung, stationäre Versorgung, Heil- und Hilfsmittel und Arzneimittel analysiert.

I   Sozialabgaben: Beitragssätze, Versicherungspflicht, Beitragsbemessungsgrenze
und Beitragsbemessungsgrundlage in der GKV
   1) Erhöhung der Beitragssätze;
   2) Erweiterung der Versicherungspflicht
      a) Ausdehnung der Versicherungspflicht/Zahl der Mitglieder,
      b) Erhöhung der Versicherungspflichtgrenze,
      c) Abschaffung/Einschränkung beitragsfreier Mitversicherung;
   3) Anhebung der Beitragsbemessungsgrenze;
   4) Verhältnis von Arbeitgeberbeitrag zu Arbeitnehmerbeitrag
      a) Umwandlung der Arbeitgeberanteile in höhere Löhne: volle Zahlung der
         Krankenversicherungsbeiträge durch den Versicherten,
      b) Erhöhung des Arbeitgeberanteils nach § 384 RVO;
   5) Verbreiterung der Beitragsbemessungsgrundlage
      a) Erweiterung des versicherungspflichtigen Bruttoarbeitsentgelts bzw. der
         versicherungspflichtigen Alterseinkünfte
         – weitere Einkunftsarten über das Lohneinkommen hinaus,
         – Familieneinkommen anstelle von Mitgliedseinkommen,
      b) Wertschöpfungsbezogene Arbeitgeberzahlungen.

II.   Erstattungen und Zuweisungen
   1) Erstattungen von GKV-Leistungen durch Gebietskörperschaften,
   2) Zuschüsse der Gebietskörperschaften,
   3) Überweisungen von anderen Sozialversicherungsträgern
      a) höhere Überweisungssätze,
      b) breitere Bemessungsgrundlage.

III.   Einnahmen aus einer verhaltenslenkenden Beitrags- und Steuerpolitik?

IV   Selbstbeteiligung (einschließlich Herausnahme von nicht notwendigen Leistungen
aus der Erstattungspflicht).

Abb. 2. Ausgewählte Handlungsparameter zur langfristigen Sicherstellung der Aufbringung des Finanzbedarfs in der GKV

Dieser Vorschlag sieht eine Anhebung der Versicherungspflichtgrenze vor. Zur Zeit haben Angestellte mit einem Gehalt oberhalb der Versicherungspflichtgrenze die Möglichkeit, ihre Krankenkasse zu wechseln, nicht aber die Arbeiter. Hier ist sicherlich Reformbedarf angezeigt. Die gegenwärtige Regelung führt dazu, daß sich Versicherte mit relativ schlechten Gesundheitsrisiken in der GKV freiwillig versichern oder dort bleiben und daß kinderreiche Versicherte dort ebenfalls ihren Krankenversicherungsschutz suchen, da der Familienlastenausgleich in der Gesetzlichen Krankenversicherung zu vergleichsweise günstigen Beiträgen führt. Bei Anhebung der Versicherungspflichtgrenze würde die Zahl der guten Risiken in der GKV tendenziell erhöht und die Finanzierung des Solidarausgleichs erleichtert werden. Diese Tendenz verstärkt sich, wenn gleichzeitig die Beitragsbemessungsgrenze erhöht würde. Diese Maßnahme würde die Regressionswirkungen, die derzeit aufgrund der Beitragsbemessungsgrenze bestehen, mindern.

Diesem Vorschlag entgegengesetzt ist die Forderung nach einer Senkung der Versicherungspflichtgrenze oder einer Erhöhung der Beitragsbemessungsgrenze ohne gleichzeitige Anhebung der Versicherungspflichtgrenze. Diese zweite Strategie würde die PKV im gegliederten Krankenversicherungssystem erheblich stärken. Die Gleichstellung von Arbeitern mit Angestellten hätte tendenziell einen gleichgerichteten Effekt. Seit 1969 wurden die sog. Friedensgrenzen akzeptiert, und daran scheint man bei den derzeitigen Reformüberlegungen auch nichts ändern zu wollen; sie werden als Konstante angesehen, die sich historisch ergeben hat.

Als eine zweite Finanzierung, die in der Praxis eine größere Bedeutung haben wird, möchte ich den Abbau von Leistungen im weitesten Sinn nennen. Ich denke, daß hier a priori schnell Konsens zu erzielen ist, wenn es darum geht, versicherungsfremde Leistungen abzubauen. Das Problem besteht jedoch darin, daß man klar definieren muß, was zum Fremdleistungskatalog der GKV zu zählen ist. Dann sind nichtversicherbare Risiken vor dem Hintergrund des versicherungstechnischen Äquivalenzprinzips von sozialpolitischen Leistungen zu trennen, die aus politischen Gründen zu dem Leistungskatalog einer sozialen Krankenversicherung zählen. Dementsprechend gibt es auch unterschiedliche Listen mit versicherungsfremden Leistungen, die von den verschiedensten Organisationen aufgestellt worden sind. Schwierig wird es m. E., wenn man diese Listen zur Kenntnis nimmt und sich dann fragt, wie die Finanzierung von auszugrenzenden, versicherungsfremden Leistungen ausfallen soll. Auf der einen Seite könnte man dann über Bundeszuschüsse finanzieren – nur braucht man hierzu einen Finanzminister, der die Finanzierung übernimmt – und auf der anderen Seite kann man über den privaten Konsum finanzieren, d. h. über eine Form der Selbstbeteiligung in Höhe von 100%. Nur diese 2 Möglichkeiten existieren, und ich finde, diese Listen aufzustellen, ohne gleichzeitig genau zu sagen, wie die Finanzierung erfolgen soll, ist unehrlich. Hinzu kommt, daß eine Ausgrenzung dieser versicherungsfremden Leistungen als Bundesaufgabe a priori nur eine Kostenverlagerung darstellt. Diese Ausgaben, die sich im Bundeshaushalt niederschlagen, müßten rein rechnerisch in der GKV zu Beitragssenkungen führen. Doch die Selbstverwaltung wird diese Erleichterung als Finanzierungspotential ansehen. Hier sehe ich die Gefahr, daß wir über Kostenverlagerungen sprechen – rechnerisch Beitragssenkungen –, obwohl wir aus der Vergangenheit wissen, daß Leistungsausgrenzungen bzw. Kostenerstattungen nicht notwendigerweise zur Kostendämpfung in der GKV beitragen. Ich denke in diesem Zusammenhang auch an Erfahrungen mit der Einführung der Lohnfortzahlung im Krankheitsfall.

Gelegentlich wird mit dem Abbau der versicherungsfremden Leistungen die Ausgliederung des Familienlastenausgleichs gefordert. Wenn sich auch die Kosten, die auf den Familienlastenausgleich zurückgehen, als Beitragssatzanteil rechnerisch bestimmen lassen – zwischen 2,5 und 3,0 Prozentpunkte –, dann muß man sich vor Augen führen, daß eine Herausnahme dieses Teils des Solidarausgleichs das Ende der einkommensbezogenen Finanzierung darstellt. Die Beitragsbemessung in ihrer derzeitigen Form würde sich in Richtung einer stärker risikoproportionalen Kalkulation entwickeln, und damit würde ein zentrales Element der GKV an Bedeutung verlieren.

Eine größere Bedeutung messe ich dem Ausschluß von Leistungen bei, die nicht zur medizinischen Versorgung im engeren Sinne zählen. Leistungen, die ganz aus dem Versicherungsschutz ausgeschlossen werden können, finden wir z. B. im Bereich des Zahnersatzes, der Physiotherapie, des Kuraufenthalts, der Hör- und Sehhilfen, im Bereich der Heil- und Hilfsmittel, der orthopädischen

Hilfsmittel sowie der Leistungen, die im Zusammenhang mit den naturgegebenen Begleiterscheinungen des Alters stehen. Als Beispiel möchte ich den Fall der nichtkrankheitsgebundenen Pflege anführen. Die konkrete Ausgrenzung solcher Leistungen wäre eine Aufgabe des Gesetzgebers, ist aber nach geltendem Recht vorrangig Aufgabe der Krankenkassen bzw. der gemeinsamen Selbstverwaltung. Sie ist z. T. den Bundesausschüssen übertragen. Ich denke hier z. B. an die Prothetikrichtlinien im zahnmedizinischen Bereich. Teilweise gibt es vertraglich vereinbarte Gremien, wie etwa den Untersuchungs- und Heilmethodenausschuß nach dem Bundesmanteltarifvertrag. Insbesondere die zuletzt genannte Möglichkeit wird nicht genügend genutzt: Der Konditionenwettbewerb der Krankenkassen steht der Anwendung dieser Möglichkeiten entgegen.

Als nächsten Punkt möchte ich kurz das kontrovers diskutierte Thema der Selbstbeteiligung ansprechen. Selbstbeteiligung ist ein politisches Reizwort geworden. Wenn wir über die Abgrenzung medizinisch nicht mehr notwendiger Leistungen sprechen, dann stehen diesem Vorschlag auch diejenigen aufgeschlossen gegenüber, die gegen die Einführung einer Selbstbeteiligung sind. Ich meine, man könnte Gegner und Befürworter in dieser Diskussion einander näherbringen, wenn man Rechenschaft darüber ablegt, was eigentlich mit der Selbstbeteiligung erreicht werden soll. Habe ich primär prozeßpolitische Ziele vor Augen, oder wird ordnungspolitisch argumentiert? Will ich also zur Kostendämpfung beitragen oder aus ordnungspolitischen Überlegungen das Kostenbewußtsein der Bevölkerung verbessern? Das ist etwas, was ich von heute auf morgen nicht erreichen kann. Wenn jeder einzelne finanziell mehr in die Pflicht genommen wird, kann ich damit nicht nachweisen, daß ich eine Kostendämpfung erreiche, es läßt sich aber sehr wohl zeigen, daß dadurch ein sorgsamerer Umgang mit der eigenen Gesundheit erreicht werden kann. Ich würde unter dem Begriff Selbstbeteiligung einen leistungsbezogenen finanziellen Eigenanteil des Patienten beim Kauf oder bei der Inanspruchnahme von Gesundheitsgütern und Dienstleistungen verstehen, deren angemessene Behandlung ein eigenes Referat verlangt. Dort müßten die Ziele der Selbstbeteiligung, die erhofften Wirkungen und die vielfältigen Erscheinungsformen genau dargestellt werden. Auch Art und Struktur der gegenwärtigen Selbstbeteiligung wären zu prüfen; sie beträgt immerhin schon rund 5 Mrd. DM.[7]

Nunmehr komme ich zu den Zuweisungen und Erstattungen. Ich habe im Rahmen der Diskussion zu diesem Thema den Eindruck gewonnen, daß es vollkommen aussichtslos ist, auf einen Bundeszuschuß zur Gesetzlichen Krankenversicherung zu hoffen. Und es erscheint genauso aussichtslos zu sein, für die nächsten 3, 4 Jahre mit Geld für den zu reformierenden Bundeszuschuß zur gesetzlichen Rentenversicherung zu rechnen. Die Forderung nach einer Reform der Krankenversicherung der Rentner läuft in meinen Augen darauf hinaus, wenn ich einmal von wichtigen technischen Details absehe, daß der GKV für die Rentner über die Rentenversicherung mehr Geld zufließen soll. Das kann von der Anpassung her nur höhere Beiträge oder sinkende Leistungen in der Rentenversicherung oder einen höheren Bundeszuschuß bedeuten. Letzter Punkt steht für die

---

[7] Siehe im einzelnen Schulenburg 1987.

nächsten 3–5 Jahre nicht zur Diskussion. Daher wird wohl nichts anderes übrig
bleiben, als im System Wirtschaftlichkeitsreserven zu mobilisieren oder andere
Finanzierungswege zu suchen.

In der Literatur wird z. B. darauf hingewiesen, daß die Arbeitgeberanteile zugunsten höherer Löhne umgewandelt werden sollten. In einer Einmalaktion sollen die Arbeitgeberanteile auf die Löhne aufgeschlagen werden. Wir hätten dann
ein lohnbezogenes System, das vollständig von den Arbeitnehmern finanziert
werden würde. Das ist ebenfalls ein Vorschlag, bei dem man ganz genau analysieren muß, was er für die paritätische Selbstverwaltung und für die zukünftige Entwicklung der Ausgaben im Gesundheitswesen bedeutet. Es gilt zu prüfen, welche
Bedeutung die Umsetzung dieses Vorschlags für die Tarifpolitik hat, wenn – was
zu erwarten ist – Ausgabensteigerungen in einem überwiegend aus Löhnen finanzierten Gesundheitswesen auftreten. Das würde das Gesamtkonzept der paritäti-
schen Selbstverwaltung erheblich beeinflussen.

Ich möchte im folgenden 2 Instrumente vorstellen, die sich auf die Erweiterung der lohnbezogenen Bemessungsgrundlage beziehen. Zunächst der Vorschlag, der aus der Diskussion um die Finanzierung der Rentenversicherung bekannt ist, nämlich einen „Maschinenbeitrag" einzuführen bzw. den Arbeitgeberbeitrag so umzugestalten, daß man ihn nicht mehr nur von der Lohn- und Gehaltssumme erhebt, sondern vom gesamten Volkseinkommen. Dieser Vorschlag
eines Wertschöpfungsbeitrags, wie es ökonomisch korrekt heißen muß, will u. a.
das Einkommen aus Unternehmertätigkeit und Vermögen mit in die Beitragsbemessungsgrundlage einbeziehen, um den Arbeitgeberanteil langfristig auf eine
breitere Bemessungsgrundlage zu stellen. Das ist ein Vorschlag, der ursprünglich
aus dem Bereich der Finanzierung und Konsolidierung der Rentenversicherung
kommt. Er würde, wenn er tatsächlich Unterstützung fände, in andere Systeme
der sozialen Sicherung übertragen werden. Unter wirtschaftspolitischen Aspekten ist eine solche Umbasierung nicht angezeigt. Die Bemessungsgrundlage, die
wir derzeit vorfinden, sollte beibehalten werden. Wenn es dennoch zum Maschinenbeitrag in der GKV käme, hätte dieser Vorschlag auch Konsequenzen für die
paritätische Selbstverwaltung, die in ihrer Wirkung noch gar nicht abzuschätzen
sind, da dann das „50 : 50-Prinzip" sehr schwer aufrechtzuerhalten wäre.

Ein zweiter Punkt bei der Erweiterung der lohnbezogenen Bemessungsgrundlage bezieht sich auf die Erweiterung des versicherungspflichtigen Bruttoarbeits-
entgelts bzw. der versicherungspflichtigen Alterseinkünfte. Man möchte entweder über den Lohn hinaus weitere Einkunftsarten hinzunehmen oder auf das
Haushalts- bzw. Familieneinkommen zurückgreifen. Es sollen demnach auch
Kapitaleinkünfte und Transfereinkommen miteinbezogen werden. Analog zur
Besteuerung könnte man auch ein Splittingverfahren einführen. Es wird behauptet, daß die alleinige Anknüpfung an das Arbeitseinkommen, wie wir es derzeit
vorfinden, deswegen nicht sachgerecht ist, weil es Versicherte gibt, die über hohe
Einkünfte verfügen, aber nur ein geringes Arbeitseinkommen aufweisen. Sie können sich dann mit relativ geringen Beiträgen den vollen Krankenversicherungsschutz „kaufen". Wenn ich allerdings alle Einkunftsarten zugrunde legen will,
brauche ich die Einkommensteuererklärung bzw. den Lohnsteuerjahresaus-
gleich, um den Beitragssatz errechnen zu können. Wegen der notwendigen Rückmeldungen vom Finanzamt zum Arbeitgeber und zur Krankenkasse müssen die

rein administrativen Durchführungsprobleme bedacht werden; ich glaube daher, daß ein solcher Vorschlag seine Grenzen hat.

Ich möchte abschließend noch auf die Zahlungen der gesetzlichen Rentenversicherung zur Krankenversicherung der Rentner (KVdR) und die Möglichkeiten einer verhaltenslenkenden Beitrags- und Steuerpolitik eingehen. Die Beitragseinnahmen der KVdR in Höhe von 11,8 % der Rentenzahlungen und durchschnittlich 5,9 % der Versorgungsbezüge und Arbeitsentgelte der in der GKV versicherten Rentner deckten im Jahr 1985 nur 44,1 % der Ausgaben der KVdR. Da nun bei der absehbaren demographischen Entwicklung insbesondere Probleme bei der Finanzierung der Krankenversicherung der Rentner auftreten werden, schlägt der Sachverständigenrat für die Konzertierte Aktion im Gesundheitswesen vor, den derzeitigen Beitragssatz in Höhe von 11,8 % an den durchschnittlichen allgemeinen Beitragssatz zu koppeln. Ich glaube, dieser Vorschlag findet vielfältige Unterstützung, aber er löst nicht das Problem. Denn die Finanzmittel, die erforderlich sind, sind nicht allein durch eine Erhöhung von 11,8 % auf den durchschnittlichen allgemeinen Beitragssatz zu erzielen. Bei der ohnehin anstehenden Reform des Bundeszuschusses an die gesetzliche Rentenversicherung sollte m. E. das Verhältnis zwischen Rentenversicherung und gesetzlicher Krankenversicherung neu geregelt werden mit dem Ziel, den Solidarbeitrag für die KVdR nicht weiter ansteigen zu lassen. Da es für derartige Neuregelungen seit langem an ordnungspolitischen und versicherungssystematischen Leitvorstellungen fehlt, sollte den Problemen einer systematischen Abgrenzung der Risiken zwischen den verschiedenen Trägern der sozialen Sicherung in Zukunft mehr Aufmerksamkeit geschenkt werden. Eines steht jedoch fest: Eine Finanzierung ist nur über höhere Beiträge in der Rentenversicherung, über Leistungskürzungen oder über Bundeszuschüsse möglich. Andere Möglichkeiten gibt es nicht.

Bei dem Vorschlag einer verhaltenslenkenden Beitrags- und Steuerpolitik geht es darum, daß man Versicherungsprämien so ausgestaltet, daß sie den Lebensstil der Versicherten berühren. Soll z. B. die Tabaksteuer erhöht und das Aufkommen für die Krankenversicherung zweckgebunden werden? Sollen überhaupt Versichertengemeinschaften zugelassen werden mit „gesundlebenden Personen" (Nichtraucher, Sportler, bestimmte religiöse Gruppen) oder sollen Risikoaufschläge eingeführt werden? Sollen Steuerabschläge bei Gütern erlaubt werden, deren Konsum erwünscht ist (z. B. Steuerabschläge für zuckerarme und kalorienarme Getränke)? Man könnte auch Steueraufschläge auf gesundheitsschädigende Verbrauchsgüter legen (Zigaretten, Salz, stark zuckerhaltige Getränke, tierische Fette oberhalb bestimmter Grenzen). Bei gefährlichen Sportarten könnten ähnliche Überlegungen angestellt werden. Ebenso könnte man Steuervergünstigungen beim Nachweis von gesundheitlichem Wohlverhalten einräumen oder bei Vorlage eines Sportabzeichens, Blutdruckpasses, Freizeitpasses etc. Prämien gewähren. Um zu dieser verhaltenslenkenden Gesundheitspolitik abschließend Stellung nehmen zu können, sind Sozialmediziner und Epidemiologen aufgerufen zu zeigen, ob dies ein Weg in die Richtung einer verbesserten, präventiven Gesundheitspolitik wäre. Es sei jedoch die Frage erlaubt, wie weit die Fürsorgepflicht des Staates in einem Wirtschaftssystem wie dem der Bundesrepublik Deutschland gehen soll oder darf. Man wäre, außer bei der Zulassung der genannten Versichertengemeinschaften, stets dem Vorwurf ausgesetzt, die Freiheit des Einzelnen durch bestimmte Maßnahmen einer verhaltenslenkenden Gesundheitspolitik zu manipulieren. Hinzu kommt, daß die fiskalischen Konsequenzen nur Nebenprodukt einer grundsätzlich nichtfiskalisch ausgerichteten Gesundheitspolitik sind und auch nur im Fall von Risikoaufschlägen bzw. Steuererhöhungen zu Einnahmen führen würden.

Die Finanzierbarkeit der GKV im Rahmen der langfristigen Weiterentwicklung der Gesundheitsversorgung

Die einnahmenorientierte Ausgabenpolitik nach § 405 a RVO

Derzeit wird versucht, die Finanzierbarkeit der GKV durch die Anbindung der Ausgaben an die Entwicklung der Grundlöhne zu garantieren. Diese Politik läßt sich am besten am Beispiel von Abb. 3 illustrieren. Dort zeigt sich, daß die Zuwachsrate der Leistungsausgaben um 1,1 % über der Zuwachsrate der Grundlohnsumme lag und insoweit gegen die einnahmenorientierte Ausgabenpolitik verstoßen wurde. Weiter läßt sich aus Abb. 3 entnehmen, wie die einzelnen Leistungsbereiche bei dieser Betrachtung liegen. Vereinfacht ausgedrückt soll die Lohnnebenkostenkonstanz als politisches Ziel dadurch verwirklicht werden, daß sämtliche Ausgaben im Gesundheitswesen der Grundlohnsummenentwicklung folgen bzw. Strukturausschläge nur zugelassen werden, wenn die Zuwachsraten

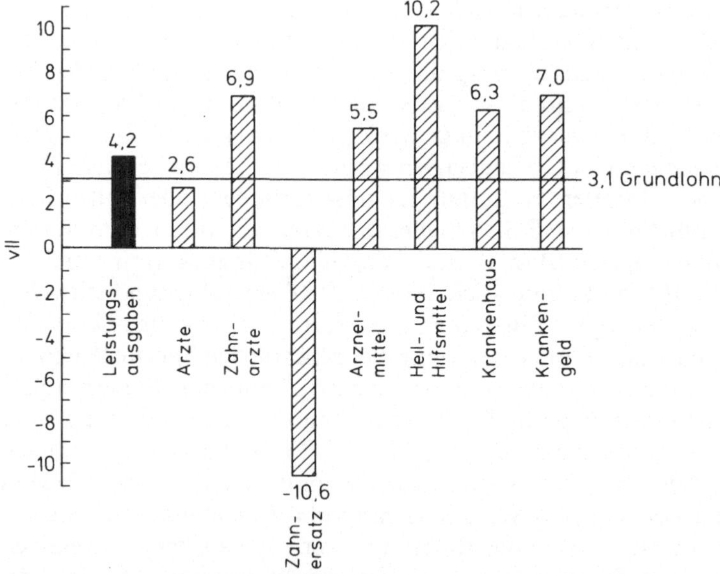

Abb. 3. Ausgaben- und Grundlohnentwicklung je GKV-Mitglied, 1986. (Arbeits- und Sozialstatistik BMA; s. im einzelnen Sachverständigenrat für die Konzertierte Aktion im Gesundheitswesen, Jahresgutachten 1987, Medizinische und ökonomische Orientierung, Baden-Baden 1987, Kapitel IV)

von Grundlohn und Leistungsausgaben übereinstimmen. Diese Budgetierung bzw. Globalsteuer soll mit Hilfe der Konzertierten Aktion im Rahmen der Selbstverwaltung mit Hilfe medizinischer und ökonomischer Orientierungsdaten verwirklicht werden (s. im einzelnen § 405a RVO sowie die Aufgabenstellung des Sachverständigenrates für die Konzertierte Aktion im Gesundheitswesen).[8]

Der Gesetzgeber spricht im § 405a RVO von einer ausgewogenen Verteilung der Belastungen und nimmt damit zur Finanzierung der GKV-Ausgaben im Rahmen der einnahmenorientierten Ausgabenpolitik Stellung. Allerdings wird weder der Belastungsbegriff konkretisiert, noch wird ausgeführt, was unter Ausgewogenheit im Zusammenhang mit der Verteilung von Belastungen gemeint sein könnte. So bleibt offen, ob mit der Verteilung von Belastungen das Verhältnis von Beiträgen zu Steuern oder von Arbeitgeber- zu Arbeitnehmerbeiträgen gemeint ist oder ob sich die Aufteilung auf die Belastungen zwischen den verschiedenen Krankenkassen oder aber zwischen verschiedenen Versichertengruppen bezieht. Unabhängig davon, an welche Verteilung finanzieller Belastungen man denkt, bleibt offen, wann eine Aufteilung als „ausgewogen" anzusehen ist. Hierzu sind nicht nur Kenntnisse über die formale und effektive Inzidenz der Finanzierung erforderlich, sondern auch Normen, wie z. B. das Äquivalenz- oder das Leistungsfähigkeitsprinzip, mit denen der empirische Befund verglichen werden kann.

Der Versuch der Budgetierung bzw. Globalsteuerung im Rahmen der einnahmenorientierten Ausgabenpolitik nach § 405a RVO kann als die Antwort der Praxis auf die Probleme der Finanzierbarkeit der GKV angesehen werden. Die enge Anbindung an die Grundlohnsummenentwicklung soll die langfristige Finanzierbarkeit der Gesetzlichen Krankenversicherung sicherstellen.

Reformperspektiven und Finanzierbarkeit der GKV

Ohne an dieser Stelle die verschiedenen Reformmodelle im einzelnen zu diskutieren, lassen sie sich danach unterscheiden, ob sie expressis verbis die Finanzierbarkeit, z. B. in Form der Beitragssatzstabilität, garantieren sollen oder ob es sich um Reformmodelle handelt, in denen sich die Frage nach der Finanzierbarkeit nicht stellt, sondern ein entsprechender Ordnungsrahmen mit den neu zu setzenden Anreizen hinsichtlich der bewirkten Ergebnisse akzeptiert wird. Eine bedarfsgerechte und kostengünstige Versorgung würde sich automatisch einstellen, wobei auch höhere Beitragssätze in einem solchen „freien" System akzeptiert würden.

Wichtiger als die Frage nach der Finanzierbarkeit erscheint dann die Analyse der allokativen und distributiven Wirkungen unterschiedlicher Reformansätze. Hierzu werden in der Literatur extreme Marktmodelle, modifizierte Marktmodelle, staatliche Versorgungssysteme und duale Systeme unterschieden; bei all diesen Reformansätzen handelt es sich nicht um Patentrezepte, sondern um Konzeptionen, bei denen insbesondere offenbleibt, wie die vielfältigen Übergangsprobleme geregelt werden sollen. Übergreifend gilt jedoch für nahezu alle Reforman-

---

[8] Siehe hierzu Henke 1988.

sätze, daß mehr Transparenz in der Finanzierung gefordert wird, daß allokative Gesichtspunkte in den Vordergrund treten sollen, daß der Wettbewerb auf der Angebotsseite und zwischen den Kassen intensiviert werden sollte und daß Trägerstrukturen in der Gesundheitspolitik zumindest der Koordinierung bedürfen. Schließlich werden neuartige Versicherungs-, Vergütungs- und Versorgungsformen gefordert, um das System der Gesundheitsversorgung langfristig zu erneuern und den Herausforderungen anzupassen.

Zusammenfassend ergibt sich, daß die langfristige Finanzierbarkeit der gesetzlichen Krankenversicherung zwar gewährleistet ist; es fragt sich nur, unter welchen Bedingungen und mit welchen allokativen und distributiven Wirkungen der Einnahmen-Ausgaben-Ausgleich herbeigeführt wird. Die optimale Gesundheitsquote ist unbekannt und damit auch die Höhe des Finanzbedarfs. Entscheidend sind die von den verschiedenen Finanzierungsebenen ausgehenden Anreize, die der weiteren Analyse, getrennt nach den verschiedenen Leistungssektoren, bedürfen. Darüber hinaus sind die eingangs genannten Einflüsse auf die Ausgabenentwicklung abzuschätzen und ist insbesondere der im Rahmen der RVO sozialversicherungsrechtlich sanktionierte Anspruch auf eine Gesundheitsversorgung nach den Regeln der ärztlichen Kunst angesichts der zunehmenden Versorgungsdichte neu zu interpretieren.

Literatur

Aaron H, Schwartz WB (1984) The painful prescription, rationing hospital care. The Brookings Institution, Washington

Behrens C (1987) Einkommensumverteilungen der Gesetzlichen Krankenversicherung (GKV) – Anmerkungen zum methodischen Ansatz –, Diskussionspapier Nr. 109, Universität Hannover, Fachbereich Wirtschaftswissenschaften

Bundesminister für Arbeit und Sozialordnung (1983) Gutachten zur Neuordnung der Krankenhausfinanzierung. Bonn

Fuchs VR (1974) Who shall live? Health, economics and social choice. New York

Graßmann PH (1985) Medizintechnik: Nutzen und Kosten, Antworten zur Wirtschaftlichkeit, Vortrag auf der 19. Jahrestagung der Deutschen Gesellschaft für Biomedizinische Technik. Stuttgart

Hamm W (1980) Irrwege der Gesundheitspolitik. Tübingen

Henke K-D (1983) Beitragsunterschiede in der gesetzlichen Krankenversicherung aus allokativer und distributiver Sicht. In: Hansmeyer K-H (Hrsg) Staatsfinanzierung im Wandel. Schriften des Vereins für Socialpolitik, N. F. Bd 134. Berlin, S 66ff

Henke K-D (1986) A „concerted" approach to health care financing in the Federal Republic of Germany. In: Health policy, Bd 6, S 341ff.

Henke K-D (1988) Funktionsweise und Steuerungswirksamkeit der Konzertierten Aktion im Gesundheitswesen (KAiG). In. Gäfgen G (Hrsg) Neokorporatismus im Gesundheitswesen, Baden-Baden

Henke K-D, Adam H (1983) Die Finanzlage der sozialen Krankenversicherung 1960–1978. Eine gesamtwirtschaftliche Analyse, Köln

Henke K-D, Adam H (1987) Risikovorsorge im Gesundheitswesen. In: Holzheu S, Kaufmann F-X et al. (Hrsg) Gesellschaft und Unsicherheit. Karlsruhe, S 192ff.

Henke K-D, Metze I (Hrsg) (1986) Finanzierung im Gesundheitswesen, Beitrage zur Gesundheitsökonomie, Bd 10. Robert Bosch Stiftung, Gerlingen

Kath D (1981) Sozialpolitik. In: Bender D et al. (Hrsg) Vahlens Kompendium der Wirtschaftstheorie und Wirtschaftspolitik. Bd 2. München, S 191

OECD (1987) Financing and delivering health care, A comparative analysis of OECD countries. Paris

Russel L (1986) Is prevention better than cure? The Brookings Institution, Washington

Sachverständigenrat für die Konzertierte Aktion im Gesundheitswesen (1987) Jahresgutachten 1987, Medizinische und ökonomische Orientierung. Baden-Baden

Schmähl W (1987) Demographischer Wandel und Finanzierung der Gesetzlichen Krankenversicherung – Auswirkungen und Finanzierungsalternativen –, Diskussionsunterlage für das 18. Colloquium Gesundheitsökonomie der Robert Bosch Stiftung. Stuttgart

v. d. Schulenburg J-M (1981) Systeme der Honorierung frei praktizierender Ärzte und ihre Allokationswirkungen. Tübingen

v. d. Schulenburg J-M (1987) Selbstbeteiligung – Theoretische und empirische Konzepte für die Analyse ihrer Allokations- und Verteilungswirkungen. Tübingen

Statistisches Bundesamt (Hrsg) (1987) Fachserie 12. Gesundheitswesen, Reihe 52, Ausgaben für Gesundheit 1970 bis 1985. Stuttgart Mainz

Thurow LC (1984) Learning to say „No“. N Engl J Med 311/24:1569ff.

Weltbank (Hrsg) (1987) Financing health services in developing countries. An agenda for reform. Washington

Zimmermann H, Henke K-D (1987) Finanzwissenschaft. Eine Einführung in die Lehre von der öffentlichen Finanzwirtschaft, 5. Auflage. München

Theoretische Grundlagen der Produktspezifikation im Krankenhaus und angrenzende Fragen *

R. Leidl

Dieser Beitrag beschäftigt sich mit grundlegenden Fragen der Spezifikation dessen, was ein Krankenhaus „produziert". Er beschränkt sich dabei auf den Hauptbereich der Produktion: Die direkte Versorgung von Krankenhauspatienten. „Im Mittelpunkt der betrieblichen Betätigung im Krankenhaus steht die stationäre Vollversorgung ..." (Eichhorn 1982, S. 219). Darüber hinaus werden von Krankenhäusern noch weitere Produkte erstellt. Hier sind aber nicht die selbsterstellten Vorleistungen im Rahmen der Patientenversorgung gemeint, wie beispielsweise die eigene Arzneimittelherstellung oder die eigene Wäscherei, sondern über die stationäre Patientenversorgung hinausführende Krankenhausprodukte wie die medizinische Forschung und Lehre, Ausbildung von Krankenhauspflegepersonal, Vorhaltung von Versorgungskapazitäten für Notfälle, ambulante Versorgung von Patienten und Betreiben des Rettungsdienstes.[1] Diese Teile im Produktspektrum des Mehrproduktunternehmens Krankenhaus dürfen bezüglich der Versorgungsfunktion des Krankenhauses wie des daraus entstehenden Ressourcenverbrauchs nicht übersehen werden.[2] Sie stehen aber nicht im Zentrum der Versorgung der eigentlichen Krankenhausfälle und werden für die Zwecke dieser Untersuchung vernachlässigt. Zum Teil können sie, wie das Beispiel einer unterschiedlichen Bewertung von Produkten in Universitätskliniken und Häusern ohne Lehraufgaben zeigt, später ohne grundsätzliche Veränderung der Produktspezifikation mit eingebaut werden. Eine Differenzierung der verschiedenen Typen von Patientenversorgung nach Fällen mit gleichen, charakteristischen Merkmalen der Versorgung wird als fallbezogene Produktspezifikation verstanden. Sie ist das Thema der weiteren Abhandlungen.

Im folgenden Abschnitt sollen ein Einblick in die konkreten Anwendungsgebiete einer fallbezogenen Produktspezifikation, wie etwa bei der Krankenhausfinanzierung, gegeben und die theoretischen Grundlagen für eine empirische Produktspezifikation im Krankenhausbereich erarbeitet werden. So wird die Beziehung zwischen Krankenhausversorgung und Gesundheit diskutiert und ein erster Überblick zu den Konzepten und Lösungsansätzen eines Einbezugs der Fallmischung gegeben. Die speziell ressourcenorientierten Fallklassifikationen werden

---

* Erstmals veröffentlicht in: Leidl R (1987) S. 19–36.

[1] Zum Leistungsspektrum im Krankenhaus vgl. z. B. Oettle (1984), S 322f

[2] Fragen nach der Zugehörigkeit von Produkten zum regulären Krankenhausbetrieb sind wegen der daraus erwachsenden unterschiedlichen Finanzierungsverpflichtungen im Rahmen der deutschen Krankenhausfinanzierung immer wieder rechtlich umstritten, vgl. z. B. zu Ausbildungsstätten, Personalwohnheimen und Kindertagesstätten Behrends (1981).

an anderer Stelle („Beschreibung einiger ressourcenorientierter Patientenklassifikationsverfahren", Leidl 1987, S. 37–50) behandelt.

Einsatzgebiete einer Spezifikation des Krankenhausprodukts

Spezifikationen von Krankenhausprodukten können in vielen verschiedenen Zusammenhängen eingesetzt werden. Für eine nähere Beschreibung werden 3 Bereiche herausgegriffen: Der Krankenhausfinanzierungsbereich wegen seiner umfassenden Bedeutung sowie, als Anwendungsgebiet von mehr analytischem Interesse, aber teilweise auch in engem Zusammenhang mit Finanzierungsfragen, die beiden Bereiche Schätzungen von Krankenhauskostenfunktion und Hypothesen über das „Krankenhausverhalten". In der Folge wird die Funktion der Mengenkomponente dargestellt und auf die Einsatzmöglichkeit der Produktspezifikation eingegangen. Eine Reihe weiterer Anwendungsgebiete, bei denen fallbezogene Produktspezifikationen nützlich oder gar notwendig sind, wird nur beispielhaft aufgeführt:

— Im betrieblichen Management der Krankenhäuser können spezifizierte Fälle als Bezugspunkt für Kostenträgerrechnungen dienen, als ein Instrument der innerbetrieblichen Wirtschaftlichkeitskontrolle, aber auch der Mittelallokation oder, längerfristig gesehen, des Produktmanagements, d. h. Planung und Beeinflussung der Fallmischung sowie der Durchführung der entsprechenden Behandlung.[3]
— Im zwischenbetrieblichen Wirtschaftlichkeitsvergleich[4] ermöglicht die fallbezogene Produktspezifikation den fallstandardisierten Krankenhausbetriebsvergleich.
— Fallbezogene Daten können zur Analyse von Marktstrukturen verwendet werden. Dazu gehören Untersuchungen über die Wettbewerbslage eines Krankenhauses,[5] aber auch Auswertungen der Informationen im Rahmen von Krankenhausbedarfsplanungen, z. B. bei fallbezogenen Nutzungsvergleichen[6] oder Aufschlüsselungen der regionalen Krankenhausnachfrage.[7]
— Schließlich bieten die fallorientierten Spezifikationen differenzierte Ansatzpunkte für Analysen und Vergleiche der Produktivität (d. h. der Faktorein-

---

[3] Die Orientierung der Krankenhausführung in Richtung eines industriellen Managements, insbesondere auch mit der Einbeziehung der Ärzteschaft, wurde bei der Einführung des fallbezogenen Systems der Diagnosis-Related Groups (DRGs) in New Jersey als einer der wesentlichen Effekte angesehen; May u. Wassermann (1984), S. 553; als Beispiele eines Produktmanagementansatzes, der sich auf die diagnostischen Kategorien der behandelten Patienten bezieht, s. Benz u. Burnham (1985).

[4] Zur Diskussion von Wirtschaftlichkeitsindikatoren im Krankenhaus s. Siebig (1980), S. 69f.

[5] Vgl. Reif et al. (1985), die eine fallbezogene Analyse eines Krankenhausmarkts mit 6 Wettbewerbern als Grundlage für ein strategisches Planungsmodell für das Krankenhausmanagement vorstellen.

[6] Siehe Thompson (1982), S. 55ff., der die Verwendung einer fallbezogenen Nutzungsanalyse für Qualitätskontrollzwecke beschreibt.

[7] Zur Methodik regionaler Analyse der Krankenhausnachfrage, allerdings ohne Falldifferenzierungen s. Zwerenz (1982).

satz/Produktoutput Relationen) und deren Veränderung oder auch der Faktoreinsatzverhältnisse selbst.[8]

Unter den Einsatzgebieten ragt die Krankenhausfinanzierung besonders heraus. Aufgrund der potentiellen kostendämpfungspolitischen, gesundheitspolitischen, aber auch der betriebsinternen Implikationen unterschiedlicher Spezifikationen des zu finanzierenden Krankenhausprodukts kann die Krankenhausfinanzierung als das Anwendungsgebiet mit der größten praktischen Relevanz angesehen werden. Die Krankenhausfinanzierung läßt sich vereinfachend mit einem System aus 4 institutionellen Akteuren, welche die entscheidenden ökonomischen Funktionen wahrnehmen, beschreiben:[9] Krankenhäuser erbringen Leistungen an Patienten, diese Leistungen werden von den Krankenversicherungen, die sich wiederum über Mitgliederbeiträge finanzieren, entgolten. Gegebenenfalls kontrolliert eine Regulierungsinstanz den eigentlichen Finanzierungsprozeß, der sich aus den beiden Komponenten Menge (der Abrechnungseinheit) und „Preis" (der monetären Bewertung, die sich freilich in den meisten Fällen auf die Kosten bezieht) zusammensetzt. Diese abstrahierende Beschreibung, die sich auch auf das Finanzierungssystem der Bundesrepublik Deutschland anwenden läßt,[10] macht deutlich, daß eine Produktspezifikation neben dem Bewertungselement die zweite instrumentelle Determinante für den Erlös ist, und dementsprechend über die Mengenkomponente bzw. ihre Definition ebenso wie über die Bewertung Steuerungsfunktionen ausgeübt werden können. Zu den komparativen Anreizwirkungen verschiedener Definitionen der Mengenkomponente liegen systematisierte Überblicke vor.[11]

Für eine vollständige Ableitung der Wirkungen eines Finanzierungssystems, auch der Differentialeffekte eines Übergangs von einer anderen Mengenkomponente zu fallbezogenen Produktspezifikationen, muß jedoch die konkrete Ausgestaltung des Finanzierungsverfahrens, das in der abstrahierenden Beschreibung ausgespart wurde, berücksichtigt werden. So dürften sich die Wirkungen der Einführung einer fallbezogenen Finanzierung danach unterscheiden, ob z. B. regional einheitliche Fallpauschalen administrativ festgelegt werden oder ob Krankenversicherungen mit einzelnen Krankenhäusern über die Fallpreise verhandeln. Eine Beurteilung des effektiven Wirkungspotentials einer Definition der Mengenkomponente kann daher letztlich nur unter der Berücksichtigung der Bewertungs- und Verfahrensaspekte erfolgen. Generalisierend läßt sich aber feststellen, daß fallbezogenen Produktspezifikationen, die als Abrechnungseinheit im Krankenhausfinanzierungssystem eingesetzt werden, auch als (temporäre) Vereinbarungen über Mengeneinheiten aufgefaßt werden können und die Bestimmung wie die Verwendungsregeln von Produktdefinitionen als finanzielle Steuerungspotentiale, die über die Festlegung einer Erlöskomponente zur Wirkung kommen, anzusehen sind.

---

[8] Vgl. beispielsweise zur Hypothese geringerer Kapitalintensitäten bei gewinnorientierten Krankenhäusern Schweitzer u. Rafferty (1976); allerdings muß bei Produktivitätsuntersuchungen besonders auf die gleiche Versorgungsqualität geachtet werden; die Problematik dieser Operationalisierung wird unterstrichen durch den Hinweis von Sloan u. Steinwald (1980), S. 19, daß Leistungsintensität pro Fall, d. h der reziproke Wert der Produktivität, gerne als Qualitätsindikator verwendet wurde.

[9] Vgl. Leidl (1983), S 136f.

[10] Ebd., S. 137ff.

[11] Für den Krankenhausbereich s. z. B. die modelltheoretisch fundierten Analysen von Sloan u. Steinwald (1980), Kap. 2, ferner Cleverly (1979) und Dowling (1974); für den ambulanten Bereich die ausführliche, auch formale Darstellung von Schulenburg (1980).

Bezüglich der konkreten Bedeutung fallbezogener (und anderer) Krankenhausfinanzierungssysteme für die Bundesrepublik Deutschland gibt es eine breite Diskussion, auf die hier nur verwiesen wird.[12] Im Vergleich zu der systemgestaltenden Bedeutung der Verfahrensaspekte und der institutionellen Funktionszuordnung in der Krankenhausfinanzierung besitzt die Definition der Abrechnungseinheit einen eher instrumentellen, gleichwohl nicht zu unterschätzenden Charakter. Dennoch soll an dieser Stelle keine theoretische Analyse der potentiellen allokativen, distributiven oder ausgabenwachstumsbezogenen Wirkungen einer fallorientierten Produktspezifikation vorgenommen werden; es war lediglich die Relevanz fallbezogener Produktspezifikationen für die Krankenhausfinanzierung aufzuzeigen.

Ein zweiter Bereich betrifft den Einsatz der Produktspezifikationen als Maß der Outputstandardisierung bei der Schätzung von Krankenhauskostenfunktionen. Die Kontrolle vergleichbarer Outputs kann als ein zentraler Punkt der Kostenschätzfunktionen erachtet werden. Kostenfunktionsschätzungen und ihre Verbesserungsmöglichkeiten durch eine Produktstandardisierung sind als ein Hilfsmittel des Krankenhausbetriebsvergleichs, d. h. für Wirtschaftlichkeitsanalysen, von Bedeutung,[13] können aber auch zur Ermittlung von (Durchschnitts)kostennormen, die wiederum Finanzierungszwecken dienen, eingesetzt werden.[14] Außerdem wurden Kostenfunktionsschätzungen zur Prüfung von Skalenerträgen (d. h. zur Ermittlung der optimalen Krankenhausgröße)[15] sowie zur Analyse der Kostenwirkungen kurzfristiger Auslastungsschwankungen (also dem Verhältnis von Grenz- und Durchschnittskosten)[16] verwendet. Die ökonomische Diskussion hat unter den Bestimmungsfaktoren der Krankenhauskosten auch eine Reihe von Fallklassifikationen mit einbezogen.[17]

Grundsätzlich lassen sich folgende Vorgehensweisen unterscheiden, wie eine fallbezogene Produktspezifikation eingesetzt werden kann.[18] Die Kostenschätzung kann jeweils nur für einen bestimmten Produkttyp erfolgen, oder sie kann als eine „Stückkostenschätzung" mit einer mit einem Fallmischungsindex gewichteten abhängigen Variablen, also den zu schätzenden Kosten,

---

[12] Vgl. die Beiträge in dem Sammelband der Studienstiftung der Verwaltungsleiter deutscher Krankenanstalten (1984), den Zwischenbericht der Kommission Krankenhausfinanzierung der Robert-Bosch-Stiftung (1983) oder den zusammenfassenden Überblick von Neubauer u. Unterhuber (1985).

[13] Vgl. zu diesem Thema die wenigen deutschen empirischen Beiträge von Henning u. Paffrath (1978), Siebig (1980) sowie die kritische Stellungnahme von Goetzke (1980); die Praxis des Krankenhausbetriebsvergleichs in der Bundesrepublik Deutschland, die sich freilich nicht auf Kostenschätzungen, sondern auf Gruppenvergleiche der Selbstkostenblätter stützt, beleuchten aus Sicht der Krankenkassen Gerdelmann (1976, 1979), seitens der Krankenhausverbände Müller (1981).

[14] Siehe dazu den theoretischen Beitrag von Beyer (1985), der sich auch speziell mit der Fallzusammensetzung befaßt.

[15] Zu diesem beliebten, ungelösten Thema s. die Überblicke von Schellhaas (1971), S. 54–56, Migue u. Belanger (1974), S. 31–39, Cullis u. West (1979), S. 144–163 oder Feldstein (1983), S. 205–213.

[16] Breyer (1986), S. 263, der eine Reihe von Arbeiten aufzählt und in einem Anhang auch einen Ansatz zur Schätzung der Grenzkosten einer Verweildauerausdehnung bzw. eines zusätzlichen Behandlungsfalls anführt.

[17] Siehe dazu die Überblicke von Breyer (1986), S. 267–272 oder Barer (1982), S. 57–65.

[18] Vgl. zur Fallstandardisierung von Kostenschätzfunktionen Barer (1982), S. 57.

144   R. Leidl

durchgeführt werden. In beiden Fällen dient die Produktspezifikation als Standardisierungsgrö-
ße. Bei einer weiteren Möglichkeit werden die Produkte als Konstrukt zu den unabhängigen, er-
klärenden Variablen aufgenommen, d. h. als Kostendeterminante verwendet. Fast alle Arbeiten
zur Kostenschätzung folgten dem letzten Ansatz. Einige empirische Beispiele von Kostenschätzstudien werden im letzten Unterpunkt (S. 154–156), der sich mit Konzeptionen der Produktspezifikation beschäftigt, berücksichtigt.

In einem dritten Bereich können fallbezogene Produktspezifikationen bei empirischen Prüfungen von Hypothesen des Krankenhausverhaltens als differenzierte
Operationalisierungen für den Handlungsparameter oder (je nach Art der Mo-
dellformulierung) die Nachfragerestriktion „Krankenhausfälle eines bestimmten
Typs" eingesetzt werden. Die auf ihre Wirkungen zu untersuchenden Restriktionen können dabei aus dem Bereich der Krankenhausfinanzierung stammen (vgl.
„Wirkungsanalyse fallbezogener Produktspezifikation", Leidl 1987, S. 85–98),
müssen es aber nicht. Ein anderes Beispiel wäre die Veränderung der Nachfragerestriktion des Krankenhauses durch eine gesundheitspolitische Maßnahme, beispielsweise zur Substitution stationärer durch ambulante Versorgung,[19] wie sie
auch im Bayern-Vertrag intendiert war.[20]

Die Vermutungen über die Wirkungen der Restriktionsänderung sind bezüglich des Krankenhausverhaltens als Hypothesen zu formulieren. Am deutlichsten zum Ausdruck kommen die
dabei gemachten Annahmen wie die abgeleiteten Ergebnisse in einem formalen Modell des
Krankenhausverhaltens.[21] Zur damit erforderlichen Ausgestaltung des Verhaltensmodells gibt
es eine langjährige Diskussion, die davon beherrscht war, wer als ökonomische Handlungsein-
heit des Krankenhauses anzusehen ist und welche Zielfunktionen unterstellt werden können.[22]
Die einzelnen Falltypen und die Analyse der Verweildauer als Verhaltensparameter spielen jedoch in diesen Modellen i. allg. eine ebenso untergeordnete Rolle wie die empirische Prüfung der
Erklärungskraft der Modelle oder gar der zugrundegelegten Annahmen über die Entscheidungs-
abläufe im Krankenhaus.[23] Im Rahmen gesundheitsökonomischer Politikevaluationen, die eine
Vielzahl von Variablen (seien es verschiedene Zielsetzungen oder multiple Restriktionen mit
wechselseitigen Abhängigkeiten) zu beachten haben, kann es aber hilfreich und notwendig sein,
auf die formale Ableitung aus einem mikroökonomischen Verhaltensmodell zu verzichten, da
die Berücksichtigung von zu vielen Variablen kaum mehr eine Interpretation der formal abgelei-

---

[19] Vgl. zu diesem Thema z. B Davis u. Russel (1972), Elnicki (1976) oder Luft (1981).

[20] Der Bayern-Vertrag bezeichnet eine mit gesundheits- und kostendämpfungspolitischen Zielsetzungen verknüpfte Honorarvereinbarung zwischen den Selbstverwaltungskörperschaften
der Krankenkassen und der niedergelassenen Ärzte aus dem Jahr 1979; zu seiner umfassenden
Evaluation s. Schwefel et al. (1986).

[21] Sloan u. Steinwald (1980), S. 34.

[22] Beispielhaft seien die vielzitierten Beiträge von Harris (1977), der das Krankenhaus als Orga-
nisationseinheit zweier verschiedener Firmen (nämlich der Ärzteschaft und der Verwaltung)
interpretiert, und von Pauly u. Redish (1973), die das Krankenhaus als Unternehmensrahmen
einer Ärztekooperative auffassen, genannt, einen älteren Überblick zu den unterschiedlichen
Zielfunktionen des Krankenhauses gibt Davis (1972), neuere Überblicke zu den Krankenhausverhaltensmodellen finden sich bei McGuire (1985), Hornbrook u. Goldfarb (1983) oder
Sloan u. Steinwald (1980), S. 12–18.

[23] Ausnahme bilden zum ersten Punkt z. B. der Beitrag von Gäfgen (1983), der in einer eigen-
tumsrechtlichen Analyse die Verhaltensparameter Verweildauer und Qualität der Versorgung
berücksichtigt, oder das Modell von Hornbrook u. Goldfarb (1983), die Fallmischungspolitik
und Verweildauerpolitik des Krankenhauses berücksichtigen und ihr Modell auch empirisch
testen, oder das LISREL-Modell von Hornung u. Massagli (1980), zur Notwendigkeit einer
empirischen Fundierung der Modellannahmen s. Schwefel (1986a).

teten Terme zuläßt.[24] Die Ableitung eines Hypothesengeflechts kann dann in vereinfachter Form, etwa einer theoretischen Fundierung der Wirkungen der gesundheitspolitischen Maßnahme auf ein repräsentatives Krankenhaus unter der Berücksichtigung der Verhaltensparameter Fallzahlen und Fallmischung sowie der Verweildauer erfolgen.[25] Zur empirischen Prüfung ist entsprechend eine fallbezogene Definition der Patientenschaft notwendig.

Die Nützlichkeit von fallbezogenen Produktspezifikationen wurde anhand verschiedener Einsatzgebiete aufgezeigt. Dabei wurden verschiedene wichtige Funktionen der Produktspezifikation unterschieden:

– als Definition der Mengenkomponente aus Fallcharakteristiken in der Finanzierung oder bei produktbezogenen Kostenschätzungen,
– als Kostendeterminante, d. h. als Unabhängige in Kostenschätzfunktionen,
– als Operationalisierung des Verhaltensparameters „Fälle eines Typs" oder als Nachfragerestriktion in Krankenhausverhaltensmodellen.

Die nächsten beiden Unterpunkte behandeln die Fragen, was aus dem Prozeß der Produktion von Gesundheit als Produkt spezifiziert wird und mit welchen Konzepten an die Fallmischung herangegangen werden kann.

Gesundheit, Gesundheitsleistungen und Krankenhausversorgung

Die erste und intuitiv naheliegendste Spezifikation dessen, was im Krankenhaus eigentlich produziert wird, ist zweifellos die Gesundheit. Ein entsprechender Ansatz würde die Messung des Gesundheitszustands eines Patienten vor Beginn der diagnostischen und therapeutischen Maßnahmen, der Veränderung dieses Zustandes und Identifikation des Anteils, der auf die Krankenhausleistungen zurückzuführen ist, erfordern. Angesichts dieser Aufgabenstellung mag ein solches Unterfangen utopisch erscheinen. Gewöhnlich führt dies zu dem Schluß, als Endprodukt der Gesundheitsversorgung nicht die zurechenbare Änderung des Gesundheitszustandes selbst, sondern die dafür erbrachten Leistungen, also Zwischenprodukte im Produktionsprozeß von Gesundheit, anzusehen. Mit dem Abrücken von Gesundheit als Spezifikationsziel wächst tendenziell auch die Operationalisierbarkeit und Meßbarkeit der Konzepte, freilich auf Kosten der Interpretierbarkeit des Beitrags zum Gesundheitsversorgungsprozeß.[26]

Die pragmatische Nützlichkeit einer Verwendung von Gesundheitsleistungen als Produkte bei empirischen Analysen der Angebotsseite, etwa für Kostenfunktionsschätzungen oder Untersuchungen des Anbieterverhaltens, ist evident. In der Konsumtheorie findet die Verwendung von Gesundheitsleistungen als Output ihre theoretische Begründung in der Übertragung des Ansatzes von Becker[27] – der Güter ähnlich Vorprodukten erst zusammen mit eigenen Inputs des

---

[24] Auf die Notwendigkeit, sich in den formalen Analysen auf ganz wenige Variablen zu beschränken, verweisen z. B. Sloan u. Steinwald (1980), S. 19 oder U. Reinhardt in seinem Diskussionsbeitrag zu Gäfgen (1982), S. 167.

[25] Für ein solches Hypothesengeflecht bei der empirischen Prüfung, allerdings ohne Daten zur Fallmischung, s. z. B. Leidl (1986), S. 269ff.; zu einem (rudimentären) diagnosebezogenen Ansatz der Analyse des Krankenhausverhaltens mit Hilfe der Krankheitsartenprofilblätter s. Tischmann (1983).

[26] Münnich (1984), S. 23.

[27] Becker (1965).

Konsumenten, insbesondere der zum Verbrauch notwendigen eigenen Zeitverwendung, als nutzenstiftend ansieht – auf die Nachfrage nach Gesundheit durch Grossmann.[28] Die Gesundheitsleistungen, bei den Krankenhausleistungen beispielsweise Operationen, verabreichte Medikamente, Pflege- und Hotelleistungen, gehen dabei als Vor- oder Zwischenprodukt neben Inputs des Patienten, wie etwa einer gesunden Lebensweise oder der Befolgung ärztlicher Ratschläge, in die individuelle Gesundheitsproduktionsfunktion ein. Dieser Ansatz hat sich bei der Erklärung der Nachfrage nach Gesundheitsleistungen theoretisch und empirisch als fruchtbar erwiesen.[29]

Nachteilig bei der Verwendung von Gesundheitsleistungen als Output der Versorgung ist jedoch, daß zwar die technische Effizienz der Leistungserstellung, nicht aber ohne weiteres die allokative Effizienz dieser Art von Gesundheitsversorgung überprüft werden kann. Gesundheitsleistungen als Indikatoren der unterschiedlichen, zu versorgenden Fälle vermengen die beiden, für analytische Zwecke strikt zu trennenden Komponenten exogen vorgegebene, morbiditätsbedingte Fallmischung und Zusammensetzung der für die Versorgung eingesetzten Leistungsmischung im Krankenhaus.[30] Typischerweise führt die Verwendung leistungsbezogener Outputspezifikationen in der Finanzierung zu einer sich selbst legitimierenden Leistungsexpansion und besitzt außerdem den grundlegenden Nachteil, daß kostensparende Leistungssubstitutionen bei der Versorgung von Krankenhausfällen nicht finanziell honoriert werden und somit keine Anreize für fallbezogene Produktivitätsfortschritte gesetzt werden. Bei Kostenschätzungen lassen Vorleistungen als Output letztlich „die Schätzgleichung zu einer Beziehung zwischen Kosten und Inputmengen degenerieren".[31] Dieses Argument läßt Spezifikationsansätze, die Gesundheitsleistungen zur Erklärung einer Ressourcenverbrauchsvariablen verwenden, in einem besonders kritischen Licht erscheinen.

Die Anwendung leistungsbezogener Konzepte für eine Produktspezifikation implizieren ferner – wenn man die Verbesserung, Erhaltung oder Förderung des Gesundheitszustands als das eigentliche Ziel der Gesundheitsversorgung nicht völlig aus den Augen verlieren will – zumindest eine gleichbleibende Qualität dieser "Outputs". Diese qualitative Dimension der Gesundheitsleistungen kann mit Hilfe der Konzepte der medizinischen Effektivitätsmessung, Qualitätsbeurteilung und Qualitätssicherung präzisiert werden: Nach einem inzwischen schon klassisch gewordenen Konzept teilt Donabedian[32] die Gesundheitsversorgung ein in die Strukturkomponente (in die der quantitative und qualitative Faktoraufwand eingeht), in die Prozeßkomponente (der Durchführung der eigentlichen Versorgungsleistungen) und in die Ergebnis- oder Outcomekomponente (welche die Änderung des Gesundheitszustands des Patienten betrifft). Diese analytische Trennung der Gesundheitsversorgung macht deutlich, daß ein reiner Prozeßvergleich von leistungsbezogen spezifizierten Zwischenprodukten zumindest implizit von einer gleichen Ergebniswirkung auf den Gesundheitszustand des Patienten, d. h. einer identischen Qualität der Leistungen, ausgehen muß bzw. bei Vorliegen von über ein festzusetzendes Maß hinaus unterschiedlichen Leistungsqualitäten eine Vergleichbarkeit der Zwischenprodukte nicht mehr vorgenommen werden kann. Eine identische Spezifikation würde sonst unvergleichbare

---

[28] Grossmann (1972).

[29] Für einen 10-Jahres-Rückblick auf seine Theorie s. Grossmann (1982), zur Verallgemeinerung Muurinen (1982).

[30] Vor allem bei Kostenschätzungen wurde die Leistungsmischung auch als Fallmischungsindikator eingesetzt; vgl. zu den beiden Komponenten und zu Beiträgen mit den verschiedenen Konzepten Barer (1982), S. 55ff. oder Zaretzky (1977).

[31] Breyer (1986), S. 270.

[32] Donabedian (1966); zur Bedeutung des Konzepts in der Qualitätssicherungsdiskussion s. den Überblick in Bundesminister für Arbeit und Sozialordnung (1981).

(End)produkte nebeneinanderstellen. Letztlich sind in der empirischen Untersuchung der Versorgung von Patienten somit Prozeß- und Ergebniskomponente, Gesundheitsvorleistungen und Gesundheitsproduktion nicht mehr vollständig zu trennen. Standardisierungen von Versorgungsleistungen zu Vergleichszwecken, wie es Produktspezifikationen u. a. sein können, bedürfen damit potentiell immer einer Kontrolle der Vergleichbarkeit ihres "outcomes". Dies verdeutlicht die analytische Verwandtschaft medizinischer Qualitätsuntersuchungen und ökonomischer Effizienzanalysen.

Die sachliche und, wie gezeigt wurde, ökonomische Interdependenz von Gesundheitsleistungen und Gesundheit läßt es sinnvoll und notwendig erscheinen, sich vor den Produktspezifikationen kurz mit dem Stand und den Möglichkeiten der Messung und Bewertung von Gesundheit auseinanderzusetzen. Wenn man auch nicht von einem generell akzeptierten Konzept der Messung des Gesundheitsstatus sprechen kann, so hat doch die Gesundheitsindikatorenforschung in den letzten 1 ½–2 Jahrzehnten beträchtliche Fortschritte in Richtung der vorhin als utopisch bezeichneten Aufgabenstellung gemacht. Die Gesundheitsstatusmessung geht über die rein diagnostische Identifizierung von Krankheiten, die aus ärztlicher Perspektive an erster Stelle einer Patienteneinordnung stehen,[33] hinaus auf die Dimensionen der physischen und sozialen Funktionseinschränkungen und der subjektiven Befindlichkeiten ein.[34] Gesundheitsstatusmessung kann damit als Verallgemeinerung und als Komplement zu den herkömmlichen, ausschließlich diagnostischen Definitionen von Krankheit angesehen werden. Die Gesundheitsindikatorenforschung begreift Gesundheit als eine vieldimensionale Größe,[35] die mit einer Vielzahl von Meßinstrumenten erfaßt und für mannigfache Ziele eingesetzt werden kann, darunter auch zu Finanzierungszwecken.[36] Die potentielle Bedeutung dieser Ansätze für die Produktspezifikation im Krankenhausbereich liegt besonders dort, wo Falldefinitionen über Diagnosen hinaus führen sollen. Dabei spielt, wie Beispiele einer versuchten Integration von Schweregradkonzepten in die Produktspezifikation im Krankenhaus zeigen, fast ausschließlich die Dimension der Funktionseinschränkungen eine Rolle, während bislang keine Ansätze einer expliziten Integration der eben nicht objektivierbaren Befindlichkeiten bekannt sind. Die operationalen Konzepte der Gesundheitsstatusmessung, insbesondere der Funktionseinschränkungen, sind daher auch für patientenbezogene Spezifikationen im Krankenhausbereich von Bedeutung.

Neben der bloßen Messung der vielen Dimensionen von Gesundheit liegt das zweite große Problem in der Bewertung der verschiedenen Zustände beziehungsweise ihrer Veränderung.

---

[33] Siehe Schröder (1983), S. 29, der in seinem Beitrag unterschiedliche Prioritäten im Krankheitskonzept aus der Sicht von Patienten, der medizinischen Wissenschaft und der Prävention beleuchtet.

[34] Eine neuere Zusammenfassung zur Gesundheitsindikatorenforschung gibt der Sammelband von Culyer (1983) mit einer ausführlichen Bibliographie (ausgewählte Werke sind kurz kommentiert); eine gute Einführung gibt Siegmann (1977); einen Überblick zu Konzepten, Maßen und ihren Anwendungsmöglichkeiten Holland et al. (1979); zum Konzept von Krankheit und Gesundheit aus der Perspektive verschiedener Fachdisziplinen s. Caplan et al. (1981), ein Kurzsurvey bei Bergner (1985).

[35] Vgl. auch zur Vieldimensionalität die lexikographisch geordnete Zusammenfassung von 7 Gesundheitsdimensionen Münnich (1984), S. 20.

[36] Culyer (1983), S. 18.

Torrance[37] unterscheidet dabei Ansätze einer Ad-hoc-Bewertung einzelner Meßwerte mit numerischen Skalen, die monetare Bewertung mit der maximalen Zahlungsbereitschaft und die von ihm favorisierte Bewertung mit Nutzwerten ("utilities"), welche die qualitativen Aspekte des Gesundheitsstatus kardinal bewerten, sich in der eindimensionalen Vergleichsgröße der sog. "Quality Adjusted Life Years" verrechnen lassen und somit ein direktes Maß der gesundheitlichen Effekte einer Maßnahme bieten. Auch wenn solchermaßen präzisierte Konzepte noch weit von einer praktischen Verwendbarkeit in der allgemeinen Krankenhausversorgung entfernt sein mögen, liegen über die rein theoretischen Konzepte hinaus für eine ganze Reihe von Krankheiten auch Operationalisierungen, Messungen und entsprechende Anwendungen vor. Bewertete Gesundheit als Output wurde hauptsächlich, je nach dem Typ der Bewertungsdimension, in Kosten-Effektivitäts-, Kosten-Nutzen- und Kosten-Nutzwert-Analysen gesundheitlicher Maßnahmen und Programme verwendet.[38]

Ein Einsatz von Gesundheitsstatusvariablen bei der Produktspezifikation im Krankenhaus macht, soweit sie nur zur Beschreibung eines zu versorgenden Falles, nicht aber zur Bemessung des tatsächlichen Beitrags zur Gesundung dient, keine weiteren Probleme. Nahezu unlösbar erscheint aber der Ansatz, die eigentliche Produktionsfunktion von Gesundheit für ein Krankenhaus, d. h. die ursächlich den Krankenhausleistungen zurechenbare Gesundheitsverbesserung zu ermitteln: So fehlt zum einen in den allermeisten Fällen die medizinisch-theoretische Fundierung der „technologischen Beziehung zwischen medizinischen (und sozialmedizinischen) Maßnahmen einerseits und ihren gesundheitlichen Folgen andererseits".[39] Zum anderen wird der Gesundungsprozeß von einer Vielzahl weiterer, teilweise schwer oder gar nicht faßbaren Faktoren wie den Lebensbedingungen, dem Lebensstil oder der psychischen Disposition des Patienten mitbestimmt.[40] Ein weiteres Hindernis in der Identifikation technologischer Relationen liegt darin, daß die Versorgungsaufgabe häufig selbst erst in einem Suchprozeß festgestellt werden muß, d. h. das Produkt von sich selbst nicht unabhängig ist, und der Suchprozeß – und eine genaue Produktbestimmung – in manchen Fällen auch im nachhinein ungeklärt bleibt.

Auf der Ebene des Gesundheitssystems hat McKeown[41] beeindruckende Beispiele über den ausbleibenden Einfluß des Auftretens neuer medizinischer Produktionstechnologien, speziell der Chemotherapie, auf die Mortalitätsentwicklung bei Infektionskrankheiten gezeigt. Bezüglich des Einflusses der Lebensbedingungen auf die Gesundheit liegen z. B. zum Zusammenhang von Arbeitslosigkeit und Gesundheit mikro- wie makroökonomisch ausgerichtete Studien mit signifikanten Ergebnissen vor.[42]

Somit lassen sich über die technologische Relation von Krankenhausleistungen und Gesundheit schwerlich umfassende Aussagen machen. Der Ansatz einer Produktspezifikation über die Identifikation der Produktionsfunktion für Gesundheit wird noch weiter problematisiert, wenn an Stelle einer theoretisch begründbaren technologischen Relation aus Patientenvariablen und Krankenhauslei-

---

[37] Torrance (1986).
[38] Als eine Pionierarbeit auf diesem Gebiet kann der Beitrag von Fanshel u. Bush (1970) gelten; eine der wenigen empirischen deutschen Arbeiten stammt von Kriedel (1980) zur Effizienzanalyse von Epilepsieambulanzen. Weitere Beiträge finden sich in dem genannten Überblicksartikel von Torrance (1986).
[39] Münnich (1984), S. 22.
[40] Ebd.
[41] McKeown (1976).
[42] Einen umfassenden Überblick über die Studien auf diesem Gebiet gibt Schwefel (1986b).

stungscharakteristiken das Produkt „Beitrag des Krankenhauses zum Gesundheitsstatus" aus der Analyse real beobachtbarer Produktionsprozesse ermittelt werden soll: Einmal kann nicht von einer Beobachtung effizienter Produktion ausgegangen werden,[43] und zweitens unterliegen die Beobachtungen zusätzlich den Restriktionen des Versorgungssystems. Produktionsrechte (z. B. für die Vorhaltung einer Fachrichtung gemäß der Krankenhausplanung oder, funktionell gesehen, Möglichkeiten zur Nachsorge von Krankenhauspatienten), Finanzierungsbeschränkungen und Zeitrestriktionen (etwa bei privatversicherten Selbständigen), aber auch alle Aspekte des substitutiven Angebots, insbesondere im ambulanten Bereich und bei der Pflegeversorgung, gehen in die Ausgestaltung der Produktionsprozesse mit ein. Da die Krankenhausversorgung innerhalb der Gesundheitsversorgung selbst nicht exakt technologisch abgrenzbar ist, wirkt sich unter den Nebenbedingungen des Gesundheitssystems die Ausgestaltung des substitutiven Angebots auf die beobachtbaren (nicht die technologischen) Relationen von Faktoreinsatz und Gesundheitseffekten besonders stark aus. Bei einer unterschiedlichen Rolle des Krankenhauses in der Gesundheitsversorgung werden gleiche Patienten unter der Annahme technologisch identischer Produktionsfunktionen zumindest an verschiedenen Stellen einer über den Krankenhausbereich hinaus definierten Gesundheitsproduktionsfunktion versorgt.

Ein Beispiel macht die Auswirkungen einer (Nicht)berücksichtigung der systembedingten Einflüsse auf die Gesundheitsproduktionsfunktion deutlich: Gibt es in einer Region I eine Unterversorgung mit Plätzen in Pflegeeinrichtungen, so kann dies – zur Sicherung eines Gesundheitszustands, welcher einer im Pflegebereich voll versorgten Region II vergleichbar ist – für eine Fallgruppe mit ausschließlich pflegebedürftigen Krankenhauspatienten zu einer Ausweitung der Akutkrankenhausversorgung über die medizinisch notwendige Verweildauer führen. Eine Produktspezifikation nach der Produktionsfunktion vom Typ (der Region) II führt bei technologisch effizienter Produktion in der Region I zur Schlechterstellung der pflegebedürftigen Krankenhauspatienten, nach dem Typ I in der Region II möglicherweise zur Förderung ineffizienter Belegung.

Aus diesen Überlegungen stellt sich einer empirischen Produktspezifikation, sei sie allgemein fallbezogen oder direkt auf den Gesundheitsstatus gerichtet, die zentrale Frage, welche Elemente der schwerlich identifizierbaren technologischen Relation von Krankenhausleistungen und Gesundheit, aber auch welche institutionellen und welche systembedingten Elemente der realen Ausgestaltung des Versorgungsprozesses in der Produktspezifikation berücksichtigt werden.

Abbildung 1 illustriert die Unterschiede der beobachtbaren Produktionsprozesse am Beispiel der markanten Unterschiede in der Verweildauer deutscher und amerikanischer Patienten in Akutkrankenhäusern.[44] Deutlicher noch als Mittelwertunterschiede (bundesrepublikanische Patienten: 15,1 Tage; amerikanische Patienten: 6,9 Tage) zeigt die prozentuale Häufigkeitsver-

---

[43] Im Zusammenhang mit dem gleichen Phänomen bei empirischen Kostenfunktionsschätzungen, die keine Minimalkostenkombination beobachten, hat Evans (1971) die Bezeichnung "behavioral cost function" geprägt; konsequenterweise fehlt diesem Funktionstyp auch die Eigenschaft der Dualität zur technisch effizienten Produktionsfunktion, vgl. Grannemann et al. (1986), S. 109f.

[44] Die beiden Datensätze werden detailliert besprochen in Leidl 1987, S. 62–63 u. S. 108

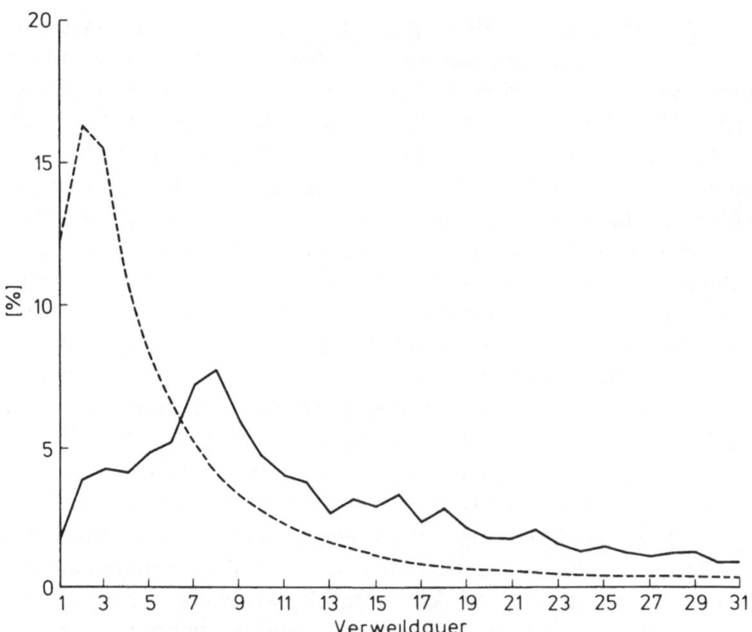

Abb. 1. Prozentuale Verteilung der Verweildauer deutscher (——) und amerikanischer (----) Krankenhauspatienten. Datenquellen: Diagnose- und Therapie-Index (DTI) von Infratest Gesundheitsforschung, 1982, 6082 Fälle; National Hospital Discharge Survey (NHDS) des US National Center for Health Statistics, 1983, 206 027 Fälle; jeweils ungewichtete Berechnung aus den nationalen Stichproben, d. h. nicht landesrepräsentativ

teilung, daß der Großteil der amerikanischen Patienten signifikant weniger lang im Krankenhaus versorgt wird (und nicht einige Langzeitfälle den Mittelwert der deutschen Patienten bestimmen). Über die Hälfte (53,4 %) der amerikanischen Patienten blieb weniger als 5 Tage im Krankenhaus. Der entsprechende Anteil für die bundesrepublikanischen Patienten beträgt etwa ein Siebtel (13,8 %). Auf die möglichen Ursachen dieser Unterschiede braucht an dieser Stelle nicht weiter eingegangen zu werden; sie mögen in der unterschiedlichen Abgrenzung zum ambulanten Bereich,[45] in anderen Finanzierungs- und Versicherungsbedingungen oder in einem unterschiedlichen Angebot an Nachsorge- und Pflegeeinrichtungen zu suchen sein. Ausschließlich in Morbiditätsunterschieden sind sie sicherlich nicht begründet.[46] Schon wegen der unterschiedlichen Aufenthaltsdauer dürften sich jedoch die Faktorintensitäten im Krankenhaus unterscheiden. Die Akutkrankenhausversorgung, so läßt sich folgern, spielt in den USA eine andere Rolle bei der Gesundung der Patienten als in der Bundesrepublik Deutschland. Eine entsprechende Vorsicht bei der Übertragung von Produktspezifikationen, die anhand des beobachteten Produktionsprozesses empirisch entwickelt wurden, scheint angebracht. Fetter et al. fanden im Vergleich französischer und amerikanischer Daten, daß die Verweildauer der französischen Krankenhauspatienten generell 1,5fach über den amerikanischen Vergleichswerten lag, daß die

---

[45] Die Verbindung zwischen ambulantem und stationärem Sektor in den USA ist dem bundesrepublikanischen Belegarztsystem vergleichbar, s. Münnich (1983), S. 67.
[46] Vgl. dazu Tabelle A1 (Leidl 1987, S. 165–167), in der diagnosespezifische Verweildauern mit analogen hohen Unterschieden ausgewiesen werden.

(DRG-)Spezifikationsstruktur bezüglich der Operationen und Diagnosen ähnlich war, sich aber die Alters- und Multimorbiditätseffekte auf die Verweildauer zwischen beiden Ländern unterschieden.[47]

Faßt man die bisherige Diskussion zum Output des Krankenhauses zusammen, so erscheint weder eine Verwendung der durch die Krankenhausleistungen erbrachten, zusätzlichen Gesundheit möglich, da selbst nach einer generell akzeptierten Lösung einer Messung und Bewertung des Gesundheitsstatus die Problematik der Zurechenbarkeit verbleibt, noch stellt die Verwendung von Krankenhausleistungsvariablen aus den oben angeführten Gründen eine Lösung der Outputspezifikation dar. Als Alternative zu diesen Vorgehensweisen bietet sich die Spezifikation des Produkts durch die patientenbezogene Versorgungsaufgabe, d. h. als eine vom Aufgabenumfang, nicht vom Ergebnis her definierte personenbezogene Dienstleistung an. Theoretisch läßt sich diese Spezifikation der Krankenhausprodukte interpretieren als Spezifikation von Fällen, in denen gleiche Eigenschaftsbündel, die aber technologisch durchaus aus unterschiedlichen Leistungsbündeln hervorgehen können, zu produzieren sind.[48] Medizinisch mehr oder weniger ähnliche Fälle, in deren Definition im übrigen durchaus verschiedene Elemente des Gesundheitsstatus als Problem-, nicht als Outputdefinition mit eingehen können, werden bei einem ähnlichen („homogenen") Ressourcenverbrauch als Produkte, als Fälle eines Typs von Versorgungsaufgaben spezifiziert. Wegen der impliziten Annahme eines qualitativ gleichen Beitrags der für die Versorgungsaufgabe erbrachten Leistungen zum "outcome" muß diese Definition eines Krankenhausprodukts freilich ebenfalls als ein Hilfskonstrukt gelten. In der praktischen Anwendung macht dies zusätzlich zur Prüfung, ob gleich spezifizierte Produkte wirklich homogen sind, eine Qualitätskontrolle der Versorgungsleistung erforderlich.

Da in die Versorgung der Fälle neben den unmittelbar patientenbezogenen Merkmalen auch unterschiedliche Versorgungsbedingungen in den Untersuchungsgebieten mit eingehen, sind auch diese als potentielle Elemente der Spezifikation oder ihrer späteren Bewertung anzusehen, obwohl sie nicht zu den technologischen Relationen einer Produktionsfunktion zu rechnen sind. Die folgende Übersicht zeigt ohne Anspruch auf Vollständigkeit eine Zusammenfassung von wichtigen potentiellen Spezifikationsvariablen.

Die Entscheidung, welche der Determinanten der Versorgung bzw. der Ressourcenverbrauchsvariablen mit in die Spezifikation eingehen, ist auch eine Entscheidung darüber, welche Determinanten als berücksichtigungsfähig (d. h. bei einer produktbezogenen Finanzierung als erstattungsfähig) gelten, und welche Determinanten demgegenüber als nicht integrierte Versorgungsrisiken neben der

---

[47] Fetter et al. (1983).

[48] Gleiche Eigenschaften sind im Sinn einer gleichen Outcomequalität zu verstehen; vgl. zum Eigenschaftsansatz ("characteristics") Lancaster (1979), Kap. 2; der Lancaster-Ansatz wurde auch in der ökonomischen Diskussion zur Produktqualität aufgegriffen; s. White (1977) oder Leland (1977); in einem Integrationsversuch der ökonomischen und medizinischen Qualitätsdiskussion verwenden ihn Doessel u. Marshall (1985) als konzeptionelle Basis einer – leider nur theoretischen gezeigten – ergebnisorientierten Qualitätsmessung von Gesundheitsversorgung.

Verschiedene Variablentypen zur Beschreibung eines Versorgungsfalls

---

1) Patientenvariablen:
Alter, Geschlecht, sozioökonomische Variable, Diagnosen, Multimorbidität (Diagnosenzahl, Begleiterkrankungen, Komplikationen), Funktionseinschränkungen, Befindlichkeit, Pflegebedürftigkeit, Veränderungen des Gesundheitsstatus, Stand der Vorbehandlungen, Krankheitsepisode.

2) Krankenhausvariablen:
Versorgungsstufe, Personal- und Sachausstattungsindikatoren, Lehrstatus, Belegarzt-, Beteiligungs-, Ermächtigungsstatus.

3) Systemvariablen:
Angebot an substitutiven Versorgungseinrichtungen (z. B. Dichte von Pflegebetten, Anteil der Belegärzte etc.).

Spezifikation verbleiben.[49] Die nichtberücksichtigten Einflußfaktoren des Ressourcenverbrauchs können z. B. bei fallpauschalierter Finanzierung Anbieter wie Nachfrager treffen, wie folgende Überlegung verdeutlicht:

> Durch die prä- und poststationäre Betreuung sei bei einem bestimmten Falltyp eine Verkürzung der Krankenhausverweildauer bei belegärztlicher Behandlung möglich. Liegt in diesem Falltyp der Anteil belegärztlicher Fälle hoch genug, um auch die als Norm verwendete durchschnittliche Verweildauer zu senken, führt eine Nichtberücksichtigung der Belegarzttätigkeit zu finanziellen Anreizen, die nicht belegärztlich versorgten Fälle qualitativ schlechter zu versorgen bzw. bei dennoch gleicher Versorgungsqualität zu Defiziten für das Krankenhaus.

Das Beispiel zeigt nochmals die generelle ökonomische Bedeutung unterschiedlicher Lösungen der bereits bei der Gesundheitsproduktion erwähnten Zurechenbarkeitsproblematik von Systemrestriktionen bei der Spezifikation von Produkten auf. Die Bestimmung der Ressourcenverbrauchsdeterminanten, die bei einer Produktspezifikation berücksichtigt werden, ist daher letztlich auch als eine gesundheits- und kostendämpfungspolitische Frage anzusehen.

Ansätze zum Einbezug der Fallmischung im Krankenhaus

Die vorangegangenen Überlegungen gingen bereits von einer fallbezogenen Produktspezifikation im Krankenhaus aus, ohne daß im einzelnen die möglichen Konzeptionen eines Einbezugs der Fallmischung näher geprüft wurden. Im folgenden wird das fallbezogene Konzept der Fallmischung seinen konzeptionellen Alternativen in systematisierender und methodisch präzisierender Weise gegenübergestellt. Eine über den pauschalen Pflegetag hinaus differenzierende Erfassung der Struktur der zu versorgenden Patientenschaft des Krankenhauses (in der amerikanischen Literatur auch als "case mix" bezeichnet) muß nämlich nicht grundsätzlich in einer mehrdimensionalen Größe, d. h. vektoriell, erfolgen und

---

[49] Auf diesen Risikoaspekt weist auch – im Zusammenhang mit dem Honorierungssystem im ambulanten Bereich – Schulenburg (1980), S. 266 hin.

Tabelle 1. Konzeptionelle Dimensionen des Einbezugs der Fallmischung

Bezugspunkt	Typ des Fallmischungsmaßes/-indikators			
	Vektoriell[a]		Skalar[b]	
Institutionen	Krankenhaus Gruppierungsverfahren	(I)	Informations- theoretische Maße	(II)
Patienten	Patientenklassifikations- verfahren	(III)	Patientenbezogene Indizes	(IV)

[a] Im Fall mehrdimensionaler und hierarchisch untergliederter Maße wäre es exakter, von Matrizentypen zu sprechen.

[b] Hierunter sind metrische und ordinal skalierte Maße einzuordnen.

sich auch, abhängig von der jeweiligen Fragestellung, nicht zwangsläufig auf einzelne Patienten beziehen.[50] So wurden in der Literatur neben den eigentlichen Patientenklassifikationsverfahren auch eine Reihe von anderen Größen als Indikatoren der Fallmischung verwendet. Teilweise verarbeiten die Maße auch die in Patientenklassifikationen erstellte Information weiter und können als „Instrumente zweiter Ordnung" bezeichnet werden.

Tabelle 1 verdeutlicht die verschiedenen konzeptionellen Ansatzmöglichkeiten, die im weiteren anhand von Beispielen aus der Literatur erläutert werden. Dabei ist zu beachten, daß bei der Einteilung Institutionen bzw. Patienten die Bezugspunkte, d. h. die letztlich verwendeten Beobachtungseinheiten, darstellen und nicht die im Maß verwendeten Variablentypen. So können etwa Krankenhausgruppierungsverfahren sowohl auf institutionellen Indikatoren der Fallmischung (z. B. dem Vorhandensein der Personal- und Sachkapazitäten für Operationen am offenen Herzen) als auch auf institutionell aggregierten Patientenvariablen (z. B. Diagnosen) beruhen. Nicht alle Maße bzw. einzelne Indikatoren sind auch direkt und für sich genommen zur Produktspezifikation, etwa zu Finanzierungszwecken, einsetzbar. Sie können aber als Standardisierungsverfahren der Fallmischung in die Spezifikation des zu produzierenden Outputs oder in seine Bewertung mit eingehen.

Zu I:

Zu den vektoriellen, institutionenbezogenen Maßen sind im weitesten Sinn alle krankenhausspezifischen Variablen zu zählen, die Hinweise auf die tatsächlich versorgte oder zumindest die potentiell versorgbare Fallmischung geben, etwa die quantitative Struktur der Fachabteilungen (nach ihrer Bettengröße oder der behandelten Fallzahl) oder Charakterisierungen durch einzelne Ausstattungsmerkmale wie das Vorhandensein bestimmter medizinisch-technischer Großgeräte oder Personalqualifikationen, aber letztlich auch Bettengröße des Krankenhauses insgesamt, Versorgungsstufe (die, wie die Versorgungsstufen I–III der

---

[50] Zur Unterscheidung patienten- und institutionsbezogener Maße der Fallmischung vgl. Office of Technology Assessment (1983), S. 13 oder Breyer (1986), S. 267f., der auch noch „leistungsbezogene" Maße unterscheidet; letztlich mussen aber auch diese wieder auf die Beobachtungseinheiten Patient oder Krankenhaus bezogen werden.

bayerischen Krankenhausbedarfsplanung,[51] gegebenenfalls auch als ordinal skalierte Maße unter der Kategorie (II) einzuordnen wären), der Lehrstatus des Krankenhauses und ähnliche Variablen. Die Grenzen für die Beispiele möglicher Fallmischungsindikatoren, die in manchen Studien auch ohne ausdrücklichen Bezug auf ihre Funktion als Indikatoren unterschiedlicher Produktspektren verwendet werden, sind hier sehr weit gezogen, um diesen Ansatztyp zu verdeutlichen. Exemplarisch wird daher auf den meistverwendeten Indikator, nämlich die Fachabteilungsstruktur, eingegangen.

Die Quantifizierung der Fachabteilungsstruktur ist, ohne weitere, aufwendige Verfahren in Anspruch zu nehmen, eine naheliegende, oft verwendete und auch heute noch gebräuchliche Form der Operationalisierung der Fallmischung im Krankenhaus. Mit das bekannteste Beispiel sind die ersten Kostenschätzungen Feldsteins.[52] Diese Methode wurde aber auch in den jüngsten amerikanischen Beiträgen zur Kostenschätzung[53] sowie bei Schätzungen von Krankenhauskostenfunktionen in der Bundesrepublik Deutschland verwendet und in Arbeiten zur Krankenhausbedarfsplanung[54] als Hilfsgröße für einen Einbezug von Morbidität eingesetzt. Freilich ist die Fachabteilungsstruktur nur ein sehr grober Indikator, vor allem im Längsschnitt und auf der Aggregationsebene des gesamten Krankenhaussystems, da qualitätsverbessernde Spezialisierungen im Zeitablauf, wie beispielsweise die Eröffnung weiterer Intensivabteilungen, als Morbiditätsverschlechterung gedeutet werden könnten. Letztere Überlegung verdeutlicht auch generell Einschränkungen der Nützlichkeit von leistungsbezogenen Maßen als Fallmischungsindikatoren.

Am Rande erwähnt seien noch Ansätze, die aus mehreren institutionenbezogenen Indikatoren eigene Taxonomien der Krankenhäuser entwickelt haben, um über die Erfassung der Zusammensetzung des Leistungspotentials auf die Fallmischungskomplexität zu schließen. So ermittelte Berry eine hierarchische Krankenhausgruppierung mit 5 Kategorien. Spätere Wiederholungen dieses clusteranalytischen Ansatzes konnten die von Berry gefundene Gruppierung jedoch nicht mehr bestätigen.[55]

Zu den Krankenhausgruppierungsverfahren ist ferner noch die "Grade of Membership Analysis" zu zählen, ein nichtparametrischer Ansatz zur Beschreibung der stochastischen Zugehörigkeit von Krankenhäusern zu (mit dem Ansatz ebenfalls ermittelten, und sich gegenseitig auch überlappenden) Idealtypen. Der Ansatz verwendet medizinische wie soziale, patientenbezogene Klassifikationsvariablen und hat sich eine einzelkrankenhausspezifische Anpassung des Preisniveaus bei der monetären Bewertung von klassifizierten Fällen zum Ziel gesetzt.[56]

Zu II:

Exemplarisch für den zweiten Ansatz, den skalaren institutionenbezogenen Fallmischungsmaßnahmen, werden 2 Größen, die jedoch beide patientenbezogene

---

[51] Bayerisches Staatsministerium für Arbeit und Sozialordnung (1986), S. 8.
[52] Feldstein (1967).
[53] Grannemann et al. (1986).
[54] Schäfer u. Wachtel (1986) und (1985).
[55] Berry (1973) sowie Klastorin u. Watts (1982).
[56] Vertrees u. Manton (1986) sowie Manton u. Vertrees (1984).

Diagnosedaten benötigen, diskutiert: ein informationstheoretisches Maß und ein Ressourcenbedarfsindex.

Das informationstheoretische Fallmischungsmaß wird auch als ein Entropiemaß bezeichnet und geht auf eine Entwicklung von Theil[57] zurück. Es wurde von Evans und Walker[58] erstmalig im Krankenhausbereich eingesetzt. Das Maß wurde zu Kostenschätzungen eingesetzt und basiert auf der vereinfacht formulierten Annahme, daß besonders schwere und ausgefallene Krankenhausfälle in nur wenigen Krankenhäusern konzentriert sind und, im Umkehrschluß, die Konzentration der Fälle über die Krankenhäuser selbst als Indikator für die Schwere der institutionellen Fallmischung verwendet werden kann. Die Validität dieses Instruments steht und fällt mit der Gültigkeit seiner Annahmen.[59] Krankenhäuser mit starker Spezialisierung müssen aber nicht notwendigerweise auch besonders ressourcenaufwendige Fälle behandeln. Es liegen auch Arbeiten vor, die ressourcenorientierte Patientenklassifikationen anstelle einfacher Diagnosen verwendeten.[60]

Ein zweiter skalarer Index ist der Resource-Need-Index (RNI), der von der amerikanischen Commission on Professional and Hospital Activities entwickelt wurde.[61] Der RNI könnte teilweise auch zu den Patientenklassifikationssystemen gerechnet werden, da er auf einem solchen Verfahren aufbaut. Er hat jedoch einen institutionenbezogenen Index zum Ziel. Der RNI basiert auf einer Klassifikation nach 351 diagnostischen Kategorien, 5 Altersgruppen und dem (Nicht)vorliegen einer Operation; er resultiert in 3490 Kategorien. Für jede der einzelnen Kategorien wurde ein standardisierter Ressourcenverbrauchsbedarf empirisch ermittelt. Dabei wurden allerdings keine Kosten, sondern "charges", d. h. Entgelte, die von den Krankenhäusern für Versorgungsleistungen berechnet werden und in die ihre unternehmerische Politik mit eingeht, verwendet. Dies wird als ein entscheidender Mangel im Verfahren der Ressourcenbedarfsbestimmung angesehen.[62] Der RNI ist mit anderen monetär bewerteten Maßen hoch korreliert[63] und wurde als Fallmischungsindex bei Analysen der Verweildauer und bei Kostenschätzungen eingesetzt.[64]

Zu III:

Zu den Patientenklassifikationen gehören einmal alle rein medizinisch orientierten Taxonomien, also krankheitsartenbezogenen Klassifikationen, mit der International Codification of Diseases als dem bekanntesten Klassifikationssystem,

---

[57] Theil (1971), S. 636ff.

[58] Evans u. Walker (1972); zur technischen Beschreibung s auch Horn u. Schumacher (1979) sowie Klastorin u. Watts (1980).

[59] Office of Technology Assessment (1983), S. 14.

[60] Zur Kostenschätzung z. B. Barer (1982), zur Kombination mit den DRGs Horn u. Schumacher (1979).

[61] Zur Beschreibung des RNI z. B. Sloan u. Becker (1981), S. 230 sowie Office of Technology Assessment (1983), S. 14.

[62] Office of Technology Assessment (1983), S. 14.

[63] Vgl. Watts u. Klastorin (1980) zur nahezu vollständigen Korrelation mit dem alten DRG-System (vgl. hierzu Leidl 1987, S. 38–40).

[64] Sloan u. Valvona (1986); Becker u. Sloan (1983) und (1981).

die v. a. für Mortalitätsstatistiken konzipiert waren.[65] Patientenklassifizierende Ansätze reichen von Verfahren, die auf anderen Krankheitsdefinitionen beruhen (s. oben), oder solchen, die speziell auf Qualitätssicherungsaspekte ausgerichtet sind, bis zu den ressourcenorientierten Fallklassifikationen, in denen Patientencharakteristika als Determinanten einer Ressourcenverbrauchsgröße in Klassen zusammengefaßt werden. Die einzelnen Krankheitsklassen sind dann die spezifizierten Produkte. Diese Verfahren werden im Detail an anderer Stelle (s. Leidl 1987, S. 37–49) behandelt.

Ansätze, die unmittelbar diagnostische Variablen z. B. für Kostenschätzungen verwenden, haben sich häufig mit Problemen wie einer zu geringen Anzahl von Freiheitsgraden oder starker Kollinearität (Korrelationen unter den unabhängigen Variablen) zu befassen. In Kostenschätzstudien wurden daher auch multivariate statistische Methoden, speziell die Faktorenanalyse zu einer Vorabverdichtung der diagnostischen Informationen eingesetzt. Dieses Vorgehen hat jedoch den Nachteil, zu inhaltlich schwer interpretierbaren Spezifikationen zu führen: beispielsweise enthält ein diagnostischer Faktor aus der Arbeit von Goodisman u. Trompeter die Diagnosen normale Entbindung, Diabetes und Magengeschwür.[66]

Zu IV:

Bei den Patientenklassifikationen dienten die Patientencharakteristiken der Zuordnung zu einer Gruppe (mit dem Mittelwert als Normmaß). Stetige Ressourcenverbrauchsdeterminanten wie etwa das Alter brauchen jedoch in einem funktional-erklärenden Spezifikationsmodell nicht klassifiziert zu werden. In diesem Fall wird anstelle von diskreten Klassen eine kontinuierliche Folge von Produkten spezifiziert und für jeden Patienten eine eigene Norm, der patientenbezogene Indexwert ermittelt. Klassifikationen von stetigen Variablen sind stets mit einem Informationsverlust verbunden; die in einem Datensatz enthaltene Information wird bei einer Klassifikation a priori reduziert. Der „Lineare Verweildauer-Index" (s. Leidl 1987, S. 99–137) versucht dies zu vermeiden und aus kontinuierlichen Variablen ein Fallmischungsmaß mit unklassifizierten Zuordnungen für einzelne Patienten zu entwickeln.

Literatur

Afifi AA, Azen SP (1979) Statistical analysis. A computer oriented approach. 2nd edn. New York San Francisco London

Ament RP, Dreachslin JL, Kobrinski EK, Wood RW (1982) Three case-type classifications: suitability for use in reimbursing hospitals. MC 20/5:460ff.

Anderson GF, Steinberg EP (1984) Hospital readmissions in the medicare population. N Engl J Med 311/21:1349ff.

Arnett III, RH, Cocotas C, Freeland M, Kowalczyk G (1984) A framework for analyzing prospective payment system rate increase factors. Health Care Finan Rev 6/4:135ff.

---

[65] Zur Geschichte der Morbiditätsklassifikation s. Statistisches Bundesamt (1968), Einleitung.

[66] Goodisman u. Trompeter (1979), S. 49; vgl. auch die Zusammenstellung von Kostenschätzungen, die mit faktorenanalytischen Verdichtungen von Diagnosen arbeiten, bei Breyer (1986).

Barer ML (1982) Case mix adjustment in hospital cost analysis: information theory revisited. J Health Eco 1/1:53ff.

Barnes CA (1985) Disease staging: a clinically oriented dimension of case mix. J Am Med Rec Assoc 22ff.

Bay KS, Leatt P, Stinson SM (1982) A patient classification system for Long-term care. Med Care 20/5:468ff.

Bay KS, Leatt P, Stinson SM (1983) Cross validation of a patient classification procedure: an application of the U method. Med Care 21/1:31ff.

Bayerisches Staatsministerium für Arbeit und Sozialordnung (Hrsg) (1986) Krankenhausbedarfsplan des Freistaates Bayern. München

Becker ER, Sloan FA (1983) Utilization of hospital services: The roles of teaching, case mix, and reimbursement. Inquiry 20:248ff.

Becker GS (1965) A theorem of the allocation of time. EJ 75:493ff.

Behrends B (1981) Das Pflegesatzrecht. Ortskrankenkasse 63/19:761ff.

Belsley DA, Kuh E, Welsch RE (1980) Regression diagnostics. New York Chichester Brisbane Toronto

Bentley JD, Butler PW (1982) Measurement of case mix. Top Health Care Fin 8/4:1ff.

Benz PD, Burnham J (1985) Case study. developing product lines using ICD-9-CM-Codes. Health Care Fin Man 38ff.

Bergner M (1985) Measurement of health status. Med Care 23/5:696ff.

Berg-Schorn E (1982) Vergleich der Todesursachenstatistik in Abhängigkeit von der Verschlüsselung nach der 8. und 9. Revision des ICD. Deutsches Institut für Medizinische Dokumentation und Information. 2. Fassung, Mai. Manuskript

Berki SE, Ashcraft MLF, Newbrander WC (1984) Length of stay variations within ICDA-8 diagnosis related groups. Med Care 22/2:126ff.

Berry RE (1973) On grouping hospitals for economic analysis. Inquiry 10/4:5ff.

Boese J, Eimeren W van, Schuller A, Schwefel D (1979) Verfahrensweisen zur Analyse der Wirtschaftlichkeit ambulanter Versorgung. In: Schwefel D, Brenner G, Schwartz FW (Hrsg) Beiträge zur Analyse der Wirtschaftlichkeit ambulanter Versorgung. Köln

Bölke G (1979) Die Krankenhausgesetzgebung des Bundes und der Länder. Arzt Krankenh 1:9ff.

Bölke G (1981) Entwicklung der Krankenhausfinanzierung bis zur Gegenwart. In: Studienstiftung der Verwaltungsleiter deutscher Krankenanstalten (Hrsg) Zentrallehrgang 1981. Solingen, S 11ff.

Bortz J (1985) Lehrbuch der Statistik für Sozialwissenschaftler, 2. Auflage. Springer, Berlin Heidelberg New York Tokyo

Brewster AC, Jacobs CM, Bradbury RC (1984) Classifying severity of illness by using clinical findings. HCFR, Ann Suppl (November):107f.

Breyer F (1985) Ökonometrisch geschätzte Krankenhaus-Kostenfunktionen und ihre Verwendung in der Krankenhausvergütung. Referat 3 im Arbeitskreis 4 der Jahrestagung „Ökonomie des Gesundheitswesens" des Vereins für Socialpolitik, Saarbrücken, 16.–18. September.

Breyer F (1986) Krankenhaus-Kostenstudien. Z Betriebswirtschaft 56/3:25ff.

Broyles RW, Rosko MD (1985) A qualitative assessment of the medicare prospective payment system. Soc Sci Med 20/11:1185ff.

Bundesgesetzblatt (1985) Verordnung zur Regelung der Krankenhauspflegesätze (Bundespflegesatzverordnung-BPflV) 44:1666ff.

Bundesminister für Arbeit und Sozialordnung (Hrsg) (1981) Effektivitätsmessung und Qualitätsbeurteilung im Gesundheitswesen. Bd 51 der Reihe Gesundheitsforschung. Bonn

Bundesminister für Jugend, Familie und Gesundheit (Hrsg) (1979) Internationale Klassifikation der Krankheiten (ICD) 1979, 9. Revision. Bd 1 Systematisches Verzeichnis. Bonn

Cameron JM (1985) Case mix and resource use in long-term care. Med Care 23/4:296ff.

Caplan AL, Engelhardt HT, McCartney JJ (eds) (1981) Concepts of health and disease. Don Mills, London Amsterdam Sydney Tokyo

Carter GM, Ginsburg PB (1985) The medicare case mix index increase. Health Care Fin Res

Catania HF, Ibrahim OM, Guasco SL, Catania N (1984) Analyzing pharmacy charges using DRGs. Am J Hosp Pharm 41:920ff.

Caterinicchio RP, Davies RH (1983) Developing a client-focused allocation statistic of inpatient nursing resource use: an alternative to the patient day. Soc Sci Med 17/5:259ff.

Cavaiola LJ, Young JP (1980) An integrated system for patient assessment and classification and nurse staff allocation for long-term care facilities. Health Serv Res 15/3:281ff.

Chamberlin EH (1933) The theory of monopolistic competition. Cambridge

Chamberlin EH (1953) The product as an economic variable. Q J Eco 67/1:1ff.

Cleverly WD (1979) Evaluation of alternative payment strategies for hospitals. A conceptual approach. Inquiry 16:108ff.

Conklin JE, Liebermann JV, Barnes CA, Louis DZ (1984) Disease staging: implications for hospital reimbursement and management. Health Care Fin Rev [Suppl]:13ff.

Connell F, Blide L, Hanken MA (1984) Ambiguities in the selection of the principal diagnosis: impact on data quality, hospital statistics und DRGs. J Am Med Rec Assoc February: 18ff.

Corn RF (1980) Quality control of hospital discharge data. Med Care 18/4:416ff.

Cooney LM, Fries BF (1985) Validation of use of resource utilization groups as a case mix measure for long-term care. Med Care 23/2:123ff.

Coulton CJ, McClish D, Doremus H, Powell S, Smookler S, Jackson DL (1985) Implications of DRG payments for medical intensive care. Med Care 23/8:977ff.

McCullagh P, Nelder JA (1983) Generalized linear models. London New York

Cullis JG, West PA (1979) The economics of health. Oxford

Culyer AJ (ed) (1983) Health indicators. Oxford

Davis K (1972) Economic theories of behavior in nonprofit, private hospitals. Eco Bus Bull 24/2:1ff.

Davis K, Russel L (1972) The substitution of hospital outpatient for inpatient care. Rev Eco Stud 54/2:1ff.

Davis K, Anderson G, Steinberg E (1984) Diagnosis related groups prospective payment: implications for health care and medical technology. Health Policy 4:139ff.

Deutsche Krankenhausgesellschaft (Hrsg) (1981 a) Stellungsnahmen und Empfehlungen der DKG. Ergänzungsband zum Geschäftsbericht 1980/81. Dusseldorf

Deutsche Krankenhausgesellschaft (Hrsg) (1981 b) Krankenhaustarif für ambulante Leistungen und stationäre Nebenleistungen (DKG-NT '80), 12. Aufl. Stuttgart

Deutsches Ärzteblatt (1986) Tätigkeitsbericht zum 89. Deutschen Ärztetag. Entschließungen zu aktuellen gesundheitspolitischen Problemen. Dtsch Ärztebl 83/21:1520

Dienst für Gesellschaftspolitik (1986) Krankenhäuser: Vorstudie zu diagnoseabhängigen Fallpauschalen. 28/7:7ff.

Dobson A (1984) Prospective payment: current configuration and future direction. Unpublished manuscript presented to the Prospective Payment Assessment Commission, February 2

Doessel DP, Marshall VJ (1985) A rehabilitation of health outcome in quality assessment. Soc Sci Med 21/12:1319ff.

Donabedian A (1966) Evaluating the quality of medical care. Millbank Mem Fund Q 43:166ff.

Doremus HD, Michenzi EM (1983) Data quality: an illustration of its potential impact upon a diagnosis related group's case mix index and reimbursement. Med Care 21/10:1001ff.

Dowling WL (1974) Prospective reimbursement of hospitals. Inquiry 11:163ff.

Doyle JC (1952) Unnecessary ovarectomies. JAMA 148/13:1105ff.

Doyle JC (1953) Unnecessary hysterectomies. JAMA 151/5:360ff.

Eichhorn S (1974) Zielkonflikte zwischen Leistungsfähigkeit, Wirtschaftlichkeit und Finanzierung des Krankenhauswesens. Krankenhaus 5:186ff.

Eichhorn S (1982) Systemplanung im Krankenhaus- und Gesundheitswesen. In: Herder-Dorneich P, Sieben G, Thiemeyer T (Hrsg) Wege zur Gesundheitsökonomie II. Bd 2 der Reihe Beiträge zur Gesundheitsökonomie. Bleicher, Gerlingen, S 11ff.

Eichhorn S (1985) Einordnung des Projekts in die Diskussion zur Gesundheitsökonomie und zur Krankenhausfinanzierung. In: Bertelsmann Stiftung (Hrsg) Aufbau eines entscheidungsorientierten Informations- und Berichtswesens im Krankenhaus. Pilotstudie im Städtischen Krankenhaus Gütersloh. Bertelsmann, Gütersloh, S 8ff.

Eimeren W van (1976) Multimorbidität in der Allgemein-Praxis. Deutscher Ärzte-Verlag GmbH, Köln-Lövenich

Ellis RP, McGuire TG (1986) Provider behavior under prospective reimbursement; cost sharing and supply. J Health Eco 5/2:219ff.

Elnicki RA (1976) Substitution of outpatient for inpatient hospital care: a cost analysis. Inquiry 13:245ff.

McElwee JW (1985) Medical staff relations and physician practice in the DRG environment. Top Health Care Financ 11/3:22ff.

Ernst & Whinney (1983) The medicare prospective payment system. Ernst & Winney (No J58475), Princeton

Evans RG (1971) Behavioral cost functions for hospitals. Can J Eco 4/4:198ff.

Evans RG, Walker HD (1972) Information theory and the analysis of hospital cost structure. Can J Eco 5/3:398ff.

Fanshell S, Bush JW (1970) A health status index and its application to health services outcomes. Operations Res 18:1021ff.

Federal Register (1983) 48/Sept. 1: 39752ff.

Federal Register (1985) 50/Sept. 3: 35646ff.

Feldstein MS (1967) Economic analysis for health services efficiency. Amsterdam

Feldstein PJ (1983) Health care economics. 2nd edn. New York Chichester Brisbane Toronto Singapur

Fetter RB (1984) Diagnosis related groups: the product of the hospital. Paper presented at the Public Policy Symposium der American Federation of Clinical Research, 41. Annual Meeting, Washington D.C., May 4

Fetter RB (1985) The DRG methodology: pittfalls and adverse effects. Paper presented at the V. Journadas Economica Saude

Fetter RB, Shin Y, Freeman JL, Averill RF, Thompson JD (1980) Case mix definition by diagnosis related groups. Med Care [Suppl]:18/2

Fetter RB, Freeman JL, Mullin R, Elia R, Newbold R (1983) Comparing hospital productivity by diagnosis related groups: United States and the European Experience. Paper presented at the Annual Meeting of the American Public Health Association, Dallas, November

Fetter RB, Averill RF, Lichtenstein JL, Freeman JL (1984) Ambulatory visit groups: a framework for measuring productivity in ambulatory care. Health Serv Res 19/4:415ff.

Flanagan JG, Sourapas KJ (1984) Preparing for prospective payment. J Am Med Rec Assoc:11ff.

Fomby TB, Hill RC, Johnson SR (1984) Advanced econometric methods. Springer, Berlin Heidelberg New York Tokyo

Frank RG, Lave JR (1985) The psychiatric DRGs: are they different? Med Care 23/10:1148ff.

Fries BF, Cooney LM (1985) Resource utilization groups: a patient classification system for long-term care. Med Care 23/2:110ff.

Fuhs PA, Martin JB, Hancock WM (1979) The use of length of stay distributions to predict hospital discharges. Med Care 17/4:355ff.

Furubotn EG, Pejovich S (1972) Property rights and economic theory: a survey of recent literature. J Law Eco 10:1137ff.

Gaensslin H, Schubö W (1973) Einfache und komplexe statistische Analyse. München Basel

Galtung J (1967) Theory and methods of social research. Oslo

Gäfgen G (1981) Die Allokationswirkungen verschiedener Eigentumsrechte im Krankenhauswesen. In: Herder-Dorneich P, Sieben G, Thiemeyer T (Hrsg) Wege zur Gesundheitsökonomie I. Band 1 der Reihe Beiträge zur Gesundheitsökonomie. Gerlingen, S 101ff.

Gäfgen G (1983) Entwicklung und Stand der Property Rights: Eine kritische Bestandsaufnahme. Referat 3P auf der Arbeitstagung ‚Ansprüche, Eigentums- und Verfügungsrechte' des Vereins für Socialpolitik, Basel, 26. September

Garg ML, Louis DZ, Gliebe WA, Spirka CS, Skipper JK, Parekh RR (1978) Evaluating inpatient costs: the staging mechanism. Med Care 16/3: 191A

Gerdelmann W (1976) Krankenhausbetriebsvergleich. Ortskrankenkasse 58:649ff.

Gerdelmann W (1979) Möglichkeiten und Grenzen des Betriebsvergleichs der Spitzenverbände der gesetzlichen Krankenkassen. Krankenh Ums 7:563ff.

Gertmann PM, Lowenstein S (1984) A research paradigm for severity of illness: issues for the diagnosis related groups system. Health Care Fin Rev [Suppl]:79ff.

Gevers JKM (1983) Issues in the acceptability and confidentiality of patient records. Soc Sci Med 17/16:1181ff.

Ginsburg PG (1985) Hospital reimbursement in the United States. In: Adam D, Zweifel P (Hrsg) Preisbildung im Gesundheitswesen. Bd 9 der Reihe Beiträge zur Gesundheitsökonomie. Gerlingen, S 71ff.

Goetzke W (1980) Der Krankenhausbetriebsvergleich als Grundlage für Wirtschaftlichkeitsprüfung und Pflegesatzermittlung? Krankenhaus Ums 9:712ff.

Goldfarb MG, Hornbrook MC, Higgins CS (1983) Determinants of hospital use: a cross-diagnostic analysis. Med Care 1:48ff.

Gonnella JS, Louis DZ, McCord JJ (1976) The staging concept – an approach to the assessment of outcome of ambulatory care. Med Care 14/1:13ff.

Gonnella JS, Hornbrook MC, Louis DZ (1984a) Staging of disease: a case mix measurement. In: Eimeren W van, Engelbrecht R, Flagle CD (ed) Third international conference on system science in health care. Springer, Berlin Heidelberg New York Tokyo, pp 1090

Gonnella JS, Hornbrook MC, Louis DZ (1984b) Staging of diseases. JAMA 251/5:637ff.

Goodisman LD, Trompeter T (1979) Hospital case mix and average charge per case. Health Serv Res 14/1:44ff.

Grannemann TW, Brown RS, Pauly MV (1986) Estimating hospital costs. Effec Health Care 5/2:107ff.

Graves EJ (1984) 1983 summary: national hospital discharge survey. Advancedata 101

Grimaldi P, Micheletti JA (1983) Diagnosis related groups. A practitioners guide. Chicago

Grossman M (1972) The demand for health. A theoretical and empirical investigation. National Bureau of Economic Research, New York

Grossman M (1982) The demand for health after a decade. J Health Eco 1/1:1ff.

Gruenberg LW, Willemain TR (1982) Hospital discharge queues in Massachusetts. Med Care 20/2:188ff.

McGuire A (1985) The theory of the hospital. A review of the models. Soc Sci Med 20/11:1177ff.

Harris JE (1977) The Internal Organization of Hospitals: some economic implications. Br J Eco 8:467ff.

Hartung J, Elpelt B, Klösener KH (1982) Statistik. München Wien

Health Care Financing Administration (U.S. Department of Health and Human Services) (1980) ICD-9-CM The international classification of diseases. 9th Revision, Clinical Modification; vol 1: Diseases: Tabular List, n p (September)

Health Care Financing Administration (U.S. Department of Health and Human Services) (1983) Health Care Financing, grants and contracts report. The New ICD-9-CM Diagnosis Related Groups Classification Scheme. Baltimore

Health Research and Educational Trust (New Jersey) (1984) DRG Evaluation, vol III, case mix classification. Data, and Management, Princeton, (February)

Health Systems International DRGs (1985) Diagnosis related groups. Second Revision, Definitions Manual 2nd edn, New Haven Connecticut (October)

Henderson DP, Sullivan TV (1984) Diagnosis related groups: effects on nursing. J Emerg Nurs 10/2:117ff.

Henning J, Paffrath D (1978) Der Krankenhausbetriebsvergleich. Ortskrankenkasse 60:567ff.

Herder-Dorneich P (1981) Problemgeschichte der Gesundheitsökonomik. In: Herder-Dorneich P, Sieben G, Thiemeyer T (Hrsg) Wege zur Gesundheitsökonomie I. Band 1 der Reihe Beiträge zur Gesundheitsökonomie. Gerlingen, S 11ff.

Hockking RR (1976) The analysis and selection of variables in linear regression. Biometrics 32:1ff.

Hocking RR, Pendelton OJ (1983) The regression dilemma. Comm Stat Theor Meth 12/5:497ff.

Holland WW, Ipsen J, Kosterzewski J (eds) (1979) Measurement of levels of health. Publication of the World Health Organisation, Copenhagen

Horn SD (1981) Validity, reliability and implications of an index of inpatient severity of illness. Med Care 19/3:354ff.

Horn SD (1983) Measuring severity of illness: comparisons across institutions. Am J Publ Health 73/1:25ff.

Horn SD (1985) Hospital planning for profit. The importance of measuring severity of illness. Alabama J Med Sci 22/1:21ff.

Horn SD, Schumacher DN (1979) An analysis of case mix complexity using information theory and diagnostic related grouping. Med Care 17/4:382ff

Horn SD, Schumacher DN (1982) Comparing classification methods: measurement of variations in charges, length of stay, and mortality. Med Care 20/5:489ff.

Horn SD, Sharkey PD (1983) Measuring severity of illness to predict patient resource use within DRGs. Inquiry 20:314ff.

Horn SD, Horn RA (1986) Reliability and validity of the severity of illness index. Med Care 24/2:159ff.

Horn SD, Chachich B, Clopton C (1983) Measuring severity of illness: a reliability study. Med Care 21/7:705ff.

Horn SD, Sharkey PD, Bertram DA (1983) Measuring severity of illness: homogenous case mix groups. Med Care 21/1:14ff.

Horn SD, Horn RA, Sharkey PD (1984) The severity of illness index as a severity adjustment to diagnosis related groups. Health Care Fin Rev [Suppl]:33ff.

Horn SD, Sharkey PD, Chambers AF, Horn RA (1985) Severity of illness within DRGs: impact on prospective payment. Am J Publ Health 75/10:1195ff.

Horn SD, Bulkey G, Sharkey PD, Chambers AF, Horn RA, Schramm CS (1985) Interhospital differences in severity of illness. Problems for prospective payment based on diagnosis related groups (DRGs). N Engl J Med 313/1:20ff.

Horn SD, Horn RA, Sharkey PD, Chambers AF (1986) Severity of illness within DRGs. Homogenity Study. Med Care 24/3:225ff.

Hornbrook MC (1982) Hospital case mix: its definition, measurement, and use: part II, review of alternative measures. Med Care Rev 34:75ff.

Hornbrook MC, Goldfarb MG (1983) A partial test of a hospital behavioral model. Soc Sci Med 17/10:667ff.

Hornung CA, Massagli MP (1980) A hospital's output as a function of supply and demand characteristics. J Health Soc Behav 21/4:302ff.

Hutter M (1979) Die Gestaltung von Property Rights als Mittel gesellschaftlicher Allokation. Göttingen

Infratest (Hrsg) (1984) Sozialatlas Bundesrepublik 1983/84. Bevölkerung und Privathaushalte. München

Jeffers JR, Siebert CD (1974) Measurement of hospital cost variation: case mix, service intensity, and input productivity factors. Health Serv Res 9:293ff.

Jencks SF, Dobson A, Willis P, Feinstein PH (1984) Evaluating and improving the measurement of hospital case mix. Health Care Fin Rev [Suppl]:1ff.

Jenkins L (ed) (1986) Diagnosis related groups newsletter. CASPE Research, 14 Palace Court, London W2 4HS (June)

Jenkins L, Sanderson H (1985) (eds) Diagnosis related groups newsletter. CASPE Research, 14 Palace Court, London W2 4HS (June)

Judge GG, Hill RC, Griffith WE, Lütkepohl H, Lee TC (1982) Introduction to the theory and practice of econometrics. New York Chichester Brisbane Toronto Singapur

Katz S, Ford AB, Moscowitz RW, Jackson BA, Jaffe WM (1963) Studies of illness in the aged – The index of ADL: a standardized measure of biological and physiological function. JAMA 185/1:914ff.

McKeown T (1976) The modern rise of population. London

Kitagawa EM (1955) Components of difference between two rates. Am Stat Assoc J 50:1168ff.

Klastorin TD, Watts CA (1980) On the measurement of hospital case mix. Med Care 18/6:675ff.

Klastorin TD, Watts CA (1982) A current reappraisal of Berry's hospital typology. Med Care 20/5:441ff.

Koutsoyiannis A (1977) Theory of econometrics. 2nd edn. London Basingstoke

Koutsoyiannis A (1979) Modern microeconomics. 2nd edn. London

Kramer AM, Shaugnessy PW, Pettigrew ML (985) Cost-effectiveness implications based on a comparison of nursing home and home health case mix. Health Serv Res 20/4:387ff.

Kriedel T (1980) Effizienzanalysen von Gesundheitsprojekten. Springer, Berlin Heidelberg New York

Lancaster K (1979) Variety, equity, and efficiency. New York

Lave JR (1984) Hospital reimbursement under medicare. Health Care Fin Man 62ff.

Leidl R (1983) The hospital financing system of the Federal Republic of Germany. Effec Health Care 1/3:133ff.

Leidl R (1986) Entwicklungen im Krankenhaussektor im Lichte des Bayern-Vertrags. In: Schwefel D, Eimeren W van, Satzinger W (Hrsg) Der Bayern-Vertrag. Evaluation einer Kostendämpfungspolitik im Gesundheitswesen Heidelberg, S 269ff.

Leidl R (1987) Die fallbezogene Spezifikation des Krankenhausprodukts: ein methodischer und empirischer Beitrag. Springer, Berlin Heidelberg New York Tokyo

Leidl R, John J, Potthoff P (1986) Indikatorensysteme zur versorgungsgerechten Krankenhausplanung. In: Behrends B, Hölzer KH, Lohmann H (Hrsg) Morbiditätsorientierte Krankenhausbedarfsplanung. Scharbeutz, S 147ff.

Leland HE (1977) Quality choice and competition. Am Eco Rev 67/2:127ff.

Lienert GA (1967) Testaufbau und Testanalyse. Weinheim Berlin

Lloyd SS, Rissing P (1985) Physician and coding errors in patient records. JAMA 254/10:1330ff.

Lück HE (1976) Testen und Messen von Eigenschaften und Einstellungen. In: Koolwijk J van, Wieken-Mayser M (Hrsg) Techniken der empirischen Sozialforschung. Band 5, Testen und Messen. München Wien, S 77ff.

Luft HS (1981) How do health maintenance organizations achieve their savings? N Engl J Med 1336ff.

Magee JM, Pathak DS, Schneider D (1985) ABC analysis of the relationship between pharmacy charges and DRGs. Am J Hosp Pharm 42:571ff.

McMahon LF, Newbold R (1986) Variations in resource use within diagnosis related groups. Med Care 24/5:388ff.

Manton KG, Vertrees JC (1984) The use of grade of membership analysis to evaluate and modify diagnosis related groups. Med Care 22/12:1067ff.

May JJ, Wassermann J (1984) Selected results from an evaluation of the New Jersey Diagnosis Related Group System. Health Serv Res 19/5:547ff.

Maynard A (1984) Budgeting in health care systems. Effec Health Care 2/2:41ff.

Meiners MR, Coffey RM (1985) Hospital DRGs and the need for long-term care services: an empirical analysis. Health Serv Res 20/3:359ff.

Mendenhall S (1985) DRG winners and losers affect profits under prospective payment. Health Fin Man 62ff.

Meyer M, Wohlmannstetter V (1985) Effizienzmessung in Krankenhäusern. Z Betriebswirtschaft 55/3:262ff.

Migue JL, Belanger G (1974) The price of health. Toronto

Mills R, Fetter RB, Riedel D, Averill R (1976) AUTOGRP: An interactive computer system for the analysis of health care data. Med Care 14/7:603ff.

Müller U (1981) Aufbereitung und Auswertung der Selbstkostenblätter. Krankenh Ums 3:135ff.

Müller U (1983) DKG-Erhebung über Patientenstrukturen. Krankenhaus 10:414ff

Münnich FE (1970) Verallgemeinerung eines Tests von Chow. Stat Hefte 11:153ff.

Münnich FE (1983) Der Kostendruck macht das Medizin-Management erfinderisch. Dtsch Ärztebl 80/41:65ff.

Münnich FE (1984) Kosten- und Allokationswirkungen des technischen Fortschritts im Gesundheitswesen. In: Münnich FE, Oettle K (Hrsg) Ökonomie des technischen Fortschritts. Band 6 der Reihe Beiträge zur Gesundheitsökonomie. Gerlingen, S 13ff

Muurinen JM (1982) Demand for health. A generalized Grossman model. J Effec Health Care 1/1:5ff.

Napoleoni C (1972) Grundzüge der modernen ökonomischen Theorien. 4. Aufl. Frankfurt

National Center of Health Statistics (1983) 1983 NHDS Data Tape Documentation (unpublished manuscript). Hyattsville/MD

Neipp J (1984) Der optimale Gesundheitszustand der Bevölkerung. Methodische und empirische Fragen einer Erfolgskontrolle gesundheitspolitischer Maßnahmen. Habilitationsschrift, Universität Heidelberg

Neubauer G, Unterhuber H (1985) Failures of the hospital financing system of the Federal Republic of Germany and reform proposals. Effec Health Care 2/4:162ff.

Neubauer G, Unterhuber H (1986) Ökonomische Beurteilung einer Fallgruppenbildung im Krankenhaus. In: Neubauer G, Sonnenholzner-Roche A, Unterhuber H (Hrsg) Fallbezogene Krankenhausvergütung mit Hifle von DRGs. Diskussionsbeiträge des Instituts für Volkswirtschaftslehre. Hochschule der Bundeswehr München (29) August

Neubauer G, Sonnenholzner-Roche A, Unterhuber H (1986) Die Problematik einer Fallgruppenbildung im Krankenhaus. In: Neubauer G, Sonnenholzner-Roche A, Unterhuber H (Hrsg) Fallbezogene Krankenhausvergütung mit Hilfe von DRGs. Diskussionsbeiträge des Instituts für Volkswirtschaftslehre. Hochschule der Bundeswehr München (29) August

Neuhauser D (1983) DRGs in Jersey. Effec Health Care 1/3:153

Nunamaker TR (1983) Measuring routine nursing services efficiency: a comparison of costs per patient day and data envelopment analysis models. Health Serv Res 18/2:183ff.

Oettle K (1984) Vergleichende mikroökonomische Analyse des Steuerungsmechanismus auf der Allokations- und Produktionsebene im stationären Bereich des Gesundheitswesens. In: Neubauer G (Hrsg) Alternativen der Steuerung des Gesundheitswesens. Bd 13 der Reihe Beiträge zur Gesundheitsökonomie. Gerlingen, S 309ff.

Oettle K (1986) Steuerung durch Selbstverwaltung, insbesondere im Krankenhauswesen. Vortrag auf der Tagung ‚Aus- und Fortbildung in Gesundheitsökonomie' der Weltgesundheitsorganisation und des MEDIS-Instituts, Neuherberg, 26. Juni

Office of Technology Assessment (U.S. Congress) (1983) Diagnosis Related Groups (DRGs) and the medicare program: implications for medical technology – a technical memorandum. Washington

Omenn GS, Conrad DA (1984) Implications of DRGs for clinicians. N Engl J Med 311/20:1314ff.

Ott AE (1974) Grundzüge der Preistheorie. 2. Aufl. Göttingen

Pauly MV, Redisch M (1973) The not-for-profit hospital as a physician's cooperative. Adv Enzyme Regul 87ff.

Pettengill J, Vertrees J (1982) Reliability and validity in hospital case mix measurement. Health Care Fin Rev 4/2:101ff.

Plomann MP (1982) Case mix classification systems: development. Description and testing. Chicago

Plomann MP, Shaffer FA (1983) DRGs as one of nine approaches to case mix in transition. Nurs Health Care 438ff.

Pokras R, Kubishke KK (1985) Diagnosis Related Groups using data from the National Hospital discharge survey: United States, 1982. Advancedata 105 (January)

Polissar L, Diehr P (1982) Regression analysis in Health Services Research: the use of dummyvariables. Med Care 20/9:959ff.

Prahl G (1986) Ein Kassenarzt senkt Krankenhauskosten. Selecta 17:1326ff.

Rafferty JA (1972) Hospital output indices. Eco Bus Bull 24/2:21ff.

Reif RA, Bickett PA, Halberstadt DE (1985) Case study: analyzing the market using DRGs and MDCs HFM 44ff.

Rines JT (1985) Prospective payment: unanswered ethical questions. J Am Med Rec Assoc March: 20ff.

Robert Bosch Stiftung (Hrsg) (1983) Zwischenbericht der Kommission Krankenhausfinanzierung der Robert Bosch Stiftung. Materialien und Berichte Nr. 12. Stuttgart

Robinson J (1933) The economics of imperfect competition. London

Rogerson CL, Stims DH, Simborg DW, Charles G (1985) Classification of ambulatory care using patient-based timeoriented indexes. Med Care 23/6:780ff.

Roos LL, Roos NP, Cageorge SM, Nicol JP (1982) How good are the Data. Med Care 20/3:266ff.

Rüschmann HH (1986) Kieler Krankenhausstudie: Kostendämpfung durch „diagnosebezogene Festpreise". Dtsch Ärztebl 24:1760ff.

Rupp A, Steinwachs M, Salkever DS (1985) Hospital payment effects on acute inpatient care for mental disorders. Arch of Gen Psychiatry 42:552ff.

SAS (Institute Inc) (1985a) SAS users guide basics. Version 5 Edn. Cary/NC

SAS (Institute Inc) (1985b) SAS users guide statistics. Version 5 Edn. Cary/NC

SAS (Institute Inc) (1985c) SAS/GRAPH users guide. Version 5 Edn. Cary/NC

Salkever DS, Skinner EA, Steinwachs DM, Katz H (1982) Episode-based efficiency comparisons for physicians and nurse practitioners. Med Care 20/2:143ff.

Satzinger W (1986) Der Bayern-Vertrag. Ziele, Hintergrund, Programm. In: Schwefel D, Eimeren W van, Satzinger W (Hrsg) Der Bayern-Vertrag. Evaluation einer Kostendämpfungspolitik im Gesundheitswesen. Heidelberg, S 1ff.

Schäfer T, Wachtel HW (1985) Krankenhausbedarfspläne. Ortskrankenkasse 12:493ff.

Schäfer T, Wachtel HW (1986) Die Ermittlung der Bedarfsdeterminanten für die Krankenhausbedarfsplanung in Baden-Württemberg. In: Behrends B, Hölzer KH, Lohmann H (Hrsg) Morbiditätsorientierte Krankenhausbedarfsplanung. Scharbeutz, S 62ff.

Schellhaass U (1971) Ökonomische Probleme des Krankenhauses und seiner Finanzierung. Soz Fortschr 3:54ff.

Schlenker RE, Shaugnessy PW, Yslas I (1985) Estimating patient-level nursing home costs. Health Serv Res 20/1:103ff.

Schneeweiss H (1978) Ökonometrie. 3. Aufl. Würzburg Wien
Schneeweiss R, Rosenblatt RA, Cherkin DC, Kirkwood CR, Hart G (1983) Diagnosis clusters:
    a new tool for analyzing the content of ambulatory medical care. Med Care 21/1:105ff.
Schneider D (1979) An ambulatory care classification system: design, development and evalua-
    tion. Health Serv Res 14/1:77ff
Schroeder E (1983) Concepts of health and illness. In· Culyer AJ (ed) Health indicators. Oxford,
    pp 23
Schüller A (1983) Property Rights und ökonomische Theorie. München
Schulenburg JM Graf von der (1980) Systeme der Honorierung frei praktizierender Ärzte und
    ihre Allokationswirkungen. Dissertation, Universität München
Schwartz FW (1981) Zur Validität von Diagnosen auf Krankenscheinen. In: Eimeren W van,
    Redler E (Hrsg) Probleme der Sekundäranalyse von Routinedaten der Gesetzlichen Kran-
    kenversicherung. Bericht der Gesellschaft für Strahlen- und Umweltforschung. München
    (MD 468), S 15ff.
Schwefel D (1986a) Explorative Forschung in der Gesundheitsökonomie Vortrag auf der Ta-
    gung ,Aus- und Fortbildung in Gesundheitsökonomie' der Weltgesundheitsorganisation
    und des MEDIS-Instituts. Neuherberg, 26. Juni
Schwefel D (1986b) Unemployment, health and Health Services in German speaking countries.
    Soc Sci Med 22/4:409ff.
Schwefel D, Schwartz FW (1978) Aussagefähigkeit und Auswertbarkeit von Diagnosen in der
    ambulanten medizinischen Versorgung – Ein Problemüberblick. In: Schwartz FW, Schwefel
    D (Hrsg) Diagnosen in der ambulanten Versorgung. Köln-Lövenich, S 7ff.
Schwefel D, Eimeren W van, Satzinger W (Hrsg) (1986) Der Bayern-Vertrag. Evaluation einer
    Kostendämpfungspolitik im Gesundheitswesen. Springer, Berlin Heidelberg New York To-
    kyo
Schwefel D, John J, Potthoff P, Eimeren W van (1986) Diagnosenstruktur in der ambulanten
    Versorgung. Explorative Auswertungen. Heidelberg
Schweitzer SD, Rafferty JA (1976) Variations in hospital product: a comparative analysis of
    proprietary and voluntary hospitals. Inquiry 3:158ff.
Scitovsky A (1985) Changes in the costs of treatment of seleceted illnesses, 1971–1981. Med Care
    23/12:1345ff.
Sherman HD (1984) Hospital efficiency measurement and evaluation: empirical test of a new
    technique. Med Care 22/10:922ff.
Siebig J (1980) Beurteilung der Wirtschaftlichkeit im Krankenhaus. Stuttgart Berlin Köln Mainz
Siegel C, Alexander MJ, Lin S, Laska E (1986) An alternative to DRGs. A clinically meaningful
    and cost-reducing approach. Med Care 24/5:407ff.
Siegmann AE (1977) Readiness of sociomedical sciences to measure health status. In: Elinson J,
    Mooney A, Siegmann AE (eds) Health goals and health indicators: policy, planning, and
    evaluation. Boulder/CO, pp 65ff.
Simborg DW (1981) DRG creep. A new hospital acquired disease. N Engl J Med 304/26:1602ff.
Sloan FA, Becker ER (1981) Internal organization of hospitals and hospital costs. Inquiry
    18:224ff.
Sloan FA, Steinwald B (1980) Insurance, regulation and hospital costs. Lexington
Sloan FA, Valvona J (1986) Why has hospital length of stay declined? An evaluation of alterna-
    tive theories. Soc Sci Med 22/1:63ff.
Smits HL (1984) Incentives in case mix measures for long-term care. Health Care Fin Rev
    6/2:53ff.
Smits HL, Fetter RB, McMahon LF (1984) Variation in resource use within diagnosis related
    groups. Health Care Fin Rev [Suppl]:71ff.
Sommer JH (1983) Kostenkontrolle im Gesundheitswesen. Diessenhofen
Statistisches Bundesamt (Hrsg) (1968) Internationale Klassifikation der Krankheiten (ICD)
    1968. 8. Revision, Bd 1, Systematisches Verzeichnis. Stuttgart Mainz
Stern RS, Epstein AM (1985) Institutional responses to prospective payment based on diagnosis
    related groups, implications for cost, quality and access. N Engl J Med 312/10:621ff.
Studienstiftung der Verwaltungsleiter deutscher Krankenanstalten (Hrsg) (1984) Zentrallehr-
    gang 1984. Berlin 3.–5. April
Tamura H, Lauer LW, Sandorn FA (1985) Estimating "reasonable costs" of medicaid patient
    care using a patient mix index. Health Serv Res 20/1:27

Theil H (1971) Principles of Econometrics. Amsterdam

Thompson JD (1984) The measurement of nursing intensity. Health Care Fin Rev [Suppl]:47ff.

Thompson JS (1982) Diagnosis related groups and quality assurance. Top Health Care Fin 8/4:43ff.

Thurmayr R, Potthoff P, Diehl R (1986) Schweregradbestimmung chronischer Erkrankungen. I. Ergebnisüberblick zum VDR-Gesamtprojekt. Rentenversicherung 7/8:493ff.

Tischmann P (1983) „Selbsteinweisungen der Krankenhäuser". Ortskrankenkasse 14/15:629ff.

Torrance GW (1986) Measurement of health status utilities for economic appraisal. J Health Eco 5/1:1ff.

Unterhuber H (1986) Preissteuerung in der Krankenhausversorgung. Möglichkeiten und Grenzen der Anwendung von Preisen zur Steuerung der Versorgung mit Krankenhausleistungen. Dissertation, Universität Neubiberg

Vertrees JC, Manton KG (1986) A multivariate approach for classifying hospitals and computing blended payment rates. Med Care 24/4:283ff.

Wagner DP, Draper EA (1984) Acute physiology and chronic health evaluation (APACHE II) and medicare reimbursement. Health Care Fin Rev [Suppl]:91ff.

Watts CA, Klastorin TD (1980) The impact of case mix on hospital costs: a comparative analysis. Inquiry 17:357ff.

Wennberg JE, McPherson K, Caper P (1984) Will payment based on diagnosis related groups control hospital costs? N Eng J Med 311/5:295ff.

White LJ (1977) Market structure and product varieties. Am Eco Rev 67/2:179ff.

Williams SV, Kominski GF, Dowd BE, Soper KA (1984) Methodological limitations in case mix hospital reimbursement, with a proposal for change. Inquiry 21:17ff.

Young WW (1984) Incorporating severity of illness and comorbidity in case mix measurement. Health Care Fin Rev [Suppl]:23ff.

Young WW, Swinkola RB, Hutton MA (1980) Assessment of the AUTOGRP patient classification system. Med Care 18/2:228ff.

Young WW, Swinkola RB, Zorn DM (1982) The measurement of hospital case mix. Med Care 20/5:501ff.

Zaretsky HW (1977) The effects of patient mix and service mix on hospital costs and productivity. Top Health Care Fin 4/2:63ff.

Zellas A (1984) Some remarks on criteria for the selection of regressors in econometric models. In: Gruber E (ed) Multicollinearity and biased estimation. Heft 27 der Reihe ‚Angewandte Statistik und Ökonometrie'. Göttingen, pp 11ff.

Zwerenz K (1982) Nachfrage und Angebot im stationären Bereich des Gesundheitswesens. Bochum

Weiterführende Literatur zum Thema „Gesundheitsökonomie"

Andersen HH, Schulenburg JM Graf von der (1987) Kommentierte Bibliographie zur Gesundheitsökonomie. Sigma, Berlin
Robert-Bosch-Stiftung (Hrsg) (1982 ff.) Beiträge zur Gesundheitsökonomie. Bleicher, Gerlingen
Verein für Socialpolitik (1984) Tagungsband der Jahrestagung 1984

5 Gesundheits- und Sozialpolitik, Verwaltung und Recht im Gesundheitswesen

Gesundheitsziele – Chancen
für ein ge-/zergliedertes Gesundheitswesen *

B.-P. Robra

In führenden Industriestaaten gewinnen in den letzten Jahren explizit formulierte Gesundheitsziele als Leitlinien einer nationalen Gesundheitspolitik an Bedeutung. Für die Bundesrepublik Deutschland besonders relevant sind die 226 Gesundheitsziele, die Ende der 70er Jahre in den Vereinigten Staaten in einem mehrstufigen Prozeß erarbeitet wurden (US-Department of Health, Education and Welfare 1979 und 1980), und die 38 Ziele des Regionalbüros für Europa der Weltgesundheitsorganisation, die 1985 als Einzelziele zur Unterstützung der europäischen Regionalstrategie für „Gesundheit 2000" erschienen sind.

Beide Zielkataloge (genauer: Daten-, Ziel-, Maßnahmen- und Indikatorkataloge) befürworten präventive Ansätze, die über den engeren Rahmen der medizinischen Versorgung hinausgehen. Versorgungs- oder Prozeßziele und Forschungsziele sind aber durchaus konform integriert. Beide versuchen, ein ergebnisorientiertes Gesundheitswesen dadurch zu fördern, daß sie Resultatziele spezifizieren. Ein einfaches, nicht untypisches Beispiel lautet: „Bis zum Jahr 2000 sollte die Säuglingssterblichkeit in der Region weniger als 20 pro 1000 Lebendgeburten betragen" (WHO 1985, Ziel Nr. 7).

Derartigen Zielkatalogen geht eine intensive Analyse verfügbarer Datenquellen zum Gesundheitszustand der Bevölkerung voraus. Regionale, zeitliche und soziale Unterschiede im Gesundheitszustand, ergänzt um weitere klinische und epidemiologische Evidenz und strukturierte Expertenbefragungen, werden systematisch auf Potentiale vermeidbarer Morbidität und Mortalität in der Bevölkerung geprüft.[1] Ein solcher Prozeß ist bereits eine gesundheitspolitische Aktivität aus eigenem Recht. Er hat natürlich normative Wertvorstellungen zu berücksichtigen (Robra et al. 1984) und ist grundsätzlich offen. Besonders die Weltgesundheitsorganisation hat deutlich gemacht, daß die Beteiligung einer „aufgeklärten und kooperativen Öffentlichkeit" über die professionelle Medizin (und ihre Verbände) hinaus ein Bürgerrecht und überdies ein essentieller Teil der Umsetzung der Ziele ist.

Um naheliegende Mißverständnisse zu vermeiden: ein solches "management by objectives" ist eine Führungstechnik westlichen Ursprungs (McGinnis 1985) und nicht mit zentralen Ziel- und Finanzplanvorgaben anderer Gesellschaftsordnungen zu verwechseln. Sie eignet sich besonders für komplexe Strukturen, in de-

---

* Erstmals veröffentlicht in: *Arbeit und Sozialpolitik* 12/1988–1/1989, S. 378–382.

[1] Vgl. die Ausführungen des Sachverständigenrates für die Konzertierte Aktion im Gesundheitswesen zum Thema „vermeidbare Mortalität", SVR 1987, Ziffer 31, sowie zu Mortalitätsunterschieden nach sozialer Schicht und Region, SVR 1987 A II. Ziffer 2.2ff.

nen auf verschiedenen (aus guten Gründen dezentralisierten) Ebenen über Entwicklungen entschieden wird und deren Teileinheiten unterschiedliche (oder sogar konflikthafte) Partikularziele verfolgen. Definiert wird der gemeinsame Zielkonsens.

In der Bundesrepublik Deutschland hat eine „Projektgruppe Prioritäre Gesundheitsziele" von der Bundesregierung und der Selbstverwaltung der deutschen Ärzte und Zahnärzte den Auftrag erhalten, Materialien zu erarbeiten, die als Entscheidungsgrundlagen zur Auswahl prioritärer Gesundheitsziele in der Bundesrepublik Deutschland dienen sollen. Ein Zwischenbericht mit dem Titel *Vorrangige Gesundheitsprobleme in den verschiedenen Lebensabschnitten* liegt vor (Projektgruppe Prioritäre Gesundheitsziele 1987). Er enthält in einer strengen Gliederung nach Altersgruppen Daten zum gegenwärtigen Zustand zahlreicher Gesundheitsprobleme, es werden (vermeidbare) gesundheitliche Risiken und denkbare Maßnahmen für gesundheitspolitisches Handeln aufgeführt. Zu jedem dargestellten Gesundheitsproblem sind ein oder mehrere Gesundheitsziele formuliert.[2] Wenn sinnvolle Trend- und Vergleichsdaten vorlagen und/oder Sachverständige einen definierten Zielwert als erreichbar einschätzen, wurden die Ziele im oben genannten Sinn für eine Zeitperspektive von ca. 10–15 Jahren quantifiziert. Die Auswahl der bearbeiteten Gesundheitsprobleme wurde durch die Kriterien Verbreitungsgrad, Schweregrad und Beeinflußbarkeit geleitet. Gesundheitliche Problembereiche, zu denen keine oder keine ausreichenden Daten vorliegen, können naturgemäß nicht in gleicher Weise berücksichtigt werden. Sie brauchen aber nicht ausgeblendet zu werden, solange sie einen „Advokaten" haben, der ihre Bedeutung im genannten Sinn plausibel machen kann.

Die Projektgruppe hat ihre Arbeit mit dem Untertitel „Entscheidungsgrundlagen für eine realistische Gesundheitspolitik in der Bundesrepublik Deutschland" gekennzeichnet. Entscheidungen über gesundheitspolitische Prioritäten selbst will sie den gesundheitspolitisch Verantwortlichen überlassen.

In der speziellen Situation der Bundesrepublik Deutschland sind Gesundheitsziele nicht nur eine Chance für die funktionelle Reintegration eines teils parallel, teils sequentiell, teils antagonistisch gegliederten Gesundheitswesens und damit Hilfsmittel einer rationalen Gesundheitspolitik. Sie sind auch eine Chance für das Gesundheitswesen, den sozialen Rang der Gesundheit der Bevölkerung – und damit den eigenen Stellenwert – im Konzert anderer gesellschaftlicher Teilsysteme[3] zu verbessern. In einer Zeitschrift für Sozialpolitik kann ein Beitrag über Gesundheitsziele daher vorrangig 2 Fragen nachgehen:

1) Wie können wir die Entwicklung des Gesundheitswesens (als gesellschaftliches Teilsystem) so fördern, daß sie im Einklang mit gesellschaftlichen Werten und Prioritäten steht?

2) Wie können wir die Entwicklung der Gesellschaft so fördern, daß sie im Einklang mit der Erhaltung und Förderung der Gesundheit ihrer Mitglieder steht (Leitbild Gesundheit)?

---

[2] Eine umfassende Darstellung der Zielvorschläge würde diesen Beitrag sprengen. Der Zwischenbericht ist erhältlich beim Zentralinstitut für die kassenärztliche Versorgung, Herbert-Lewin-Str. 5, 5000 Köln 41.

[3] Bildungswesen, Verteidigung, Recht, Verkehr, privater Konsum ...

Diese Fragen sind im Ringen um vordergründig operationalisierte Finanzierungsziele vielen aus dem Blick gekommen, die Verantwortung für die ökonomische Entwicklung im Gesundheitswesen und in der Gesellschaft tragen. Sie werden auch auf der Seite derer, die Verantwortung für die medizinische Entwicklung tragen,[4] nicht auf der übergeordneten sozialen Ebene gestellt und beantwortet.

Gesellschaftliche Prioritäten für das Gesundheitswesen

Die je eigene Identität der Sektoren, Körperschaften, Verbände und Professionen im Gesundheitswesen ist stark, gestützt auf Tradition, Gesetz und Markt. Keine Mitgliederversammlung, kein Hauptgeschäftsführer, kein engagierter Beamter will die Leistungskürzungen, die mit restriktiven ökonomischen Rahmenbedingungen assoziiert werden, im je eigenen Bereich hinnehmen – unabhängig davon, ob er den „Leistungsträgern" oder den „Kostenträgern" zugerechnet wird. Ein positives Engagement für bessere Versorgungs- und Arbeitsmöglichkeiten lohnt sich nicht mehr. Der Status quo ist der beste erreichbare. Es gilt, Schlimmeres zu verhüten. Knappheitsentscheidungen sollen die anderen vertreten. Ein Wachstum im Rahmen der Grundlohnsumme gibt immerhin jedes Jahr einige Milliarden mehr zum Verteilen. Damit kann man angesichts steigender Personalkosten und neuer Technologien zwar keine Sprünge machen, dafür entsteht aber auch kein konflikthafter Begründungsbedarf.

Daß auch ein solches – jegliches realistisches – Wachstum unausweichliche Knappheit von Ressourcen bedeutet, kann Lehrbuchwissen bleiben. Sich sektorübergreifend auf gemeinsame Ziele zu besinnen, wird im Rahmen eines verbandlich gegliederten Gesundheitswesens leicht eher als Störfaktor denn als Herausforderung für die Erfüllung der je eigenen Aufgaben angesehen. Dies aber ist offensichtlich das Szenarium einer immer nur unter partikularen Interessen innovationsfähigen und letztlich verantwortungslosen „Nichtpolitik". Sie bedeutet ungebremste Dominanz der ökonomischen Rahmenbedingungen und konzeptlose Weitergabe von Knappheit – ohne den Versuch, sie durch Einflußnahme auf Strukturen und Entwicklungen aktiv für eine Steigerung der gesundheitlichen Produktivität des Gesundheitswesens zu nutzen. Auch die in den einzelnen Sektoren des Gesundheitswesens vorhandene Sachkunde kann nicht sektorübergreifend gesellschaftlich nützlich werden. Bestenfalls findet der Versuch eines (einseitigen) Verdrängungswettbewerbs statt (z. B. à la „Bayernvertrag").

Glücklicherweise ist die Lage nicht ganz hoffnungslos. Positiv ist die Bereitschaft wichtiger Kassenverbände, neue Aufgaben in der Prävention zu übernehmen. Selbst wenn sich diese Tendenz erkennbar aus Marketingmotiven speist, läßt sich dahinter doch ein entwicklungsfähiges Menschen- und Gesellschaftsbild erkennen, das den sozialen Stellenwert der Gesundheit stärkt.

Die ambulante kassenärztliche Versorgung hat mit der Umstellung auf den EBM in ihrem Bereich einen erkennbaren Schritt getan, der einerseits mit einer gerechteren[5] internen Verteilung von Einkommen einhergeht, andererseits wegen

---

[4] Ärzte und andere Professionen, Institutionen und Verbände, darunter auch die Krankenkassen, Unfallversicherungsträger, Reha-Träger, Gebietskörperschaften und die Industrie.

[5] Jedenfalls von den Selbstverwaltungsgremien mit Vorbehalt der Korrektur akzeptierten und durch Kontingentierungen innerhalb des Honorarvolumens abgefederten.

der damit verbundenen Eingriffe in die Leistungsbewertung das Arbeitsprofil der Praxen verändern wird. Die angestrebten gesundheitlichen Konsequenzen sind mit dem Schlagwort „sprechende Medizin" knapp umschrieben, wenn auch nicht explizit operationalisiert. Diese medizinische Zielstellung, die von Apparateärzten vorhersehbar kritisiert wird, greift Änderungen des Krankheits-, Beschwerde- und Belastungspanoramas auf. Sie fördert Entwicklungen in Richtung auf persönlich erbrachte (damit nicht in Menge delegationsfähige), beratende und begleitende Leistungen der niedergelassenen Ärzte. Sie ist damit klientenorientiert. Auch dem schon genannten Bayernvertrag kann man eine klientenorientierte Zielsetzung nicht absprechen. Klientenorientierung ist in einem Nichtmarkt, den der Gesundheitssektor darstellt, allerdings noch keine Garantie für eine bedarfsgerechte, wirksame und wirtschaftliche Leistungsstruktur.

In einem expliziten Auftrag des Parlaments an die in der Konzertierten Aktion versammelten Träger des Gesundheitswesens, Gesundheitsziele[6] zu entwickeln, manifestiert sich zunächst der Vorrang des demokratischen Souveräns über den Verbändeegoismus. Gleichzeitig ist ein solcher Auftrag eine hervorragende Chance, bewährte Selbstverwaltungsstrukturen zu aktivieren, um eine Reihe von defizitären Bereichen im Gesundheitswesen zu bearbeiten, darunter die Resultatorientierung, Verfahren der Evidenzbewertung, Allokationsmechanismen, die Priorität der Primärversorgung, eine präventive Orientierung und Evaluationsansätze.

Resultatorientierung im Gesundheitswesen

Die große Mehrheit aller Daten, die im Gesundheitswesen erhoben werden, sind Prozeßdaten, ein großer Teil der Konflikte betrifft Zuständigkeiten bei der Leistungserbringung – damit ist die Perspektive der Gesundheitspolitik mehr als zuträglich auf eine Prozeßorientierung verengt. Gesundheitsziele können eine Resultatorientierung im Gesundheitswesen fördern. Dazu müssen sie quantifiziert und nachprüfbar gemacht werden. Prämissen und Annahmen, unter denen sie formuliert worden sind, müssen offengelegt werden. Eine Aufstellung guter Absichten und guter Zwecke allein ist keine ausreichend konkrete Zielformulierung. Auch eine allgemeine („konzeptionelle") Definition von Gesundheit[7] ist kein Er-

---

[6] „... die einzelnen Versorgungsbereiche nach der Vorrangigkeit ihrer Aufgaben ... bewerten" heißt es im § 150 GRG-Entwurf (Bundestagsdrucksache 11/2237 vom Mai 88) mit Blick auf den Abbau von Überversorgung und den Ausgleich von Unterversorgung (zwei ohne inhaltliche Vorgaben und normative Wertungen leere – wenn auch für das BMA offensichtlich zentrale – Begriffe); nach der Begründung zum Gesetz ist die Bundesregierung „der Auffassung, daß die Orientierung von Leistungen und Ausgaben an gesundheitlichen Prioritäten und Zielen verbessert werden muß" (allgemeiner Teil der Begründung, S. 147). Sie erläutert im besonderen Teil der Begründung zum § 150, daß die Konzertierte Aktion im Gesundheitswesen „gesundheitspolitische Prioritäten und Wirtschaftlichkeitsreserven" aufzuzeigen habe. Der Begriff „Orientierungsdaten" vermengt im übrigen empirische und normativ bewertende Aspekte, er wird besser durch die eindeutigeren Begriffe „Daten" und „Ziele" ersetzt.

[7] Z. B. ist nach einer Formulierung der deutschen Ärzteschaft Gesundheit „die aus der personellen Einheit von subjektivem Wohlbefinden und objektiver Belastbarkeit erwachsende körperliche und seelische, individuelle und soziale Leistungsfähigkeit der Menschen" (im sog. „Blauen Papier", in dem die gesundheits- und sozialpolitischen Vorstellungen der deutschen Ärzteschaft zusammengestellt sind. Bundesärztekammer 1986 und früher).

satz für konkrete Entscheidungen mit Ordnungs- oder Vorrangcharakter. Eine
Resultatorientierung verlangt auch eine ernsthafte Auseinandersetzung mit Fragen der Lebensqualität in unterschiedlichen Altersgruppen und Lebenslagen. Die
Sterblichkeit reicht als Resultatmaß nicht aus, sondern muß durch Indikatoren
des funktionellen Gesundheitszustands und des subjektiven Befindens ergänzt
werden. Es ist a priori klar, daß die Wahl des Resultatindikators die abgeleiteten
Versorgungsprioritäten dominiert.

Kriterien und Verfahren der Evidenzbewertung

Die Kriterien und Verfahren einer Bewertung von Evidenz im Bereich der Krankenversorgung und der Prävention sind derzeit weitgehend informell und damit
offen für zufällige, nicht sachgerechte Einflüsse.[8] Die Verhandlungen und Entscheidungen im Bereich der GKV werden mit ihren Begründungen nicht ausreichend offengelegt.[9] Damit wird eine Chance verschenkt, die Qualität der Bewertung in diesem Bereich zu forcieren und Maßstäbe für die Begründung zukünftiger Technologien[10] zu setzen. Obsolet gewordene Technologien und Programme
werden nicht unverzüglich aus dem Leistungskatalog der GKV ausgemustert
oder in der Indikation klar beschränkt.[11] Der Diffusionsprozeß medizinischer
Innovationen wird nicht erforscht und kann daher auch nicht gezielt beschleunigt
werden. Die Aufstellung eines Katalogs von Gesundheitszielen ist ein Mittel, die
Bewertung und Verbreitung vorhandener Evidenz zu verbessern und eine Analyse vorrangig fehlender Evidenz zu erstellen.

Intersektorale Allokation

Die Aufstellung von Gesundheitszielen kann zu einer begründeten Fachdiskus-
sion über die Abgrenzung der wichtigsten Bruchkante im Gesundheitswesen führen, den Übergang zwischen der ambulanten und der stationären Versorgung in
beide Richtungen. Wir brauchen nicht nur eine Flexibilisierung von
Finanzierungs- und Arbeitsmöglichkeiten des einen Sektors auf Kosten und in
der Domäne des anderen, sondern auch fachlichen Konsens über gesundheits-
problemspezifische Vorgehensweisen, die quer zu den ständischen Interessen der
Versorger liegen. Die Selbstverwaltung wird durch die Aufgabe, dreiseitige Ver-

---

[8] Ein Auftrag zur Ex-ante-Bewertung neuer Untersuchungs- und Behandlungsmethoden in
§ 144 GRG-Entwurf muß inhaltlich und formal gefullt werden (gegenwärtig z. T. Aufgaben
des U- und H-Ausschusses).

[9] Vgl das bewußt auf Öffentlichkeit angelegte Prozedere der amerikanischen "Consensus-
Conferences".

[10] Unter Technologie wird nach amerikanischem Vorbild jedes Arzneimittel, medizinische Hilfsmittel und jedes diagnostische und therapeutische Verfahren verstanden, also nicht nur die
"hardware", sondern auch die "software" medizinischer Leistungen; die Anforderungen an
die Qualität der Evidenz in den genannten Bereichen sind erkennbar inkonsistent.

[11] Die Art und Weise, wie im Rahmen der EBM-Reform einzelne Leistungslegenden aus- und
(bei Widerstand) auch wieder eingemustert wurden, stützt die These mangelnder Klarheit bei
der Evidenzbewertung.

träge zu schließen (§ 123 GRG-E, § 372 RVO), *inhaltlich* gefordert. Als positive Beispiele in diesem Bereich sind Vereinbarungen über die (pauschale) Kostenübernahme einer befristeten Hauspflege unmittelbar nach Entlassung aus dem stationären Bereich (wie in Berlin) oder die Regelungen für Anschlußheilverfahren (AHB) bei wichtigen Krankheitsgruppen an der Bruchkante zwischen stationärer Versorgung und Rehabilitationsmaßnahmen zu nennen. Auch die Diskussion über Anhaltszahlen für die stationäre Verweildauer sollte datengestütztfachlich und unter Vorrang häufiger Behandlungsanlässe erfolgen, nicht administrativ unter einer pauschalen Heckenschnittperspektive geführt werden.

Die Vorstellungen der KBV für den Anteil der Allgemeinärzte an der kassenärztlichen Versorgung – als Beispiel einer Übernahme struktureller Verantwortung durch die Profession – müssen sektorübergreifend um Anhaltszahlen für die fachliche Struktur der Weiterbildungsstellen ergänzt werden, und dies unter expliziten gesundheitlichen Zielsetzungen und einem klaren Modell von Krankenversorgung und gesundheitlicher Betreuung, auf das nicht nur Konkurrenzdenken Einfluß nimmt. Der relative Abbau von Leistungen im Gesundheitswesen, der bei faktisch konstanten Ressourcen aus steigendem Anspruchsniveau, demographischer Alterung und medizinischem Fortschritt folgt, kann nicht mit realistischer Hoffnung auf großen Erfolg dem Gesundheitswesen als interne Optimierungsaufgabe überlassen werden (nach Art eines Dampfdrucktopfs). Er bedarf fairerweise erkennbarer gesellschaftlicher Prioritäten (auf der Basis gesellschaftlicher Präferenzen), welche Leistungen reduziert, verzögert oder in der Wachstumsrate gemindert werden sollen und wo besonderer „Problemdruck" gespürt wird. Hier liegt eine Grenze für „Selbstverwaltungslösungen". Die Übernahme *politischer* Verantwortung ist erforderlich.

Intrasektorale Allokation

In einer Lage, in der Konkurrenzkämpfe bestimmter Fachgruppen im Gesundheitswesen immer stärker werden (müssen), muß jede am Gemeinwohl orientierte Körperschaft (KVen, Kassen, Kammern, Gemeinden, Länder, Bund) sehen, daß sich nicht nur die zahlreichsten und/oder lautesten durchsetzen, sondern gesundheitsbezogen argumentiert wird. Dies aber kann nur in einem Kontext klarer gesundheitlicher Ziele und Prioritäten und mit Resultatorientierung geschehen.

Priorität der Primärversorgung

In Analogie zum Sport ist auch in der medizinischen Versorgung ein ausgewogenes Verhältnis von Spitzen- zu Breitenversorgung[12] zu entwickeln. Die Wirksamkeit der Breitenversorgung findet in der Medizin – darüber klagen insbesondere Vertreter der Allgemeinmedizin – weniger fachliche Aufmerksamkeit als die Spitzenversorgung. Hier liegt ein leicht erkennbares Prioritätendefizit. Gesundheitsziele können es korrigieren. Die steigende Zahl der Hypertoniker, die von ihrem

---

[12] Ein Begriff aus der Begründung des GRG, Bundestagsdrucksache 11/2237, S. 143.

Hochdruck wissen und erfolgreich kontrolliert sind, ist in diesem Sinn ein gesundheitlicher Fortschritt der letzten Jahre, der viele andere Errungenschaften der Hochleistungsmedizin bei seltenen Erkrankungen in den Schatten stellt.

Präventive Orientierung

Gesundheitsziele helfen, der Prävention einen angemessenen, d. h. größeren Stellenwert im Gesundheitswesen, aber auch in anderen Bereichen des Lebens einzuräumen. Wir brauchen eine stärkere Zusammenschau und Integration gesundheitlicher mit sozialen Entwicklungen.

Evaluation

Gesundheitsziele sind als Evaluationsrahmen der medizinischen Versorgung nötig. Damit schließt sich der Kreis zur oben angeführten „Resultatorientierung". Der Verzicht auf die Formulierung quantitativer Gesundheitsziele verschenkt eine Chance, mit ökonomischem und sozial verträglichem (weil erkennbar begründetem) Aufwand Daten für die Beobachtung des Gesundheitszustands der Bevölkerung und seiner beeinflußbaren Determinanten zu erheben. Gesundheitsziele – nicht Fiskalziele – müssen die Datenerhebung im gesundheitlichen Bereich und die Gesundheitsberichterstattung vorrangig bestimmen.

Gesundheitliche Prioritäten für die Gesellschaft

Sind Gesundheitsziele nun ein Mittel der Politik nur in einer Knappheitsgesellschaft, sozusagen für Entwicklungsländer? Sind sie auch in entwickelten Industriegesellschaften hilfreich, in denen Gesundheit als superiores Gut konsumiert wird? Natürlich hat auch eine reiche, entwickelte Gesellschaft ein Recht, von ihren Experten Antworten auf die Frage zu verlangen, wie die Gesundheit am besten zu erhalten und zu fördern sei, eine sonst auf Effizienz und Effektivität ausgerichtete Leistungsgesellschaft allemal. § 1 der Bundesärzteordnung[13] faßt diese gesellschaftliche Norm verpflichtend zusammen. Mehr noch: Ist es nicht legitim, daß Ärzte (als dominante Gruppe im Gesundheitswesen) die Richtlinien der Politik zu beeinflussen suchen, damit die Gesundheit einen hohen (höchsten?) Stellenwert in politischen Entscheidungen hat (bekommt, behält)?[14]

Für Ärzte ist die gegenwärtige Dominanz ökonomischer vor medizinischen Rahmenbedingungen für die Entwicklung des Gesundheitswesens in besonderem Maß unerträglich. Die Medizin selber muß daher gesellschaftliche Perspektiven für mehr Gesundheit aufzeigen, einerseits durch methodisch strenge Analyse vermeidbarer Morbidität und Mortalität (s. oben), andererseits durch eine positive

---

[13] § 1(1) der Bundesärzteordnung lautet: „Der Arzt dient der Gesundheit des einzelnen Menschen und des gesamten Volkes." BGBl. 1.I S. 1885ff. vom 20. Oktober 1977.

[14] Ein schlechtes Verhältnis zwischen dem größten Ärzteverband und dem Bundeskanzler ist in diesem Sinn nicht nur schlechte Verbandspolitik, sondern auch schlechte Gesundheitspolitik.

Utopie der Gesundheit als gesellschaftlichem Leitbild. Dies ist eine Bringschuld. Sie muß – gerade unter den Bedingungen entwickelter Gesellschaften – Antennen, Mittel und Organisationsformen (Institutionen) entwickeln, die die angesprochenen Perspektiven vermitteln. Zu diesen Mitteln gesellschaftlicher Einflußnahme kann ein jährlicher Gesundheitsbericht gehören. Eine systematische Gesundheitsberichterstattung[15] legt Rechenschaft ab und schafft Legitimation, zeigt aber auch Defizite auf und meldet Forderungen an.

Dem zunehmenden Druck, die Verwendung von Mitteln im Gesundheitswesen zu rechtfertigen, ist nicht nur mit ökonomischen Argumenten zu begegnen.[16] Dies würde die gesellschaftliche Legitimation des Gesundheitswesens keinesfalls ausschöpfen. Es ist auch eine gesundheitsbezogene Argumentation nötig. Sie setzt aber operationalisierte Ziele voraus. Ohne Gesundheitsziele gibt es keine faßbaren Erfolgskriterien und damit keine am Resultat orientierten Erfolge, sondern nur erbrachte „Leistungen". Die aber werden – wie die Erfahrung zeigt – gleichgesetzt mit verzehrten Ressourcen und Lohnnebenkosten. In dem Maße, wie der gesundheitliche Sektor darauf verzichtet, an der Definition und gesellschaftlichen Verankerung von Gesundheitszielen mitzuwirken, verkürzt er seine eigene gesellschaftliche Legitimation und Gestaltungskraft. Die Medizin ist dann erfolgreich, wenn die Gesellschaft als ganzes die Gesunderhaltung/Gesundheitsförderung als gesellschaftliche Aufgabe wahrnimmt (im doppelten Sinn), und zwar systemübergreifend und vorrangig.

Nun gibt es mehr als ein Beispiel für Fehlleistungen, zu denen es kommt, wenn die Medizin sich unter Verlassen überkommener (d. h. auch individualzentrierter) Grundsätze in den Dienst bestimmter gesellschaftlicher Zwecke und Systeme stellen läßt. Es ist Medizinern also deutlich zu machen, daß das Aufstellen von Gesundheitszielen kein Verrat an den alten Werten der Medizin ist. Dafür reicht der Hinweis auf den demokratisch gebildeten gesellschaftlichen Willen vorhersehbar nicht aus. Es muß mehr herauskommen, als eine Triage auf den verschiedenen Allokationsebenen. Als Voraussetzung für ein Engagement der Medizin bei der Entwicklung von Gesundheitszielen muß klar sein, daß die Medizin die Gesellschaft immer wieder auf ungelöste und/oder zu wenig bearbeitete Gesundheitsprobleme aufmerksam machen darf (muß), und zwar auch außerhalb des Gesundheitswesens im engeren Sinne; dies mit dem Ziel der erfolgreichen Mobilisierung zusätzlicher Ressourcen für das Gesundheitswesen im Konkurrenzkampf mit den anderen gesellschaftlichen Teilsystemen (Gesundheitsadvokatur) und mit der Möglichkeit eines Nachweises des gesundheitlichen Erfolgs. Hier muß also ein sachgerechter Konflikt mit der pauschalen politischen Vorgabe einer Beitragssatzstabilität entstehen. Gesellschaftliche Prioritäten für das Gesundheitswesen müssen gleichzeitig gesundheitliche Prioritäten für die Gesellschaft sein.

---

[15] Vgl. die „Stellungnahme des Sachverständigenrates für die Konzertierte Aktion zum Aufbau einer Gesundheitsberichterstattung", SVR 1988, S 192ff

[16] Z. B. Gesundheitswesen als arbeitsintensive, Beschäftigungskrisen stabilisierende Wachstumsbranche mit großer Investitionskraft und positiven Auswirkungen auch auf schwache regionale Teilarbeitsmärkte, Ausbau von Kosten-Wirkungs-Analysen und Kosten-Nutzen-Analysen.

Gesundheitsziele – Katalysator und Instrument der Gesundheitspolitik

Prioritäre Gesundheitsziele sind mehr als ein technokratisches Optimierungsinstrument zum Schmieren von Budgetierungen. Sie haben eine Leitbildfunktion für die Gestaltung einer gesundheitsförderlichen und humanen Gesellschaft, in der alle Teilsysteme und Institutionen an der Beseitigung krankmachender Einflüsse mitarbeiten und die Auswirkungen ihrer Handlungen auf die Gesundheit berücksichtigen müssen (gesundheitliche Folgekosten). Gesundheitsziele mobilisieren Ideen und Kräfte, harmonisieren partikulare Interessen und fokussieren zersplitterte Kompetenzen – und das mit einem vergleichsweise geringen Aufwand.

Sie sind auf einen gesellschaftlichen Grundkonsens angewiesen, aber Konsens in jedem Detail braucht nicht zu sein. Man hätte sonst wieder die alte partikulare Situation mit umgekehrten Vorzeichen (der letzte dominiert). Es kann durchaus Bereiche geben, in denen es (noch) nicht zu einem Zielkonsens gekommen ist. Wenn in einer Zieldiskussion Minderheitenpositionen vertreten werden, bleibt nicht nur die Pluralität gewahrt, sondern auch die Gesundheit im gesellschaftlichen Diskurs thematisiert. Je klarer der Dissens beschrieben ist, desto fruchtbarer ist die Situation für die Entwicklung von konkreten Alternativen und Maßnahmen.

Wenn die Politik nicht selber detaillierte Ziele entwickeln will, muß sie Kriterien für die Zielauswahl vorgeben, wie z. B. individuelle und kollektive Krankheitslast, Vermeidbarkeit von Morbidität und Mortalität, auch Gleichheit in Gesundheitsfragen.[17] Sie kann auf konkrete Quantifizierungen von Zielproblemen drängen,[18] sie muß die Mittel für vorrangige Ziele und Aufgaben bereitstellen und verteidigen helfen, und sie kann die Zielerreichung periodisch überprüfen lassen. Dabei ist es vielleicht noch wichtiger, die Ziele zu identifizieren, die nicht erreicht werden, als jene Zielbereiche, die auf dem richtigen Weg sind. In den USA ist beispielsweise das Ziel, die Zahl unerwünschter Teenagerschwangerschaften zu reduzieren (und als Folge davon eine Reihe weiterer gesundheitlicher und sozialer Probleme zu vermeiden), offensichtlich hinsichtlich seiner Umsetzbarkeit unterschätzt worden. Die Häufigkeit von Tennagerschwangerschaften hat sich nicht vermindert. Das Ziel bleibt, die Mittel und Wege dahin sind revisionsbedürftig.

Wird das Verhältnis von Selbstverwaltung und Politik über einen Zielkonsens bestimmt, erhält die Selbstverwaltung innerhalb eines politisch verantworteten Rahmens den größten möglichen Spielraum. Die Alternative wäre ein inhaltliches Hineinregieren in fachliche, großen interdisziplinären Sachverstand erfordernde Bereiche des Gesundheitswesens. Dies wäre auch deswegen ungünstig, weil die *Mobilität* von Ressourcen eine wichtige Voraussetzung von Effektivität und Effizienz der medizinischen Versorgung ist. Vertragliche Fixierungen verdienen daher grundsätzlich den Vorzug vor gesetzlichen. Gesundheitsziele sind so-

---

[17] Es gibt verschiedene Definitionen für „Gleichheit" im Gesundheitswesen (vgl. Robra u. a. 1984).

[18] „eine den Stand der medizinischen Wissenschaft berücksichtigende bedarfsgerechte Versorgung..." ist z. B. weder resultatorientiert quantifiziert noch prioritär gestaffelt.

mit kein Instrument, das die Struktur im Gesundheitswesen revolutioniert. Sie setzen das gegliederte System voraus.

Man könnte einen Konflikt zwischen gesellschaftlichen Gesundheitszielen und der Freiheit des einzelnen Bürgers sehen, sich in gesundheitlichen Fragen mündig selbst zu bestimmen – einschließlich der Freiheit, sich gesundheitsriskant oder ungesund zu verhalten. Ein solcher Konflikt wäre aber nicht anders zu bewerten als bei anderen sozialen Entscheidungsprozessen auch.[19] Im Gegenteil, ein gesellschaftlicher Konsens über prioritäre Gesundheitsziele (nicht nur Versorgungsziele) *hilft*, die individuelle Arzt-Patienten-Beziehung vom direkten Zwang zu Knappheitsentscheidungen frei zu halten und fördert daher die Anwaltsfunktion des Arztes sowie die Beratung und Entscheidung des Einzelnen in seinen individuellen gesundheitlichen Problemen. Im übrigen umfassen Gesundheitsziele ausdrücklich eine Stärkung der Eigenverantwortung, wo dies problemadäquat ist, und erleichtern dem mündigen Bürger die Kenntnis von Prioritäten und Handlungsalternativen (d. h. die „Marktübersicht").

Das Zieldefizit, das Informationsdefizit und das Steuerungsdefizit unseres Gesundheitswesens bedingen sich gegenseitig, aber das Defizit expliziter Ziele steht am Anfang dieser Politikdefizite.

Literatur

Bundesärztekammer (Hrsg) (1986) Gesundheits- und sozialpolitische Vorstellungen der Deutschen Ärzteschaft, beschlossen vom 89. Deutschen Ärztetag 1986 in Hannover (Das Blaue Papier). Köln

McGinnis JM (1985) Setting nationwide objectives in disease prevention and health promotion: the United States experience. In: Holland WW, Detels R, Knox G (eds) Oxford textbook of public health, vol 3. Oxford, pp 385–401

Projektgruppe Prioritäre Gesundheitsziele (Hrsg) (1987) Vorrangige Gesundheitsprobleme in den verschiedenen Lebensabschnitten – Entscheidungsgrundlagen für eine realistische Gesundheitspolitik in der Bundesrepublik Deutschland, Köln

Robra B-P, Meye MR, Schwartz FW (1984) Positive Gesundheitsziele – normative und pragmatische Positionen. MMG 9·170–176

Sachverständigenrat für die Konzertierte Aktion im Gesundheitswesen (1987) Medizinische und ökonomische Orientierung – Vorschlage für die Konzertierte Aktion im Gesundheitswesen (Jahresgutachten 1987), Baden-Baden

Sachverständigenrat für die Konzertierte Aktion im Gesundheitswesen (1988) Medizinische und ökonomische Orientierung – Vorschläge für die Konzertierte Aktion im Gesundheitswesen (Jahresgutachten 1988), Baden-Baden

US-Department of Health, Education and Welfare (ed) (1979) Healthy People, the Surgeon General's Report on Health Promotion and Disease Prevention. Washington

US-Department of Health, Education and Welfare (ed) (1980) Promoting Health, Preventing Disease – Objectives for the Nation. Washington

Weltgesundheitsorganisation (WHO) Regionalbüro für Europa (Hrsg) (1985) Einzelziele für „Gesundheit 2000". Kopenhagen

---

[19] Niemand sieht die Freiheit der Berufswahl allein dadurch eingeschränkt, daß nicht für jedes Fach überall Lehrstühle eingerichtet sind. Niemand sieht die Freiheit der Konsumenten durch die staatliche Wohnungsbauförderung oder den halben Mehrwertsteuersatz auf bestimmte Produkte tangiert, niemand die Freiheit der Forschung durch Schwerpunktprogramme der DFG; und niemand sieht das Leben der Seefahrer mehr als ethisch vertretbar bedroht, wenn nicht in jedem Priel vorsorglich ein Seenotrettungskreuzer dümpelt, solange die Rettungsflottille insgesamt nach vernünftigen und transparenten Kriterien disloziert ist.

Finanzausgleich als Voraussetzung für funktionsfähigen Kassenwettbewerb in der Gesetzlichen Krankenversicherung [*]

W.-D. Leber

Freie Kassenwahl für Angestellte und gleichzeitig die Zwangsmitgliedschaft für Arbeiter – dies stößt in einer modernen, demokratischen Gesellschaft zunehmend auf Widerspruch. Gleichwohl baut die „bewährte" Kassenartenstruktur der GKV gerade auf diesem Anachronismus auf. Die Forderungen nach einem einheitlichen Sozialrecht für alle Arbeitnehmer werden immer häufiger. Kann aber die GKV ihre wesentlichen Aufgaben – Absicherung gegen Gesundheitsrisiken zu vertretbaren Kosten und sozialer Ausgleich – noch erfüllen, wenn nicht nur die Angestellten, sondern auch die Arbeiter ihre Kasse frei wählen dürfen?

Die folgenden Ausführungen zeigen, daß die Einführung von freier Kassenwahl für alle Versicherten im gegenwärtig bestehenden System zu erheblichen Ineffizienzen führen kann – von den sozialen Konsequenzen infolge auseinanderdriftender Beitragssätze[1] einmal ganz abgesehen. Ein funktionsfähiger Wettbewerb zwischen den Kassen kann erst durch eine zusätzliche Maßnahme entstehen, die manchen als das Gegenstück zum Wettbewerb erscheint: kassenübergreifender Finanzausgleich. Ein Finanzausgleich zur Berücksichtigung der unterschiedlichen Risikostrukturen der konkurrierenden Kassen muß nicht der Weg in die Einheitsversicherung bedeuten, sondern ist geradezu die Voraussetzung für freie Kassenwahl und mehr Wettbewerb in der GKV. Dazu muß er allerdings – anders als der bestehende KVdR-Ausgleich – als Risiko- bzw. Finanzmittelausgleich und nicht als Ausgabenausgleich gestaltet werden.

Die Problematik ist von zentraler Bedeutung für die angekündigte Strukturreform. Da es in der Regel einige Überwindung erfordert, sich mit den Wirkungen und mathematischen Feinheiten verschiedener Ausgleichsmechanismen auseinanderzusetzen, werden im folgenden eine einfache Darstellung gewählt und die komplexen wohlfahrtstheoretischen Zusammenhänge auf die simple Frage reduziert: Setzen sich im Wettbewerb bei freier Kassenwahl die effizientesten Kassen durch, oder sind die Rahmenbedingungen derart, daß die „falschen" Kassen auf der Strecke bleiben? Eine Antwort wird anhand eines überschaubaren Vierkassenbeispiels vorgeführt.

---

[*] Erstmals veröffentlicht in: *Arbeit und Sozialpolitik* 10/1987, S. 266–272.

[1] Zum Ausmaß der Beitragssatzdifferenzen vgl. Sachverständigenrat für die Konzertierte Aktion im Gesundheitswesen: Jahresgutachten 1987 – Medizinische und ökonomische Orientierung. Baden-Baden 1987, S. 281; zur Diskussion der Beitragssatzunterschiede vgl. Kops, M./Jaschke, H.: Ein Kausalmodell zur Erklärung der Beitragssatzunterschiede zwischen den Gesetzlichen Krankenkassen, in: Jahrbuch für Sozialwissenschaften 1987, S. 85–112, und die dort angegebene Literatur.

GKV-Beitragssätze: Irrlichter als Preissignale

Die Wahl einer Kasse ist für den Versicherten eine Beitrags-Nutzen-Abwägung: Zu welchem Preis ist bei den verschiedenen Kassen eine Absicherung gegen Gesundheitsrisiken möglich? Die Kassen versuchen eine bedarfsgerechte Versorgung zu möglichst geringen Kosten anzubieten, und die Versicherten geben durch ihre Kassenwahl eine Beurteilung dieser Bemühungen. Die „besten" Kassen erhalten aber nur dann Zulauf, wenn die Beitragsdifferenz zwischen den Kassen deren unterschiedliche Effizienz widerspiegelt, ein niedriger Preis also – bei entsprechender Leistung – hohe Effizienz signalisiert. Im momentanen GKV-System sind die Preissignale jedoch Irrlichter. Die Beitragssätze spiegeln im wesentlichen die Risikostruktur der Versicherten wider, so daß effiziente Kassen unter Mitgliederschwund leiden, wenn sie zufällig schlechte Risiken haben, und Kassen mit günstiger Risikostruktur (z.B. viele junge Leute mit hohem Einkommen) können unabhängige von ihrer Effizienz einen Mitgliederzuwachs verzeichnen. Ein Beispiel mag dies verdeutlichen.

Die 4 fiktiven Kassen A, B, C und D unterscheiden sich in

- Altersstruktur (vereinfacht zu 5 Altersgruppen),
- Grundlohn je Versicherten,
- Ausgabenprofil,
- Gesamtzahl der Versicherten und
- Beitragssatz.[2]

Zunächst ein Blick auf die Versichertenstruktur und die Ausgaben in den einzelnen Altersgruppen. Aus der ersten Spalte der Tabelle 1 ist die Stärke der 5 Altersgruppen in den jeweiligen Kassen zu ersehen. Die zweite Spalte gibt die Ausgaben je Altersstufe, Versicherten und Jahr wieder. Die Kasse B hat zum Beispiel pro Versicherten in der zweiten Altersgruppe durchschnittliche Ausgaben von jährlich 700 DM. Die dritte Spalte ergibt sich aus der Multiplikation von erster und zweiter Spalte und zeigt die Gesamtausgaben je Altersgruppe.

Es wird angenommen, daß das Versorgungsangebot der Kassen auf gleichem Niveau liegt. Außerdem soll die Morbiditätsstruktur in allen Kassen identisch sein.[3] Geringere Ausgaben einer Kasse sind dann in der Effizienz der Kasse begründet und können z.B. auf ein besonders dynamisches Management zurückzuführen sein: Durch geschickt geführte Preisverhandlungen und wirksame Wirtschaftlichkeitskontrolle ist eine kostengünstige Versorgung erreicht worden, durch ein Netz ambulanter Dienste einschließlich häuslicher Krankenpflege werden weniger teure stationäre Aufenthalte notwendig etc.

Die Effizienz der einzelnen Kassen A–D ist aus der zweiten Spalte ersichtlich: Der Kasse C ist es z.B. möglich, für 2500 DM einen Versicherten der obersten Altersgruppe zu versorgen, die Kasse B hingegen benötigt 2900 DM. Abbildung 1 zeigt die Ausgabenprofile für alle Kassen. Die Kassen A und C haben in der Beispielkonstruktion gleiche Ausgaben pro Altersstufe; Kasse B arbeitet am unwirtschaftlichsten. In einem funktionsfähigen Markt müßte der Beitragssatz

---

[2] Zur Vereinfachung wird von möglichen Unterschieden in der Geschlechtsstruktur abgesehen. Der Ausgleich unterschiedlicher Männer- bzw. Frauenquoten in den einzelnen Altersgruppen wird anhand einer Heilbronner Kasse weiter unten demonstriert.

[3] Zur Problematik dieser Annahme vgl. den Abschnitt „Weitere Risikofaktoren".

Tabelle 1. Alters- und Ausgabenstruktur der 4 Kassen

Kasse	Alters- gruppe	Anzahl der Versicherten (in Tausend) (1)	Ausgaben je Versicherten (DM/Jahr) (2)	Ausgaben gesamt (Mio. DM) (3) = (1)·(2)
A	1	200	600	120
	2	200	650	130
	3	200	900	180
	4	200	1 300	260
	5	200	2 500	500
Gesamt:		1 000		1 190
B	1	600	650	390
	2	500	700	350
	3	400	1 100	440
	4	300	1 500	450
	5	200	2 900	580
Gesamt:		2 000		2 210
C	1	170	600	102
	2	160	650	104
	3	170	900	153
	4	160	1 300	208
	5	140	2 500	350
Gesamt:		800		917
D	1	50	500	25
	2	100	600	60
	3	250	800	200
	4	300	1 200	360
	5	300	2 400	720
Gesamt:		1 000		1 365
A–D	1	1 020	625	637
	2	960	671	644
	3	1 020	954	973
	4	960	1 331	1 278
	5	840	2 560	2 150
Gesamt:		4 800		5 682

genau dieses widerspiegeln. Kasse D sollte den niedrigsten Beitrag haben und dem Kassenwählenden hohe Effizienz signalisieren, die Kassen A und C müßten gleich hohe Beitragssätze aufweisen und Kasse B am teuersten sein.

Tabelle 2 zeigt, daß bei einer Beitragssatzberechnung analog zum bestehenden GKV-System[4] die Wirtschaftlichkeit der Kasse nicht aus den Beitragssätzen abzulesen ist. Durch die Altersstruktur und die unterschiedlichen Grundlöhne sind die Beitragssätze so verzerrt, daß A und C unterschiedliche Beiträge haben und die unwirtschaftliche Kasse den günstigsten. Die Versicherten wählen alle die falsche Kasse! Das Gesamtsystem tendiert zu wachsender Unwirtschaftlichkeit!

---

[4] Hier allerdings ohne KVdR-Ausgleich.

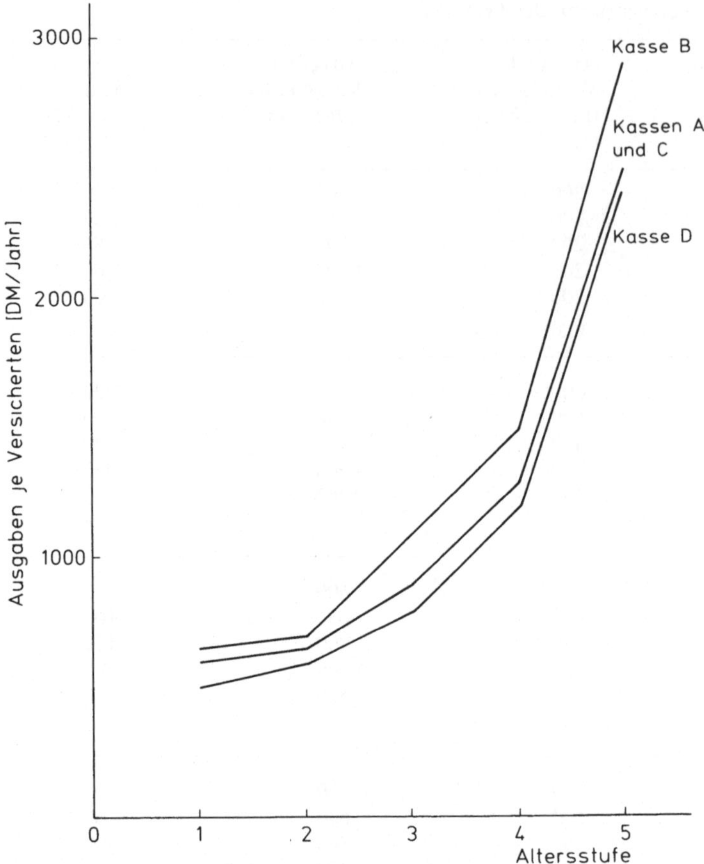

Abb. 1. Ausgabenprofile der Kassen A–D

Tabelle 2. Beitragssätze vor Finanzausgleich

Kasse	Ausgaben Mio. DM (1)	Grundlohn Mio DM (2)	Grundlohn je Versicherten in DM (3)	Beitragssatz [%] (4) = 100·(1)/(2)
A	1 190	11 000	11 000	10,8
B	2 210	26 000	13 000	8,5
C	917	7 200	9 000	12,7
D	1 365	9 000	9 000	15,2

Alternative: PKV?

Der Einfluß der Versichertenstruktur auf den Beitrag könnte durch Übergang zu risikoproportionalen Beiträgen eliminiert werden. Dies erfordert wegen des mit dem Alter anwachsenden Risikos entweder steigende Beiträge mit steigendem Alter (jeweils befristete Risikoübernahme) oder die Bildung einer Alterungsrücklage – also eine Kapitaldeckung des im Zeitablauf steigenden Risikos – bei konstanten Beiträgen über das ganze Leben hinweg. Mit risikoproportionalen Beiträgen, bei denen es weder zu intergenerativen noch zu sozialen Transfers kommt, arbeitet momentan die PKV. Da die gebildete Alterungsrücklage nicht in die neu gewählte Versicherung übernommen werden kann und die Eingangsbeiträge mit zunehmendem Alter steigen, ist allerdings derzeit ein Wechsel der Versicherung in fortgeschrittenem Alter für den Versicherten mit hohen Verlusten verbunden.

Von diesem – behebbaren – Mangel abgesehen, gilt das PKV-System mit Kapitaldeckung und risikoproportionalen Beiträgen als „ideales Marktmodell" für die Absicherung gegen Gesundheitsrisiken. Die effizientesten Kassen können den günstigsten Tarif anbieten und sich am Markt durchsetzen. Durch Umwandlung der gegenwärtigen GKV in ein Krankenversicherungssystem mit risikoproportionalen Beiträgen (verbunden mit Kontrahierungszwang und Übernahme der Alterungsrücklage bei Kapitaldeckungsverfahren) könnte ein funktionierender Wettbewerb entstehen. Umverteilungsziele müßten dann jedoch durch das bestehende Einkommensteuersystem erreicht werden. Dies wäre die immer wieder vorgeschlagene Trennung von Versicherung und Verteilung, bzw. die Trennung von allokativen und distributiven Aufgaben.[5]

Der „idealtypischen Marktlösung" fehlt es u. a. an Überzeugungskraft, weil die Übergangsprobleme vom jetzigen System zu dieser Wettbewerbslösung kaum lösbar sind. Die wesentliche Schwierigkeit stellt das mit dem Alter steigende Gesundheitsrisiko dar: Der Übergang vom bestehenden Umlageprinzip mit intergenerativem Ausgleich hin zum Kapitaldeckungsverfahren ist quasi unmöglich. Die bislang nichtgebildete Alterungsrücklage könnte von den Rentnern nicht aufgebracht werden und auch ein langsamer Übergang hätte kaum Chancen im politischen Prozeß. Angesichts der Schwierigkeiten, schon den bestehenden Generationenvertrag in der Kranken- und Rentenversicherung einzuhalten, ist die zusätzliche Belastung durch Bildung einer Kapitaldeckung illusorisch.

Ein weiteres Argument gegen einen Übergang zu risikoproportionalen Beiträgen sind die schwierigen komplementären Reformen im Einkommensteuerrecht, die zur Erhaltung der bestehenden Umverteilung notwendig würden. Ein Blick auf die gegenwärtig geführten Auseinandersetzungen um die angekündigte Steuerreform läßt die Schwierigkeiten erahnen, die eine Übernahme der größtenteils zur Zeit gar nicht erfaßbaren, GKV-internen Umverteilung zwischen Einkommensgruppen, Familien und Generationen in das bestehende Steuersystem mit sich bringen würde.

KVdR-Ausgleich – oder: Wie man es nicht machen sollte!

Wenn ein Übergang zu risikoproportionalen Beiträgen ausgeschlossen wird, dann bietet sich als zweiter Weg zu unverzerrtem Wettbewerb ein kassenübergreifender Ausgleich der Risiken an. Der bestehende Ausgleich innerhalb der

---

⁵ Vgl. Frankfurter Institut für wirtschaftspolitische Forschung e. V. (Kronberger Kreis): Mehr Markt im Gesundheitswesen. Bad Homburg 1987.

GKV – der Ausgleich innerhalb der Krankenversicherung der Rentner – ist allerdings für ein Wettbewerbssystem gänzlich ungeeignet. Der KVdR-Ausgleich gleicht nicht Risiken, sondern Ausgaben aus.[6] Da die Ausgaben vollständig ausgeglichen werden, besteht finanziell gesehen für die Rentner eine Einheitsversicherung. Eine Konsequenz daraus ist die Herausbildung von Konditionenwettbewerb als vorherrschende Form des Kassenwettbewerbs. Für die Rentner kann eine Kasse Leistungsverbesserungen auf Kosten aller Kassen vornehmen, Einsparungen andererseits versickern im allgemeinen GKV-Durchschnitt. Der ausgabentreibende Effekt der Krankenversicherung der Rentner ist bisher zu wenig in der Diskussion über eine Strukturreform berücksichtigt worden. Bedenkt man, daß die KVdR-Ausgaben inzwischen mehr als ein Drittel aller Ausgaben der Kassen umfassen (und stetig steigen!), so wird der lähmende Effekt auf die Geschäftsführung der Kassen zu einer nicht mehr zu vernachlässigenden Systemschwäche.[7] Aus der Sicht des einzelnen Kassenmanagers fließt ein Großteil mühsam erwirtschafteter Einsparungen in den Finanzausgleich der Rentner. Ein Beispiel gibt der Heil- und Hilfsmittelbereich: Wie groß ist die Motivation, etwa einen Preisnachlaß bei Hörgeräten auszuhandeln, wenn nur 30 Prozent der Einsparungen bei der Kasse verbleiben, weil 70 Prozent der Aufwendungen für Hörgeräte Ausgaben der Krankenversicherung der Rentner sind? Daß in einem solchen System der Wettbewerb nicht kostensenkend wirkt, ist nicht verwunderlich: In einem Wettbewerb mit Ausgabenausgleich gewinnt derjenige, der am meisten ausgibt!

Eine Verminderung des Ausgabenausgleichs (z. B. nur noch 50 %iger Ausgleich) würde zwar den ausgabensteigernden Effekt lindern, auf der anderen Seite jedoch wieder den wettbewerbsverzerrenden Effekt unterschiedlicher Alterslasten hervorbringen. Es würde lediglich eine Verzerrung durch eine andere ersetzt. Deshalb ist ein grundsätzlich anderes Vorgehen vonnöten: Der Finanzausgleich im Kassenwettbewerb muß ein vom Ausgabeverhalten der einzelnen Kasse unabhängiger Ausgleich der Risiken sein. Wie dies möglich ist, wird anhand des oben eingeführten Vierkassenbeispiels demonstriert.

Altersstrukturausgleich

Höhere oder niedrigere Beitragssätze aufgrund der Alterslast existieren bei der einzelnen Kasse immer dann, wenn das Altersprofil dieser Kasse vom durchschnittlichen Altersprofil aller Kassen (quasi dem Bevölkerungsaufbau) abweicht. Wenn verhindert werden soll, daß Kassen schon allein aufgrund ihres hohen Altenanteils einen hohen Beitrag haben, dann müssen Kassen mit vergleichsweise jungen Versicherten in den Finanzausgleich zahlen und Kassen mit hohem Altenanteil Zuweisungen erhalten. Kassen mit durchschnittlichem Altersaufbau bleiben vom Ausgleich unberührt. Der folgende Vorschlag zielt darauf ab, die

---

[6] Zur Funktionsweise vgl. Mess, E.: Die schwierigen Finanzierungsprobleme in der Krankenversicherung der Rentner, in: Die Ersatzkasse 9/1986, S. 353–359; und Mathew, H.: Das KVdR-Abrechnungsverfahren mit der BfA, in: Die Ersatzkasse 9/1986, S. 359–367

[7] Vgl. Kübler, G.: KVdR-Finanzausgleich ist korrekturbedürftig, in: Die Krankenversicherung 3/1986, S. 77–80.

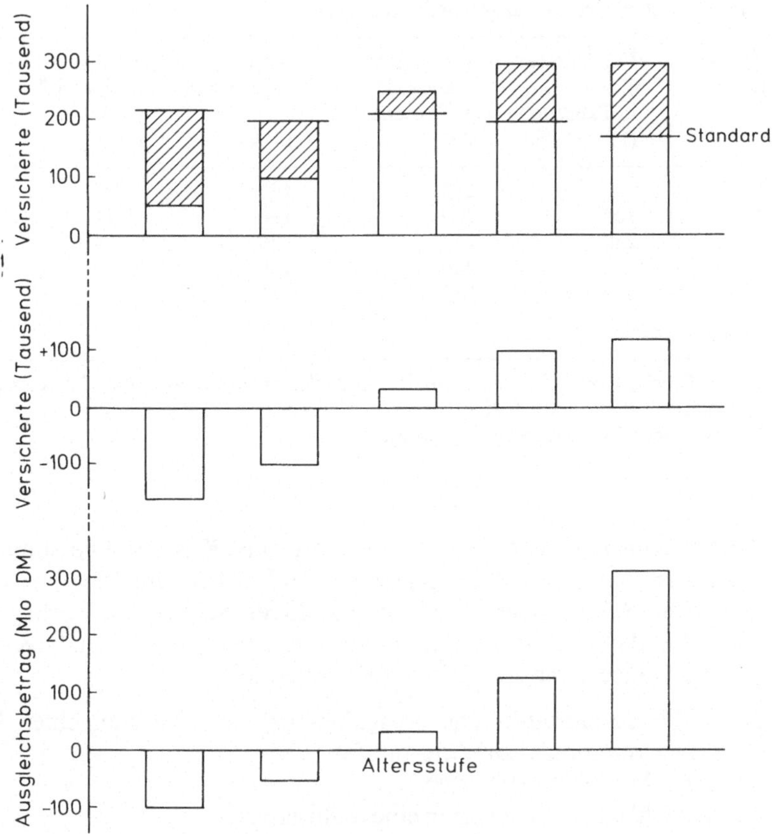

Abb. 2. Altersstrukturausgleich für Kasse D

durchschnittlichen Mehr- oder Minderausgaben auszugleichen, die sich aus den Abweichungen von der Standardaltersstruktur ergeben. Hat eine Kasse überdurchschnittlich viele Versicherte in der teuren Altersgruppe 5 und entsprechend weniger in der billigen Gruppe 1, dann sollen ihr die daraus resultierenden Mehrausgaben erstattet werden.

Zunächst müssen die Abweichungen von der Standardverteilung berechnet werden. Dazu wird die Altersverteilung im gesamten System (vgl. Tabelle 1, erste Spalte, alle Kassen) auf die jeweilige Kassengröße bezogen. Abbildung 2 zeigt für Kasse D im oberen Teil die Altersgruppenstärke im Vergleich zum Standardaufbau. Der mittlere Teil der Abb. 2 gibt die Abweichungen wieder: In der Altersgruppe 1 hat Kasse D 163 000 Versicherte weniger, in Gruppe 5 125 000 mehr, als es dem allgemeinen Kassendurchschnitt entspricht. Die Abweichungen vom Standardaltersprofil addieren sich notwendigerweise zu null (Summe der Flächen über der Linie ist gleich Summe der Flächen unter der Linie). Die Mehr- oder Minderausgaben, die aus den Abweichungen resultieren (unterer Teil der Abb. 2), ergeben sich nach Multiplikation mit den durchschnittlichen Ausgaben

Tabelle 3. Altersstrukturausgleich der Kasse D

Alters-gruppe	Versicherte Kasse D in Tausend (1)	Versicherte Standard[a] in Tausend (2)	Abweichung in Tausend (3)=(1)-(2)	Standard-ausgaben[b] DM/Jahr (4)	Ausgleichs-betrag in 1 000 DM (5)=(3)·(4)
1	50	213	-163	625	-101 483
2	100	200	-100	671	- 64 083
3	250	212	38	954	35 772
4	300	200	100	1 331	133 125
5	300	175	125	2 560	319 940
Ausgleichszahlung an Kasse D:					320 271

[a] Aus Tabelle 1 (alle Kassen, 1. Spalte) multipliziert mit dem Anteil der Kasse D an allen Versicherten: $1\,000/4\,800 = 0{,}209$.

[b] Aus Tabelle 1 (alle Kassen, 2. Spalte).

je Altersstufe (vgl. Tabelle 1, zweite Spalte, alle Kassen). Die Summation über alle Altersstufen zeigt, ob die Kasse per saldo Mittel im Finanzausgleich einzahlt (negativer Saldo) oder empfängt (positiver Saldo). Im vorliegenden Beispiel (Abb. 2, Tabelle 3) führt die Summation zu einer Zahlung an die Kasse D.

Das Ganze in mathematischer Kürze; es sei:

A_j　GKV-durchschnittliche Ausgaben pro Versicherten einer Jahrgangsstufe (hier vereinfacht zur Altersstufe),

V　Anzahl aller Versicherten,

V_j　Anzahl aller Versicherten eines Jahrgangs,

V_k　Anzahl aller Versicherten einer Kasse,

V_{jk}　Anzahl aller Versicherten einer Kasse und eines Jahrgangs.

Der Zahlungs- bzw. Zuweisungsbetrag F_k einer Kasse K im Finanzausgleich berechnet sich dann zu:

$$F_k = \sum_j A_j \left(V_{jk} - \frac{V_k}{V} V_j \right) \qquad (1)$$

Der Klammerausdruck ist dabei die Abweichung vom Standardaltersprofil. Er ist gleich Null, wenn die Jahrgangsstärke dem Standardprofil entspricht (vgl. Kasse C).

Das Beachtenswerte an dieser Formel (Gl. 1) ist, daß eine Größe nicht vorkommt: die Ausgaben der einzelnen Kasse. Mehr- oder Minderausgaben der einzelnen Kasse haben keinen Einfluß auf die Höhe des Ausgleichsbetrags. Unwirtschaftliches Verhalten wird nicht belohnt. Damit verbleiben Einsparungen in voller Höhe bei den effizienten Kassen und können sich im Beitrag niederschlagen. Dieser Beitragssatz BS_k errechnet sich bei Grundlohnsumme GL_k und Ausgaben in Höhe von A_k wie folgt:

$$BS_k = \frac{A_k - F_k}{GL_k} \qquad (2)$$

Grundlohnausgleich

In einem System mit Beitragssätzen gemäß Gl. 2 hat nach wie vor die Finanzkraft (genauer: die Grundlohnsumme) der Versicherten Einfluß auf den Beitragssatz. Kassen mit gut verdienenden Versicherten haben vergleichsweise niedrige Beiträge. Bei einem Grundlohnausgleich erfolgt die Beitragsberechnung so, als ob die Mitglieder aller Kassen gleichviel verdienen würden. Der korrigierte Beitragssatz KBS_k einer Kasse K ergibt sich dabei aus den Ausgaben, der Versichertenzahl und einem fiktiven durchschnittlichen Grundlohn DGL:

$$KBS_k = \frac{A_k}{V_k \cdot DGL} \tag{3}$$

Dabei muß die Summe der Ausgaben aller Kassen gleich der Summe der Einnahmen (Grundlohnsumme · korrigierter Beitragssatz) sein:

$$\sum_k A_k = \sum_k KBS_k \cdot GL_k \tag{4}$$

Einsetzen von Gl. 3 in Gl. 4 und Umstellen führt zum Wert von DGL, eine mit den Ausgaben gewichtete Grundlohnsumme:

$$DGL = \frac{\sum_k \frac{A_k}{V_k} \cdot GL_k}{\sum_k A_k} \tag{5}$$

Für den gesamten Alters- und Grundlohnausgleich gilt damit folgende Beitragssatzberechnung:

$$BS_k = \frac{A_k - F_k}{V_k \cdot DGL}$$

$$\text{mit } DGL = \frac{\sum_k (A_k - F_k) \cdot \frac{GL_k}{V_k}}{\sum_k A_k}$$

Der Grundlohnausgleich wird in der Regel für Mitglieder diskutiert und für die kostenlos Mitversicherten ein gesonderter Familienlastenausgleich erwogen. Da die Familienquoten sehr unterschiedlich sind – sie reichen von 4–175 Mitversicherten je 100 Mitgliedern (ohne Rentner) –, da außerdem die Zusammensetzung der Mitversicherten aus Ehepartnern und Kindern (mit sehr unterschiedlichen Ausgaben) ebenfalls schwankt, ist ein Ausgleich der Familienlast ohne Ausgabenausgleich kaum zu bewerkstelligen.

Der hier vorgeschlagene Grundlohnausgleich für Versicherte umgeht diese Schwierigkeiten. Für den Beitragssatz ist das Verhältnis der erwarteten Ausgaben für Mitglied und Mitversicherte zum Grundlohn entscheidend. Statt nun den Grundlohnausgleich auf Mitglieder zu beziehen und die (Ausgaben der) Mitversicherten gesondert zu behandeln, werden die Mitversicherten einfach als Mitglieder mit besonders geringem Grundlohn (nämlich null) behandelt. Der Grundlohnausgleich für Versicherte ist damit gleichzeitig ein vollständiger Familienlastenausgleich!

Mit gleicher Eleganz löst sich das Problem der unterschiedlichen Rentneranteile. Auch die Rentner werden zu „Grundlöhnern". Ihr Grundlohn setzt sich aus ihren eigenen Beiträgen und den Zahlungen der Rentenversicherung an die Krankenversicherung zusammen. Es bleibt zwar das „Verschiebebahnhofproblem" – Generationenausgleich in der Kranken- oder in der Rentenversicherung –, aber der wettbewerbsverzerrende Effekt unterschiedlicher Rentneranteile und unterschiedlicher Rentenhöhen entfällt.

Der momentan existierende, ausgabentreibende KVdR-Ausgleich würde also durch ein vom Ausgabenverhalten der einzelnen Kasse unabhängiges Verfahren ersetzt: Der Altersstrukturausgleich korrigiert die unterschiedlichen Ausgabenbelastungen der Kassen, die sich beim Umlageverfahren aus dem hohen Durchschnittsalter der Rentner ergeben. Der Grundlohnausgleich für Mitglieder, Mitversicherte und Rentner verteilt die Grundlohnsumme so, daß der Kasse für jeden Versicherten die gleiche Finanzkraft zur Verfügung steht.

Es muß betont werden, daß der Grundlohnausgleich Vorteile kleiner Solidargemeinschaften nicht beeinträchtigt. Solidarisches Verhalten der Versicherten durch Vermeidung überflüssiger Inanspruchnahme findet nach wie vor seinen vollen Niederschlag im Beitragssatz der Kasse. Durch den Grundlohnausgleich wird lediglich der Einfluß des Grundlohns und der verzerrende Effekt unterschiedlicher Familienlastquoten auf den Beitrag eliminiert.

Der gesamte Finanzausgleich im Vierkassenmodell

Zurück zum Beispiel: Tabelle 4 zeigt die Berechnung der Beitragssätze nach komplettem Finanzausgleich; Abb. 3 skizziert die Beitragssatzverschiebungen, die sich durch einen Altersausgleich (1. Schritt) und einen Grundlohnausgleich (2. Schritt) ergeben.

Tabelle 4. Beitragssätze vor und nach Finanzausgleich

Kasse	A	B	C	D
(1) Ausgaben (Mio DM)	1 190	2 210	917	1 365
(2) Altersausgleich	44	− 364	0	320
(3) Altersbereinigte Ausgaben (1)–(2)	1 146	2 574	917	1 045
(4) Grundlohn	11 000	26 000	7 200	9 000
(5) Korrigierter Grundlohn	11 216	22 431	8 973	11 216
(6) Beitragssatz vor Ausgleich (1)/(4)	10,8	8,5	12,7	15,2
(7) Beitragssatz nach Altersausgleich (3)/(4)	10,4	9,9	12,7	11,6
(8) Beitragssatz nach Alters- und Grundlohnausgleich (3)/(5)	10,2	11,5	10,2	9,3

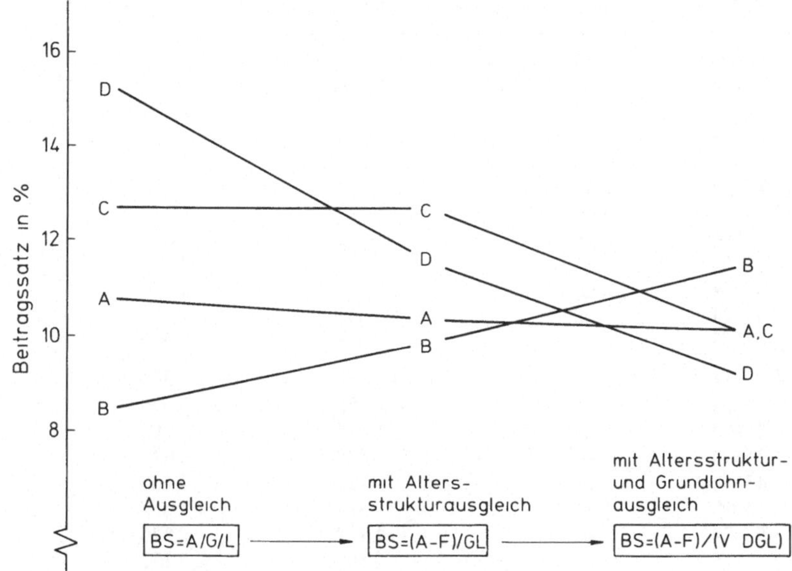

Abb. 3. Beitragssätze mit und ohne Finanzausgleich

Der Sinn der vielen Zuweisungen und Zahlungen wird beim Vergleich von Abb. 3 mit Abb. 1 deutlich. Nach kassenübergreifendem Finanzausgleich entspricht die Beitragsstruktur genau der Ausgabenstruktur:

– Kasse D hat als effizienteste Kasse den niedrigsten Beitrag.
– Die Kassen A und C haben einen Beitrag in gleicher Höhe.[8]
– Die unwirtschaftliche Kasse B hat verdientermaßen den höchsten Beitragssatz.

Die Beitragssätze erfüllen wieder ihre Funktion als Preissignale.

Geschlechtsstruktur

Im Vierkassenbeispiel wird vernachlässigt, daß Männer und Frauen Gesundheitsleistungen in sehr unterschiedlichem Umfang in Anspruch nehmen. Da die Geschlechtsstruktur vieler Kassen – insbesondere bei Betriebskrankenkassen – stark vom Durchschnitt abweicht, ist in der GKV ein Ausgleich für den „Risikofaktor Geschlecht" erforderlich. Dies geschieht zweckmäßigerweise analog zum dargestellten Altersstrukturausgleich. So wie ein ungünstiger Altersaufbau Zuweisungen im Altersstrukturausgleich begründet, so sollen auch Belastungen

---

[8] Es können sich geringfügige Abweichungen vom Ausgleichsideal – „Gleiche Ausgabenstrukturen führen nach Ausgleich zu gleichen Beitragssätzen" – ergeben. Diesem Ideal könnte nur dann entsprochen werden, wenn im Altersstrukturausgleich nicht mit durchschnittlichen, sondern mit den jeweils kassenspezifischen Ausgaben je Altersstufe ausgeglichen würde, dann aber addieren sich Zahlen und Zuweisungen nicht notwendigerweise zu null.

Tabelle 5. Alters- und Geschlechtsausgleich am Beispiel einer Heilbronner Kasse

Alters-gruppe	m.: männlich w.: weiblich	Abweichung vom Standard-aufbau[a]	Ausgaben je Versicherten[a] DM	Ausgleichs-betrag 1 000 DM
$\leqq$ 14	m.	−1 633	659	− 1 076
15–24	m.	171	420	72
25–34	m.	−1 149	610	− 701
35–44	m.	− 931	878	− 818
45–54	m.	962	1 153	1 109
55–64	m.	− 67	1 750	− 118
65–74	m.	665	2 749	1 828
$\geqq$ 75	m.	686	3 010	2 064
$\leqq$ 14	w.	−1 576	550	− 867
15–24	w.	− 256	596	− 152
25–34	w.	−1 815	966	− 1 753
35–44	w.	− 679	1 024	− 695
45–54	w.	781	1 263	987
55–64	w.	314	1 652	519
65–74	w.	1 962	2 546	4 996
$\geqq$ 75	w	2 565	3 232	8 290
Ausgleichszahlung an die Kasse				13 684

[a] Berechnet nach den Werten aus den Anhangtabellen 1, 2 und 3
[Nach Ministerium für Arbeit, Gesundheit, Familie und Sozialordnung des Landes Baden-Württemberg (Hrsg.): Leistungs- und Kostentransparenz – Erste Ergebnisse eines Modellversuchs in der gesetzlichen Krankenversicherung, Stuttgart 1987]

ausgeglichen werden, die auf eine vom Durchschnitt abweichende Geschlechtsstruktur zurückzuführen sind. Tabelle 5 zeigt in Spalte 4 anhand von Heilbronner Daten[9] aus dem Jahre 1984, daß der Umfang der Mehrausgaben durch Frauen- bzw. Männerüberschuß altersabhängig ist, eine einfache formelmäßige Berücksichtigung der Frauen- bzw. Männerquote also nicht ausreichen würde, um Beitragssatzverzerrungen zu eliminieren. Vielmehr müssen die Abweichungen für jeden einzelnen Jahrgang gesondert berechnet werden. Dazu wird der Altersausgleich nach Gleichung 1 zu einer Doppelsumme erweitert, wobei der Index g für das Geschlecht steht:

$$F_k = \sum_g \sum_J A_{gJ} \left(V_{gJk} - \frac{V_k}{V} V_{gJ} \right) \tag{7}$$

Die Doppelsumme besagt nichts anderes, als daß sowohl die Daten aller Altersstufen als auch die Werte von Männern und Frauen summiert werden. Zur Verdeutlichung wird in Tabelle 5 eine Berechnung mit den jüngst veröffentlichten Daten der Transparenzstudie Heilbronn durchgeführt.

---

[9] Ministerium für Arbeit, Gesundheit, Familie und Sozialordnung des Landes Baden-Württemberg (Hrsg.): Leistungs- und Kostentransparenz – Erste Ergebnisse eines Modellversuchs in der gesetzlichen Krankenversicherung. Stuttgart 1987.

Weitere Risikofaktoren

In der bisherigen Darstellung wurden die „großen" GKV-Risikofaktoren Alter, Geschlecht, Grundlohn sowie Anzahl, Alter und Geschlecht der Mitversicherten ausgeglichen. Verbleibende Unterschiede in der Kostenstruktur je Versicherten wurden der Effizienz des Kassenmanagements zugeschrieben. Die Liste der Risikofaktoren ist natürlich beliebig erweiterbar.[10] Ein in den einzelnen Kassen unterschiedlich hoher Anteil von Rauchern, Alkoholikern oder Blutern würde ähnliche Beitragssatzverzerrungen nach sich ziehen wie abweichende Geschlechts- und Altersstrukturen. Durch Übergang zu Dreifach- oder gar Mehrfachsummen (vgl. Gl. 1 und 7) kann theoretisch jeder Grad an Ausgleichsperfektion erreicht werden. Aber lohnt sich das?

Um verzerrte Beitragssätze zu vermeiden, müssen nur diejenigen Risikofaktoren ausgeglichen werden, für die gleichzeitig 3 Bedingungen gelten:

1) Die sog. schlechten Risiken müssen nachweisbar höhere Ausgaben verursachen. Entscheidend ist nicht die Morbidität, sondern die Inanspruchnahme von Gesundheitsleistungen.
2) Es muß ein bedeutender Anteil von Versicherten betroffen sein, damit die Ausgaben überhaupt auf den Beitrag der gesamten Kassen durchschlagen.
3) Der Anteil der schlechten Risiken muß in den Kassen unterschiedlich sein, da sich ansonsten keine Verschiebung der Wettbewerbspositionen ergibt.

Wie stark die Beitragssatzverzerrung ist, wenn ein Risikofaktor nicht berücksichtigt wird, läßt sich unter Vernachlässigung von Alter und Geschlecht grob abschätzen. Es sei:

A_r Ausgaben der Risikogruppe,
A_d GKV-durchschnittliche Ausgaben,
R/V_k Anteil der Risikogruppe an allen Versicherten V der Kasse K,
N/V Anteil der Risikogruppe in der gesamten GKV,

dann ist die Abweichung des verzerrten Beitragssatzes ZBS vom durchschnittlichen Beitrag BS:

$$\frac{ZBS - BS}{BS} = \frac{A_r}{A_d}\left(\frac{R}{V_k} - \frac{N}{V}\right) \tag{8}$$

Dazu ein Beispiel: Wenn Arbeitslose 50 % mehr Gesundheitsleistungen in Anspruch nehmen als andere Versicherte und in einer Kasse die Arbeitslosenquote bei 6 % der Versicherten (nicht der Mitglieder!) liegt – bei einem GKV-Durchschnitt von 4 % –, dann beträgt die Abweichung 1,5 % (0,06–0,04) = 0,03, was bei Beitragssätzen in der Höhe von 12 % ungefähr 0,4 Prozentpunkten entspricht.

---

[10] Zu anderen Risikofaktoren vgl. Henke, K.-D./Adam, H.: Risikovorsorge im Gesundheitswesen, in: Holzheu, F./Kaufmann, F.-X. u. a. (Hrsg.): Gesellschaft und Unsicherheit, Karlsruhe 1987.

Die eigentliche Hürde für ein differenzierteres Ausgleichsverfahren ist die Erfassung der Risiken:

1) Die Mehrausgaben eines Risikofaktors müssen repräsentativ für die GKV getrennt für Männer und Frauen und für jede Altersstufe ermittelt werden.
2) Für alle Kassen muß der Anteil jeder Risikogruppe an der gesamten Versichertengemeinschaft bekannt sein. Bedenkt man, daß 1986 überhaupt zum ersten Mal die Altersstruktur der Versicherten je Kasse erfaßt wurde und dies bisher nur im Vierjahresturnus wiederholt werden soll, dann wird der hochdifferenzierte Ausgleich schnell zum fernen Zukunftstraum.

Wichtiger als die Erweiterung des Alters-, Geschlechts- und Grundlohnausgleichs um weitere Risikofaktoren ist die Angleichung im Mitgliedsrecht der einzelnen Kassenarten und die Beseitigung von Verzerrungen, die sich auf der Leistungsseite ergeben, so z. B. die durch die Mischkalkulation im allgemeinen Pflegesatz verursachte Subventionierung der Umlandkassen.

Umsetzungschancen

Trotz dieser Einschränkungen bleibt festzuhalten: Auch ohne risikoproportionale Beiträge und ohne Übergang zum Kapitaldeckungsverfahren kann durch kassenübergreifenden Risikoausgleich ein funktionierender Wettbewerb zwischen den Kassen organisiert werden. In einem solchen System mit GKV-Prinzipien (Familienversicherung, einkommensbezogene Beiträge) und kassenübergreifendem Finanzausgleich (Alters-, Familienlast- und Grundlohnausgleich) führt die freie Kassenwahl für alle Arbeitnehmer zu einem gesamtwirtschaftlich sinnvollen Ergebnis. Durch den Wettbewerbsdruck ist eine verstärkte Ausschöpfung von Einsparpotentialen zu erwarten. Auch sozialpolitisch hat der Finanzausgleich bedeutsame Vorteile: Die einzelne Kasse hat ein gleich starkes Interesse an Mitgliedern jeder Einkommensgruppe – an hochverdienenden freiwillig Versicherten genauso wie an Arbeitslosen. Anreize, sich vorrangig um die sog. guten Risiken zu kümmern, entfallen.

Der Vorschlag eines Grundlohnausgleichs und einer weitgehenden Neuordnung des Alterslastenausgleichs zwischen den Kassen klingt natürlich zunächst wie ein gewaltiger, den Reformwillen überfordernder Schritt – was nicht zuletzt an der schwer durchschaubaren Materie liegt. Gleichwohl sind nur geringfügige institutionelle Änderungen notwendig. Das Bundesversicherungsamt würde statt des KVdR-Ausgleichs künftig einen Grundlohn-, Geschlechts- und Altersausgleich vornehmen, die bestehenden Kassen blieben erhalten. Auch der Aufwand zur Beschaffung der erforderlichen Daten ist überschaubar: Die Grundlohndaten sind vorhanden und neben dem längst überfälligen GKV-Ausgabenprofil (Ausgaben in Abhängigkeit von Alter und Geschlecht) sind lediglich Alter und Geschlecht der Versicherten (einschließlich Rentner) vollständiger zu erfassen als bisher.

Die Kassenlandschaft würde sich durch freie Kassenwahl und Mitgliederwanderung nur allmählich ändern. Damit das System offenbleibt für neue Ideen, sollte mittelfristig die Bildung neuer Kassen ermöglicht werden. Parallel dazu müßten die Gestaltungsmöglichkeiten im Vertragsrecht erweitert werden, um den Kassen mehr Chancen zu geben, Einsparungen zu erwirtschaften.

Wie sind also die Umsetzungschancen einzuschätzen? Zunächst einmal bedarf es der Gewöhnung, daß Finanzausgleich – richtig konstruiert – den Wettbewerb fördern kann. Dann aber spricht alles für das vorgeschlagene Modell:

1) Der Finanzausgleich ist aus Gründen der Effizienz genauso geboten wie aus Gründen der sozialen Gerechtigkeit.
2) Die wesentlichen Prinzipien der Gesetzlichen Krankenversicherung – Sachleistungsprinzip, Familienversicherung, einkommensbezogene Beiträge – bleiben erhalten.
3) Komplementäre Reformen im Einkommensteuerrecht sind nicht erforderlich.

Trotz aller Argumente: Es wird natürlich Widerstand geben – von all jenen nämlich, die im Finanzausgleich zahlen müssen. Vielleicht sollte man Konsens herbeiführen, bevor alle notwendigen Daten erhoben sind und errechnet wird, wer zu dieser Gruppe gehört.[11] Die Hoffnung auf baldigen Konsens gründet sich v. a. auf den Mangel an Alternativen: Wenn die Wahlfreiheit, die bisher Privileg der Angestellten war, auch für Arbeiter gelten soll, wenn man die Einheitsversicherung aus guten Gründen ablehnt, wenn der Übergang zu risikoproportionalen Beiträgen nicht möglich ist, wenn man des weiteren verzerrten Wettbewerb für unsozial und unwirtschaftlich hält, was bleibt dann noch – außer Finanzausgleich?

---

[11] Vgl. das Vorgehen in: Rawls, J.: Eine Theorie der Gerechtigkeit, Frankfurt 1971. Zur Diskussion der Grundsätze einer gerechten Gesellschaftsordnung nimmt Rawls einen hypothetischen Urzustand an, in dem sich die einzelnen Parteien auf Regeln einigen, ohne ihren jeweiligen Platz in der Gesellschaft zu kennen.

Zur Verfassungsmäßigkeit
unterschiedlicher Beitragssätze
in der Gesetzlichen Krankenversicherung

W. Gitter

Die Entwicklung der Beitragssätze
in der Gesetzlichen Krankenversicherung (GKV)

Die heftigen Diskussionen um das Gesundheitsreformgesetz sind nach dessen Inkrafttreten abgeklungen. Es hat sich trotz weiterbestehender kritischer Einwände eine objektivere Sicht durchgesetzt, die die positiven Auswirkungen des Gesetzes, insbesondere die dadurch veranlaßte Stabilisierung der Beitragssätze und teilweise sogar deren Reduzierung,[1] anerkennt. Allerdings haben sich im Hinblick auf die Beitragssätze einzelner Kassen neue Probleme ergeben. Diese Probleme sind darauf zurückzuführen, daß im Gesundheitsreformgesetz bewußt auf eine grundsätzliche Neuregelung der Organisationsstruktur verzichtet wurde, so daß wie bisher die verschiedenen Kassenarten mit unterschiedlichen Risikostrukturen nebeneinander bestehen. Diese Situation hat sich in letzter Zeit dadurch verschärft, daß einige große Unternehmen, wie z. B. Audi Ingolstadt, BMW in München, das Drägerwerk in Lübeck, Preußen Electra in Hannover, beabsichtigen, eigene Betriebskrankenkassen zu gründen. Die Ortskrankenkassen der entsprechenden Regionen befürchten, daß durch diesen „Akt der Entsolidarisierung" ihre Beitragssätze erneut deutlich ansteigen werden.

Betrachtet man die Entwicklung der Beitragssätze in der GKV, so lassen sich 2 grundlegende Tendenzen festhalten:

Zum einen hat sich bei allen Kassenarten der durchschnittliche Beitragssatz seit Bestehen der GKV ständig erhöht, von minimalen Schwankungen einmal abgesehen.[2]

Zum anderen driften die Beitragssatzunterschiede zwischen den einzelnen Kassenarten, aber auch kassenartintern, immer weiter auseinander.

Extremwerte sind z. B. der Beitragssatz der AOK Papenburg mit 16%, hingegen liegt der Beitragssatz bei der Betriebskrankenkasse der Waagenfabrik Sauter bei 8,0%. Innerhalb einer Stadt wie Hamburg sind extreme Unterschiede in der Höhe der zu zahlenden Beiträge zu verzeichnen: Ein Durchschnittsverdiener in Hamburg kann mit einem monatlichen Krankenversicherungsbeitrag von 285 DM zu einer Betriebskrankenkasse oder auch mit 465 DM zur AOK belastet

---

[1] Vgl. dazu Jung OK (1989) Neues Kapitel in der Krankenversicherung, BArbBl 2/1989, S 11ff.; Standfest OE (1988) Tatsachen und Fiktionen um das Gesundheitsreformgesetz, KrV 1988, S 231ff.; Zipperer OM (1989) Die Gesundheitsreform: Änderungen des Leistungsrechts, KrV 1989, S 4ff.

[2] Vgl. Anlage 2 zu BT-Drcks. Nr. 11/2237.

sein, erhält aber die gleichen Leistungen, und dies zu einem Unterschiedsbetrag von 180 DM.[3] Zudem ist ein Nord-Süd-Gefälle auch innerhalb ein- und derselben Kassenart zu verzeichnen: So liegt z. B. der Beitragssatz der AOK Hamburg bereits bei 15,5%, während Versicherte der AOK Bad Tölz 11,0% für ihre Krankenversicherung aufbringen müssen.

Mitglieder der AOK Steinfurt haben bereits gegen einen Beitragssatz von 15,4% Verfassungsbeschwerde beim Bundesverfassungsgericht eingelegt.

Ursachen für die bestehenden Beitragssatzunterschiede

Es stellt sich nun die Frage, worin die Ursachen für die unterschiedlichen Beitragssätze in der Gesetzlichen Krankenversicherung zu suchen sind.

Argumente der Spitzenverbände der Gesetzlichen Krankenkassen

Die Verbände der Träger der GKV bestreiten derzeit hauptsächlich die öffentliche Diskussion um Ursachenforschung und Lösungsansätze. Bestimmt wird das Diskussionsbild v. a. durch gegenseitige Schuldzuweisungen. Der Bundesverband der Ortskrankenkassen beklagt seit Jahren den Abzug sog. positiver Risiken durch die Neugründung von Betriebskrankenkassen und Innungskrankenkassen sowie einen steten Zuwachs von schlechten Risiken wie Arbeitslose, chronisch Kranke, Rehabilitanden, Sozialhilfeempfänger, Asylanten, Aussiedler usw. Die Betriebs- und Innungskrankenkassen und ihre Spitzenverbände werfen den Ortskrankenkassen hingegen vor, durch Unwirtschaftlichkeit sowohl im Leistungsbereich als auch im Verwaltungs-, Personal- und Sachaufwand ihre Misere selbst herbeigeführt zu haben und – statt sich von innen zu erneuern – sich auf die Hilfe des Gesetzgebers zu verlassen, wohl wissend, daß sie im System der Gesetzlichen Krankenversicherung eine Sonderstellung innehaben; sie sind vom Gesetz bisher und auch weiterhin mit der Aufgabe betraut, Basis- und Auffangsystem in der GKV zu sein, so daß den Gesetzgeber auch die Verpflichtung trifft, die Ortskrankenkassen bestands- und leistungsfähig zu erhalten. Die Ortskrankenkassen würden aber stets die Schuld bei anderen suchen, nur nicht bei sich selbst.

Man kann diese Argumente der Spitzenverbände um die Ursachen für unterschiedliche Beitragssätze in der GKV, die derzeit die Diskussion bestimmen, wohl nicht einfach als unzutreffend vom Tisch wischen, weder die der Ortskrankenkassen noch die der Betriebs- und Innungskrankenkassen. Aber eine von gegenseitigen Schuldzuweisungen geprägte Diskussion trägt zur Lösung der Problematik nicht gerade bei.

---

[3] Vgl. zur Gesamtproblematik auch den Zwischenbericht der Enquetekommission (1988) „Strukturreform der gesetzlichen Krankenversicherung" vom 31.10.1988, BT-Drcks. Nr. 11/3267, S 372ff.

Gesetzliche Regelungen über die Beitragsbemessung

Näheren Aufschluß über die eigentlichen Ursachen für unterschiedliche Beitragssätze in der GKV kann gegebenenfalls eine Betrachtung der gesetzlichen Regelungen über die Beitragsbemessung bringen.

Das SGB-V enthält keine Vorschrift, die für alle Kassen der gesetzlichen Krankenversicherung den gleichen Beitrag vorschreiben würde, etwa in der Form, daß für den Bundesminister für Arbeit und Sozialordnung eine Ermächtigungsgrundlage vorhanden wäre, den Beitragssatz jährlich durch Erlaß einer Rechtsverordnung neu festzusetzen. Vielmehr werden nach dem Grundsatz der Beitragsbemessung in § 220 SGB-V die Mittel der Krankenversicherung durch Beiträge und sonstige Einnahmen der Kassen aufgebracht, wobei die Beiträge so zu bemessen sind, daß sie zusammen mit den sonstigen Einnahmen die im Haushaltsplan vorgesehenen Ausgaben und die vorgeschriebene Auffüllung der Rücklagen decken.

Dieser Grundsatz gilt allgemein für alle Kassenarten in der GKV. Weil aber – verkürzt gesagt – die Ausgaben jeder einzelnen Kasse durch Einnahmen gedeckt werden müssen, die Einnahmen sich wiederum hautpsächlich aus den Beitragszahlungen der Mitglieder zusammensetzen, setzt jede Krankenkasse ihren Beitragssatz unter Berücksichtigung ihrer Ausgaben fest. Die einzelnen Krankenkassen sind also bei der Festsetzung ihres Beitragssatzes autonom, wenngleich sie an die Vorschriften der §§ 220 ff. SGB-V gebunden sind. Damit scheidet zwar eine willkürliche Handhabung der Beitragssatzbemessung durch die Krankenkassen aus, dennoch bestimmt die Höhe der Ausgaben der einzelnen Kasse wesentlich deren Beitragssatz.

Die Höhe dieser Ausgaben der einzelnen Krankenkasse wird von den Vorschriften der §§ 220 ff. SGB-V über die Beitragsbemessung nicht tangiert. Diese gelten für alle Kassen gleichermaßen. Auch Unterschiede im Leistungsrecht können für unterschiedlich hohe Leistungsausgaben und damit für unterschiedlich hohe Beiträge nicht mehr (allein) verantwortlich gemacht werden: Schon vor Inkrafttreten des SGB-V wurden die bisher nach § 179 Abs. 3 RVO möglichen satzungsmäßigen Mehrleistungen Schritt für Schritt abgebaut, so daß in der Regel von den Krankenkassen der Gesetzlichen Krankenversicherung nur noch die Regelleistungen im Falle der Krankheit gewährt wurden. In § 11 SGB-V sind seit dem 1.1.1989 satzungsmäßige Mehrleistungen gesetzlich nicht mehr vorgesehen.[4]

Die Ursachen für unterschiedlich hohe Ausgaben der Krankenkassen werden deshalb in 2 Bereichen zu suchen sein: Entweder im Bereich der Wirtschaftlichkeit, sei es bei der Leistungserbringung, bei den Verträgen mit Leistungserbringern, Krankenhäusern und Apotheken usw., sei es bei dem Verwaltungsaufwand der einzelnen Kasse; oder aber in den hinter den Vorschriften über die Beitragsbemessung liegenden Strukturmerkmalen der Gesetzlichen Krankenversicherung.

---

[4] Vgl. dazu auch den Zwischenbericht der Enquetekommission (1987/88/89) BT-Drcks. Nr. 11/3267, S 374–375.

Über die Frage der Wirtschaftlichkeit bei der Leistungserbringung als Ursache für unterschiedliche Beitragssatzhöhen in der GKV kann an dieser Stelle nur spekuliert werden. Allein die Tatsache, daß der Gesetzgeber durch die Neuregelungen des SGB-V das Wirtschaftlichkeitsgebot bei der Leistungserbringung stärker als bisher betont und auch verstärkte Kontrollen über die Einhaltung des Wirtschaftlichkeitsgebots durch die Krankenkassen gesetzlich angeordnet hat, spricht dafür, daß die Wirtschaftlichkeit durchaus eine Rolle für die Beitragssatzhöhe spielt. Die Effizienz dieser Neuregelungen und der darauf beruhenden Kontrollmechanismen muß abgewartet werden, ein positiver Einfluß auf die Wirtschaftlichkeit der Leistungserbringung und damit auch auf die für die Beitragssatzbemessung relevante Höhe der Ausgaben kann aber wohl durchaus erwartet werden. Im übrigen wäre es jedoch Aufgabe einer eingehenden wissenschaftlichen Untersuchung, Unterschiede in bezug auf die Wirtschaftlichkeit verschiedener Kassenarten herauszuarbeiten, um Spekulationen darüber den Boden in Zukunft zu entziehen.

Mit Sicherheit haben jedoch auch die Strukturprinzipien der GKV, die hinter den Regelungen über Mitgliedschaft und Beitragsbemessung stehen, Einfluß – wenn nicht sogar entscheidende Auswirkungen – auf die Beitragssatzentwicklung bei den einzelnen Kassenarten.

Strukturprinzipien der GKV

Betrachtet man die Vorschriften der GKV über ihren Aufbau und ihre Organisation – wobei die rechtshistorische Entwicklung dieser Regelungen in keinem Fall außer acht gelassen werden darf –, so wird deutlich, daß der Gesetzgeber bereits bei Schaffung der Gesetzlichen Krankenversicherung nicht mit dem Ziel tätig geworden ist, eine weitestgehende Beitragssatzgleichheit zu schaffen, sondern daß er andere Strukturprinzipien in den Vordergrund gerückt hat.

Zu nennen ist hier einmal das soziale Schutzprinzip, denn ursprünglich ging es bei Schaffung der sozialen Sicherung v. a. darum, den Arbeitern, die aufgrund ihres geringen Einkommens und noch fehlender Arbeitsplatzschutzgesetzgebung dieses Schutzes am dringendsten bedurften, eine Absicherung für existentielle Notfälle zu gewähren. Durch die ständige Erweiterung des Kreises der pflichtversicherten Personen und die Ausweitungen der Leistungsansprüche im Fall der Krankheit im Lauf der Jahrzehnte seit Bestehen der GKV ist das soziale Schutzprinzip in den Hintergrund gedrängt worden, wenngleich Rechtsprechung und Gesetzgeber formal noch daran festhalten.

Weiteres Strukturprinzip ist die Solidargemeinschaft der in der GKV Versicherten. Dazu gehört der Familienlastenausgleich ebenso wie die Heranziehung der Mitglieder zur Finanzierung der GKV durch Beiträge entsprechend ihres Einkommens, also unabhängig von persönlichen Risikofaktoren, Dauerkrankheiten oder chronischen Erkrankungen. Auch die Absicherung von solchen Personen, die aufgrund ihrer sozialen Situation nicht in der Lage sind, mit ihrem Einkommen Beiträge an die GKV zu entrichten, wie z. B. Sozialhilfeempfänger und Arbeitslose bei Bezug von Arbeitslosenhilfe, gehört zum solidarisch geprägten System der sozialen Sicherung.

Weiteres wesentliches Strukturmerkmal der GKV ist schließlich noch das gegliederte Kassenorganisationssystem.

Die Gliederung der Träger der Gesetzlichen Krankenversicherung erfolgte bereits seit ihren Ursprüngen im 19. Jahrhundert nach einer Vielzahl unterschiedlicher Gesichtspunkte, nämlich einmal nach örtlichen Kriterien (AOK), nach Berufszweigen (IKK, Ersatzkassen, Bundesknappschaft, Seekrankenkasse), nach Betriebszugehörigkeit (BKK) oder nach Wirtschaftszweigen (Landwirtschaftliche Krankenkasse). Der Gesetzgeber hat dabei in den Anfängen der gesetzlichen Sozialversicherung teils an bereits bestehende Einrichtungen angeknüpft, teils neue Kassen geschaffen. Die Dezentralisierung und damit auch die Versichertennähe stand bei der Gliederung der GKV ebenso im Vordergrund wie der Aspekt, daß durch möglichst kleine Versichertengemeinschaften, deren Mitglieder mehr oder weniger von denselben Risiken bedroht waren, die gegenseitige Verantwortung für das Versicherungssystem stärker sei. Die Versichertengemeinschaften wurden dadurch – auf Dauer gesehen – für leistungsfähiger gehalten und man hoffte, dadurch auch der Gefahr des Mißbrauchs von Versicherungsleistungen „bei Simulation" am besten entgegenwirken zu können.

Bereits in den Jahren 1909/1910 – während der Diskussionen um den Entwurf der RVO – erwiesen sich diese Risikogemeinschaften aber als zu klein und nicht leistungsfähig genug; schließlich hatten damals 44,6% der Kassen weniger als 100 Mitglieder, 92,1% weniger als 1000 Mitglieder und nur 1,1% der Kassen verfügten über mehr als 5000 Mitglieder. Die Folge war eine Kassenorganisationsreform, die eine Mindestgröße für Krankenkassen vorschrieb, Ortskrankenkassen wurden zu größeren Einheiten verschmolzen und die Bildung besonderer Kassen, zu denen die Betriebskrankenkassen und die Innungskrankenkassen zählten, wurde vorübergehend erschwert. Dadurch reduzierte sich die Zahl der Krankenkassen auf die Hälfte. Diese Tendenz hat sich bis zum Jahre 1988 fortgesetzt: 1938 war noch ein Bestand von 4510 Kassen zu verzeichnen, während 1950 nur noch 1996 Kassen existierten. 1985 gab es 1215 Kassen, was im wesentlichen auf eine deutliche Abnahme bei der Zahl der Betriebskrankenkassen zurückzuführen war (1950: 1320 BKK; 1985: 754 BKK). 1988 bestanden insgesamt noch 1164 Gesetzliche Krankenkassen, davon 268 Ortskrankenkassen und 706 Betriebskrankenkassen.[5]

Der Trend zu größeren Versichertengemeinschaften bei jeder einzelnen Kasse hat sich also über Jahrzehnte hinweg fortgesetzt. Dagegen sind aber – trotz zahlreicher gesetzlicher Neuregelungen auf dem Gebiet der gesetzlichen Krankenversicherung – die Merkmale, nach denen die GKV gegliedert ist, unverändert beibehalten worden. Auch durch die Neuregelungen der §§ 173 ff. SGB-V hat sich diesbezüglich keine Änderung ergeben. Dies kann als – bereits mehrfach wiederholte – Entscheidung des Gesetzgebers angesehen werden, das gegliederte Kassenorganisationsprinzip als Wesensmerkmal der Gesetzlichen Krankenversicherung beibehalten zu wollen und diesem Prinzip – ebenso wie dem Solidaritätsprinzip – den Vorrang vor einer Beitragssatzgleichheit für alle Mitglieder der GKV einzuräumen.

---

[5] Vgl. Zwischenbericht der Enquetekommission (1987/88/89) BT-Drcks. Nr. 11/3267, S 370.

Gerade aber das Solidaritätsprinzip wie auch das gegliederte Kassenorganisationsprinzip haben unverkennbar nicht unerheblichen Einfluß auf die Beitragssatzhöhe in der GKV bzw. auf die Beitragssatzunterschiede zwischen den einzelnen Kassenarten und auch kassenartintern, wie dies z. B. im Nord-Süd-Gefälle zum Ausdruck kommt. Ein hohes Grundlohnniveau der Versicherten ermöglicht höhere Beitragseinnahmen; sog. „gute Versichertenrisiken" verursachen weniger Ausgaben; hingegen verursacht ein hoher Anteil an Familienmitversicherten eine höhere Familienlastquote, d. h. weniger Beitragseinnahmen müssen höhere Leistungsausgaben decken. Nachgewiesen ist auch, daß z. B. bei Arbeitslosen mit der Dauer der Arbeitslosigkeit auch die Krankheitshäufigkeit zunimmt und somit höhere Leistungsausgaben anfallen. Auch bei Rentnern decken die Beitragsleistungen bei weitem nicht die auf diesen Versichertenkreis entfallenden Leistungsausgaben.

Auch der Zwischenbericht der Enquetekommission zur Strukturreform der Gesetzlichen Krankenversicherung kommt zu dem Ergebnis, daß die bestehende Kassenorganisationsstruktur und damit das traditionell gegliederte System der GKV ein wesentliches Ursachenbündel für die wachsenden Beitragssatzunterschiede in der GKV darstellt: Ausschlaggebende Bedeutung erlangen dabei das durch die gegliederte Struktur verursachte unterschiedliche Grundlohnsummenniveau sowie die ebenfalls dadurch bedingten unterschiedlichen Risikostrukturen innerhalb der bestehenden Versichertengemeinschaften. Die Enquetekommission kommt dabei zu der Feststellung, daß die Ortskrankenkassen bei einem niedrigeren Grundlohnsummenniveau eine schlechtere Risikozusammensetzung der Versichertengemeinschaft hinnehmen muß und somit bei einem schlechteren Finanzierungspotential einen höheren Finanzbedarf als die übrigen Kassen abdecken muß.[6] Herausragend ist dabei, daß der Anteil der bei der AOK versicherten Arbeitslosen drei mal so hoch ist wie bei den Betriebskrankenkassen und daß die Ortskrankenkassen 68,65% der Behinderten sowie 70,13% der Rehabilitanden versichern.

Unterschiede im Finanzierungspotential und im Finanzbedarf sind also bei den einzelnen Kassenarten der GKV nicht von der Hand zu weisen.

Andererseits ermöglicht die Vielzahl nebeneinander bestehender Kassen oft gerade den sog. guten Risiken mit hohem Grundlohnniveau die Wahl zwischen mehreren Kassen, z. B. zwischen AOK, BKK oder IKK und Ersatzkassen. Zu beachten ist hierbei gleichzeitig, daß auch ein gravierender Wandel in der sozioökonomischen Struktur der Gesellschaft eingetreten ist. Überwiegte seit Bestehen der GKV zunächst die Gruppe der Arbeiter, so sind mittlerweile ca. 50% der Versicherten dem Kreis der Angestellten mit Wahlmöglichkeit zu den einzelnen Kassenarten zuzurechnen. Die Ortskrankenkassen haben aber in der Regel den höchsten Beitragssatz der Kassen einer Region. Es ist deshalb kaum wahrscheinlich, daß ein Versicherter, der die Möglichkeit zu einem Wechsel zu einer Krankenkasse mit niedrigerem Beitragssatz hat, unter Besinnung auf das Solidaritätsprinzip bei der AOK verbleibt. Der sog. „Entsolidarisierungseffekt" ist deshalb

---

[6] Vgl. Tabelle 4.9 zu den Grundlohnsummen sowie Tabellen 4.10–4.19 zu den Risikostrukturen der RVO- und Ersatzkassen im Zwischenbericht der Enquetekommission (1987/88/89) BT-Drcks. Nr. 11/3267, S 377ff.

nicht nur ein Gespenst, das die AOK in der Diskussion um die Kassenorganisationsreform an die Wand malt. Zwar kann nicht behauptet werden, daß die Entsolidarisierung durch andere Krankenkassen und der damit verbundene Mitgliederschwund bei den Ortskrankenkassen die einzige Ursache für unterschiedliche Beitragssätze ist, sie spielt aber doch eine wesentliche Rolle in einem ganzen Bündel von Ursachen.

Verfassungsmäßigkeit der Beitragssatzunterschiede in der Gesetzlichen Krankenversicherung

Berührte Grundrechte

Sicherlich kommt hier zunächst Art. 3 Abs. 1 GG, also eine denkbare Verletzung des Gleichbehandlungsgrundsatzes in Betracht, wenn ein Versicherter für die gleichen Leistungen im Falle der Krankheit mehr an Beiträgen entrichten muß als ein vergleichbarer Versicherter mit gleichem Einkommen. Im Rahmen des Art. 3 Abs. 1 GG müßte auch das Sozialstaatsgebot aus Art. 20 Abs. 1 GG beachtet werden.

Denkbar wäre aber auch evtl. eine Verletzung von Art. 14 GG (Eigentum) bzw. – als Auffangtatbestand[7] – eine Verletzung des Art. 2 Abs. 1 GG, des allgemeinen Freiheitsrechts.

Das BVerfG wird sich in naher Zukunft mit der Frage der Verfassungsmäßigkeit unterschiedlicher Beitragssätze in der GKV zu beschäftigen haben, da – wie oben bereits angedeutet – Mitglieder der AOK Steinfurt Verfassungsbeschwerde gegen einen Beitragssatz von 15,4% eingelegt haben.

Wie das BVerfG entscheiden wird, bleibt abzuwarten. Bereits im Jahre 1985 hatte sich jedoch das Bundessozialgericht in einem Verfahren mit der Frage zu beschäftigen, ob Beitragssätze von 14,2 bzw. 14,9%, die ein Versicherter einer AOK in den Jahren 1980 bzw. 1981 zu entrichten hatte, mit dem Gleichbehandlungsgrundsatz aus Art. 3 Abs. 1 GG und dem Sozialstaatsgebot aus Art. 20 Abs. 1 GG vereinbar waren.[8]

Die Entscheidung des BSG vom 22.05.1987 zur Frage der Verletzung von Art. 3 Abs. 1 GG durch unterschiedliche Beitragssätze in der GKV

Das BSG hat die Klage in dieser Entscheidung für unbegründet erachtet und keine Verletzung verfassungsmäßiger Rechte, insbesondere von Art. 3 Abs. 1 in Verbindung mit Art. 20 Abs. 1 GG, in diesen Beitragssätzen gesehen.

Das Gericht hat sich dabei auf die ständige Rechtsprechung des BVerfG bezogen: Danach verbietet der allgemeine Gleichheitssatz des Art. 3 Abs. 1 GG, wesentlich Gleiches ohne zureichende sachliche Gründe ungleich und wesentlich Ungleiches ohne sachliche Gründe gleich zu behandeln; damit enthält Art. 3

---

[7] Vgl. BVerfGE 65, 297.
[8] BSGE 58, 134ff.

Abs. 1 GG zunächst ein Willkürverbot, darüber hinaus aber auch die an Gesetzgebung und Rechtsprechung gerichtete Verpflichtung, eine Gruppe von Normadressaten im Vergleich zu anderen Normadressaten nicht anders, also nicht ungleich zu behandeln, falls zwischen beiden Gruppen keine Unterschiede von solcher Art und von solchem Gewicht bestehen, daß sie die Ungleichbehandlung rechtfertigen.[9] Welche Elemente des zu regelnden Sachverhalts dabei so bedeutsam sind, daß ihrer Gleichheit oder Verschiedenheit bei der Ausgestaltung der Regelung Rechnung getragen werden muß, hat grundsätzlich der Gesetzgeber zu entscheiden, sofern nicht schon die Verfassung selbst Wertungen enthält, die dann auch den Gesetzgeber binden. Im übrigen kann durch die Gerichte nur die Einhaltung bestimmter äußerster Grenzen überprüft und ihre Überschreitung beanstandet werden.

Eine Verletzung des Art. 3 Abs. 1 GG und damit ein Verstoß gegen den Gleichbehandlungsgrundsatz ist also nicht bereits dann gegeben, wenn der Gesetzgeber bei Regelung eines Lebenssachverhalts nicht die optimale, d. h. z. B. die gerechteste oder vernünftigste Regelung trifft. Vielmehr hat der Gesetzgeber einen sehr weiten Gestaltungsspielraum beim Erlaß von Neuregelungen.[10] Der Gesetzgeber braucht deshalb, wenn er zwischen Gruppen von Normadressaten differenzieren will, lediglich nachvollziehbare Gründe, die die Differenzierung nicht als sachwidrig und damit als willkürlich erscheinen lassen.

Dieser gesetzgeberische Gestaltungsspielraum kann jedoch zum einen aus der Verfassung selbst heraus eine Einschränkung erfahren. Zu denken wäre hierbei an das Sozialstaatsgebot aus Art. 20 Abs. 1 GG. Dessen Reichweite ist allerdings noch unklar. Nach einem Urteil des BVerfG[11] zielt die Sozialstaatsklausel überhaupt nur auf eine gerechte und ausgeglichene Gestaltung der gesellschaftlichen Verhältnisse. Hauptsächliches Ziel der Sozialstaatsklausel ist nach ständiger Rechtsprechung des Bundesverfassungsgerichts die Bewältigung sozialer Notlagen und Beeinträchtigungen, wie sie z. B. durch Krankheit, Alter, Invalidität, Arbeitslosigkeit und sonstige benachteiligende Lebensumstände herbeigeführt werden. Die gesetzliche Sozialversicherung ist dabei als konkretisierte Ausprägung des Sozialstaatgedankens anzusehen.[12] Gleichwohl verpflichtet die Sozialstaatsklausel den Gesetzgeber nicht, am traditionellen System der sozialen Sicherung festzuhalten und hierin keine Änderungen vorzunehmen. Vielmehr ist der Gesetzgeber nur gehalten, ein Grundsystem zur Absicherung für existenzielle Notlagen bereitzustellen. Das bestehende System der Sozialversicherung und damit auch das der gesetzlichen Krankenversicherung ist jedoch an keiner Stelle der Verfassung garantiert. Grundlegende Reformen des Systems der GKV sind deshalb mit dem Sozialstaatsgebot ebenso vereinbar wie unterschiedliche Beitragsleistungen zur Erreichung dieses existenziellen Schutzes.

Eine weitere Einschränkung des gesetzgeberischen Gestaltungsspielraums kann jedoch dadurch eintreten, daß das Gesetz, für das der Gesetzgeber Neuregelungen vorgesehen hat, mehrere Strukturprinzipien nebeneinander aufweist, so

---

⁹ BVerfGE 55, 72, 88f.
¹⁰ BVerfGE 49, 260, 271; E 61, 138, 147
¹¹ BVerfGE 22, 204.
¹² BVerfGE 28, 348.

wie dies in der GKV der Fall ist. Ein derartiges System bedarf nach Ansicht des Bundessozialgerichts[13] wegen der Fülle von – häufig rein zufälligen – Überschneidungen, zu deren Erklärung auf jeweils andere Kriterien zurückgegriffen werden muß, eher eines Ausgleichs als ein in sich geschlossenes, also homogen gegliedertes System.

Die Ausgleichsbedürftigkeit in diesem Sinne gilt nach Ansicht des BSG besonders für die Unterschiede in den Beitragssätzen der Krankenkassen, jedenfalls dann, wenn die Sätze erheblich voneinander abweichen, die Versicherten jedoch in vieler Hinsicht Gemeinsamkeiten aufweisen und zwar gerade solche versicherungsrechtlich relevanter Art, wie etwa die Höhe des Grundlohns oder in örtlicher oder beruflicher Beziehung.[14]

Trotz dieser Ausführungen hat das BSG eine Verletzung von Art. 3 Abs. 1 GG durch unterschiedlich hohe Beitragssätze in der GKV verneint, diese vielmehr als eine notwendige Folge des gegliederten, d. h. dezentralen Aufbaus der Gesetzlichen Krankenversicherung angesehen. Wollte man sie vermeiden, so müßte nach – zutreffender – Ansicht des BSG der Aufbau der GKV grundlegend in Richtung auf eine Einheitsversicherung geändert werden. Ob dies allerdings wünschenswert sei, ob insbesondere die Vorteile einer Einheitsversicherung deren Nachteile überwiegen würden, habe in erster Linie der Gesetzgeber zu entscheiden. Der Gesetzgeber ist weder unter dem Gesichtspunkt des Art. 3 Abs. 1 GG noch unter dem Aspekt der Sozialstaatsklausel gehalten, bei seiner Entscheidung über die Neuregelungen in der GKV allein oder vorrangig die Herstellung von Beitragssatzgleichheit zum Ziel zu haben; vielmehr kann er im Rahmen seiner Gestaltungsfreiheit auch anderen sachlichen Erwägungen Raum geben und ihnen damit die Einheit der Versicherung und die Gleichheit der Beitragssätze bis zu einem „gewissen Grad opfern".[15] Das BSG hat sich aber nicht einmal andeutungsweise zu diesen „Opfergrenzen" geäußert.

Man wird aber – wenn man die Formel des Bundesverfassungsgerichts zugrunde legt – von einer Verletzung des Art. 3 Abs. 1 GG (ggf. unter Berücksichtigung des Sozialstaatsgebots aus Art. 20 Abs. 1 GG) erst dann sprechen können, wenn die Beitragssatzunterschiede so gravierend sind, daß es praktisch als sachwidrig und damit als willkürlich angesehen werden muß, wenn der Gesetzgeber bei seinen Neuregelungen trozdem weiterhin andere Strukturprinzipien in den Vordergrund stellt und einen dringend notwendigen Ausgleich gravierender Beitragssatzunterschiede unterläßt. Dies wird aber erst dann angenommen werden können, wenn die Gesetzliche Krankenversicherung, so wie sie jetzt strukturiert ist, nicht mehr funktionsfähig wäre und nur durch unverhältnismäßig hohe Beitragssätze aufrechterhalten werden könnte.

Für die Versicherten von Kassen mit hohen Beitragssätzen dürfte dieses Ergebnis wenig erfreulich sein und ebenso wenig weiterhelfen wie die vom BSG in seiner Entscheidung aus dem Jahre 1985 gemachten Feststellungen, daß es bereits seit Bestehen der GKV Beitragssatzunterschiede gegeben habe und sich die relativen Abweichungen vom Mittelwert – von extremen Ausnahmen abgesehen – zu-

---

[13] Vgl. BSGE 58, 142.
[14] BSGE 58, 142.
[15] BSGE 58, 144.

mindest prozentual verringert hätten. Ebenso wenig hilfreich ist die Aussage des BSG, daß das Sozialstaatsgebot in Verbindung mit Art. 3 Abs. 1 GG dem Gesetzgeber keinesfalls auferlege, Finanzausgleichsverfahren anzuordnen. Neben einem minimalen Effekt des sozialen Ausgleichs hätten Finanzausgleichsverfahren nämlich auch den Effekt, daß Besserverdienende, die durchaus in der Lage wären, hohe Beiträge zu bezahlen, ebenfalls in den Genuß niedrigerer Beitragssätze kämen.

Man muß dem BSG an dieser Stelle jedoch entgegenhalten, daß es sich die v. a. auf die rechtshistorische Entwicklung der GKV gestützte Argumentation zu Art. 3 Abs. 1 GG etwas zu einfach gemacht hat. Zwar ist in der Tat die GKV seit ihren Anfängen ein gegliedertes System gewesen, das sich mehr oder weniger durch die Zusammenfassung von Berufsgruppen bewährt hat. Die ursprünglichen Leistungen der GKV waren aber im Versicherungsfall auf die existentielle Absicherung von Lohnausfällen begrenzt und erst allmählich wurden auch medizinische Leistungen durch die GKV erbracht. Das Lohnausfallrisiko war aber bei einer Zusammenfassung nach Berufsgruppen bei den Mitgliedern der Solidargemeinschaft relativ gleich. Darin ist z. B. auch der Grund zu sehen, daß Beamte – auch mit niedrigen Einkommen – nicht zum Kreis der schutzbedürftigen Personen gerechnet und mit in die GKV einbezogen wurden. Im Fall der Krankheit hatte der Dienstherr aufgrund seiner Fürsorgepflicht den Beamten abzusichern und ihm trotz Krankheit weiterhin Gehalt zu bezahlen.

Schon längst ist der Anteil der Leistungen für Lohnfortzahlungen bei den Ausgaben der GKV in den Hintergrund getreten, weil hier die Absicherung v. a. durch § 1 Lohnfortzahlungsgesetz bzw. durch § 616 BGB zumindest in den ersten 6 Wochen in Form der Lohnfortzahlung durch den Arbeitgeber erfolgt. Hingegen haben die medizinischen Leistungen entscheidenden Anteil an den Leistungsausgaben erlangt; sie werden sich weiter erhöhen, wenn man den Fortschritt in der medizinischen Wissenschaft und Technik berücksichtigt. Auch der Anteil von Rentnern in der GKV wird immer größer und damit verbunden auch die Leistungsausgaben, die auch für längere Zeit erbracht werden müssen, da die durchschnittliche Lebenserwartung ständig ansteigt. Wenn Rentner generell in den Genuß niedrigerer Beiträge kommen, so bedeutet dies, daß zumindest die erwerbstätigen Mitglieder der Solidargemeinschaft dafür auch mit ihren Beiträgen aufkommen müssen. Auch die Absicherung von Aussiedlern und Umsiedlern bringt Ausgabenbelastungen mit sich, die in erheblichem Maße durch die Beiträge der erwerbstätigen Versicherten abgedeckt werden müssen. Diese Belastungen sind aber auf die einzelnen Kassenarten in der GKV unterschiedlich stark verteilt und beeinflussen mit Sicherheit das Beitragssatzniveau bei der einzelnen Kasse in unterschiedlichem Maß. Hätte der Gesetzgeber durch die Neuregelungen des SGB-V nicht wenigstens einige Maßnahmen zu einer gerechteren Verteilung getroffen, wie z. B. daß Rentner in der Kasse verbleiben, bei der sie zur Zeit ihrer aktiven Beschäftigung Mitglied waren (§ 182 SGB-V) oder z. B. das Verbleiben der Arbeitslosen in ihren früheren Kassen (Art. 34 Nr. 8 GRG, der § 159 AFG geändert hat) oder auch die Einführung von obligatorischen risikostrukturbezogenen Finanzausgleichsverfahren, wenn auch nur kassenartintern (§ 266 SGB-V), so wäre wohl durchaus in der Zukunft bei weiter auseinanderdriftenden Beitragssätzen ein Verstoß gegen den Gleichbehandlungsgrundsatz in Betracht zu ziehen. Fraglich ist hierbei, wo die Grenze für eine Verletzung des Art. 3 Abs. 1 GG liegen würde. Das BSG hat hierzu nicht Stellung genommen. Man wird deshalb die Entscheidung des BVerfG abwarten müssen, denn diese Grenzziehung ist eine reine Wertungsentscheidung und kann nicht eindeutig beantwortet werden.

Verletzung anderer Grundrechte?

Wie sieht es nun mit der möglichen Verletzung anderer Grundrechte durch unterschiedlich hohe Beitragssätze in der GKV aus?

Art. 14 Abs. 1 GG

In Betracht kommt zunächst eine Verletzung des in Art. 14 Abs. 1 GG geschützten Eigentumsrechts.

Art. 14 Abs. 1 GG gewährt einen verfassungsrechtlichen Schutz des privaten Eigentums, der gleichwohl unter dem Vorbehalt der Sozialbindung steht, denn Inhalt und Schranken des Eigentums werden durch die Gesetze bestimmt. Bei der Prüfung des Schutzbereichs von Art. 14 Abs. 1 GG ist daher stets Zweck und Funktion der Eigentumsgarantie zu beachten, nämlich daß dem Träger des Grundrechts durch Art. 14 Abs. 1 GG ein Freiheitsraum im vermögensrechtlichen Bereich gesichert und ihm damit eine eigenverantwortliche Gestaltung des Lebens ermöglicht werden soll.[16]

Eine Verletzung des Eigentumsrechts aus Art. 14 Abs. 1 GG kann durch die unterschiedlichen Beitragssätze in der GKV wohl nicht bei einzelnen Versicherten eintreten. Sozialversicherungsrechtliche Positionen fallen nach ständiger Rechtsprechung des BVerfG[17] nämlich nur dann unter die Eigentumsgarantie des Art. 14 Abs. 1 GG, wenn eine Zuordnung einer vermögenswerten Rechtsposition zu einem Rechtsträger nach Art eines Ausschließlichkeitsrechts als privatnützig erfolgen kann, diese Position auf nicht unerhebliche Eigenleistungen des Versicherten zurückzuführen ist und sie ihm zur Existenzsicherung dient, in dem Sinne, daß der Fortfall oder auch nur eine Einschränkung dieser Position die freiheitssichernde Funktion der Eigentumsgarantie wesentlich berühren würde.

Bejaht hat das BVerfG den Eigentumsschutz bisher bei Anwartschaften in der gesetzlichen Rentenversicherung, jedoch nicht bei Beitragsleistungen in der Gesetzlichen Krankenversicherung. Sicherlich kommt der Möglichkeit, für maßvolle Beitragsleistungen umfassenden Krankenversicherungsschutz zu genießen, eine freiheitssichernde Funktion zu. Der einzelne Bürger wäre bei einer Vielzahl von Erkrankungen, die ggf. nur mit Einsatz hochwertiger Technik und aufgrund des neuesten Stands der medizinischen Wissenschaft geheilt werden können, wohl nicht mehr in der Lage, die dadurch verursachten Kosten zu tragen. Gleiches gilt für Krankenhausaufenthalte sowie Zahnersatz und kieferorthopädische Leistungen.

---

[16] BVerfGE 69, 299ff
[17] BVerfGE 69, 272, 300; E 72, 141ff.

Dennoch führen unterschiedlich hohe Beitragssätze in der GKV nicht zu einer Verletzung des Art. 14 Abs. 1 GG, da dieser nicht das Vermögen des Einzelnen als solches vor der Auferlegung von Abgaben oder Beiträgen schützt,[18] sondern nur das Eigentum in einem Umfang, der zu einer eigenverantwortlichen Gestaltung des Lebens erforderlich ist. Art. 14 Abs. 1 GG schützt aber gerade nicht den Erwerb an sich, sondern das Erworbene.

Zudem muß die Sozialbindung des Eigentums nach Art. 14 Abs. 1, S. 2 GG beachtet werden. Das Bundesverfassungsgericht hat hierzu mehrfach entschieden, daß Gesetzesänderungen in bezug auf Beiträge oder auch auf Leistungen stets dann als zulässig angesehen werden müssen, wenn sie erforderlich sind, um das bestehende System der sozialen Sicherung aufrechtzuerhalten und v. a. die Finanzgrundlagen dafür zu sichern.[19] Eine Grenze für derartige Leistungskürzungen wäre in Hinblick auf das Sozialstaatsgebot erst dann erreicht, wenn dadurch die Gewährleistung einer medizinischen Grundversorgung der Bevölkerung gefährdet würde.

Der Versicherte erwirbt also mit seiner Beitragsleistung zur GKV keine von Art. 14 Abs. 1 GG umfaßte Rechtsposition, d. h. keine Anwartschaft auf eine ganz bestimmte Leistung in ganz bestimmter Ausgestaltung und in bestimmter Höhe, die nur ihm und nicht einem anderen Mitglied zustehen würde; er erhält nur den Anspruch auf die Leistungen der GKV, sofern der Versicherungsfall Krankheit eintritt; diese Leistungen stehen aber jedem Mitglied der Gesetzlichen Krankenversicherung gleichermaßen zu, unabhängig von der Höhe der geleisteten Beiträge. Die Beitragsleistung an und für sich begründet deshalb keine von Art. 14 Abs. 1 GG umfaßte schutzwerte Rechtsposition. Das Bundesverfassungsgericht hat lediglich angedeutet, daß eine Verletzung des Art. 14 Abs. 1 GG allenfalls dann in Betracht käme, wenn die Beitragshöhe jegliches Maß übersteigen würde. Auch hier hat aber das Bundesverfassungsgericht keine exakte Grenze festgelegt, sondern die jeweils besonderen Gegebenheiten des Einzelfalls für wesentlich erachtet.

Eine Verletzung des Art. 14 Abs. 1 GG kommt aber auch auf seiten der Arbeitgeber nicht in Betracht, obwohl sie die Hälfte des Beitrags zur GKV für ihre Beschäftigten zu entrichten haben. Besteht keine Möglichkeit der Versicherung bei beitragsgünstigeren Krankenkassen, so müssen diese Arbeitgeber zwar einen höheren Arbeitgeberanteil entrichten als vergleichbare andere Arbeitgeber, was wiederum Auswirkungen auf ihr Unternehmen hat, sei es im Hinblick auf Gewinn, Liquidität, Wettbewerbsfähigkeit usw. Wie aber vorhin bereits ausgeführt, schützt Art. 14 Abs. 1 GG weder die Erwerbschancen, sondern nur das Erworbene, noch führt die auf einfach gesetzlichen Regelungen beruhende Verpflichtung zur Entrichtung von Abgaben und Beiträgen zu einer Verletzung des Art. 14 Abs. 1 GG. Diese Pflicht resultiert vielmehr aus dem Gedanken der Sozialpflichtigkeit von Eigentum und Vermögen.

Man wird deshalb bei den derzeitigen bestehenden Beitragssatzunterschieden in der GKV keine Verletzung des Eigentumsschutzes aus Art. 14 Abs. 1 GG annehmen können. Die Beurteilung der Frage, wann Beitragssätze in ihrer Höhe je-

---

[18] BVerfGE 14, 221ff.; E 36, 383ff.; E 10, 354, 371.
[19] BVerfGE 72, 141ff.; E 72, 175ff., 195; E 69, 299ff F 14 221ff

des Maß übersteigen und damit dann doch zu einer Verletzung des Art. 14 Abs. 1
GG führen könnten, hat das Bundesverfassungsgericht in einer wertenden Entscheidung zu treffen.

Art. 2 Abs. 1 GG

Letztendlich bleibt noch zu fragen, ob die unterschiedlichen Beitragssätze in der
GKV zu einer Verletzung des durch Art. 2 Abs. 1 GG geschützten allgemeinen
Freiheitsrechts führen.

Art. 2 Abs. 1 GG schützt die persönliche Handlungsfreiheit, auch in Form einer wirtschaftlichen Betätigungsfreiheit. Deshalb wäre es durchaus denkbar, daß
der Schutzbereich des Art. 2 Abs. 1 GG berührt wird, wenn ein Versicherter in der
GKV für die gleichen Leistungen mehr an Beiträgen entrichten muß als ein anderer Versicherter in der gleichen Situation. Die höhere Beitragszahlung bedeutet
einen Einkommensverlust für diesen Versicherten, der seine wirtschaftliche Betätigungsfreiheit durchaus beeinträchtigen kann. Ebenso denkbar ist auch, daß die
Wettbewerbsfähigkeit von Unternehmen durch unterschiedlich hohe Lohnnebenkosten, zu denen auch der Arbeitgeberanteil zur GKV zu rechnen ist, verzerrt
wird.

Bei Art. 2 Abs. 1 GG, dem allgemeinen Freiheitsrecht, handelt es sich – wie
bereits angedeutet – um einen Auffangtatbestand innerhalb der Grundrechte.
Deshalb ist für die Frage nach dem Umfang des Schutzes der persönlichen Handlungsfreiheit im Rahmen der Beurteilung sozialgesetzlicher Neuregelungen vorab
erst zu klären, ob nicht Art. 14 GG als das speziellere Grundrecht zum Schutz
vermögensrechtlicher Positionen vorrangig ist. Art. 2 Abs. 1 GG ist deshalb nur
bei solchen Beschränkungen der allgemeinen Handlungsfreiheit einschlägig, die
nicht bereits in den Schutzbereich des Art. 14 Abs. 1 GG fallen. Dies ist – wie
oben bereits festgestellt – hier nicht der Fall, so daß durch unterschiedlich hohe
Beitragssätze in der GKV durchaus eine Verletzung des Art. 2 Abs. 1 GG in Betracht kommen kann.

Art. 2 Abs. 1 GG schützt jedoch nicht bereits vor jeder Beeinträchtigung der
allgemeinen Handlungsfreiheit, sondern ist vielmehr erst dann verletzt, wenn die
Beeinträchtigung ein unerträgliches Maß erreichen würde. Das BVerfG hat hierzu jedoch ausgeführt,[20] daß der Gesetzgeber in der unaufhebbaren und grundsätzlichen Spannungslage zwischen dem Schutz des einzelnen und den Anforderungen einer sozialstaatlichen Ordnung einen weiten Raum freier Gestaltung hat,
innerhalb dessen er Maß und Art der im Interesse des Gemeinwohls notwendigen
oder doch vertretbaren Eingriffe in die Freiheit des Einzelnen zu bestimmen hat.
Für die verfassungsrechtliche Beurteilung der Vereinbarkeit einer Regelung mit
Art. 2 Abs. 1 GG genügt bereits die Feststellung, daß der Gesetzgeber nicht aus
dem Bereich des eingeräumten Ermessens herausgetreten ist und daß er Verfas-
sungsgrundsätze nicht verletzt hat.

Eine solche Überschreitung des gesetzgeberischen Ermessensspielraums oder
gar eine Verletzung von Verfassungsgrundsätzen kann aber dem Gesetzgeber im

---

[20] Vgl. BVerfGE 10, 354ff.

Hinblick auf die Vorschriften über Mitgliedschaft und Beitragsbemessung – zumindest derzeit – (noch) nicht vorgeworfen werden, so daß die unterschiedlichen Beitragssätze in der GKV mit Art. 2 Abs. 1 GG vereinbar sein werden. Auch diese Frage muß letztlich durch eine Wertungsentscheidung des BVerfG beantwortet werden.

Zwischenergebnis

Die obige Analyse der Schutzbereiche von Art. 3 Abs. 1 (in Verbindung mit Art. 20 Abs. 1 GG - Sozialstaatsprinzip), Art. 14 Abs. 1 sowie Art. 2 Abs. 1 GG bringt kaum Antworten zur Frage, bis zu welcher Höhe Beitragssatzunterschiede in der GKV noch als verfassungsgemäß anzusehen wären. Das Bundesverfassungsgericht hat bisher – von den Entscheidungen zu den Neuregelungen im Recht der gesetzlichen Rentenversicherung einmal abgesehen – stets die Erhaltung des bestehenden Systems der gesetzlichen Sozialversicherung vor die Belange des einzelnen Versicherten gestellt. Dies bedeutet aber keineswegs, daß dies in Zukunft auch so bleiben wird. Wie bereits ausgeführt, wird an keiner Stelle der Verfassung das bestehende System der sozialen Sicherung garantiert, eine Bestandsgarantie ergibt sich auch nicht aus dem Sozialstaatsgebot des Art. 20 Abs. 1 GG. Dieses Sozialstaatsgebot gebietet dem Gesetzgeber lediglich die Schaffung oder Erhaltung einer sozialen Mindestversorgung gegen existenzielle Notlagen, wobei die gesetzliche Sozialversicherung durchaus als anerkannte Ausprägung des Sozialstaatsgebots angesehen werden muß.

Vorschläge zur Neuregelung des Kassenorganisationsrechts

Auch der Gesetzgeber hat mittlerweile Handlungsbedarf erkannt und will ein weiteres Auseinanderdriften der Beitragssätze in der GKV verhindern. Dazu soll nach der Reform des Leistungsrechts durch das SGB-V die Struktur des Kassenorganisationsrechts in einem zweiten Reformschritt eine Neuregelung erfahren. Die Vorschriften des SGB-V bieten ersten Ansätze für eine positivere Beeinflussung der unterschiedlichen Risikostrukturen in den Versichertengemeinschaften. Weitere Änderungen im Kassenorganisationsrecht sind aber in jedem Falle notwendig und werden auch bereits diskutiert.

So hat z. B. der Hamburger Senat einen „Entwurf eines Gesetzes über Notmaßnahmen für den Erhalt der gegliederten Krankenversicherung als Überbrückung bis zur Organisationsreform" im Bundesrat eingebracht. Dieser Gesetzentwurf sieht auf der Grundlage bestimmter Beitragssatzschwellenwerte alljährlich einen bundesweiten kassenartinternen Finanzausgleich vor. Dadurch würden jedoch lediglich die Beitragssätze bei den Ortskrankenkassen, die zwar intern selbst um mehrere Prozentpunkte variieren, einander angeglichen werden. Die vorgeschlagene Regelung hätte jedoch nicht den Effekt, die Beitragssatzdifferenzen zwischen den einzelnen Kassenarten einzuebnen. Gerade hier liegt aber eine wesentliche Schwäche des bestehenden Systems der gegliederten Krankenversicherung.

Auch der Sachverständigenrat für die Konzertierte Aktion im Gesundheitswesen hat mittlerweile bereits konkrete Vorschläge ausgearbeitet, die die Problemlage grundsätzlicher angehen. Das Jahresgutachten 1989 des Sachverständigenrats wiederholt seine bereits aufgestellten Forderungen, eine einheitliche Regionsabgrenzung für alle Kassen vorzunehmen, um das gegenwärtige unkoordinierte Nebeneinander von bundesweiten und regionalen Verhandlungen mit den Leistungserbringern, Krankenhäusern und Apotheken zu beenden. Der Rat empfiehlt, in einer neugegliederten Gesetzlichen Krankenversicherung den bereits bestehenden interregionalen Ausgleich beizubehalten, allerdings nicht als Ausgaben- sondern als Risikostrukturausgleich. Die neugegliederte GKV wäre dann durch regionale Beitragssätze und einen bundesweiten Risikostrukturausgleich gekennzeichnet. Nach den Vorstellungen des Rats sollen folgende Grundsätze den systemkonkurrierenden Kassen zugrunde liegen:

– Die derzeitigen Finanzierungsprinzipien der GKV (einkommensproportionale Beiträge und kostenlose Mitversicherung bei nichtverdienenden Familienmitgliedern) sollen erhalten bleiben.
– Rentner sollen beitragsrechtlich wie Erwerbstätige behandelt werden.
– Jeder Versicherte soll ein Wahlrecht zwischen den in seiner Region tätigen Kassen erhalten, die Kassen ihrerseits sollen einem Kontrahierungszwang unterstellt werden.
– Zwischen den Kassen einer Region soll ein allgemeiner Risikostrukturausgleich durchgeführt werden, der neben dem Grundlohnausgleich je Versicherten auch einen nach Alter und Geschlecht differenzierten Morbiditätsausgleich enthalten soll.
– Zwischen den Kassen verschiedener Regionen soll ein bundesweiter Risikostrukturausgleich stattfinden, der mit dem kommunalen und bundesstaatlichen Finanzausgleich abzustimmen sein soll.[21] Die Vorschläge des Sachverständigenrats der Konzertierten Aktion im Gesundheitswesen zielen damit genau auf die wesentlichen Ursachen der unterschiedlichen Beitragssätze in der GKV ab, nämlich einmal auf die Einnahmenseite, d. h. auf das Finanzierungspotential durch Einwirkung auf die Grundlohnsummen, zum anderen auf eine ausgeglichenere Zusammensetzung der Risikostrukturen in der jeweiligen Versichertengemeinschaft.

Auch die Enquetekommission „Strukturreform der Gesetzlichen Krankenversicherung" hat mittlerweile einen umfassenden Zwischenbericht zur Problematik der Beitragssatzunterschiede vorgelegt. Die Enquetekommission kommt darin zu dem Ergebnis, daß die Konstruktion des traditionellen Systems der gegliederten Krankenversicherung und die Intentionen des historischen Gesetzgebers in zunehmendem Maße in einem erheblichen Widerspruch sowohl zur sozioökonomischen Entwicklung der Bundesrepublik Deutschland als auch zu den Ansprüchen an eine zukunftsorientierte Organisation des Krankenversicherungssystems

---

[21] Vgl. DOK (1989) S 179; Leber W (1988) Konkurrierende Regionalkassen – Ein Konzept zur Neuordnung des gegliederten Kassensystems, Arbeit Sozialpol 10, 313ff ; Brunkhorst J (1988) Risikoausgleich und regionale Krankenversicherung, Arbeit Sozialpol 8, 234ff., Töns OH (1989) Kassenwahlrechte, DOK, S 104ff.

selbst stehen. Handlungsbedarf wurde dabei v. a. in 3 Punkten erkannt, nämlich erstens bezüglich der Zweiklassenschichtung der Versicherten mit unterschiedlichen Rechten im System, nämlich Arbeiter mit Zwangskassenzugehörigkeit auf der einen Seite, Angestellte mit Kassenwahlrecht auf der anderen Seite; zweitens den Abbau der in einem vielschichtigen Zusammenwirken von Grundlohnunterschieden und schiefen Risikostrukturen bei Kassen und Kassenarten entstehenden Beitragssatzunterschiede; drittens Marktanteilsverschiebungen zwischen den Kassenarten, die zu Lasten der Zwangskasse AOK verlaufen und deren Wettbewerbsfähigkeit negativ beeinflussen.[22]

Als Lösungsansätze kommen nach Ansicht der Enquetekommission 3 gegensätzliche Strategien in Betracht:

1) das gegliederte System wird durch eine regional organisierte Einheitsversicherung ersetzt;
2) es kommt zur Neukonstruktion eines Zuweisungssystems, das die heutigen Strukturdefekte durch generellen Verzicht auf Wahlmöglichkeiten und Wettbewerb zu beseitigen versucht;
3) es wird eine grundsätzliche Öffnung der verschiedenen Kassen und Kassenarten für alle Versicherten und die gleichzeitige Implementation von mehr (und unverzerrtem) Wettbewerb in das System vorgenommen. Verfassungsrechtliche Schranken werden diesbezüglich – zu Recht – nicht gesehen. Da aber das gegliederte System der gesetzlichen Krankenversicherung beibehalten werden soll, kommen nach Ansicht der Enquetekommission lediglich die letzten beiden Möglichkeiten näher in Betracht. Die Mitglieder der Enquetekommission selbst haben sich nicht auf einen bestimmten Reformvorschlag einigen können. Vorgestellt wurden vielmehr 2 Modelle: Nämlich erstens die Wahlfreiheit mit wettbewerblicher Orientierung (Reformoption I) und zweitens ein Wahlfreiheitsmodell mit sozialpolitischer Orientierung (Reformoption II). Beiden Vorschlägen ist gemeinsam, daß die Versicherten zwischen allen Kassenarten frei wählen dürfen, daß diese Kassen einem Kontrahierungszwang und einem Diskriminierungsverbot gegenüber allen Versicherten unterliegen und die Einhaltung dieser Prinzipien durch die Aufsichtsbehörde gewährleistet wird.

Die Reformoption I setzt dabei des weiteren darauf, daß ein unverzerrter Wettbewerb zwischen den Kassenarten auf Dauer gesehen zu einer Minderung der Beitragssätze und der Beitragssatzunterschiede führen wird. Aus beschäftigungspolitischen und auch aus wettbewerbspolitischen Gründen soll jedoch als Übergangslösung ein zeitlich und nach dem Grundlohn bemessener, und damit inhaltlich begrenzter Risikoausgleich stattfinden. Ein weitergehender Risikoausgleich, etwa im Hinblick auf die unterschiedlichen Risikofaktoren bei einer Kassenart wird hingegen abgelehnt.

Die Reformoption II lehnt demgegenüber einen Wettbewerb auf der Leistungsseite ab. Es sollen vielmehr gleiche Finanzierungsbedingungen hergestellt werden, indem die Beiträge von allen Kassenarten entweder regional oder auf Basis bundesweiter Berechnungen erhoben werden. Des weiteren wird ein Risi-

---

[22] Vgl. dazu BT-Drcks. Nr. 11/3267, S 385.

koausgleich gefordert, der auf die unterschiedlichen Risikostrukturen der Versichertengemeinschaften und auf das unterschiedliche Grundlohnsummenniveau Einfluß nimmt.

Die soeben dargestellten Vorschläge des Sachverständigenrats der Konzertierten Aktion im Gesundheitswesen sowie der Enquetekommission „Strukturreform der Gesetzlichen Krankenversicherung" sind aber nur mögliche Lösungsansätze in einer Vielzahl von Strategien. Genausogut wäre aber auch eine grundlegende Strukturreform hin zu einer Art Einheitsversicherung denkbar. Der Gesetzgeber dürfte jedoch bemüht sein, den Eingriff in das bestehende Kassenorganisationssystem so gering wie möglich auszugestalten. Wie diese Entwicklung weitergehen wird, muß abgewartet werden. Gesetzgeberische Maßnahmen sind jedoch unerläßlich, damit nicht doch noch eines Tages die Beiträge zur GKV und insbesondere die Beitragssatzunterschiede eine Höhe erreichen, die nicht mehr verfassungsgemäß wäre.

Weiterführende Literatur zum Thema „Gesundheitspolitik, Verwaltung, Management und Recht im Gesundheitswesen"

Gesundheitspolitik

Abelin T, Brzezinski ZJ, Carstairs VDL (eds) (1987) Measurement in health promotion and protection. WHO, Regional Office for Europe, Copenhagen (WHO Regional Publications. European Series; No. 22)
Smith A, Jacobson B (eds) (1988) The nation's health: a strategy for the 1990s. King's Fund Publishing Office, London
U.S. Department of Health and Human Services (1986) The 1990 health objectives for the nation: a midcourse review. U.S. Gouvernment Printing Office, Washington/D.C.
WHO (1986) Targets for health for all: Targets in support of the European regional strategy for health for all. 2. impr. WHO Regional Office for Europe, Copenhagen

Verwaltung und Management im Gesundheitswesen

Bundesministerium für Arbeit und Sozialordnung. Reihe Gesundheitsforschung: Forschungsberichte
Fottler MD, Hernandez SR, Joiner CL (eds) (1988) Strategic management of human resources in health services organizations. Wiley & Sons, New York
Fox PD, Goldbeck WB, Spies JJ et al. (1984) Health care cost management: private sector initiatives. Health Administration Press, Ann Arbor
Koff SZ (1988) Health systems agencies: a comprehensive examination of planning and process. Human Sciences Press, New York
MacStravic RES (1986) Managing health care marketing communications. Aspen, Rockville
Sachverständigenrat für die Konzertierte Aktion im Gesundheitswesen (1987) Medizinische und ökonomische Orientierung: Vorschläge für die Konzertierte Aktion im Gesundheitswesen, Jahresgutachten 1987. Nomos, Baden-Baden
Sachverständigenrat für die Konzertierte Aktion im Gesundheitswesen (1988) Medizinische und ökonomische Orientierung: Vorschläge für die Konzertierte Aktion im Gesundheitswesen, Jahresgutachten 1988. Nomos, Baden-Baden
Sachverständigenrat für die Konzertierte Aktion im Gesundheitswesen (1989) Qualität, Wirtschaftlichkeit und Perspektiven der Gesundheitsversorgung: Vorschläge für die Konzertierte Aktion im Gesundheitswesen, Jahresgutachten 1989. Nomos, Baden-Baden
Sachverständigenrat für die Konzertierte Aktion im Gesundheitswesen (1990) Herausforderungen und Perspektiven der Gesundheitsversorgung: Vorschläge für die Konzertierte Aktion im Gesundheitswesen, Jahresgutachten 1990. Nomos, Baden-Baden
Scheyer WL (ed) (1985) Handbook of health care material management. Aspen, Rockville
Suver JD, Kahn III CN, Clement JP (eds) (1986) Cases in health care financial management. Health Administration Press, East Huron
U.S. Department of Health and Human Services (1985ff.) Research Activities

Recht im Gesundheitswesen

Gitter W (1986) Sozialrecht: ein Studienbuch, 2. neubearb. Aufl. Beck, München (Juristisches Kurzlehrbuch)
Lauter H, Schreiber HL (Hrsg) (1981) Rechtsprobleme in der Psychiatrie, 2. überarb. Aufl. Rheinland, Pulheim

6 Geschichte des Gesundheitswesens

Entstehung und Ausdehnung der Gesetzlichen Krankenversicherung bis zum Inkrafttreten der Reichsversicherungsordnung 1914 *

C. Huerkamp

Nachdem in Preußen durch die Kassengesetzgebung von 1845 bis 1854 das System der sog. „Zwangskassen" institutionalisiert und ausgebaut worden war, war seit den späten 50er Jahren eine immer deutlichere liberale Kritik am Kassenzwang und den Zwangskassen zu beobachten.[1] Die Gewerbeordnung von 1869 formulierte einen Kompromiß zwischen Anhängern und Gegnern des Kassenzwangs, indem sie die Zwangskassen zwar nicht grundsätzlich beseitigte, ihnen aber die freien Kassen der Gewerk- und Arbeitervereine gleichberechtigt zur Seite stellte. Während so 1869 und auch noch im Hilfskassengesetz von 1876 die freien und eingeschriebenen Hilfskassen im Sinne liberaler politischer Forderungen gefördert wurden, knüpfte das Reichsgesetz von 1883 über die Krankenversicherung der Arbeiter wieder deutlich an die Prinzipien der Zwangsversicherung an.[2] Es sah einen Beitrittszwang für Arbeiter in Gewerbe und Industrie vor, die unter 2000 Mk. jährlich verdienten, staffelte die Beiträge der Versicherten nach der Lohnhöhe und nicht nach dem Krankheitsrisiko, verzichtete auf ein Gesundheitsattest beim Eintritt in die Versicherung und erhob von den Unternehmern einen Beitrag zu den Versicherungskosten, der sich auf die Hälfte des Beitrags der versicherten Arbeiter belief.

Auch was die Stellung des Arztes in den neugeschaffenen Kassen angeht, orientierte sich die Gesetzliche Krankenversicherung an den „Zwangskassen" der Zeit vor 1880 und nicht an dem zweiten Strang in der Tradition der Versicherung gegen Krankheit, den freien Hilfskassen. § 6 des Krankenversicherungsgesetzes (KVG) von 1883 bestimmte, daß die Kassen ihren Mitgliedern im Krankheitsfall

---

* Erstmals veröffentlicht in: Huerkamp C (1985) Der Aufstieg der Ärzte im 19. Jahrhundert: vom gelehrten Stand zum professionellen Experten: das Beispiel Preußens. Vandenhoeck & Ruprecht, Göttingen (Kritische Studien zur Geschichtswissenschaft, Bd 68, Kap 6, S 194–199).

[1] Frevert U (1984) Krankheit als politisches Problem 1770–1880. Soziale Unterschiede in Preußen zwischen medizinischer Polizei und staatlicher Sozialversicherung, Göttingen, S 174ff.

[2] Auf die Motive und Interessen, die bei der Entstehung des KVG von 1883 eine Rolle spielten, kann an dieser Stelle nicht eingegangen werden, vgl. dazu an neuerer Literatur: Tennstedt F (1981) Sozialgeschichte der Sozialpolitik in Deutschland. Vom 18. Jahrhundert bis zum Ersten Weltkrieg. Göttingen, S 135ff.; Tennstedt F (1981) Vorgeschichte u. Entstehung der Kaiserlichen Botschaft vom 17. November 1881. Z Sozialref 27:663–710. Ritter GA (1983) Sozialversicherung in Deutschland und England. Entstehung u. Grundzüge im Vergleich. München, S 18–49; Zöllner D (1981) Landesbericht Deutschland. In: Köhler PA, Zacher HF (Hrsg) Ein Jahrhundert Sozialversicherung in der Bundesrepublik Deutschland, Frankreich, Großbritannien, Österreich u. der Schweiz. Berlin, S 57–96. Als ältere Darstellung v. a.: Kleeis F (1981, 1928) Die Geschichte der sozialen Versicherung in Deutschland. Berlin

freie ärztliche Hilfe und freie Arznei in natura zu gewähren hatten. Sie konnten daher nicht wie die Hilfskassen diese Verpflichtung durch Zahlung eines Geldbetrags an das erkrankte Mitglied ersetzen, von dem dieses dann selber einen Arzt bezahlen konnte.

Die große Mehrzahl der neugebildeten Kassen schloß daraufhin zunächst privatrechtliche Verträge mit einem oder mehreren Ärzten ab, denen sie in der Regel gegen Zahlung einer jährlichen Pauschalsumme die Versorgung ihrer erkrankten Mitglieder übertrugen. Im großen und ganzen bildeten sich die gleichen Modi heraus, wie sie die ärztliche Versorgung auch schon in den Kassen vor 1883 gekennzeichnet hatten. Die zahlreichen kleineren Kassen – noch 1900 betrug die Durchschnittsmitgliederzahl je Kasse nur 423 Personen[3] – hatten meist nur einen Vertragsarzt, an den sich die Mitglieder im Fall einer Erkankung zu wenden hatten. Bei einem Teil der größeren Kassen bestand ein Distriktarztsystem, d. h. der Einzugsbereich der Kasse wurde nach Wohnbezirken in bestimmte Distrikte eingeteilt; für jeden war ein von der Kasse bestimmter Arzt zuständig, von dem sich die Patienten im jeweiligen Bezirk im Krankheitsfall behandeln lassen mußten. Auch dieses System war schon aus der Frühzeit der Kassen im zweiten Drittel des 19. Jahrhunderts bekannt; in dieser Weise war beispielsweise die ärztliche Versorgung im Berliner Gewerkskrankenverein, der 1856 bereits 42000 Mitglieder zählte, organisiert.[4] Auch den von den Knappschaften angestellten Knappschaftsärzten wurden bestimmte Bezirke zugeteilt, in denen sie die kranken Knappschaftsmitglieder zu versorgen hatten.

Ein anderer Teil der größeren Kassen hatte die „beschränkte freie Arztwahl", wobei die Patienten unter den bei der Kasse tätigen Ärzten frei wählen konnten. Wieder andere Kassen hatten die später von den Ärzteverbänden allgemein geforderte „freie Arztwahl" eingeführt, d. h. jeder Arzt, der die Zulassung bei der Kasse beantragte, wurde auch zugelassen, teilweise aber mit der Auflage, daß er schon eine Zeitlang am Ort praktiziert haben müsse (Karenzzeit). Auch die freie Arztwahl hatten vor 1883 schon einzelne Kassen praktiziert, z. B. eine Reihe von Betriebs- und Fabrikkrankenkassen in Barmen.[5]

Dem Arzt war innerhalb der Gesetzlichen Krankenversicherung (GKV), wie in den meisten frühen Fabrik- und Ortskrankenkassen auch schon, eine zentrale Machtposition gegenüber dem erkrankten Versicherten zugewiesen: Dieser mußte, um Krankengeld beziehen zu können, erst eine Erwerbsunfähigkeitsbescheinigung vorlegen, die nur der Arzt ausstellen konnte; er mußte sich in regelmäßigen Abständen wieder beim Arzt vorstellen, und er war gehalten, alle ärztlichen Anordnungen strikt zu befolgen.

Seine Machtbefugnisse gegenüber dem Patienten bezahlte der Kassenarzt mit weitgehender Abhängigkeit vom Kassenvorstand, der seinen therapeutischen

---

[3] Übersichten nach Kassenarten über die Ergebnisse der Krankenversicherung im Deutschen Reiche in den Jahren 1885–1901, in: Statistik des Deutschen Reiches, N. F., Bd 147, Die GKV im Jahre 1901, Berlin 1903, S 11*.

[4] Koblank (1858) Notizen über den Gewerks-Krankenverein in Berlin ., in: Congrès International de Bienfaisance de Francfort-sur-le-Mein, Session de 1857, Bd. 2, Frankfurt, S 166f., 177.

[5] Artikel im Ärztlichen Vereinsblatt 1902, Nr. 477, S 324–48 über die Entwicklung der Barmener Kassenverhältnisse, hier S 343.

Handlungsspielraum empfindlich einengen konnte, etwa durch Direktiven zur sparsamen Arzneimittelverordnung und durch die Kontrolle seiner Krankschreibungstätigkeit.

Der Berliner Gewerksverein hatte schon 1856 eine Instruktion für die bei ihm angestellten Ärzte erlassen, in der die Pflichten der Gewerksärzte genau festgehalten waren, insbesondere wie oft sie Sprechstunden abhalten, wann sie Besuche machen, unter welchen Bedingungen sie den Kranken in ein Krankenhaus einweisen mußten und ähnliche Einzelheiten mehr. Der Gewerksverein erwartete von seinen Ärzten, „daß dieselben für das Wohl der Kranken jederzeit ordentlich sorgen werden, jedoch dabei auch das Interesse der Kranken-Kasse, namentlich bei Anweisung auf Unterstützungsgelder berücksichtigen".[6] Die Instruktion endete mit den Worten: „Jeder bei dem Gewerks-Kranken-Vereine angestellte Arzt muß die vorstehenden Instruktionen genau befolgen. Verstöße dagegen werden, wenn dieselben zur Kenntnis des Verwaltungs-Comités kommen, von demselben streng gerügt oder ... durch Ausscheiden als Vereins-Arzt geahndet werden."[7]

Auch in finanzieller Hinsicht saß die Kasse in der Regel am längeren Hebel. Besonders in den größeren Gemeinden, wo mehrere Ärzte gleichzeitig praktizierten, die an einer Tätigkeit als Kassenarzt Interesse hatten, konnten die Kassenvorstände mühelos die Honorare drücken und sich billige ärztliche Hilfe für ihre Mitglieder verschaffen.

Zwar gab es Klagen über diese beiden hauptsächlichen Nachteile kassenärztlicher Tätigkeit – Unterbezahlung der ärztlichen Arbeit und Einmischung des Kassenvorstandes in rein ärztliche Aufgabenbereiche – auch schon in den Jahrzehnten vor 1883, doch drang sie bis zum Erlaß des KVG kaum jemals bis in die Spalten der ärztlichen Vereinspresse vor, sondern ist nur verstreut in verschiedensten Quellen und Stellungnahmen zum Versicherungswesen der Zeit vor 1883 nachzuweisen.[8] Das änderte sich schlagartig mit Inkrafttreten des KVG zu Beginn des Jahres 1884. Die angemessene Honorierung der ärztlichen Arbeit für die Kassen sowie eine dem Arzt zukommende unabhängige Position von den Direktiven eines mit Laien besetzten Kassenvorstands, seit Beginn der 90er Jahre auch die Forderung nach „freier Arztwahl" – das waren Themen, die fortab in Dutzenden von Vorträgen in den lokalen ärztlichen Vereinen, in ungezählten Artikeln im Ärztlichen Vereinsblatt als dem zentralen Organ der Ärzteorganisationen und auf nahezu jedem Ärztetag öffentlich erörtert wurden.

Daß die Stellung der Ärzte zu den Krankenkassen plötzlich zu einem die gesamte Ärzteschaft tangierenden Problem wurde, lag sowohl am schieren Größenwachstum der Versicherung – Schwierigkeiten, die vordem einige wenige Kassenärzte in ihrem Verhältnis zum Kassenvorstand gehabt hatten, wurden nun von einer großen und stets wachsenden Zahl von Ärzten erfahren – als auch an Veränderungen in der Organisationsstruktur der Kassen und der Zusammensetzung der Kassenvorstände, die diese Probleme schärfer hervortreten ließen. Außerdem wurde durch die Zunahme der Versichertenzahlen der Markt für ärztliche Dienstleistungen grundlegend umgeformt. Damit wurden neue Reibungsflächen

---

[6] Koblank, S 174.
[7] Ebd., S 175.
[8] Diesen Quellen ist Ute Frevert in ihrer Arbeit nachgegangen. Frevert (s. Fußnote 1), S 236ff.

geschaffen, welche die alten bei weitem in den Schatten stellten[9] und die „Kassenarztfrage" immer mehr zu einem Kardinalproblem für die gesamte Ärzteschaft
werden ließen. Im folgenden soll versucht werden, die Verschärfung der im Prinzip schon vor 1883 existierenden Konfrontationslinien und das Entstehen neuer
Konfliktzonen nachzuzeichnen.

Die quantitative Ausdehnung des Versicherungswesens spielte hierfür, wie
schon gesagt, eine entscheidende Rolle. 1883 waren durch das Krankenkassengesetz alle Personen, die als Arbeiter in Bergbau, Industrie und Handwerk arbeiteten und unter 2000 Mk. im Jahr verdienten, der Versicherungspflicht unterworfen worden. Das waren 1885 4,29 Mio. Menschen, 9,2 %, und wenn man die
Knappschaftskassen mit ihren 377 000 Mitgliedern dazu rechnet, ziemlich genau
10 % der Bevölkerung. Schon dadurch war gegenüber dem Zustand vor 1883 die
Zahl der Versicherten nach einer Schätzung von Theodor Lohmann, einem der
geistigen Väter des KVG, annähernd verdoppelt worden.[10]

Exakte Zahlen existieren zwar nur für einzelne Städte, diese aber scheinen
Lohmanns Schätzung zu bestätigen. In Dresden etwa waren bei Erlaß des KVG
schon 10,9 % der Bevölkerung (25 030 Personen) bei Innungskrankenkassen, eingeschriebenen Hilfskassen, Genossenschaftskassen oder auf sächsischer Gewerbegesetzgebung beruhenden Krankenkassen versichert.[11] Im Hinblick auf das
KVG war aber eine Zahl von 45 000 versicherungspflichtigen Personen ermittelt
worden, so daß 20 000 Personen, die bislang noch keiner Krankenkasse angehört
hatten (8,7 % der städtischen Bevölkerung) neu versichert werden mußten. Auch
in der Reichshauptstadt Berlin, wo am Schluß des Jahres 1883 schon fast 100 000
Personen in Pflichtkassen versichert waren, wuchs die Zahl der Versicherten
rasch an: Mitte 1885 zählten die 68 Berliner Ortskrankenkassen bereits 180 000
Mitglieder.[12]

Durch die erste Novelle zum Krankenversicherungsgesetz vom 28. Mai 1885
wurde der Versicherungszwang auf alle Arbeiter bei den Post-, Telegraphen- und
Eisenbahnverwaltungen, auf den gewerbsmäßigen Fuhrwerks- und Binnenschifffahrtsbetrieb und auf alle sonstigen (bei Speditionen etc. tätigen) Transportarbeiter ausgedehnt;[13] die Novelle vom 5. Mai 1886 gab den Einzelstaaten bzw. den
Gemeinden und weiteren Kommunalverbänden die Möglichkeit, in ihrem Bezirk
die Versicherungspflicht für land- und forstwirtschaftliche Arbeiter einzuführ-

---

[9] So konnte sich der spätere Kreisphysikus Oskar Schwartz, der in den 50er Jahren Fabrikarzt
  bei 2 Krankenkassen wurde, nicht erinnern, daß damals „Streitigkeiten bei der Besetzung von
  Kassenarztstellen" – wie sie seit den 90er Jahren gehäuft auftraten (dazu Abschnitt 3. in diesem Kapitel) vorgekommen seien; Schwartz O (1907) 60 Jahre ärztlicher, amtlicher u. schriftstellerischer Tätigkeit, 1846–1907. Köln, S 9.
[10] Vgl. Lohmanns Ausführungen in der Reichstagssitzung vom 20. 4. 1883, Stenographische Berichte über die Verhandlungen des Deutschen Reichstags, Bd 71, S 1993. Vgl. auch Tennstedt
  F (1983) Die Errichtung von Krankenkassen in deutschen Städten nach dem Gesetz betr. die
  Krankenversicherung der Arbeiter vom 15. Juni 1883. Z Sozialreform 29:316.
[11] Hesse G (1909) Ein Vierteljahrhundert deutscher Krankenversicherung. Bericht über die Entwicklung der Krankenversicherung in Dresden in den Jahren 1884 bis 1909. Dresden, S 16.
[12] Dierks A (1922) Entstehung und Entwicklung der deutschen Krankenversicherung bis zum
  Jahre 1909, Dissertation, Universität Gießen (veröffentlicht im Zentralblatt der Reichsversicherung 1922, Nr. 15/16), Sp. 484.
[13] Dierks (1922) Sp. 485 f.

Tabelle 6. Die Ausdehnung der Gesetzlichen Krankenversicherung 1885–1914

Jahr	Mitgliederbestand jeweils am Ende des Jahres (in Tausend)	In % der Reichsbevölkerung
1885	4294	9,2
1886	4570	9,7
1887	4842	10,2
1888	5516	11,5
1889	6071	12,5
1890	6343	12,9
1891	6531	13,1
1892	6514	13,0
1893	6755	13,3
1894	6939	13,5
1895	7289	14,0
1896	7696	14,6
1897	8123	15,2
1898	8503	15,6
1899	8787	15,9
1900	9116	16,3
1901	9152	16,1
1902	9473	16,4
1903	9897	16,9
1904	10421	17,5
1905	10940	18,1
1906	11438	18,7
1907	11722	18,9
1908	11775	18,7
1909	12244	19,2
1910	12847	19,9
1911	13357	20,4
1912	12971	19,6
1913	13091	19,5
1914	15610	23,0

Quellen: Für 1885–1901: Übersichten nach Kassenarten über die Ergebnisse der Krankenversicherung im Deutschen Reich in den Jahren 1885–1901. In: Statistik des Deutschen Reiches, N.F. Bd 147: Die Krankenversicherung im Jahre 1901, Berlin 1903, S. 10* f.
Für 1901–1914: Bde. 156, 163, 170, 177, 186, 194, 229, 238, 248, 258, 268, 277, 289 der Statistik des Deutschen Reiches.
Bevölkerungszahlen bei *Hoffmann WG* et al. (1965) Das Wachstum der deutschen Wirtschaft seit der Mitte des 19. Jahrhunderts. Berlin, S 172 ff.
Erläuterungen: Die Zahlen umfassen nur die Mitglieder in den reichsgesetzlichen Krankenkassen, nicht jedoch die Mitglieder der Knappschaftskassen.
Das Absinken der Mitgliederzahlen von 1911 nach 1912 erklärt sich daraus, daß ab 1912 die eingeschriebenen und die landesrechtlichen Hilfskassen, die Ende 1911 noch knapp 1 Mio. Mitglieder zählten, in der Statistik nicht mehr berücksichtigt wurden.
Die Bevölkerungszahl für 1914 wurde durch Extrapolation geschätzt. Für 1914 ist die Mitgliederzahl im Jahresdurchschnitt, nicht am Ende des Jahres erfaßt.

ren;[14] durch eine weitere Novelle wurden 1892 die Handlungsgehilfen und Lehrlinge sowie alle in den Geschäftsbetrieben der Anwälte, Notare, Krankenkassen, Berufsgenossenschaften und Versicherungsanstalten beschäftigten Personen, sofern ihr jährliches Einkommen 2000 Mk. nicht überstieg,[15] in die Versicherung einbezogen.

Durch diese Novellen und mehr noch durch die weitere Ausdehnung von Gewerbe und Industrie weitete sich der Kreis der Versicherten rasch aus. Schon 1895 gehörten den reichsgesetzlichen Kassen 7,3 Mio. Mitglieder an, 1900 waren es 9,1 Mio. und 1905 10,9 Mio. (14 bzw. 16,3 bzw. 18,1 % der Bevölkerung).

In dieser Zahl sind jedoch die Mitglieder der Knappschaftskassen nicht enthalten, da die Knappschaftsversicherung nicht unter die Bestimmungen der GKV fiel, auch wenn sie ihren Mitgliedern im wesentlichen die gleichen Leistungen unter den gleichen Bedingungen gewährte. Schließt man daher in einer Darstellung der Ausdehnung der Versicherungspflicht auch die Knappschaftskassen ein, die 1895 480000, 1900 638000 und 1905 719000 Mitglieder zählten,[16] erhöht sich der Prozentsatz der versicherten Bevölkerung auf 14,9 % im Jahre 1895, 17,4 % 1900 und 19,3 % im Jahre 1905.

Die zum 1. Januar 1914 in Kraft tretende Reichsversicherungsordnung (R. V. O.) dehnte dann den Kreis der Versicherten noch einmal massiv aus, indem sie die Versicherungsgrenze auf 2500 Mk. heraufsetzte und die Landarbeiter, die Dienstboten und die Hausgewerbetreibenden, für die der Versicherungszwang bislang nur ortsstatutarisch festgesetzt werden konnte, auf Reichsebene der Versicherungspflicht unterwarf.

Der Anteil der Krankenversicherten an der Gesamtbevölkerung schnellte dadurch von 19,5 % im Jahre 1913 auf 23 % 1914 hoch. Hinzu kamen noch die Mitglieder der Knappschaftskassen, der Eisenbahnbetriebs-, Post- und anderen Staatskrankenkassen, und die bei immer mehr Kassen mitversicherten Familienangehörigen, so daß insgesamt schätzungsweise 50 % der Reichsbevölkerung von den Kassen erfaßt wurden und kostenlose ärztliche Behandlung erhielten.[17]

Diese rapide Ausdehnung der Versicherung bewirkte, daß die Kassenarzttätigkeit, die früher von einzelnen Ärzten mehr oder weniger als Anhängsel zur eigentlichen Praxis, der Privatpraxis, ausgeübt worden war, für mehr und mehr Ärzte die entscheidende Grundlage ihrer Existenzsicherung wurde. Nach einer Schätzung des Berliner Arztes und Reichstagsabgeordneten Otto Mugdan widmeten 1908 90 % aller praktizierenden Ärzte drei Viertel ihrer Tätigkeit der Durchführung der Arbeiterversicherung.[18] Das mußte Probleme wie etwa die Honorarfrage oder das Problem einer angemessenen Position des Arztes gegenüber dem Kassenvorstand zwangsläufig in ein neues Licht rücken.

---

[14] Aufgrund dessen führte zwischen 1887 und 1894 eine Reihe von Bundesstaaten, darunter alle größeren bis auf Preußen, Bayern und Hamburg den Versicherungszwang für land- und forstwirtschaftliche Arbeiter ein Dierks (1922) Nr. 17, Sp 509

[15] Dierks (1922) Nr. 17, Sp. 511–13

[16] Einen Überblick über die Entwicklung der Knappschaftskassen gibt Bd 177 der Statistik des Deutschen Reichs. Die GKV im Jahre 1905, Berlin 1907, S 38*f.

[17] Rumpe R (1905) Das Deutsche Krankenversicherungsgesetz nach 20jährigem Bestehen, in: Preußische Jahrbücher, S 104, schätzt schon 1905 die Zahl der gegen Krankheit versicherten Personen auf annähernd 30 Mio. Einwohner, d. h. 50 % der Reichsbevölkerung; die Schätzung von 50 % für 1913 auch bei Tennstedt F (1976) Sozialgeschichte der Sozialversicherung. In: Blohmke et al. (Hrsg) Handbuch der Sozialmedizin, Bd 3. Stuttgart, S 388.

[18] Ärztliches Vereinsblatt 1908, Nr. 678, S 755.

Öffentliche Gesundheitspflege
in der Weimarer Republik und in der Frühgeschichte
der Bundesrepublik Deutschland *

W. U. Eckart

Mit Recht ist die Zeit der Weimarer Republik, zuletzt 1985 von Labisch und Tennstedt, als „Blütezeit" der öffentlichen (kommunalen) Wohlfahrts- und Gesundheitspflege[1] unter der Leitwissenschaft der Sozialhygiene bezeichnet worden. Das gesamte Farbspektrum dieser Blütezeit in einem kurzen Beitrag wiedergeben zu wollen, ist unmöglich. Ich kann mich daher nur auf Umrisse des angeschnittenen Themas beschränken, wobei ich ausgehen werde von den theoretischen Voraussetzungen der Leitwissenschaft öffentlicher Gesundheitspflege jener Zeit, der Sozialhygiene, um mich dann der didaktischen Vermittlung und anhand einiger Beispiele auch der praktischen Umsetzung dieser Leitwissenschaft zu widmen. Vom Verlust der Leitwissenschaft, der Zerschlagung ihrer Institutionen und der Vertreibung ihrer Träger in den Monaten nach dem 30. Januar 1933 will ich abschließend einen kurzen Blick auf die Determinanten öffentlicher Gesundheitspflege in den ersten Jahren unserer Republik richten, der freilich mehr Fragen aufwerfen als Ergebnisse präsentieren soll.

Anfänge der deutschen Sozialmedizin im 19. Jahrhundert

Die Anfänge des Wissenschaftszweigs, der nach der Jahrhundertwende in Deutschland als Sozialhygiene breiteste Resonanz finden sollte, lagen bereits in der Mitte des 19. Jahrhunderts. Sie waren eng verknüpft mit den sozialpolitischen Ideen des bürgerlichen Revolutionsversuchs um 1848 und verbinden sich mit den Namen Salomon Neumann (1819–1908) und Rudolf Virchow (1821–1902).

Neumann hatte in seiner 1847 erschienenen Schrift über *Die öffentliche Gesundheitspflege und das Eigentum*[2] zum ersten Male in aller Deutlichkeit die „soziale Natur der Heilkunst" unterstrichen. Auch Virchow hat in der von ihm und Rudolf Leubuscher herausgegebenen Wochenschrift *Die medizinische Reform*

---

* Erstmals veröffentlicht in: Öff. Gesundheitswesen 51/1989:213–221. Vortrag anläßlich der 24. Wissenschaftlichen Jahrestagung der Deutschen Gesellschaft für Sozialmedizin und Prävention „Sozialmedizin in Gesundheit und Krankheit", Hannover, MHH, 15.–17.09.1988.

[1] Labisch A, Tennstedt F (1985) Der Weg zum „Gesetz über die Vereinheitlichung des Gesundheitswesens" vom 3. Juli 1934. Entwicklungslinien und -momente des staatlichen und kommunalen Gesundheitswesens in Deutschland, 2 Teile Schriftenreihe der Akademie für öffentliches Gesundheitswesen in Düsseldorf, Bd 13.1,2, Düsseldorf, S 139f.

[2] Neumann S (1847) Die öffentliche Gesundheitspflege und das Eigentum. Kritisches und Positives mit Bezug auf die preußische Medicinalverfassungsfrage. Berlin.

wiederholt die These vom sozialen Charakter der Medizin[3] betont und vor diesem Hintergrund die Aufgaben einer öffentlichen Gesundheitspflege seiner Zeit definiert. Diese habe, „indem sie in ihren Forschungen den Lebensverhältnissen der verschiedensten Volksklassen" nachgehe „und die feinen, gleichsam geheimen Schwankungen des Massenlebens" verfolge, „bei den meisten sozialen Schwierigkeiten eine entscheidende Stimme". „Allein, so Virchow weiter, ‚darauf' beschränke ‚sich ihre Wirksamkeit nicht. Von Zeit zu Zeit' würden jene Schwankungen größer, zuweilen ungeheuer, in dem einzelne Krankheiten in epidemischer Form" aufträten. „In solchen Fällen" werde „die öffentliche Gesundheitspflege souverän, der Arzt gebietend".[4] Obwohl hier die Bedeutung öffentlicher Gesundheitspflege mit besonderem Blick auf epidemiologische Aspekte sehr deutlich im Zusammenhang mit dem sozialen Charakter von Krankheit, dem Zusammenhang von „Krankheit und sozialer Lage", thematisiert wurde, ist es in den folgenden Jahrzehnten zu einer Verbreitung dieser Ansichten nicht gekommen.

Der beispiellose Aufschwung der naturwissenschaftlichen Medizin, an ihrer Spitze die experimentelle Hygiene, und endlich der Bakteriologie konnte eine Verfolgung der revolutionären Programme Neumanns, Virchows und anderer, die Erforschung der sozialen Determiniertheit des Menschen in Gesundheit und Krankheit, nicht begünstigen. Statt dessen entwickelten sich die experimentelle Hygiene und Bakteriologie zu unangefochtenen „Leitwissenschaften" in der ersten Entwicklungsphase des modernen öffentlichen Gesundheitswesens. Ihre Erfolge redeten eine deutliche Sprache, wie beispielhaft der Sieg über die Cholera belegt. Andere Beispiele ließen sich anreihen. Öffentliche Gesundheitspflege war dabei sowohl in unmittelbar kurativer als auch in präventiver Hinsicht in erster Linie disziplinierende Hygienisierung der Bevölkerung, v. a. der städtischen Unterschichten. Ihre Organisation und Wirkungsentfaltung entsprach einerseits dem obrigkeitsstaatlichen Muster vertikaler Intervention, ermöglichte daneben aber auch das Entstehen eines schier unüberschaubaren Dienstleistungsnetzes öffentlicher Fürsorgestellen und wohlfahrtspflegerischer Vereine, die das Signum des Karitativen einte. In dieses Interventionsmuster fügte sich auch die im europäischen Vergleich fraglos vorbildliche Sozialgesetzgebung der 80er Jahre (1883: Krankenversicherung der Arbeiter; 1884: Unfallversicherung; 1889: Alters- und Invalidenversicherungsgesetz), die zwar das Netz sozialer Sicherung enger knüpfte, als geschenkte Sozialreform von oben die gesellschaftliche Bedingtheit von Krankheit an der Basis aber zunächst wenig veränderte, zur Vermehrung des Wissens um sie kaum beitrug und sozialrevolutionäres Potential geschickt abschöpfte.[5]

---

[3] Labisch u. Tennstedt (1985) wie Anm. 1, 24; zur sozialen Funktion der Medizin, vgl. auch Sigerist HE (1954) Die Heilkunst im Dienste der Menschheit. Stuttgart, S 72–73 u. besonders Ackerknecht E (1932) Beiträge zur Geschichte der Medizinalreform von 1848, Leipzig.

[4] Virchow R (1923) Einführungsartikel der Zeitschrift *Die Medizinische Reform* (10. Juli 1848–29. Juli 1849), hier zit. nach Grotjahn A (1923) Soziale Pathologie. Versuch einer Lehre von den sozialen Beziehungen der Krankheiten als Grundlage der sozialen Hygiene. Berlin, S 3.

[5] Vgl. Hentschel V (1983) Geschichte der deutschen Sozialpolitik (1880–1980). Soziale Sicherung und kollektives Arbeitsrecht. Frankfurt.

Spätestens um die Jahrhundertwende wurden die Grenzen der wissenschaftlichen Hygiene als Leitwissenschaft öffentlicher Gesundheitspflege deutlich. Weder die technische Assanierung und Hygienisierung der Städte noch das individualisierte Krankheitskonzept der Bakteriologie oder die fortschrittliche Sozialgesetzgebung waren geeignet, isoliert die ungeheuren sozialen Probleme und in ihrer Folge die vielfältigen hygienischen Aufgabenstellungen, die die zweite Phase der Industrialisierung in den schnell expandierenden Städten mit sich brachte, zu lösen. Hinzu trat, daß die euphorischen Hoffnungen, die man im Zusammenhang mit der Bekämpfung der Volkskrankheit Tuberkulose auf die Bakteriologie allein gesetzt hatte, trogen. Es wurde bald deutlich, daß es gerade bei dieser Krankheit nicht nur biologische, sondern gerade auch die sozialen Existenzbedingungen waren, die Ausbruch und Verlauf entscheidend beeinflußten. Die erste große zusammenhängende Aufsatzsammlung, die sich den spezifischen Auswirkungen sozialer Lebensbedingungen auf die Gesundheit des Menschen widmete, erschien 1913 unter dem Titel *Krankheit und soziale Lage*. Herausgeber waren Mosse und Tugendreich.[6]

Sozialhygiene

Unter den Ärzten, die jene Zusammenhänge auch an anderen Beispielen bald nach der Jahrhundertwende erkannten und auf dem Boden dieser Erkenntnis erste theoretische Konzepte von einer neuen sozialen Hygiene entwickelten, ist an erster Stelle der sozialdemokratische Arzt Alfred Grotjahn (1869–1931) zu nennen. Seine Hauptthesen, die für die Weiterentwicklung und praktische Umsetzung einer sozialhygienisch orientierten und öffentlichen Gesundheitspflege insbesondere in der Weimarer Republik von zentraler Bedeutung sein sollten, will ich hier kurz noch einmal nach der dritten Auflage seines Hauptwerks *Soziale Pathologie* (1923)[7] zusammenfassen. Für Grotjahn stand zweifelsfrei fest, daß die „gewiß großartigen Ergebnisse der rein naturwissenschaftlich betriebenen Hygiene erst dann zu verallgemeinernden Normen verarbeitet werden (können), wenn kulturhistorische, psychologische, nationalökonomische und politische Erwägungen in die Erörterung einbezogen werden"[8] und die Hygiene damit zu einer sozialhygienischen Gesamtdisziplin werde. Ihr eigentliches Wesen bestehe darin, „alle Dinge des öffentlichen Lebens und der sozialen Umwelt im Hinblick auf ihren Einfluß auf die körperlichen Zustände zu betrachten und aufgrund dieser der sozialen Hygiene eigentümlichen Betrachtungsweise Maßnahmen zu finden, die keineswegs immer einen rein ärztlichen Charakter zu haben brauchen, sondern sehr häufig in das Gebiet der Sozialpolitik oder der Politik überhaupt hinübergreifen"[9]. Allein die soziale Hygiene sei imstande, aus ihren Untersuchungen „Maßnahmen abzuleiten", die es einem Volke, das in jeder Hinsicht solchen Re-

---

[6] Mosse M, Tugendreich G (Hrsg.) (1977) Krankheit und soziale Lage, ungekürzte photomech. Neuauflage der Ausgabe München 1913, hrsg. von J. Cromm (Vorworte v. H. P. Bahrdt u. M. Pflanz), Göttingen.
[7] Grotjahn (1923), vgl. Fußnote 4.
[8] Grotjahn (1923) S 4.
[9] Grotjahn (1923) S 5–6.

geln folge, „mit Sicherheit ermöglichen" könnten, „die körperliche Grundlage seiner Kultur, seiner Volkskraft, dauernd unversehrt zu erhalten".[10] Ausgehend von diesen Feststellungen definierte Grotjahn folgerichtig Sozialhygiene als „deskriptive" und „normative Wissenschaft".[11] Gemeint war also keineswegs nur eine Dokumentation der vielfältigen Zusammenhänge zwischen Krankheit und sozialer Lage und die auf dieser Basis erfolgende individuell-kurative ärztliche Intervention, angesprochen war auch der normsetzende, verändernde und damit erst wirklich präventive Charakter der neuen Wissenschaft.

Die Elemente, insbesondere des normativen sozialhygienischen „Kalküls", so hatte Grotjahn bereits 1912 in seiner Berliner Antrittsvorlesung[12] formuliert, seien zwar in erster Linie „kulturhistorische, psychologische, nationalökonomische und politische". Die „Zielvorstellung" aber bleibe selbstverständlich gesundheitsfürsorglich und erstrecke sich auf „die größtmögliche Verhütung der dem Körper drohenden Schädlichkeiten und die größtmögliche Herbeiführung" körperförderlicher Momente bei der größtmöglichen Bevölkerungszahl, wenn nicht bei ihrer Gesamtheit.[13] Sozialhygiene also als Methode präventiver Medizin im großen, läßt sich als das eigentlich neue Element zusammenfassen.

Neben Grotjahn, der als Hauptvertreter einer theoretisch vorwiegend aus den Sozialwissenschaften entwickelten Sozialhygiene steht, wären unter den theoretischen Begründern der neuen Disziplin auch andere, wenngleich mit teilweise unterschiedlichen Auffassungen im Detail, zu nennen. Alfons Fischer (1873–1937) etwa, Adolf Gottstein (1857–1941), Arthur Schlossmann (1867–1932) und Ludwig Teleky (1872–1957) an erster Stelle.[14] Die meisten der grundsätzlichen Überlegungen zu dem weit gespannten Aufgabenfeld einer öffentlichen Gesundheitspflege auf dem Boden der jungen wissenschaftlichen Sozialhygiene sind bereits vor dem 1. Weltkrieg entwickelt worden. Der Krieg verhinderte indes ihre frühzeitige didaktische Umsetzung und lieferte zugleich die gesundheitlichen, wirtschaftlichen und sozialen Krisen, in denen die Sozialhygiene nach 1919 ihr praktisches Bewährungsfeld fand.

An dieser Stelle muß ein kurzer Exkurs in den Gang der Darstellung eingefügt werden, der aber im Hinblick auf die theoretisch-ideologischen Determinanten sozialer Hygiene als Leitwissenschaft öffentlicher Gesundheitspflege in den 20er Jahren bedeutsam ist. Eine zweite Disziplin, die sich – in breitesten Bevölkerungskreisen zunehmend rezipiert und akzeptiert – in den 20er Jahren verselbständigen und institutionalisieren sollte, hatte sich nämlich ebenfalls vor 1914

---

[10] Grotjahn (1923) S 9.

[11] Grotjahn (1923) S 10: „Demnach läßt sich die soziale Hygiene definieren: 1. Die soziale Hygiene als *deskriptive* Wissenschaft ist die Lehre von den Bedingungen, denen die Verallgemeinerung hygienischer Kultur unter der Gesamtheit von örtlich, zeitlich und gesellschaftlich zusammengehörigen Individuen mit deren Nachkommen unterliegt. 2. Die soziale Hygiene als normative Wissenschaft ist die Lehre von den *Maßnahmen*, die die Verallgemeinerung hygienischer Kultur unter der Gesamtheit von örtlich, zeitlich und gesellschaftlich zusammengehörigen Individuen und deren Nachkommen bezwecken."

[12] Grotjahn A (1912) Die Aufgaben der sozialen Hygiene. Dtsch Med Wochenschr 38:2318–2320.

[13] Grotjahn (1912) S 2319.

[14] Vgl. Gottstein A, Schlossmann A, Teleky L (1925) Handbuch der sozialen Hygiene und Gesundheitsfürsorge, 6 Bde. Berlin, S 27.

teils unabhängig, teils der Sozialhygiene inkorporiert entwickelt: die Rassenhygiene. Die Grundlagen dieser von Alfred Ploetz (1860–1940) im Jahre 1895 zuerst benannten und umrissenen Lehre fußten in der Gedankenwelt des Darwinismus, des auf ihm errichteten Sozialdarwinismus sowie auf der jungen wissenschaftlichen Vererbungslehre.[15] Ihr Ziel richtete sich auf die „Erhaltung und Fortpflanzung der (biologischen) Rasse unter den günstigsten Bedingungen", wobei es ihr als „quantitative Rassenhygiene" um die „Mehrung", als „qualitative Rassenhygiene" oder Eugenik um die „Verbesserung" oder „Hebung" des Volksbestands ging. Als „positive" bzw. „negative" Rassenhygiene standen ihr zu diesem Zwecke die Mittel der „Auslese" bzw. der „Ausmerze" zur Verfügung.[16] Wie radikal bereits in den 20er Jahren gerade der letzte Aspekt gedacht wurde, zeigt etwa die 1920 publizierte Schrift *Die Freigabe der Vernichtung lebensunwerten Lebens* von Karl Binding (1841–1920) und Alfred Hoche (1865–1943).[17] Sowohl die quantitative als auch die qualitative Rassenhygiene fanden nach dem 1. Weltkrieg geradezu ideale Diskussions- und Betätigungsfelder. Das Menetekel des durch Kriegsverlust und Geburtenrückgang drohenden Aussterbens des deutschen Volkes sowie das Schreckgespenst drohender Entartung durch die Zunahme sog. Keimgifte (Alkohol, Tuberkulose etc.) als Folgen zunehmender Verelendung durch Krieg und Wirtschaftskrise wurden durchaus allgemein empfunden und die Verbreitung eugenisch-biologistischer Vorstellungen ging quer durch die politischen Lager in bürgerlichen und sozialistischen Ärztekreisen der Republik von Weimar. Der englische Medizinhistoriker Paul J. Weindling[18] sieht für die 20er Jahre „in Deutschland nicht nur einen Höhepunkt für Demokratie und Sozialpolitik allgemein, sondern auch für eine eugenisch begründete Sozialpolitik"[19] im besonderen. Es entwickelte sich im Schoß und neben der sozialhygienischen eine „eugenische Bewegung" der Weimarer Republik, die sich verbreiterte und in

---

[15] Vgl. aus der inzwischen umfangreichen historiographischen Literatur zum Thema u. a. Kroll J (1983) Zur Entstehung und Institutionalisierung einer naturwissenschaftlichen und sozialpolitischen Bewegung: Die Entwicklung der Eugenik/Rassenhygiene bis 1933, Dissertation, Universität Tübingen 1983; Mann G (1988) Biologismus – Vorstufen und Elemente einer Medizin im Nationalsozialismus. Dtsch Ärztebl 17:836–837. Baader G (1988) Rassenhygiene und Eugenik – Vorbedingungen für die Vernichtungsstrategien gegen sogenannte „Minderwertige" im Nationalsozialismus. Dtsch Ärztebl 27:1357–1363.

[16] Auch A. Grotjahn stand der Rassenhygiene keineswegs fern. Bereits 1912 hatte er sie in seiner Habilitationsvorlesung thematisiert und vorbehaltlos als eine „Methode" zur „Verhütung der Entartung und Verkümmerung" akzeptiert, die sich der „sozialen Hygiene zwanglos" eingliedere (Grotjahn, Aufgaben, wie Anm. 12, 2319); neben einer „qualitative(n)" und „quantitative(n) Rationalisierung der menschlichen Fortpflanzung (Grotjahn, Soziale Pathologie, wie Anm. 4, 468–532) schwebten ihm als weitere Maßnahmen die „Asylierung" Erbkranker und auch die Zwangssterilisation für Schwachsinnige und Epileptiker vor; vgl. Baader G (1984) Die Medizin im Nationalsozialismus. Ihre Wurzeln und die erste Periode ihrer Realisierung 1933–1938. In: Gross C, Wiham R (Hrsg) Nicht mißhandeln (Stätten der Geschichte Berlin, Bd 5). Berlin, S 1–106, hier 74–77; vgl. zur problematischen historischen Einordnung Grotjahns auch Deppe H.-U. (1983) Vorsicht vor Alfred Grotjahn. Sozialhygiene und Eugenik. Dem Gesundheitswes 5:23.

[17] Binding K, Hoche A (1920) Die Freigabe der Vernichtung lebensunwerten Lebens. Ihr Maß und ihre Form, Leipzig.

[18] Weindling PJ (1987) Die Verbreitung rassenhygienischen/eugenischen Gedankengutes in bürgerlichen und sozialistischen Kreisen in der Weimarer Republik. Medizinhist J 22:352–368.

[19] Weindling (1987) S 352.

großen Teilen der bürgerlichen Ärzteschaft als sozial-darwinistische Rassenhygiene zunehmend radikalisierte. Hierüber wird noch zu berichten sein. Ich komme nun zur Umsetzung der Sozialhygiene als Leitwissenschaft öffentlicher Gesundheitspflege im akademischen Unterricht und in der sozialmedizinischen Praxis der 20er Jahre.

Sozialhygienischer Unterricht

Der offizielle Beginn des sozialhygienischen Unterrichts in Deutschland ist im Jahre 1920 auf 2 institutionellen Ebenen anzusetzen. So erhielt Grotjahn 1920 an der Berliner Universität – gegen den Willen der Medizinischen Fakultät – den ersten Lehrstuhl für Sozialhygiene, den er bis zu seinem Tod 1931 innehaben sollte.[20] Seine Vorlesungen vertiefte er in seminaristischen Übungen für seine Studenten und seine Doktoranden, daneben aber auch für nichtärztliche Hörer. Mit Blick auf die aktuelle Diskussion um die Einrichtung besonderer Studiengänge für Bevölkerungsmedizin und Öffentliche Gesundheitspflege ist sowohl dieser Umstand interessant als auch das Themenspektrum der Seminarveranstaltungen, das uns zwischen 1919 und 1931 bekannt ist und in fallender Häufigkeit die Aspekte Epidemiologie, Mutter/Kind, Statistik, Hygiene der Fortpflanzung (Eugenik), Sozialwissenschaften, Gesundheitspolitik, Versicherungswesen/Sozialfürsorge, Arbeit und Freizeit sowie das Wohnungswesen abdeckte.[21]

Für die zweite institutionelle Ebene sozialhygienischer Ausbildung sollte der bereits erwähnte Theoretiker Adolf Gottstein wichtig werden. Der Charlottenburger Arzt und spätere preußische Ministerialdirektor hatte bereits während des 1. Weltkrieges den Gedanken forciert, die sozialhygienische Ausbildung für die in der öffentlichen Gesundheitspflege tätigen Kreis- und Kommunalärzte verpflichtend zu machen, was 1919 bzw. 1921 Realität werden sollte, und zu diesem Zweck besondere Ausbildungsstätten zu schaffen. Auf seine Anregung hin entstanden 1920 in Breslau, Charlottenburg und Düsseldorf „Sozialhygienische Akademien",[22] deren theoretischer Unterricht die Grundlagen der Sozialhygiene vermitteln sollte und die Fächer Sozialpathologie, Statistik, Volkswirtschaftslehre, Sozialpolitik, Verfassungs- und Verwaltungsrecht und schließlich Sozialversicherungsrecht umfaßte. Das hierauf aufbauende praktische Studium widmete sich dem breiten Spektrum der gesamten Gesundheits- und Sozialfürsorge, wobei neben die Vorlesungen praktische Übungen und Exkursionen traten. Bemerkenswert ist der Umstand, daß diese Akademien von Anfang an auch Nichtärzten of-

---

[20] Vgl. zu Biographie und Programm Grotjahns, Tutzke D (1973) Alfred Grotjahn und die Sozialhygiene. Zschr Ärztl Fortbild 67:783–788; Tutzke D (1979) Alfred Grotjahn. Leipzig; Tutzke D (1973) Alfred Grotjahn (1869–1931) und die junge Sowjetunion. Z Ges Hyg 19:596–599; Labisch A (1983) Alfred Grotjahn (1869–1931) und das gesundheitspolitische Programm der Mehrheitssozialdemokraten von 1922. Med Mensch Ges 8:192–197 sowie Labisch u. Tennstedt (1985) bes. Bd I, 140ff., 155ff., 359ff., Bd II, 419–420.

[21] Vgl. Tutzke D (1970) Die sozialhygienischen Übungen an der Berliner Medizinischen Fakultät von 1920 bis 1933. Z Ges Hyg Teilgebiete 16:335–339.

[22] Zur Vorgeschichte und ersten Arbeitsphase der Akademien vgl. Teleky L (1921) Die Aufgaben der Sozialhygienischen Akademien, in: Dtsch Med Wochenschr 47:717–719; vgl. auch Labisch u. Tennstedt (1985) S 59–60.

fen stehen sollten, worauf Ludwig Teleky, Leiter der Westdeutschen Sozialhygienischen Akademie in Düsseldorf, besonderen Wert legte: „Auch werden die Akademien", berichtet Teleky am 23. Juni 1921 in der DMW, „in ihr Tätigkeitsgebiet den sozialhygienischen Unterricht solcher Gruppen von Nichtärzten aufnehmen müssen, die sozialhygienischer Kenntnisse bedürfen: Verwaltungsbeamte, Beamte der Sozialversicherungsinstitute. Natürlich wird dieser Unterricht wesentlich verschieden sein müssen von dem für Ärzte, da ja die Vorkenntnisse der Hörer dieser Kurse sowohl nach der negativen als der positiven Seite wesentlich andere sind".[23] Ich denke, diese wenigen Hinweise sind vielleicht auch anregend, in die aktuelle Curriculardiskussion sozialmedizinischer Ausbildung historische Vorbilder stärker einzubringen, als dies bisher geschehen ist. Ich komme nun zur sozialmedizinischen Praxis der 20er Jahre.

Sozialhygiene in der Weimarer Republik und unter der nationalsozialistischen Diktatur

Die Ausrufung der Republik, der Fall der konstitutionellen Monarchien und die feste Absicht, anstelle des alten kaiserlichen Machtstaats den sozialen, wenn nicht sozialistischen Wohlfahrtsstaat zu errichten, verlangte auch für den Bereich der öffentlichen Gesundheitspflege neue Zielorientierungen und neue politische Rahmenbedingungen. Die Forderung nach einer weitgehenden Neustrukturierung des gesamten Gesundheitswesens, nach dem Aufbau eines suffizienten und einheitlichen Gesundheitsfürsorgewesens erhoben sich allenthalben. Insbesondere der alte noch aus dem Kaiserreich herrührende Kompetenzdualismus zwischen Kreis- und Stadtärzten sollte durch eine solche einheitliche, hierarchische Neustrukturierung zugunsten der Kreisärzte beseitigt werden. Aus den verschiedensten Gründen ist es hierzu freilich nicht gekommen, obwohl für eine solche Neuregelung von vielen Seiten detaillierte Pläne vorgelegt worden waren, wie die beispielhafte Studie von Alfons Labisch und Florian Tennstedt zur Vorgeschichte des Vereinheitlichungsgesetzes von 1934 zeigt.[24] Zwar hatte die Verfassung der Weimarer Republik vom 11. August 1919 dem Reich durch eine Reihe von Artikeln die Kompetenz einer Rahmengesetzgebung für die öffentliche Gesundheitspflege und die unmittelbare Kontrolle über einige zentrale Gesundheitsinstitutionen, wie etwa das Reichsgesundheitsamt, belassen.[25] Gebrauch ist hiervon jedoch cum grano salis wenig gemacht worden. Den Ländern blieb wie in der Reichsverfassung von 1871 das Recht der Gesetzgebung im einzelnen, was dazu führte, daß diese ihre historisch gewachsenen Gesetze und Einrichtungen nach ihren jeweiligen landespolitischen Gegebenheiten fortschrieben. Das vielfältige Bild, das so in der gesetzlichen Regelung der öffentlichen Gesundheitspflege entstand, kann hier nicht verglichen werden. Entscheidend ist das Ergebnis, daß nämlich durch eben dieses Regelungsdefizit der öffentlichen Gesundheitspflege im kommunalen Bereich ein bedeutsamer Aufgabenzuwachs zuteil wurde, der ei-

---

[23] Teleky (1921) S 719.
[24] Labisch u. Tennstedt (1985).
[25] Vgl. Frey G (1923) Gesundheitspflege. In: Hesse P (Hrsg) Politisches Handwörterbuch, Bd 1. Leipzig, S 706–707; Schreiber G (1926) Deutsches Reich und deutsche Medizin. Studien zur Medizinalpolitik des Reiches in der Nachkriegszeit (1818–1926), Leipzig, S 1–118.

ne „Blütezeit" öffentlicher Gesundheitsleistungen in den Städten und Gemeinden ermöglichte, die erst 1933 ihr abruptes Ende finden würde. Dies galt insbesondere für die Situation in den preußischen Großstädten, wo eine Zusammenfassung aller Maßnahmen in der Gesundheitspflege durch die Einrichtung kommunaler Gesundheitsämter realisiert werden konnte, nachdem die karitativen, privaten Zweige der Gesundheitsfürsorge durch die Inflation des Jahres 1923 finanziell ruiniert waren. Die Leiter dieser kommunalen Gesundheitsämter verstanden sich immer auch gleichzeitig als Kommunalpolitiker. „Sie haben sich", wie der bergische Sozialarzt Wilhelm Hagen (1893–1982) in seinen Erinnerungen berichtet,[26] „als Stadträte, Beigeordnete und Bürgermeister durchgesetzt. Im Rahmen dieser Gesundheitsämter wurden nicht nur die Institutionen geschaffen, sondern auch ein Stab von Kommunalärzten herangebildet, die ihre Lebensaufgabe in der Gesundheitspolitik und in der prophylaktischen Medizin sahen", ihre Motivation aber aus der jungen problembezogenen Sozialhygiene schöpften. Ihre hochmotivierten Mitarbeiter rekrutierten sich meist aus der Gruppe der Jungärzte, die während des Weltkriegs approbiert oder notapprobiert worden waren und kaum Aussichten auf eine Kassenzulassung haben durften. Insbesondere die Metropole Berlin, stellte einer großen Zahl engagierter liberaler und sozialistischer Ärzte ein ideales Experimentierfeld zur praktischen Umsetzung dieser Ideen zur Verfügung.

Ich möchte daher am Beispiel der 4,1-Mio.-Stadt Berlin um 1926/27 das Wirken kommunaler öffentlicher Gesundheitspflege anhand einiger typischer Sonderbereiche der offenen vorbeugenden Gesundheitsfürsorge skizzieren,[27] in der sich das präventive Element bevölkerungsnaher Gesundheitspädagogik mit dem der ambulanten kurativen Versorgung im Sinne einer sozialhygienischen Praxis am deutlichsten verband. Ergänzen soll dieses Bild die knappe Darstellung der mit jenen Einrichtungen eng kooperierenden Kassenambulatorien der Stadt. Sie werden Verständnis für diese Beschränkung haben, denn die ausführliche Beschreibung der Berliner Gesundheitsverwaltung, aller Einrichtungen der allgemeinen, der halboffenen und geschlossenen Gesundheitsfürsorge, des Städtischen Rettungs- und Krankentransportwesens oder der hygienischen Volksbelehrung[28] in der Berliner Funkstunde[29] wäre zwar höchst aufschlußreich aber leider auch rahmensprengend.

---

[26] Hagen W (1969) Gesundheitspolitik im 20. Jahrhundert. Off Gesundheitswes 31:53–58, 54f. Hier zit. nach Labisch u. Tennstedt (1985) Bd 1, S 60–61.

[27] Zugrunde lag, soweit nicht anders angemerkt, die vom Reichsausschuß für das ärztliche Fortbildungswesen herausgegebene Dokumentation: Gesundheitswesen und soziale Fürsorge im Deutschen Reich. Sammlung von Ausarbeitungen und Leitsätzen für die von der Hygiene-Organisation des Völkerbundes veranstaltete Internationale Studienreise für ausländische Medizinalbeamte in Deutschland 1927, zusammengestellt im Reichsgesundheitsamt, Berlin 1928.

[28] Vgl. Tugendreich G (1923) Zur Frage der hygienischen Volksbelehrung, in: Dtsch Med Wochenschr 49:193–194, Schreiber (1926) S 66–73.

[29] Vgl. Frank P (1924) Rundfunkvorträge aus dem Gebiete des Gesundheitswesens, Dtsch Med Wochenschr 50:27 (4. Juli 1924); kurz vor der Fertigstellung hierzu die Untersuchung von Biermann R Medizin im Rundfunk im ersten Jahrzehnt seines Bestehens, 1923–1933, Dissertation, Universität Münster, zum Themenfeld die Analyse von Alt K (1983) Der deutsche Zahnärzterundfunk (1926–1932) als Mittel der Zahnärztlichen Fortbildung und Volksbelehrung in der Weimarer Zeit. Dissertation, Universität Berlin.

An erster Stelle unter den Einrichtungen der offenen vorbeugenden Gesundheitsfürsorge Berlins sind sicher die knapp 100 Schwangeren-, Säuglings- und Kleinkinderfürsorgestellen[30] zu nennen, deren Arbeit untereinander sowie mit den städtischen Wohlfahrts- und Jugendämtern eng verzahnt war. Gesundheitserziehung, Problemberatung, ärztliche und wirtschaftliche Akuthilfe gingen in diesen Einrichtungen stets Hand in Hand. Die Konsultationsakzeptanz und Beratungseffizienz insbesondere der Säuglingsfürsorgestellen war auch für heutige Verhältnisse extrem hoch, weil die Standesämter Berlins alle Geburten an die jeweils zuständigen Fürsorgestellen weitermeldeten und die Auszahlung des gesetzlichen Stillgelds an eine Vorstellung in eben diesen Einrichtungen gebunden war. Neben der normalen Beratungstätigkeit behandelten alle Fürsorgestellen unmittelbar auch in Ernährungsnotfällen sowie beim Auftreten von Neugeborenensyphilis. Bei sozialer Not und mangelnder Stillfähigkeit lieferten sie verbilligte oder kostenlose Milch. Der Erfolg dieser Fürsorgeeinrichtungen läßt sich leicht an den Zahlen ablesen: So wurden 1926 insgesamt 28255 eheliche und 6003 uneheliche Säuglinge erstmalig vorgestellt, was bezogen auf alle Lebendgeborenen der Stadt im gleichen Zeitraum etwa 77% bzw. 70% entsprach. Die Zahl aller Säuglings- und Kleinkindberatungen belief sich auf nahezu 1 Mio.

Der Mütter- und Säuglingsberatung vorgeschaltet bzw. sie ergänzend arbeiteten die 1927 in Berlin existierenden 8 Eheberatungsstellen[31] der Stadt, die meist nebenamtlich von Kommunalärzten geleitet wurden. Die Aufgaben dieser Fürsorgestellen erstreckten sich auf die freiwillige Beratung von Ehewilligen und Ehepaaren in allen Fragen der Eheeignung sowie der Sexualhygiene. Die Einrichtung von Eheberatungsstellen im Sinne einer eugenisch orientierten Familienfürsorge, mit der in der Mitte der 20er Jahre in einigen größeren Städten des Reichsgebiets, so auch in Berlin, begonnen worden war, deckte sich in besonderer Weise mit sozialhygienischen Vorstellungen, und es waren wie in der sozialhygienischen Praxis überhaupt meist liberale sozialistische, kommunistische, häufig jüdische Ärztinnen und Ärzte, die, wie etwa Alfred Korach im Bezirk Prenzlauer Berg, Georg Löwenstein in Lichtenberg oder Herta Nathorff und Lilly Ehrenfried in Moabit, die Einrichtung solcher Institutionen förderten und vorantrieben. Bei der Beratung ging es dabei keineswegs nur um Fragen von Geschlechts- oder drohenden Erbkrankheiten, sondern gerade auch um Probleme des Zusammenhangs zwischen sozialer Wohnungsnot und den hieraus erwachsenden sexuellen und gesundheitlichen Notstandssituationen. Das großstädtische Mietskasernensystem brachte es mit sich, daß in einem Haus, bei einer Annahme von durchschnittlich 2,5 Kindern je Ehepaar ca. 500 Menschen, Untermieter, Schlafburschen, Woh-

---

[30] Vgl. Stöckel S (1988) Säuglingsfürsorge in Berlin zwischen sozialer Reform und Eugenik (Vortragszusammenfassung). Nachrichtenbl Dtsch Ges Gesch Med Naturwissenschaft Technik 38:65–66; Schreiber (1926) S 53–55.

[31] Vgl. Weindling (1987) S 366; Winau R (1988) Ansätze einer sozialen Medizin im Berlin der zwanziger Jahre (Vortragszusammenfassung). Nachrichtenbl Dtsch Gesellsch Gesch Med Naturwissenschaft Technik 38:65; Loewenstein G (1980) Lebenserinnerungen (Interviewzusammenfassung). In: Leibfried S von, Tennstedt F (Hrsg) Kommunale Gesundheitsfürsorge und sozialistische Ärztepolitik zwischen Kaiserreich und Nationalsozialismus – autobiographische, biographische und gesundheitspolitische Anmerkungen von Dr. Georg Loewenstein. (= Arbeitsberichte zu verschütteten Alternativen in der Gesundheitspolitik, Bd 3), Bremen, S 12.

nungslose, angeheiratete Familienangehörige nicht eingerechnet, zusammen wohnen mußten. Wie drängend die Not war, um die jene Beratungen also kreisten, wird so vielleicht deutlicher.[32]

Von sozialhygienisch außerordentlich hoher Bedeutung waren schließlich Fürsorgeeinrichtungen für Tuberkulöse und Geschlechtskranke.[33] So waren die Tuberkulosenfürsorgestellen Berlins zwar Meldestellen im Sinne des Pr. Ges. zur Bekämpfung der Tuberkulose vom 4. August 1923; ihre Dienstleistungen erstreckten sich neben der Diagnosestellung sowie der Einleitung von Heilstättenkuren, Krankenhausbehandlungen und Siechenaufnahme in erster Linie aber auf präventive Aktivitäten, die sich auf die „Sanierung der Wohnungen" sowie die „Belehrung und Überwachung des Kranken und seiner Umgebung" richteten. 25 städtische Fürsorgestellen und 5, die in Arbeitsgemeinschaft mit der Landesversicherungsanstalt Berlin unterhalten wurden, teilten sich in diese Aufgaben.

Nachdem durch das Reichsgesetz zur Bekämpfung der Geschlechtskrankheiten vom 18. Februar 1927 dieser Teil der Gesundheitspflege endgültig aus dem polizeilichen Kompetenzbereich in den gesundheitsfürsorgerischen übergegangen war, fielen gerade der kommunalen Geschlechtskrankenfürsorge[34] besondere Aufgaben im Rahmen von Diagnose, Therapie und hygienischer Belehrungsarbeit zu. Diese Leistungen verteilten sich auf je 6 Ambulatorien und 6 Fürsorgestellen, in denen zusammen allein 1927 annähernd 70 000 Beratungen durchgeführt worden sind.

Ich kann hier nicht auf alle Einzelaspekte eingehen, die das facettenreiche Bild einer kommunalen öffentlichen Gesundheitspflege im Berlin der späten 20er Jahre bot. Städtische Einrichtungen der Alkoholiker-, Psychopathen-, Sucht und Krüppelfürsorge, das Armenarztwesen oder auch die mobile Krankenversorgung im Hause durch Bezirksgemeindekrankenschwestern wären hier in der offenen Fürsorge neben Tagungskurstätten für rachitische Kinder und ebensolchen Einrichtungen, Ambulatorien und Waldschulen für Tuberkulöse in der halboffenen Fürsorge zu erwähnen. Statt dessen möchte ich abschließend einen kurzen Blick auf eine Reihe von Einrichtungen werfen, die das Berliner Stadtarztwesen mit seiner sozialhygienisch-sozialmedizinischen Orientierung seit der Mitte der 20er Jahre zunehmend ergänzten; die Rede ist von den „Ambulatorien" und „Gesundheitshäusern" der Metropole, die als Antwort der Krankenkassen Berlins auf den sog. „Ärztestreik" vom Dezember 1923 über das ganze Stadtgebiet verteilt errichtet wurden. Auf die standespolitische Vorgeschichte dieses Ärztestreiks, der den Höhepunkt des Honorar- und Zulassungskonflikts zwischen den führenden ärztlichen Standesorganisationen und den sozialdemokratisch geprägten Krankenkassen darstellte und unmittelbare Reaktion des Etablierten, um seine Pfründe fürchtenden Ärztestandes auf die kassenbegünstigende Notverordnung der Regierung Stresemann (13. Oktober 1923) war, kann ich

---

[32] Vgl. Loewenstein G (1980) Die Gefahren des Wohnungselends für die Volksgesundheit. In: Leibfried S von, Tennstedt F (Hrsg) Kommunale Gesundheitsfürsorge. Bremen, S 156–161; Loewenstein G (1931) Wohnungsnot und Sexualnot. Ärztin 7:134–137.

[33] Schreiber (1926) S 24–32; vgl. auch Gesundheitswesen und soziale Fürsorge im Deutschen Reich, wie Anm. 27.

[34] Schreiber (1926) S 32–39.

hier nicht eingehen.[35] Mit Hilfe eigener Ambulatorien hofften die Krankenkassen primär, sich aus der Abhängigkeit von den kassenärztlichen Vereinigungen und ihrem Streik zu lösen. Die Großpraxen, die mit angestellten Ärzten – sog. „Nothelfern" – verschiedener Fachrichtungen besetzt und mit modernsten medizinischen Geräten ausgestattet waren, entwickelten sich aber darüber hinaus bald zu Zentren praktischer Sozialmedizin, in denen sich individualmedizinisch-kurative aber auch präventive und gesundheitspädagogische Aspekte ärztlicher Tätigkeit ideal ergänzten. Besonderen Raum nahm die beratende aufklärerische Tätigkeit auf den Gebieten der Sexual- und Eheberatung,[36] der Schwangerenfürsorge, der Geschlechtskrankenfürsorge sowie der Alkoholikerbetreuung ein. Unterstützung und personelle Förderung erwuchs den Ambulatorien aus der „Arbeitsgemeinschaft sozialdemokratischer Ärzte" und dem „Verein sozialistischer Ärzte". Skepsis wurde ihnen aus den Reihen der Standesvertreter zuteil, die die Ambulatorien bald als „Behandlungsfabriken" mit „Massenabfertigung" und die dort arbeitenden Ärzte als „Streikbrecher" und sozialistische Feinde eines „freien und berufsfreudigen Arztseins" diffamierten, so etwa der Reichstagsabgeordnete (DNVP) Karl Haedenkamp (1889–1955) in einer Reichstagsrede vom 20. Juni 1925. Haedenkamp, der sich zwischen 1930 und 1933 maßgeblich für die Annäherung zwischen Hartmannbund und NSDAeB einsetzen sollte, zitierte seine Kritik aus einem offenen Brief an den Abgeordneten Dr. Julius Moses (SPD) (1868–1942). Den Ärzteverbänden ist es auch nach dem „Waffenstillstand" mit den Kassen vom April 1924 nicht gelungen, die Ambulatorien, deren Zahl stetig stieg, zu beseitigen, obwohl die ökonomische Situation der Kassen am Beginn der 30er Jahre zunehmend desolater, der Spielraum für sozialhygienische Aktivitäten unter dem Eindruck der Notverordnungspolitik und wachsender ideologischer Radikalisierung immer geringer wurde. Der Keim des Hasses war indes längst gesät, als sich die Zerschlagung eines richtungsweisenden Modells sozialhygienischer Gesundheitspflege 1933 in beängstigender Geschwindigkeit vollzog.[37]

Daß es meist jüdische, sozialistische oder kommunistische Ärzte waren, die in ihren Praxen, den Beratungsstellen und Kassenambulatorien gerade den Schwachen der Gesellschaft ihre Hilfe widmeten, ließ nationalsozialistischen Ärzten

---

[35] Vgl. hierzu besonders Hansen E, Heisig M, Leibfried S et al. (1981) Seit über einem Jahrhundert ... Verschüttete Alternativen in der Sozialpolitik. Sozialer Fortschritt, organisierte Dienstleistermacht und nationalsozialistische Machtergreifung: der Fall der Ambulatorien in den Unterweserstädten und Berlin. 100 Jahre Kaiserliche Botschaft zur Sozialversicherung (Wirtschafts- und sozialwissenschaftliches Institut des DGB und Forschungsschwerpunkt Reproduktionsrisiken, soziale Bewegungen und Sozialpolitik der Universität Bremen). Köln; Winter I (1971) Die KPD und der Konflikt zwischen den Ärzten und Krankenkassen 1923/24. NTM Gesch Naturwiss Technik Med 8:92–100; Winter I (1977) Ärzte und Arbeiterklasse in der Weimarer Republik. In: Kühn K (Hrsg) Ärzte an der Seite der Arbeiterklasse. Beiträge zur Geschichte des Bündnisses der deutschen Arbeiterklasse mit der medizinischen Intelligenz, Berlin, S 25–35, 33f., Baader G (1984) S 82–85.

[36] Weindling (1987) S 365–366.

[37] Vgl. hierzu v. a. Leibfried S, Tennstedt F (1981) Berufsverbote und Sozialpolitik 1933. Die Auswirkungen der nationalsozialistischen Machtergreifung auf die Krankenkassenverwaltung und die Kassenärzte. Analyse, Materialien zu Angriff und Selbsthilfe, Erinnerungen (Arbeitspapiere des Forschungsschwerpunktes Reproduktionsrisiken, soziale Bewegungen und Sozialpolitik, Nr. 2), Bremen[3].

und Gesundheitspolitikern und solchen, die sich wie viele bereits im Sog des Hitlerfaschismus befanden, die Sozialhygiene lange vor 1933 hassenswert erscheinen. Öffentliche Gesundheitspflege auf der Grundlage einer Sozialhygiene, die sich als Hilfe reichende, praktisch-fördernde, präventive und soziale Gesundheitswissenschaft und -praxis etwa im Rahmen der Ehegesundheitsberatung, der Sexualhygiene, der Säuglings- und Kleinkinderfürsorge oder in Ambulatorien für die sozialen Unterschichten mit dem Wissen um eugenische Probleme, aber unter Verzicht auf eine biologistische, sozialdarwinistische Bevölkerungsideologie und damit – in den Augen der nationalsozialistischen Kritiker – letztlich „kontraselektorisch" einzusetzen bereit war, fügte sich ins Bild des verhaßten, liberalen, gleichmacherischen Staates der „Systemzeit" und der auf diesem Humus wuchernden „Volksentartung". Der 30. Januar 1933 leitete das abrupte Ende jener fürsorgerisch-sozialhygienisch orientierten Gesundheitspflege ein. Ihre schnelle Zerschlagung ging einher mit der definitiven Umwandlung öffentlicher Gesundheitspflege in eine nationalsozialistische Erb- und Rassenpflege, wobei die Sozialhygiene als Leitwissenschaft der einen durch die rücksichtslossozialdarwinistische Rassenhygiene als Leitideologie der anderen ersetzt wurde. Das Ergebnis dieses Paradigmenwechsels, die Inauguration der neuen Leitideologie öffentlicher Gesundheitspflege, kann kaum treffender gekennzeichnet werden als durch den programmatischen Beitrag des Würzburger Arztes und Hochschullehrers Ludwig Schmidt-Kehl (1891–1941) zum Thema „Hygiene, Sozialhygiene, Rassenhygiene", der Ostern 1934 in der Zeitschrift des Nationalsozialistischen Deutschen Ärzte-Bundes *Ziel und Weg* publiziert wurde.[38] Schmidt-Kehl arbeitete in Würzburg von 1937–1941 als Direktor des dortigen Instituts für Vererbungswissenschaft und Rasseforschung. Für den überzeugten Nationalsozialisten Schmidt-Kehl war 1934 das „demokratische" gleichwertende, karitative Bemühen des Arztes um jeden Menschen[39] durch die Ergebnisse der „Erbforschung" gründlich überholt. Es könne nun nicht mehr darum gehen, ganz im Sinne des „Salus aegroti suprema lex", in der öffentlichen Gesundheitspflege nur das Wohl des einzelnen im Auge zu haben. „Sozialpolitik, Hygiene und Sozialhygiene" hätten „unbewußt die natürliche Auslese weitgehend ausgeschaltet und damit die Geburtensiege der Unerwünschten ermöglicht. Die darin liegende Gefahr" habe „die aristokratisch wertende Rassenhygiene erkannt."[40] Unter ihrer Führung heiße es nun nicht mehr „Salus aegroti", sondern „Salus populi suprema lex".[41]

---

[38] Schmidt-Kehl L (1934) Hygiene, Sozialhygiene, Rassenhygiene. Ziel Weg 4:251–252.

[39] Schmidt-Kehl (1934) S 25: „Aber etwas lag dem Arzt und Hygieniker bisher fern: sich irgend einem Hilfe-heischenden Menschen zu versagen; ihre Arbeit lag ganz im Zuge der christlichen Humanität".

[40] Schmidt-Kehl (1934) Und weiter: „Sozialpolitik, Hygiene und Sozialhygiene wird und muß es immer geben in einem Kulturvolk. Es darf aber nicht weiter aus dieser Tätigkeit Gefahr für den Bestand des Volkes drohen. Unzweckmäßig wäre es, im alten Sinne weiterzuarbeiten ... Vielmehr muß alle hygienische und damit alle sozialhygienische Arbeit im neuen Deutschland ebenso wie die sozialpolitische Arbeit den Geist des Nationalsozialismus atmen; dieser Geist aber ist auf die Rasse gerichtet. Soll das deutsche Volk leben, so muß der Individualismus überwunden werden, das Wohl des einzelnen darf nicht mehr im Vordergrund stehen."

[41] Schmidt-Kehl (1934) S 252.

Der Bruch mit dem verhaßten karitativen Individualismus in der sozialhygienisch orientierten Gesundheitspflege war aber nicht nur ein ideologischer Bruch, der Bruch mit einer Leitwissenschaft; er hatte auch unmittelbare, personale Konsequenzen. So wurden, wie der Bremer Sozialhistoriker Stephan Leibfried dokumentiert, 1933/34 innerhalb weniger Monate allein 17 von 19 leitenden Berliner Stadtärzten als „nicht arisch" oder „national unzuverlässig" entlassen, und ein Blick auf die Schicht unterhalb der leitenden Stadtärzte ergibt kein wesentlich günstigeres Bild.[42] Einer beachtlichen Gruppe dieser Ärzte gelang die Emigration, meist in die USA. Unter diesen Emigranten befanden sich etwa Georg Loewenstein, Alfred Korach, der seinen Namen änderte und zwischen 1939 und 1963 Professor of Public Health an der University of Cincinnati/Ohio war, Franz Goldmann oder Georg Wolf. Andere wurden von den Nationalsozialisten ermordet, wie etwa der Kommunist und Sozialhygieniker Georg Benjamin.[43] Damit trat zum Verlust der Leitwissenschaft öffentlicher Gesundheitspflege ergänzend und verschärfend der fast vollständige Verlust personaler Kontinuität in der theoretischen und praktischen Führungsschicht dieser Leitwissenschaft. Gesetzliche Marksteine der Zerschlagung waren das „Gesetz zur Wiederherstellung des Berufsbeamtentums" (7. April 1933), auf dessen Grundlage die Lehrer der alten Sozialhygiene beseitigt und die Ortskrankenkassen von rassisch belastetem oder national unzuverlässigem Personal „gesäubert" wurden – in Berlin belief sich der „Austausch" auf nahezu 50 %; das „Gesetz zur Verhütung erbkranken Nachwuchses" (14. Juli 1933), das das Primat der negativen Sterilisationseugenik festschrieb und schließlich das bereits in den 20er Jahren entworfene „Gesetz über die Vereinheitlichung des Gesundheitswesens" (3. Juli 1934), das die bereits „gesäuberten" kommunalen Gesundheitsämter verstaatlichte, den Weisungen des Reichsinnenministeriums unterstellte und der Organisation der auch ihm als Passus inkorporierten „Erb- und Rassenpflege" eine wesentliche Voraussetzung schuf. Mit diesem Gesetz, so kann man wohl fraglos der ebenso knappen wie präzisen Zusammenfassung von Labisch u. Tennstedt (1988)[44] zustimmen, wurde zwar der „moderne", „öffentliche Gesundheitsdienst ... gegründet", gleichzeitig aber auch die „innovative Kultur gemeindenaher Gesundheitssicherung" nachhaltig „zerstört". Es ist immer wieder versucht worden, das nach dem Krieg zwar um seinen Rassenpassus entschlackte und vielfach ergänzte oder veränderte, bis heute aber in vielen Bundesländern als Grundlage des öffentlichen Gesundheits-

---

[42] Vgl. Kröner P (1983) Vor fünfzig Jahren. Die Emigration deutschsprachiger Wissenschaftler 1933–1939. Im Auftrag der Gesellschaft für Wissenschaftsgeschichte zusammengestellt. Katalog anläßlich des 21. Symposiums der Gesellschaft für Wissenschaftsgeschichte vom 12. bis 14. Mai 1983 in der Herzog August Bibliothek. Münster, S 11.

[43] Vgl. Tutzke (1970) S 337.

[44] Labisch A, Tennstedt F (1988) 50 Jahre „Gesetz über die Vereinheitlichung des Gesundheitswesens". Der öffentliche Gesundheitsdienst wurde gegründet und die innovative Kultur gemeindenaher Gesundheitssicherung zerstört, in: Gesellschaftliche Bedingungen öffentlicher Gesundheitsvorsorge. Problemsichten und Problemlösungsmuster kommunaler und staatlicher Formen der Gesundheitsvorsorge, dargestellt am Beispiel des öffentlichen Gesundheitsdienstes. Gesammelte Aufsätze einer historisch-soziologischen Untersuchung hrsg. v. d. Deutschen Zentrale für Volksgesundheitspflege (Deutsche Zentrale für Volksgesundheitspflege, Schriftenreihe, Bd 49). Frankfurt am Main, S 63–79.

dienstes noch wirksame Gesetz als „posthumes Kind der Weimarcr Zeit", das sich letztlich, und sei es nur durch seine verschiedenen Durchführungsverordnungen, bewährt habe, zu entschuldigen.[45] Wir müssen indes ernsthaft darüber nachdenken, ob nicht gerade im Hinblick auf die vor uns liegenden Aufgaben öffentlicher Gesundheitspflege hier endlich ein klarer Trennungsstrich und konzeptionelle Neuorientierungen angebracht wären.

Von der Sozialhygiene zur Public health – Deutschland nach 1945

Ich möchte an dieser Stelle nicht tiefer in den Problemkreis öffentlicher Gesundheitspflege im Ideologiebereich nationalsozialistischer Bevölkerungspolitik eindringen. Engagierte und fundierte Analysen wurden gerade in der jüngsten Vergangenheit vorgelegt. Statt dessen möchte ich mich abschließend Problemen der konzeptionellen Neuorientierung öffentlicher Gesundheitspflege in der Frühgeschichte der Bundesrepublik Deutschland zuwenden.

Nach dem Ende des 2. Weltkriegs waren die sozialen und hygienischen Lebensbedingungen in Deutschland aufs Stärkste beeinträchtigt. Wohnungsnot, eine extreme Bevölkerungsfluktuation und die katastrophale Ernährungslage stellten dabei die wesentlichsten Determinanten für den Aufgabenbereich einer helfenden, wiederherstellenden und vorbeugenden öffentlichen Gesundheitspflege dar. Dominierende Gesundheitsstörungen waren Mangelernährung, Tuberkulose, Diphtherie, Typhus, Paratyphus, Ruhr. Hinzu kam der nahezu völlige Zusammenbruch des Krankenhauswesens. Diesen Sachzwängen hatten Reorganisation und Leistungsspektrum der öffentlichen Gesundheitsfürsorge im Sinn einer Krisenintervention zunächst sehr pragmatisch zu entsprechen, wobei die rechtliche Arbeitsgrundlage der Gesundheitsämter weiterhin das zwar um seinen Rasseparagraphen entschlackte ansonsten aber kaum veränderte Gesetz über die Vereinheitlichung des Gesundheitswesens vom 3. Juli 1934 blieb.

Die Not aktivierte heute kaum mehr nachvollziehbare Kräfte und unsere Bewunderung hat den Ärztinnen und Ärzten des öffentlichen Gesundheitsdienstes jener Zeit uneingeschränkt zu gelten. Eingesetzt wurden in erster Linie die klassischen, krisenorientierten Mittel der Gesundheitsfürsorge: Behebung des größten Nahrungsmangels, Verbesserung der Wohnverhältnisse und der allgemeinen Hygiene sowie der vorbeugende Seuchenschutz in Form von Massenimpfung gegen Pocken, Ruhr, Typhus und - seit den frühen 50er Jahren – auch gegen Tuberkulose sind hier an erster Stelle zu nennen. Die klassischen, stark hygienisch orientierten Methoden bewährten sich, und man muß trotz der überaus schwierigen Situation der ersten Nachkriegsjahre von einem überaus suffizienten praktischen Neubeginn sprechen. Im konzeptionellen Bereich lagen die Dinge freilich anders,

---

[45] Zuerst wohl von Pürckhauer F (1954) Das Gesundheitsamt im Wandel der Zeit. Off Gesundheitsdienst 6:279–296, 280; zuletzt von Pfau E (1988) Zum Gesetz über die Vereinheitlichung des Gesundheitswesens – Erhebungen zur Anamnese und Überlegungen zur Prognose. Öff Gesundheitswes 50:202–205, 203.

wenn wir Zeitzeugen Glauben schenken dürfen, wie etwa der langjährigen Senatsdirigentin beim Berliner Senator für Gesundheit, Soziales und Familie, Dr. Ruth Mattheis, die 1984 in Bremen über ihre Erfahrungen im Berliner Gesundheitsdienst der ersten Nachkriegsjahre vortrug: „Alles in allem", so Frau Mattheis, müsse „selbstkritisch" berichtet werden, „daß die Chance des Neubeginns nur sehr bedingt dazu genutzt worden" sei, auch die „Arbeitsmethoden und Arbeitsziele systematisch zu überdenken und neu zu bestimmen."[46] Gleichwohl scheint eine Bedürfnislage hierfür vorhanden gewesen zu sein. So springt bei einer Durchmusterung der reichlich vorhandenen Literatur zum Thema aus den frühen 50er Jahren immer wieder die bemühte Suche nach definitorischer Nähe und inhaltlichen Anknüpfungspunkten zur frühen Weimarer Sozialhygiene ins Auge. Wilhelm Hagen (1953) an erster Stelle, Ewald Gerfeldt (1951), Werner Fischer-Defoy, Maria Daelen (1954) und andere sind hier zu nennen. Daneben bemühten sich verschiedene Arbeitsgemeinschaften oder auch die „Alfred-Grotjahn-Gesellschaft für Sozialhygiene" um eine Renaissance der alten Disziplin. Selbst der Ruf, nach Weimarer Muster wieder „Sozialhygienische Akademien" einzurichten (1952, W. Fischer-Defoy), wurde vereinzelt laut. Zu einer wirklich bedeutsamen Rückbesinnung auf die Sozialhygiene ist es indes, anders als in der DDR,[47] nicht gekommen, und als in den 60er Jahren die Sozialmedizin begann, sich als neue Leitwissenschaft öffentlicher Gesundheitspflege zu entfalten, geschah dies fast ausschließlich am angelsächsischen Vorbild der Public health.

Mögliche Gründe für den späten Beginn einer konzeptionellen Neuorientierung öffentlicher Gesundheitspflege und für den weitgehenden Verzicht, hierbei deutsche Traditionslinien stärker zu berücksichtigen, gehören in den Aufgabenbereich historischer Forschung zu den Anfängen öffentlicher Gesundheitspflege in der Bundesrepublik Deutschland. Diese steht selbst erst in den Anfängen und ich will daher nur Leitfragen formulieren: So etwa die nach den Spätfolgen der durch den Nationalsozialismus erzwungenen Emigration und nach den Gründen der nicht stattgefundenen Remigration wichtiger Träger sozialhygienischer Theorie und Praxis. Fraglich ist in diesem Zusammenhang auch, ob eine Sozialhygiene, deren Träger um 1933 vielfach als sozialistisch identifiziert oder difamiert worden waren, nach 1945 unter den politischen Bedingungen des beginnenden Kalten Krieges in Westdeutschland ein geeignetes Wiederbelebungsklima überhaupt hätte finden können. Hinterfragenswert scheint auch der Eindruck, daß in vielen theoretischen und praktischen Beiträgen zur öffentlichen Gesundheitspflege bereits am Anfang der 50er Jahre mit Blick auf Geschichte und Effizienz US-amerikanischer "public health" einer Konzentration auf den Problemkreis individueller „Leistungs- und Konkurrenzfähigkeit" oder auf den mikrosozialen Bereich der Familie der Vorzug gegeben wurde. Bedeutsam für den Bedarf eines konzeptionellen Neubeginns scheint fernerhin die sich erst im Verlauf der 50er Jahre vollziehende Verschiebung im Spektrum epidemiologisch relevanter

---

[46] Mattheis R (1984) Der öffentliche Gesundheitsdienst in der Nachkriegszeit – Reorganisation und zukunftsorientierte Ansätze. In: Akademie für öffentliches Gesundheitswesen in Düsseldorf (Hrsg) 50 Jahre Gesetz über die Vereinheitlichung des Gesundheitswesens, Bd 12. Düsseldorf, S 44–45.

[47] Vgl. etwa Winter K (1977) Lehrbuch der Sozialhygiene. Berlin, S 13–37.

Krankheitsformen von den klassischen infektiösen zu den nichtinfektiösen Massenerkrankungen und die mit ihr verbundene Um- und Neubewertung von Prophylaxe und Prävention im Bezugsrahmen einer sozialen Medizin. Fragen knüpfen sich schließlich an äußere Determinanten wie etwa die Entwicklung eines umfassenden Krankenkassenwesens, die zunehmende Zergliederung gesundheitlicher Versorgungsbereiche oder auch die Durchsetzung des sozialstaatlichen Subsidiaritätsprinzips.[48] Eine Geschichte öffentlicher Gesundheitspflege im ersten Jahrzehnt unserer Republik[49] mangelt es wahrlich nicht an historischen Problemstellungen, deren Behandlung ein weites Aufgabenfeld zukünftiger medizinhistorischer Forschung eröffnet.

---

[48] Vgl. Zenker H-J (1984) 50 Jahre Gesetz über die Vereinheitlichung des Gesundheitswesens – Anlaß, ein Jubiläum zu feiern? Eine Einführung zur Tagung. In: Akademie für öffentliches Gesundheitswesen in Düsseldorf (Hrsg) 50 Jahre Gesetz über die Vereinheitlichung des Gesundheitswesens, Bd 12, Düsseldorf, S 7–9, 8.

[49] Für die Besatzungszeit vgl. Sons HU (1983) Gesundheitspolitik während der Besatzungszeit. Das öffentliche Gesundheitswesen in Nordrhein-Westfalen 1945–1949 (Düsseldorfer Schriften zur Neueren Landesgeschichte und zur Geschichte Nordrhein-Westfalens, Bd 7), Wuppertal.

Weiterführende Literatur zum Thema „Geschichte des Gesundheitswesens"

Eckart WU (1990) Geschichte der Medizin. Springer, Berlin Heidelberg New York Tokyo
Fischer A (1965) Geschichte des deutschen Gesundheitswesens, 2 Bde, reprogr. Nachdr. Olms, Hildesheim
Frevert U (1984) Krankheit als politisches Problem 1770–1880: soziale Unterschichten in Preußen zwischen medizinischer Polizei und staatlicher Sozialversicherung. Vandenhoek & Ruprecht, Göttingen (Kritische Studien zur Geschichtswissenschaft; 62)
Hentschel V (1983) Geschichte der deutschen Sozialpolitik (1880–1980): Soziale Sicherung und kollektives Arbeitsrecht. Suhrkamp, Frankfurt am Main
Kuclien F (1985) Ärzte im Nationalsozialismus. Kiepenheuer & Witsch, Köln
Thom A, Caregorodcev GJ (1989) Medizin unterm Hakenkreuz. VEB Verlag Volk und Gesundheit, Berlin

II Ausgewählte Texte zu speziellen Anwendungsfeldern

Einleitung

Umwelt und Gesundheit ist ein multidisziplinäres Forschungsfeld von gegenwärtig rasch wachsender Bedeutung. Im Public-health-Kontext interessieren v. a. Studien zu Auswirkungen an großen Bevölkerungsgruppen. Die Arbeit von Wichmann et al. stellt ein Beispiel der analytischen Kombination versorgungsepidemiologischer Primär- und Sekundärdaten mit Routineexpositionsdaten aus einem bundesweit installierten Erfassungsnetz am Beispiel der Smogepisode 1985 dar.

In der *Arbeitsmedizin* gewinnen neben der Darstellung gut definierter akuter Einwirkungen zunehmend Analysen zu Langzeitwirkungen kleiner, kumulierter Noxen am bereits vorgeschädigten oder anderweitig zusätzlich belasteten menschlichen Organismus an Bedeutung. Hierzu liefern epidemiologische Methodenansätze in der Arbeitsmedizin wesentliche Beiträge. Die Arbeiten von Frentzel-Beyme und Ahrens et al. stellen typische Vertreter von Forschungsansätzen auf dem Gebiet der arbeitsmedizinischen Epidemiologie ("occupational epidemiology") dar, wobei auch Stärken und Schwächen der beiden Studientypen, der Kohortenstudie einerseits und der Fall-Kontroll-Studie andererseits, zutage treten. Im Zentrum des Interesses steht die stoffliche Exposition, deren gesundheitliche Auswirkungen untersucht werden. Welche Bedeutung Formen von nichtstofflicher Belastung für die Entstehung haben, zeigen Untersuchungen zum Zusammenhang zwischen Arbeitslosigkeit und Gesundheit. Der Beitrag von Schwefel gibt eine Literaturzusammenstellung zu dieser Fragestellung von Studien im deutschsprachigen Raum.

Traditionell hat der öffentliche Gesundheitsdienst eine bedeutsame Funktion für die Gesundheitssicherung in der *Gemeinde*. Unzulänglichkeiten des öffentlichen Gesundheitsdienstes für Public health in einem umfassenden Sinne haben zu zahlreichen kritischen Bestandsaufnahmen und Reformvorschlägen geführt. Müller et al. geben in ihrem Beitrag eine Übersicht über den Stand der gesundheitspolitischen und wissenschaftlichen Diskussion mit dem Ziel einer Weiterentwicklung des öffentlichen Gesundheitsdienstes. Im Beitrag von Troschke und Riemann werden auf unterster Gemeindeebene die Erwartungen an gesunde Lebensbedingungen als Mittel lokaler Gesundheitspolitik dargestellt.

Gesundheitssystemforschung definiert sich von ihrem Objekt her und befaßt sich vorrangig mit dem Systemaspekt des Gesundheitswesens. Der Beitrag von Brecht et al. stellt die Strukturierung eines Schwerpunktes zur Prognoseforschung im Gesundheitswesen dar.

Gesundheitsberichterstattung beschreibt Determinanten (Umwelt, Lebensstile, Lebenslagen) und Indikatoren der Gesundheitszustände der Bevölkerung bzw. ihrer relevanten Teilgruppen in zeitlicher und räumlicher Verteilung und die Maßnahmen zu ihrer Beeinflussung, deren Nutzung, den dadurch bewirkten Ressourcenverzehr und gesundheitlichen Ertrag. Die Bundesregierung hat eine „Forschungsgruppe Gesundheitsberichterstattung" damit beauftragt, eine Bestandsaufnahme von in Frage kommenden Datenquellen und einen Konzeptvorschlag vorzulegen. Wesentliche Ergebnisse aus dem Abschlußbericht kommen in dem gleichlautenden Text zur komprimierten Darstellung.

Unter *Evaluationsforschung* im Gesundheitswesen verstehen wir die umfassende Bewertung von Maßnahmen, Einrichtungen oder Programmen hinsichtlich ihrer gesundheitlichen, ökonomischen, sozialen (und weiteren) Folgewirkungen. *Qualitätssicherung und Technologiebewertung* sind spezielle Anwendungen der Evaluationsforschung im Gesundheitswesen. Sie werden von den Beiträgen von Selbmann und Kirchberger repräsentiert.

Selbsthilfe- und Netzwerkforschung untersucht einen wesentlichen Teil dessen, was man als „Laiensystem" dem professionellen Versorgungssystem gegenüberstellen könnte. Es geht um die Unterstützungs- und Vorsorgeleistungen von Selbsthilfegruppen und anderen „kleinen Netzen" bei der Bewältigung von Alltagsproblemen, Lebenskrisen und chronischen Krankheiten und Behinderungen. In den Beiträgen von Kaufmann und v. Ferber wird ein Einblick in das abgeschlossene DFG-Schwerpunktprogramm „Staat, intermediäre Instanzen und Selbsthilfe" sowie in den ebenfalls abgeschlossenen BMFT-Forschungsverbund „Laienpotential, Patientenaktivierung und Gesundheitsselbsthilfe" gegeben. Trojan et al. berichten Ergebnisse aus einer Studie über die Bedeutung von lokalen Netzwerken für die Gesundheitsförderung.

Unter Versorgungsepidemiologie wird die Anwendung quantitativer epidemiologischer Methoden auf die Analyse von Nutzung, Nutzern, Ereignissen, Maßnahmen und Resultaten der Versorgung verstanden. Der Beitrag von Schach und Kerek-Bodden stellt anhand so gewonnener Daten einen internationalen Vergleich ausgewählter Fragen der ambulanten primären Versorgung dar. Versorgungsforschung untersucht die gleichen Fragen unter Einbeziehung, gelegentlich auch ausschließlicher Anwendung qualitativer Methoden. Der Beitrag von Radebold gibt dafür ein Beispiel anhand der regionalen sozialgerontologischen Versorgung; die Beiträge von Cooper et al. geben für beide Formen je ein Beispiel aus der psychiatrischen Versorgungsforschung. Die nächsten beiden Beiträge (Raspe et al., Ahrens et al.) liefern weitere Beispiele für bereichsspezifische Untersuchungen der Versorgungsforschung. Der Beitrag von Badura und Lehmann gibt einen Überblick über Rahmenbedingungen und Probleme der Rehabilitation in der Bundesrepublik Deutschland.

1 Umwelt und Gesundheit

Smogepisoden in Nordrhein-Westfalen und ihre gesundheitlichen Auswirkungen *

H.-E. Wichmann, A. Brockhaus, H. W. Schlipköter

Einleitung

In England und den USA kam es in den 50er und 60er Jahren zu mehreren Smogsituationen, bei denen die damals sehr hohen Immissionskonzentrationen mit deutlichen Auswirkungen auf die Morbidität und Mortalität der betroffenen Bevölkerungsgruppen einhergingen (Csicsaky u. Wichmann 1985). Am bekanntesten ist hierbei die Smogkatastrophe vom Dezember 1952 in London, während der 2000 Menschen zusätzlich starben (Scott 1958). Mit dem Rückgang der Schadstoffbelastung gingen auch die gesundheitlichen Auswirkungen von Smogsituationen zurück, ohne jedoch ganz zu verschwinden.

Im Ruhrgebiet fanden 1962 und 1985 zwei Smogepisoden statt, die genauer hinsichtlich möglicher Beeinträchtigungen der Gesundheit analysiert wurden (Steiger u. Brockhaus 1966, 1971; Wichmann et al. 1985, 1987, 1989; Wichmann u. Spix 1990). Angeregt durch die Behauptung, in diesen Smogsituationen habe es keinerlei gesundheitliche Auswirkungen gegeben (Hompesch 1987), sollen im folgenden diese Ergebnisse dargestellt und mit den Befunden anderer Autoren verglichen werden.

Smogepisode des Dezember 1962

Im Dezember 1962 kam es für mehrere Tage zu einer Inversionswetterlage und einer damit verbundenen Zunahme der Immission (Schlipköter 1964). In dieser Zeit wurden Aerosolkonzentrationen von 2,4 mg/m^3 und SO_2-Konzentrationen von 5 mg/m^3 gemessen (Tabelle 1). Die Zahl der Todesfälle stieg in der Phase der Inversionswetterlage (3.–7. 12. 62) im Ruhrgebiet deutlich an und fiel danach wieder ab (Abb. 1). Derartige Veränderungen waren in den ländlichen Regionen nicht erkennbar (Steiger u. Brockhaus 1971).

Dennoch war die Mortalitätserhöhung nicht auf das Ruhrgebiet beschränkt (Tabelle 2). Während die tägliche Sterbezahl im Ruhrgebiet auf 119 % anwuchs, war auch in den Regierungsbezirken Köln und Düsseldorf ein etwas schwächerer, statistisch aber abgesicherter Anstieg erkennbar. Besonders auffällig war das Anwachsen auf 125 % im Stadtgebiet von Köln. Generell zeigte bei der Gegenüberstellung von 49 Landkreisen mit einer Einwohnerdichte bis zu 500 Einwohnern pro km^2 und 18 Stadtkreisen mit Einwohnerdichten über 2500 Einwohnern

---

* Erstmals veröffentlicht in: Öff. Gesundheitswesen 50/1988:314–318.

Tabelle 1. In den Smogsituationen 1962 und 1985 erreichte Immissionswerte, verglichen mit den empfohlenen MIK-Werten (maximale Immissionskonzentrationen, VDI-Richtlinie 2310)

	Dezember 1962 $[mg/m^3]$	Januar 1985 $[mg/m^3]$	MIK-Wert $[mg/m^3]$
Schwebstaub			
3-h-Wert	–	0,85[a]	0,45
24-h-Wert	2,4[b]	0,60	0,30
SO_2			
Halbstundenwert	–	2,17	1,00
24-h-Wert	5,0	0,83	0,30
NO_2			
Halbstundenwert	–	0,41	0,20
24-h-Wert	–	0,23	0,10
CO			
Halbstundenwert	–	17	50
24-h-Wert	–	8	10

[a] Gleitender 3-h-Wert.
[b] Anderes Meßverfahren.

pro km² die Gruppe der Städte eine deutliche Zunahme der Mortalität, die in den Landkreisen wesentlich schwächer ausgeprägt war.

Die Inversionswetterlage im Dezember 1962 war großräumig über Europa wirksam, so daß die Unterschiede der Mortalität zwischen Ruhrgebiet oder Großstädten und ländlichen Gebieten nicht durch unterschiedliche Wettereinflüsse erklärt werden konnten. Andere Einflußgrößen wurden nicht untersucht. In London stiegen im übrigen die Luftschadstoffkonzentrationen ebenfalls stark

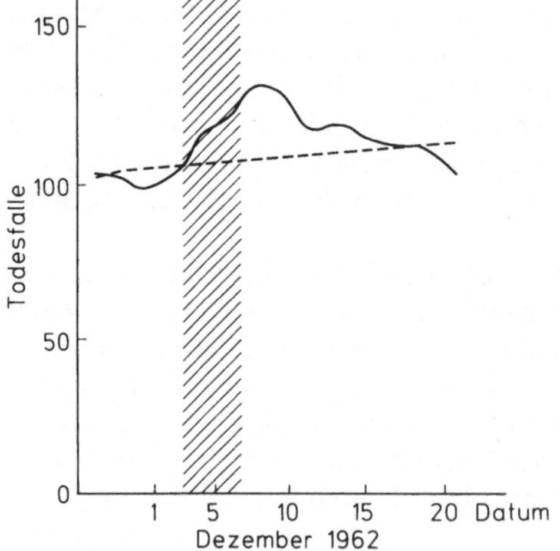

Abb. 1. Anstieg der Todesfälle im Ruhrgebiet (gleitendes 7-Tage-Mittel der täglichen Sterbeziffern) während der Smogepisode des Dezember 1962 (*schraffiert*). (Nach Steiger u. Brockhaus 1971)

Tabelle 2. Mortalitätsveränderungen in der Smogperiode des Dezember 1962. (Nach Steiger u. Brockhaus 1971)

	Mittlere Sterberate/Tag für 100 000 Einwohner		
	Smogzeitraum + Folgetage A[a]	Vergleichszeitraum B[b]	A in % von B
Kreise mit mehr als 2 500 Einwohnern/km²	3,16	2,80	113 ***
Kreise mit 500 bis 2 500 Einwohnern/km²	2,84	2,56	111 **
Kreise mit weniger als 500 Einwohnern/km²	2,85	2,66	107 *
Ruhrgebiet	3,19	2,69	119 ***
Castrop-Rauxel	3,30	1,48	223 ***
Herne	3,75	2,59	145 *
Dortmund	3,39	2,74	124 **
Essen	3,37	2,84	119 **
Regierungsbezirk Düsseldorf	3,11	2,85	109 *
Regierungsbezirk Köln	3,07	2,65	116 **
Köln	3,11	2,49	125 **
Regierungsbezirk Münster	2,62	2,50	105
Regierungsbezirk Aachen	2,88	2,76	104

[a] A: 3.–15. 12. 62.
[b] B: 1. 11.–2. 12., 16.–31. 12. 62.
[c] ohne Ruhrgebietsstädte.
* $p < 0,05$; ** $p < 0,01$; *** $p < 0,001$.

an, wobei zusätzlich 340 Personen verstarben (Scott 1963). Dies entspricht einer Sterblichkeitserhöhung von 20 %.

Smogepisode des Januar 1985

Nach 2 kleineren Smogsituationen im Januar 1979 und Januar 1982, in denen keine Veränderungen der Mortalität gefunden wurden (Wichmann et al., in Vorbereitung) kam es im Januar 1985 erneut über großen Teilen Mitteleuropas zu einer ausgeprägten Inversionswetterlage mit erhöhten Immissionskonzentrationen (Tabelle 1). Diese führte im Zeitraum vom 17. 1.–20. 1. 85 zum Smogalarm, der im westlichen Ruhrgebiet die höchste Alarmstufe erreichte. Im Auftrage des Ministers für Arbeit, Gesundheit und Soziales des Landes Nordrhein-Westfalen wurde eine umfangreiche Analyse der gesundheitlichen Auswirkungen durchgeführt (Wichmann et al. 1985). Als Ergebnis der Studie zeigte sich bei der Mortalität ein Anstieg im Belastungsgebiet (östliches und westliches Ruhrgebiet) sowie Köln und Düsseldorf auf 108 %, im Übergangsgebiet auf 107 % und im Nichtbelastungsgebiet (ländliche Teile von Nordrhein-Westfalen) auf 102 % (Tabelle 3). Im Vergleich zum Smog des Jahres 1962 war der Mortalitätsanstieg 1985 deutlich

Tabelle 3. Mortalitätsveränderungen in der Smogperiode des Januar 1985. (Nach Wichmann et al. 1985)

	Mittlere Sterberate/Tag für 100 000 Einwohner		
	Smogzeitraum + Folgetage A[a]	Vergleichs- zeitraum B[b]	A in % von B
Belastungsgebiet[c]	3,96	3,67	108**
Übergangsgebiet[d]	3,70	3,47	107
Nichtbelastungsgebiet[e, f]	3,18	3,11	102
Ruhrgebiet	3,93	3,71	106**
Duisburg, Oberhausen	3,81	3,49	109*
Bottrop, Gladbeck, Gelsenkirchen, Herne	4,21	3,99	106
Essen	4,09	4,02	102
Dortmund	3,57	3,91	91
Düsseldorf	4,19	3,86	108
Köln	3,93	3,37	117*
NRW Ost[e]	3,15	3,09	102
NRW Süd/West[f]	3,23	3,14	103

[a] A: 17. 1.–23. 1. 85.
[b] B: 3. 1.–13. 2. 85.
[c] Ruhrgebiet, Düsseldorf, Köln.
[d] Restliches NRW (ohne c, e und f).
[e] Bielefeld, Borken, Coesfeld, Gütersloh, Herford, Hochsauerlandkreis, Lippe, Münster, Minden-Lübbecke, Paderborn, Soest, Steinfurt, Warendorf.
[f] Aachen Stadt/Land, Bonn, Düren, Euskirchen, Heinsberg, Oberbergischer Kreis, Olpe, Rhein-Sieg-Kreis, Siegen.
* $p < 0,05$; ** $p < 0,01$.

niedriger; in Dortmund kam es sogar zu einem Abfall der täglichen Sterberate. Demgegenüber wurde in Düsseldorf (108%) und Köln (117%) eine ähnliche Größenordnung wie im Jahre 1962 erreicht. In den ländlichen Gebieten von Nordrhein-Westfalen wurden nur kleine Veränderungen der Gesamtmortalität beobachtet, die sich statistisch nicht absichern ließen.

Der zeitliche Verlauf der Mortalität zeigte während der Smogsituation einen Anstieg im Belastungsgebiet (Abb. 2), es gab aber einen weiteren deutlichen Mortalitätsgipfel Anfang 1985, der sich durch zwei extrem kalte Tage erklären läßt. Auch die Morbiditätsdaten stiegen z. T. in dieser kalten Phase Anfang Januar an. Sie zeichnen sich aber v. a. durch einen parallelen Anstieg in der Smogphase und einen Abfall danach aus, ein Verhalten, das außerhalb des Belastungsgebietes nicht zu finden ist. Dies gilt für Patienten mit Atemwegs- oder Herz-Kreislauf-Erkrankungen, für die umfangreiche Daten über stationäre Neuaufnahmen, Krankentransporte und ambulante Behandlungen in Krankenhäusern zur Verfügung standen. Demgegenüber war in der Smogperiode keine erhöhte Besuchsfrequenz bei niedergelassenen Internisten, Ärzten für Allgemeinmedizin und Kinderärzten festzustellen, sondern sogar ein leichter Rückgang.

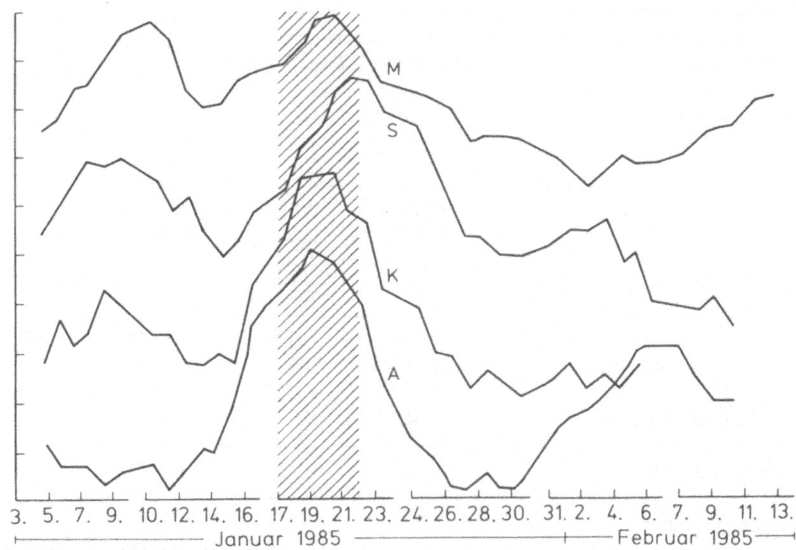

Abb. 2. Anstieg der Gesamtmortalität (*M*), der stationären Neuaufnahmen[a] (*S*), der Krankentransporte[a] (*K*), der ambulanten Behandlungen[a] (*A*) während der Smogepisode des Januar 1985 (*schraffiert*) im Belastungsgebiet (Ruhrgebiet, Köln, Düsseldorf; gleitendes 7-Tage-Mittel der täglichen Sterbeziffern bzw. Patientenzahlen). (Nach Wichmann et al. 1985)

Versuchte man, mit Hilfe der Regressionsanalyse die meteorologischen Einflüsse und die Schadstoffeinflüsse voneinander abzugrenzen (Tabelle 4), dann ergab sich ein klarer Zusammenhang zwischen den Tagesmaxima der Immissionskonzentrationen und den gesundheitlichen Veränderungen des gleichen Tages. Noch deutlichere Zusammenhänge zeigten die Tagesmittelwerte der Immissionskonzentrationen im Vergleich zu den 2 Tage später beobachteten Veränderungen von Morbidität und Mortalität. Eine Abgrenzung der Schadstoffe untereinander war wegen des nahezu parallelen Verlaufes der Schadstoffprofile nicht möglich. Die Temperatur hatte einen deutlichen Einfluß auf die Mortalität (eine erhöhte Zahl Verstorbener bei niedrigeren Temperaturen) sowie auf die Arztbesuche (vermehrte Arztbesuche bei höheren Temperaturen).

Zusammengefaßt kam es in der Smogsituation zu einem statistisch abgesicherten Anstieg der Mortalität, der Krankentransporte und der stationären Aufnahmen im Belastungsgebiet, der im Kontrollgebiet fehlte (Abb. 3). Hierbei waren nicht nur Patienten mit Atemwegserkrankungen betroffen, sondern auch Patienten mit Herz-Kreislauf-Erkrankungen, bei denen teilweise noch stärkere Einflüsse beobachtet wurden (s. Übersicht).

Die folgende Übersicht enthält die Ergebnisse weiterer Untersuchungen der Smogsituation 1985. So fanden Behrendt et al. (1985) Veränderungen der Ultrastruktur des Respirationstraktes bei Ratten, die während der Smogphase in Außenkäfigen gehalten wurden. Spirometrische Untersuchungen von Brunekreef (1985) bei Schulkindern in den Niederlanden, wo SO_2-Konzentrationen von 0,25 mg/m³ erreicht wurden, ergaben leichte, statistisch signifikante Verschlech-

---

[a] Patienten mit Atemwegs- und/oder Herz-Kreislauf-Erkrankungen.

Tabelle 4. Gesundheitliche Auswirkungen während der Smogepisode im Belastungsgebiet. Regressionsanalyse von Patienten oder Verstorbenen. Variablen für Wetter und Schadstoffkonzentrationen desselben Tages $[R^2(t)]$ oder für 2 Tage früher $[R^2(t-2)]$

Variationsursache	Partielles R^2 (t)				
	M	S	K	A	N
Temperatur[a]	0,06	0,08	0,02	0,00	0,47**
Biotropie	0,03	0,00	0,00	0,01	0,02
Temperatur und Biotropie	0,06	0,12	0,05	0,01	0,60**
Schwebstaub[+] (Tagesmaxima)	0,13*	0,09*	0,33**	0,18**	0,02
SO_2[+] (Tagesmaxima)	0,09	0,03	0,24**	0,19**	0,00
NO_2[+] (Tagesmaxima)	0,12*	0,06	0,29**	0,07	0,03
CO[+] (Tagesmaxima)	0,04	0,07	0,26**	0,06	0,05
Alle Schadstoffe	0,20	0,13	0,34*	0,35**	0,12
Gesamtmodell	0,27	0,25	0,38*	0,36*	0,72**

Variationsursache	Partielles R^2 (t-2)				
	M	S	K	A	N
Temperatur[a]	0,18**	0,05	0,10	0,01	0,51**
Biotropie	0,03	0,02	0,00	0,08	0,10
Temperatur und Biotropie	0,19*	0,15*	0,18*	0,08	0,51**
Schwebstaub[+] (Tagesmittelwert)	0,16**	0,28**	0,23**	0,35**	0,00
SO_2[+] (Tagesmittelwert)	0,17**	0,20**	0,22**	0,30**	0,00
NO_2[+] (Tagesmittelwert)	0,17**	0,26**	0,14*	0,28**	0,00
CO[+] (Tagesmittelwert)	0,19**	0,25*	0,15*	0,31**	0,00
Alle Schadstoffe	0,21*	0,31**	0,28*	0,37**	0,02
Gesamtmodell	0,40**	0,46**	0,47*	0,46**	0,53**

* $p < 0,05$; ** $p < 0,01$.

[a] Die Korrelation zwischen Temperatur und M, S, K, A ist negativ, zwischen Temperatur und N positiv.

M Gesamtmortalität, *S* stationäre Aufnahmen in Krankenhäusern AE/HKE wochentagsbereinigt, *K* Krankentransporte (AE/HKE) wochentagsbereinigt, *A* ambulante Behandlungen in Krankenhäusern (AE/HKE) wochentagsbereinigt, ohne 4.1. *N* Besuche bei niedergelassenen Ärzten, wochentagsbereinigt ohne Wochenende, *AE/HKE* Atemwegs- und/oder Herz-Kreislauf-Erkrankungen

[+] Mittelwert von 36 Meßstationen im Belastungsgebiet. Die Schadstoffe sind einzeln in der Regressionsanalyse berücksichtigt worden, zusätzlich zu Temperatur und Biotropie. Die Korrelation zwischen Luftschadstoffen und Morbidität oder Mortalität ist positiv.

terungen mehrerer Lungenfunktionsparameter. Schöttes et al. (1986) beobachteten in Gelsenkirchen eine Verdoppelung der Neuaufnahmen von Patienten mit Atemwegserkrankungen in der Smogphase, verglichen mit einem Kontrollzeitraum. Meister et al. (im Druck) konnten in einer laufenden Kohortenstudie die Smogauswirkungen bei Patienten mit chronischer Bronchitis beobachten und

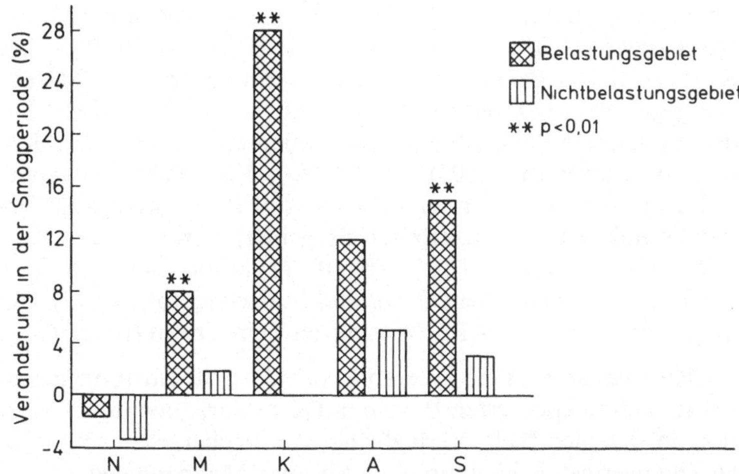

Abb. 3. Vergleich der Smogwoche (17.–23. 1. 1985) mit dem Kontrollzeitraum (3.–16. 1., 24. 1.–13. 2. 1985) im Belastungsgebiet (Ruhrgebiet, Köln, Düsseldorf) und im Kontrollgebiet (ländliche Gebiete von Nordrhein-Westfalen). *N* Besuche bei niedergelassenen Ärzten; *M, K, A, S* wie Abb. 2

stellten fest, daß im Belastungsgebiet von Nordrhein-Westfalen die Exazerbationen sich während der Smogperiode gegenüber dem Mittelwert der Wintersaison verdoppelten.

Reier et al. (1986) untersuchten die Mortalität und Morbidität in Bochum. Sie fanden einen Anstieg der Todesrate in der Smogwoche im Vergleich zur Vorperiode und eine deutliche Korrelation zwischen der täglichen Todesrate und SO_2-Konzentrationen, die auch nach Berücksichtigung der Temperatur erhalten blieb. Bei den stationären Aufnahmen in Bochum sowie beim Einsatz des Notarztwagens waren hingegen keine Auffälligkeiten in der Smogperiode erkennbar. Die Autoren schließen daraus, daß keine sicheren Beziehungen zwischen medizinischen Parametern und der Smogbelastung nachzuweisen gewesen seien. Hompesch (1987) glaubt, eine Zunahme der Sterbefälle während der Smogperioden 1962 und 1985 ausschließen zu können. Basis seiner Analyse sind die monatsweise (!) aggregierten Sterbezahlen von 30 Winterhalbjahren im Ruhrgebiet, die nach Auffassung des Autors keine wesentliche Veränderung in den Smogmonaten 1962 und 1985 gezeigt hätten, da diese innerhalb der großen Schwankungsbreite von einem Jahr zum anderen lägen.

Untersuchungen zu möglichen gesundheitlichen Auswirkungen der Smogsituation des Januar 1985 (*AE* Atemwegserkrankungen, *HKE* Herz-Kreislauf-Erkrankungen)

Wichmann et al. (1985): Erhebungen in allen Kreisen und Gemeinden von Nordrhein-Westfalen (1.1.–15.2.85): (1) Anstieg der Gesamtmortalität (24 000 Verstorbene) in der Smogwoche im Belastungsgebiet/Kontrollgebiet um +8%**/+2%. AE: +3%/−5%; HKE: +6%/+8%; (2) Anstieg der stationä-

---

** p<0,01.

ren Aufnahmen mit AE oder HKE in 186 Krankenhäusern (n = 13000 Patienten) um +15%**/+3%. AE: +7%/+0%; HKE: +19%**/+5%. (3) Anstieg der Krankentransporte von Patienten mit AE oder HKE in 7 Großstädten des Belastungsgebiets (n = 1500) um 28%**. AE: +36%**; HKE: +25%**. (4) Anstieg der ambulanten Behandlungen von Patienten mit AE oder HKE in 109 Krankenhausabteilungen (n = 5400) um +12%/+5%, (5) leichter Abfall der Besuche bei 615 niedergelassenen Ärzten im 1. Quartal 1985 (aggregierte Daten von 1250000 Arztkontakten): −1% (Belastungsgebiet) bzw. −2% (Kontrollgebiet) AE: +0%/−4%; HKE: −1%/−2%. Bei (1) bis (4) Korrelation** zwischen Patienten/Tag bzw. Verstorbenen/Tag und Luftschadstoffen des gleichen Tages oder 2 Tage vorher nach Berücksichtigung der Temperatur (r = 0,36–0,61).

Behrendt et al. (1985): Veränderung der Ultrastruktur des Respirationstrakts bei außenluftexponierten Ratten in Düsseldorf, Bochum, Gelsenkirchen: Alteration des Riechepithels, Vermehrung von Becherzellen und Clara-Zellen, partieller Zilienverlust, Schädigung von Alveolar-Makrophagen.

Brunekreef (1985): Lungenfunktionsuntersuchungen bei Kindern in den Niederlanden (IJmond-Gebiet): Verminderung** von FVC, $FEV_{0\,5}$, FEV_1, PEF, $MEF_{75\%}$, $MEF_{50\%}$, MMEF in der Smogperiode (18. 1. 85) im Vergleich zu Basismessungen im November/Dezember 84 (n = 62) sowie im Vergleich zu Kontrollmessungen im Februar 85 (n = 60 bzw. n = 41).

Schöttes et al. (1986): Stationäre Aufnahmen in der Inneren Abteilung des Marienhospitals Gelsenkirchen: Verdopplung der Neuaufnahmen von Patienten mit AE in der Smogphase 16. 1.–31. 1. 85 und danach im Vergleich zum Kontrollzeitraum (Anfang Januar und Anfang Februar 85) (n = 71). Kein entsprechender Anstieg bei Patienten mit HKE (n = 104).

Reier et al. (1986): (1) Mortalitätsdaten aus Bochum (1.–31. 1. 85, ca. n = 450 Verstorbene): Anstieg der Todesrate in der Smogperiode, im Vergleich zur Vorperiode (p < 0,05), Korrelation zwischen Todesrate/Tag + 2 Tage und SO_2-Tagesmittelwert r = 0,63*, nach Berücksichtigung der Temperatur r = 0,53. Mortalitätsrate im Januar 85 ähnlich wie im Januar 84. (2) Stationäre Aufnahmen im Krankenhaus Bergmannsheil, Bochum (13.–23. 1. 85, n = 363), kein Anstieg der stationären Aufnahmen von Patienten mit Atemwegserkrankungen bzw. Herz-Kreislauf-Erkrankungen auf Intensiv- oder Allgemeinstation erkennbar. (3) Beim Einsatz des Notarztwagens (1.–21. 1. 85, n = 215) keine Auffälligkeiten in der Smogperiode erkennbar. Zusammenfassung der Autoren: „Insgesamt sind keine sicheren Beziehungen zwischen irgendwelchen medizinischen Parametern und der Smogbelastung nachzuweisen."

Meister et al. (1987) Tagebuchprotokolle und regelmäßige ärztliche Untersuchungen bei 181 Patienten mit chronischer Bronchitis (multizentrische Kohortenstudie in Belastungsgebieten an Rhein und Ruhr, Berlin, Hamburg, Hannover, Frankfurt, München; 1.12.–31.3.85): Deutliche Zunahme der Exazerbationen Anfang Januar 85 und in der Smogphase, doppelt so hohe Exazerbations-

---

* p < 0,05, ** p < 0,01.

quote im Belastungsgebiet Nordrhein-Westfalen während der Smogperiode im Vergleich zur Wintersaison. Korrelationen** zu Tagestemperatur, SO_2- und Schwebstoffen.

Hompesch (1987): Monatliche (!) Sterbezahlen der Winterhalbjahre 1955/56 bis 1974 bzw. 1961 bis 1985 in Nordrhein-Westfalen und einzelnen Ruhrgebietsstädten: Die Schwankungsbreite (Range) der monatlichen Sterbefälle zwischen den Jahren beträgt bis zu 90% des Gesamtmittelwerts. Interpretation des Autors:

Eine Zunahme der Sterbefälle während der Smogperioden 1962 und 1985 konnte ausgeschlossen werden. Die Smogverordnung sollte umgehend als eine behördliche Maßnahme im Übermaß aufgehoben werden.

Diskussion

In den Smogsituationen des Dezember 1962 und des Januar 1985 war ein eindeutiger Anstieg der Mortalität erkennbar. Dieser war 1962 stärker als 1985, was aufgrund der erheblich höheren Immissionskonzentrationen auch erwartet werden mußte. Dies gilt insbesondere für das Ruhrgebiet. Überraschend ist allerdings, daß es in Düsseldorf und insbesondere in Köln im Januar 1985 zu ähnlich starken Veränderungen der täglichen Sterberaten wie 1962 kam. Die kleinräumige Analyse der Smogauswirkungen (Wichmann et al., in Vorbereitung) zeigt, daß hierbei stadtklimatische Faktoren und das Zusammenwirken von Kälte und Immissionsbelastung in der Smogphase 1985 von besonderer Bedeutung gewesen zu sein scheinen.

Morbiditätsuntersuchungen aus dem Jahr 1962 liegen für Nordrhein-Westfalen nicht vor, die Morbidität wurde aber in früheren Smogsituationen im Ausland untersucht (Martin u. Bradley 1960; Lawther 1958; Lawther u. Waller 1970). Die niedrigsten Konzentrationen, die zu einem signifikanten Anstieg von Krankenhausaufnahmen bzw. zur Verschlechterung von Erkrankungssymptomen führten, wurden bei Tagesmittelwerten von 0,5 mg/m³ SO_2 und gleichzeitig erhöhten Schwebstaubwerten von 0,25 mg/m³ (Britishsmoke) beschrieben. Da im Januar 1985 Tagesmittelwerte bis zu 0,83 mg/m³ SO_2 und 0,6 mg/m³ Schwebstaub erreicht wurden, waren die beobachteten Anstiege der Morbiditätsdaten auch zu erwarten.

In der umfangreichen Untersuchung (Wichmann et al. 1985) war eine vollständige Erfassung der Mortalitätsdaten möglich, und auch die Beteiligung der Krankenhäuser an der Erhebung der stationären Aufnahmen war außergewöhnlich gut. Als wichtiger Einflußfaktor war die Meteorologie zu berücksichtigen. Temperatur, Biotropie, Windgeschwindigkeit und Feuchtigkeit wurden in die Analyse einbezogen: es konnte aber nur der Einfluß niedriger Temperaturen auf die Mortalität gezeigt werden, der auch aus zahlreichen früheren Untersuchungen bekannt war. Hinweise auf den Ablauf von Epidemien, die den zeitlichen Verlauf überlagert haben könnten, gab es für diesen Zeitraum nicht. Da keine In-

---

** p < 0,01.

nenraummessungen vorlagen, konnte nicht ausgeschlossen werden, daß eine stärkere Innenraumbelastung, bedingt durch Tabakrauch, reduzierte Belüftung und stärkeres Heizen wegen der niedrigen Temperaturen, eine Rolle gespielt hat. Dies erklärt allerdings nicht den Unterschied zwischen dem Belastungsgebiet und dem Kontrollgebiet. Auch könnten psychogene Effekte der Alarmsituation die Nutzung des medizinischen Systems beeinflußt haben. Wegen der Parallelität der Kurven und der Übereinstimmung der Ergebnisse der meisten zitierten Studien (s. Übersicht) scheint ein solcher Effekt als alleinige Erklärung aber ebenfalls nicht ausreichend. Der leichte Rückgang der Besuche bei niedergelassenen Ärzten, der vor allem bei älteren Patienten zu beobachten war, hing möglicherweise mit den öffentlichen Aufrufen zusammen, im Smog das Haus nicht unnötig zu verlassen. Die Frage, ob vermehrt Hausbesuche in Anspruch genommen wurden, konnte aus den vorliegenden Untersuchungsergebnissen nicht beantwortet werden.

Unseres Erachtens muß man für die Smogsituation 1985 davon ausgehen, daß gesundheitliche Auswirkungen nachweisbar waren. Diese bewegen sich aber in einer Größenordnung, die auch durch extreme Witterungsbedingungen oder andere Einflüsse (z. B. Influenzaepidemien) erreicht werden kann. Die Tatsache, daß in 2 der zitierten Studien anderer Autoren keine Veränderungen gesehen wurden, läßt sich möglicherweise mit dem kleinen Stichprobenumfang oder dem groben Auswertungsverfahren erklären. Die offenkundige Schwäche in der Argumentation von Hompesch (1987) liegt darin, daß bei der Verwendung von Monatsmittelwerten die auf wenige Tage beschränkte Smogsterblichkeit verdeckt wird, wenn man die Sterblichkeitsziffern der zahlenmäßig weit überwiegenden smogfreien Tage eines Monats hinzuaddiert. So wäre dieses grobe Verfahren, angewandt auf die Smogkatastrophe des Dezembers 1952 in London noch nicht einmal in der Lage gewesen, die 2000 damals zusätzlich Verstorbenen innerhalb der Schwankungsbreite der monatlichen Sterbezahlen zu erkennen.

Insgesamt zeigen die Smogsituationen des Dezember 1962 und des Januar 1985, daß bei deutlicher Überschreitung der MIK-Werte (Maximale Immissionskonzentrationen) bzw. beim Überschreiten der Auslösewerte der Smogverordnung Veränderungen der Morbidität und Mortalität eingetreten sind. Ein Vergleich mit den MAK-Werten (maximale Arbeitsplatzkonzentrationen), wie er von Hompesch (1987) vorgenommen wurde, erscheint nicht gerechtfertigt. Die MAK-Werte haben die Aufgabe, gesunde Arbeitnehmer an gefährdeten Arbeitsplätzen während eines 8-Stunden-Tages zu schützen, Kranke, alte Menschen und Kinder können nur durch eine auf diese Risikogruppen zugeschnittene Smogverordnung, die bereits bei Immissionskonzentrationen deutlich unterhalb der MAK-Werte wirksam wird, vor gesundheitlichen Schäden bewahrt werden.

Literatur

Behrendt H, Seemayer NH, Rosenbauer K, Brockhaus A (1985) Tierexperimentelle Untersuchungen während der „Smog-Episode": Vorläufige morphologische und funktionelle Befunde an der Rattenlunge. Vortrag auf der Kleinkonferenz „Untersuchung der gesundheitlichen Auswirkungen der Smog-Situation im Januar 1985" am 5. 12. 1985 in Düsseldorf

Brunekreef B (1985) Lungenfunktionsuntersuchungen an Kindern. Vortrag auf der Kleinkonferenz „Untersuchung der gesundheitlichen Auswirkungen der Smog-Situation im Januar 1985" am 5.12.1985 in Düsseldorf

Csicsaky M, Wichmann H-E (1985) Grundzüge der neuen Smogverordnung Nordrhein-Westfalens. Medizinisches Institut für Umwelthygiene (Jahresbericht 1984) 17:41–78

Hompesch H (1987) Gesundheitsgefährdung und Todesfälle durch Smog. Öff Gesundheitswes 49:105–111

Lawther PJ (1958) Climate, air pollution and chronic bronchitis. Proc Roy Soc Med 51:16–18

Lawther PJ, Waller RE (1970) Air pollution and exacerbation of bronchitis. Thorax 25:525–539

Martin AE, Bradley WH (1960) Mortality, fog and atmospheric pollution. Mtl Bull Minist Health Lab Serv 19:56–75

Meister R, Dülme W, Kettrup A (1987) Einfluß von winterlicher Jahreszeit und Smog auf den Krankheitsverlauf. Prax Klin Pneumol 41:831–832

Reier W, Höltmann B, Ulmer WT (1986) Smogalarm im Ruhrgebiet: Einwirkungen auf das bronchopulmonale System (eine klinische Studie in Bochum). Inn Med 2:54–59

Schlipköter HW (1964) Vorkommen und Gefahren der Luftverunreinigungen in Großstädten von Nordrhein-Westfalen. Jahrbuch des Landesamtes für Forschung NRW. Westdeutscher Verlag, Köln, S 475–503

Schöttes C, Schweisfurth H, Thiel H (1986) Smog 1985: Morbidität von respiratorischen Erkrankungen in Gelsenkirchen. Atemw Lungenkrankh 8:341–344

Scott JA (1958) The London fog of december 1957. Med Officer 99:367–368

Scott JA (1963) The London fog of december 1962. Med Officer 109:250–252

Steiger H, Brockhaus A (1966) Untersuchungen über den Zusammenhang zwischen Luftverunreinigungen und Mortalität im Ruhrgebiet. Naturwissenschaften 19:498

Steiger H, Brockhaus A (1971) Untersuchungen zur Mortalität in Nordrhein-Westfalen während der Inversionswetterlage Dezember 1962. Staub-Reinh. Luft 31:190–192

Verein Deutscher Ingenieure (1974) Maximale Immissionswerte. VDI-Handbuch Reinhaltung der Luft 1. VDI-Richtlinie 2310

Wichmann H-E, Müller P, Allhoff P (1985) Untersuchung der gesundheitlichen Auswirkungen der Smogsituation im Januar 1985 in Nordrhein-Westfalen. Abschlußbericht im Auftrag des Ministers für Arbeit, Gesundheit und Soziales des Landes Nordrhein-Westfalen (ISBN: 3 925 840 04 4)

Wichmann H-E, Spix C, Mücke G (1987) Kleinräumige Analyse der Smogperiode des Januar 1985 unter Berücksichtigung meteorologischer Einflüsse. Untersuchung im Auftrag des Ministers für Arbeit, Gesundheit und Soziales des Landes NRW (ISBN: 3 925 840 08 7)

Wichmann H-E, Müller W, Allhoff P, Beckmann M, Bocter M, Csicsaky N, Jung MJ, Molik B, Schoeneberg G (1989) Health effects during a smog-episode in West Germany in 1985. Environmental Health Perspectives 79:89–99

Wichmann H-E, Spix C (1990) Ergänzende Betrachtungen zu den gesundheitlichen Auswirkungen der Smogepisode 1985. Öff Gesundheitswes 52:260–266

Weiterführende Literatur zum Thema „Umwelt und Gesundheit"

Eimeren W van, Faus-Kessler T, König K et al. (1987) Umwelt und Gesundheit: Statistisch-methodische Aspekte von epidemiologischen Studien über die Wirkung von Umweltfaktoren auf die menschliche Gesundheit. Springer, Berlin Heidelberg New York Tokyo
Gesellschaft zur Förderung der Lufthygiene und Silikonforschung e.V. (1989) Umwelthygiene: Jahresbericht 1988/89, Bd 21. Düsseldorf
Umweltbundesamt (1985) Deposition von Luftverunreinigungen in der Bundesrepublik Deutschland: Erste Bestandsaufnahme, Stand Mitte 1984 (Berichte 4/85). Erich Schmidt Verlag, Berlin
Umweltbundesamt (1988) UMPLIS Informations- und Planungssystem Umwelt: Umweltforschungskatalog 1988 (UFOKAT '88), 7. Ausgabe. Erich Schmidt Verlag, Berlin

2 Arbeitswelt

Fall-Kontrollstudie zu beruflichen Risikofaktoren des Larynxkarzinoms

W. Ahrens, K.-H. Jöckel, W. Patzak, G. Elsner

Einleitung

Gemessen an dem epidemiologischen Wissen über berufliche Ursachen, das man mittlerweile über Tumoren anderer Lokalisationen wie der Lunge oder Blase hat, weiß man über die beruflichen Ursachen des Kehlkopfkrebses relativ wenig. Insbesondere in der Bundesrepublik Deutschland besteht ein Defizit entsprechender Forschungsarbeiten. Internationale Studien weisen auf ein berufliches Ursachenspektrum hin, das dem des Lungenkrebses ähnelt (Simonato u. Saracci 1983; Dubrow u. Wegman 1983).

Der Kehlkopfkrebs gehört in der Bundesrepublik Deutschland zu den eher häufigen Krebsarten. Als Krebstodesursache stand dieser Tumor 1980 an 13. Stelle. Im Zeitraum 1976–1980 starben im gesamten Bundesgebiet 1004 Männer und 104 Frauen an diesem Tumor. Dies entspricht einer altersstandardisierten Mortalitätsrate von 2,45 bei Männern und 0,16 bei Frauen (pro 100 000 und Jahr) und einem Geschlechterverhältnis von 15:1 (Becker et al. 1984). Die Mortalitätsrate für Bremen entspricht mit 2,24 bei Männern und 0,17 bei Frauen dem Bundesdurchschnitt.

Im Land Bremen starben im Zeitraum 1975–1984 insgesamt 107 Männer und 8 Frauen an einem Kehlkopftumor (ICD 161); dies entspricht einem Anteil von 1,3% der in diesem Zeitraum an einer bösartigen Neubildung (ICD 140–208) verstorbenen Männer, während der Anteil bei den Frauen sogar unter 0,1% liegt.

Die Inzidenz dieses Tumors ist für die Bundesrepublik Deutschland nur durch die regionalen Krebsregister Hamburgs und des Saarlands dokumentiert. Dort betrug die Inzidenz 1973–1977 bei Frauen das 2,1fache der Mortalität, bei den Männern das 1,6fache (Hamburg) bzw. 2,7fache (Saarland). Die Krebsregister der Nachbarländer Holland, Dänemark und DDR nennen Faktoren zwischen 1,9–5,5 für Frauen und 2,2–4,3 für Männer (Comprehensive Cancer Center South 1985; Waterhouse et al. 1982).

In der Bundesrepublik Deutschland ist bei den Männern ein Anstieg der Sterblichkeit zu beobachten. Er betrug von 1952 bis 1981 ca. 76%, während die Mortalität der Frauen in diesem Zeitraum leicht abgesunken ist. Im gleichen Zeitraum hat sich die Lungenkrebsmortalität der Männer mehr als verdoppelt. Als hauptsächliche Risikofaktoren für das Larynxkarzinom sind Rauchen und Alkoholgenuß zu nennen, welche sich bei gleichzeitiger Einwirkung in ihrer Wirkung multiplizieren (Saracci 1987; Tuyns et al. 1988; Byers et al. 1988; Guenel et al. 1988)

Ziel dieser als Pilotstudie konzipierten Fall-Kontroll-Studie ist es, mehr über die beruflichen Ursachen des Larynxkarzinoms in der Bundesrepublik Deutschland zu erfahren. Dabei werden mögliche Verzerrungen durch berufsspezifische Rauch- oder Trinkgewohnheiten in der Analyse berücksichtigt.

Methode

Untersuchungskollektiv

Untersucht wurden 100 männliche Larynxkarzinompatienten, die im Jahr 1986 die HNO-Klinik des Zentralkrankenhauses (ZKH) St. Jürgen der Stadt Bremen aufsuchten. Die Patienten wurden von einem der behandelnden Ärzte persönlich interviewt. Hierfür wurde ein standardisierter Fragebogen eingesetzt, der eine detaillierte Berufsbiographie, eine Stoffliste beruflicher Expositionen sowie Fragen zu den Rauchgewohnheiten, zum Alkoholkonsum und zu demographischen Daten umfaßte. Von den 100 interviewten Fällen wurden 55 im Erhebungsjahr erstmalig diagnostiziert (inzidente Fälle), bei den übrigen Fällen reicht die Erstdiagnose bis in das Jahr 1976 zurück. Um eine mögliche Verzerrung der Fallgruppe durch Überrepräsentation von Patienten mit hoher Überlebensrate zu verringern, wurden 15 Fälle, deren Erstdiagnose zum Befragungszeitpunkt älter als 2 Jahre war, von der weiteren Analyse ausgeschlossen. Diese Subgruppe ist in Tabelle 1 getrennt ausgewiesen. Als Vergleichsgruppe wurden 100 männliche Patienten mit einer den Fällen vergleichbaren Altersverteilung mit Hilfe des standardisierten Fragebogens durch den gleichen Arzt befragt. Die überwiegende Zahl der Kontrollpatienten stammt ebenfalls aus der HNO-Klinik. Aufgrund strenger Ausschlußkriterien war es erforderlich, andere Kliniken in die Befragung mit einzubeziehen, um im Befragungszeitraum von Juli 1986 bis Januar 1987 die angestrebte Anzahl an Kontrollen zu erreichen. Um gleichzeitig den vergleichsweise großen Einzugsbereich der HNO-Klinik in der Kontrollgruppe ungefähr abzubilden, wurden die Augenklinik und die Urologische Klinik des ZKH St. Jürgen in die Befragung mit einbezogen. Neben Alter und Geschlecht war eine zu den Fällen vergleichbare Schwere der Einlieferungsdiagnose wichtigstes Selektionskriterium für die Krankenhauskontrollen. Jedoch waren alle bösartigen Neubildungen sowie Erkrankungen, die mit dem Rauchen assoziiert sind, nicht als Kontrollen zugelassen. Unter diesen Kriterien wurden mindestens 2mal pro Woche die zu befragenden Patienten aus den Neuaufnahmen der in die Erhebung einbezogenen Kliniken ausgewählt und angesprochen.

Behandlung der Befragungsdaten

Für jede Arbeitsstelle wurde die Branche, die tätigkeitsbezogene Berufsbezeichnung und – falls von der Branche abweichend – der Betriebsbereich erfaßt. Die Branchenbezeichnung wurde anhand der Systematik der Wirtschaftszweige (Statistisches Bundesamt 1979) 5stellig verschlüsselt. Die Verschlüsselung der Berufsangabe erfolgte 4stellig nach der Klassifizierung der Berufe (Statistisches Bundesamt 1975). Ausbildungs- bzw. Lehrzeiten wurden nach dem Lehrberuf kodiert. Anhand von Listenausdrucken wurden die Branchen- und Berufsangaben ohne Kenntnis des Fallstatus nachkodiert. Für die Auswertung wurden die Berufe zu 31 Gruppen mit jeweils möglichst einheitlichen Tätigkeitsmerkmalen zusammengefaßt.

Die Angaben zu den Rauchgewohnheiten umfassen den Zeitraum, eventuelle Unterbrechungszeiten von mindestens 6 Monaten Dauer, die Art der gerauchten Tabakprodukte (Zigarette, Pfeife, Zigarre) und die täglich gerauchte Anzahl. Die Anzahl Zigaretten wurde in den 4 Kategorien bis unter 5, 5–15, 16–30 und mehr als 30 Zigaretten täglich erfragt. Für Zigarettenraucher wurde die lebenslang gerauchte Menge durch Berechnung einer Variablen „Packungsjahre" abgeschätzt. Dieser kumulative Index wurde nach folgender Formel berechnet:

$$\text{Packungsjahre} = \text{tägliche Anzahl} \cdot \text{Rauchjahre} : 20$$

Die Berechnung der Rauchjahre erfolgte unter Abzug eventueller Unterbrechungszeiten bis einschließlich 1983. Die nach 1983 gerauchte Menge wurde weder bei Fällen noch bei Kontrollen berücksichtigt, da davon auszugehen ist, daß die Larynxkarzinompatienten, die ihre Diagnose bereits 1984 erfahren haben, ihre Rauchgewohnheiten daraufhin möglicherweise geändert haben. Da die tägliche Anzahl nur als kategorielle Angabe vorlag, wurde für jede Häufigkeitskategorie ein empirischer Wert in die Formel eingesetzt. Aus den Daten einer am Bremer Institut für Präventionsforschung und Sozialmedizin (BIPS) 1986 durchgeführten Fall-Kontrollstudie zum Lungenkrebs ergaben sich unabhängig vom Fallstatus für die Häufigkeitsklassen die Medianwerte 3, 10, 20, 40 Zigaretten täglich.

Jeder Proband wurde gefragt, wie häufig er Alkohol trinkt, und einer von 4 Häufigkeitskategorien zugeordnet: täglich, an weniger als 7 Tagen/Woche, weniger als einmal/Woche, selten. Weiterhin wurde das bevorzugt konsumierte Alkoholgetränk erfaßt (Bier, Sekt oder Wein, Spirituosen), wobei Mehrfachnennungen möglich waren.

Statistische Auswertungen

Die statistischen Analysen wurden mit dem Programmpaket Statistical Analysis System (SAS) durchgeführt. Für die Risikofaktoren Rauchen, Alkohol, Beruf und Arbeitsstoffe wurden Odds ratios (OR) (Rothman 1986) berechnet, die das Risiko, bei Vorliegen des entsprechenden Risikofaktors, am Larynxkarzinom zu erkranken, relativ zur Kontrollgruppe angeben. Alle OR sind um mögliche Alterseffekte bereinigt, d. h. nach Alter adjustiert. Für die Berechnung der OR in einzelnen Berufsgruppen und für Arbeitsstoffe wurde zusätzlich nach Tabakkonsum in 3 Strata (0–5 Packungsjahre oder Pfeifen-/Zigarrenraucher, 6–30 Packungsjahre, mehr als 30 Packungsjahre) und Alkoholkonsum in 3 Strata (weniger als einmal wöchentlich, 1- bis 6mal pro Woche, täglicher Alkoholkonsum) mittels Indikatorvariablen adjustiert. Die Vertrauensbereiche sind angegeben als 95%-Konfidenzintervalle (KI) für den beidseitigen Test. Die Berechnung erfolgte „ungematched" mittels logistischer Regression (SAS PROC LOGIST).

Ergebnisse

Sowohl nach der Histologie als auch nach der Lokalisation des Tumors am Kehl-
kopf entspricht die Fallgruppe der Verteilung, wie sie auch in der Literatur berichtet wird: Bis auf einen Fall mit malignem Hämangioperizytom handelte es
sich bei allen übrigen Tumoren um Plattenepithelkarzinome. Bei zwei Drittel der
eingeschlossenen Fälle war der Tumor an der Stimmritze lokalisiert (vgl. Abb. 1).

Tumoren dieser Lokalisation führen frühzeitig zu Beschwerden und haben
damit eine relativ gute Prognose. Unter den 15 von der Analyse ausgeschlossenen
Fällen, deren Überlebenszeit zum Befragungszeitpunkt 2 Jahre und mehr betrug,
wurden dementsprechend 14 glottische und 1 subglottischer Tumor beobachtet.

Die ausgeschlossenen Fälle waren durchschnittlich 6 Jahre jünger als die eingeschlossenen und die Kontrollen, deren Durchschnittsalter bei 60 Jahren lag
(Tabelle 1). Bedingt durch den Zentrumcharakter der HNO-Klinik für die Kehl-
kopftumorchirurgie kamen die Fälle aus einem weiten Einzugsbereich um Bre-

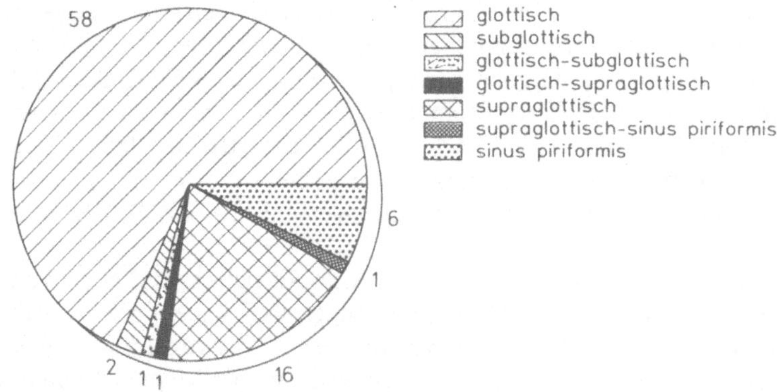

Abb. 1. Tumorlokalisation der eingeschlossenen Fälle (n = 85)

Tabelle 1. Verteilung der Patienten nach Alter und Wohnort

	Fälle		Kontrollen
	Eingeschlossen[a]	Ausgeschlossen	
n	85	15	100
Alter			
Mittelwert	60,0	54,1	60,2
Standardabweichung	9,5	12,1	10,1
Altersbereich	42–78	39–71	43–81
Letzter Wohnort			
Stadtgebiet Bremen	34%	27%	37%
< 50 km Umkreis	19%	40%	31%
> 50 km Umkreis	47%	33%	32%

[a] Vgl. Text.

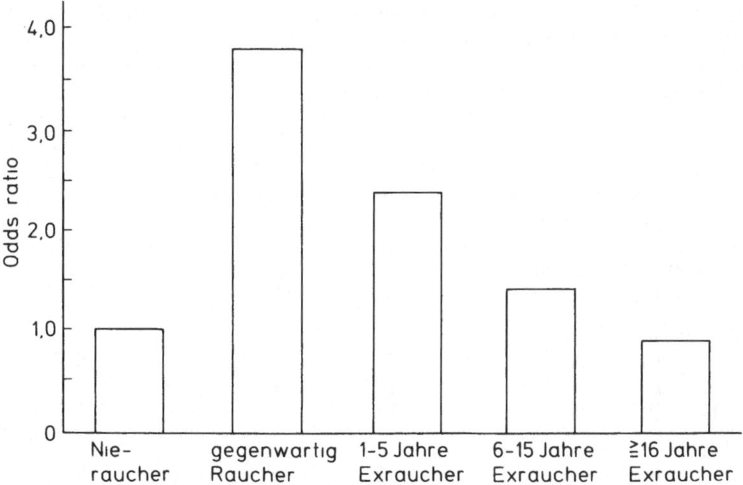

Abb. 2. Odds ratio für Exraucher nach Dauer seit Aufgabe des Rauchens

men, nahezu die Hälfte aus Orten, die weiter als 50 km von Bremen entfernt sind. Der Anteil der Kontrollen mit letztem Wohnort im Stadtgebiet ist mit dem entsprechenden Anteil der eingeschlossenen Fälle gut vergleichbar, jedoch ist der Anteil der Patienten, die mehr als 50 km von Bremen entfernt wohnen, in dieser Gruppe geringer (Tabelle 1).

Nur 3 der 85 eingeschlossenen Fälle waren Nieraucher gegenüber 9 Kontrollen; 2 Fälle und 6 Kontrollen haben nur Pfeife oder Zigarre geraucht, 60 Fälle und 67 Kontrollen nur Zigaretten und 20 Fälle und 18 Kontrollen haben sowohl Zigaretten als auch Pfeife oder Zigarre geraucht. Gegenüber Nierauchern, ausschließlich Pfeifenrauchern und Zigarettenrauchern unter 6 Packungsjahren ergeben sich für eine Rauchmenge von 6–29 Packungsjahren und für 30 und mehr Packungsjahre OR von 2,5 (KI 1,01–6,32) bzw. 3,5 (KI 1,36–9,01). Verglichen mit Nierauchern haben Exraucher ein niedrigeres Risiko als gegenwärtige Raucher. Mit zunehmender Dauer seit Aufgabe des Rauchens sinkt das Risiko beständig ab und erreicht in unserem Falle nach ca. 15 Jahren den Wert von Nierauchern (Abb. 2).

Gegenüber Personen, die angeben, weniger als einmal pro Woche Alkohol zu trinken (28 Fälle, 46 Kontrollen), ergibt sich aus unseren Daten für täglichen Alkoholkonsum ein signifikant erhöhtes OR von 3,6 (KI 1,6–8,2). Demgegenüber ergibt sich für das Alkoholtrinken an 1 bis 6 Tagen pro Woche kaum eine Risikoerhöhung (OR = 1,2, KI 0,6–2,4). Vergleicht man die Risiken in Abhängigkeit vom bevorzugt konsumierten Alkoholprodukt mit den seltenen Alkoholtrinkern (weniger als einmal pro Woche) so ergibt sich für Spirituosen ein erhöhtes OR von 2,3 (KI 1,1–5,0), nicht jedoch für Wein oder Bier (OR = 0,5, KI 0,2–2,1 respektive 1,0, KI 0,5–1,9). Unter den täglichen Alkoholkonsumenten befinden sich überproportional viele Personen, die Spirituosen als bevorzugt konsumiertes Alkoholprodukt angeben, nämlich 19 Fälle und 8 Kontrollen. Sie stellen damit ca. zwei Drittel der täglichen Alkoholkonsumenten.

Tabelle 2. Risiko für das Larynxkarzinom in Abhängigkeit von Rauchmenge (Packungsjahre) und Häufigkeit des Alkoholkonsums

Alkoholkonsum/Rauchmenge (Packungsjahre)	Anzahl		OR		95% Konfidenz-intervall
	Fälle	Kon-trollen	roh	adj. 1 [a]	
Weniger als 1mal/Woche					
0– 5 Packungsjahre [b]	5	12	1,0	1,0	–
6–29 Packungsjahre	17	23	1,8	1,8	0,5– 6,3
≥ 30 Packungsjahre	6	11	1,3	1,4	0,3– 6,1
An 1–6 Tagen/Woche					
0– 5 Packungsjahre	1	9	0,3	0,3	0,0– 2,9
6–29 Packungsjahre	15	19	1,9	2,1	0,6– 7,3
≥ 30 Packungsjahre	13	12	2,6	2,8	0,7–10,5
Täglich					
0– 5 Packungsjahre	2	2	2,4	2,6	0,3–24,6
6–29 Packungsjahre	9	6	3,6	4,2	0,9–19,6
≥ 30 Packungsjahre	17	6	6,8	7,7	1,8–32,5

[a] Altersadjustiert.
[b] Referenzkategorie inklusive Pfeifen- oder Zigarrenraucher.

Ein überproportional hoher Anteil der täglichen Alkoholtrinker ist gleichzeitig als starke Raucher (30 und mehr Packungsjahre) einzustufen. Für diese Subgruppe ergibt sich gegenüber schwachen Rauchern (0–5 Packungsjahre), die selten Alkohol trinken, ein stark erhöhtes OR von 7,7 (KI 1,8–32,5). Die Risiken für die einzelnen Kombinationen von Häufigkeit des Alkoholkonsums und Rauchmenge sind in Tabelle 2 dargestellt. Generell ergibt sich für mittlere und starke Raucher, die täglich Alkohol trinken, das 2- bis 5fache des Risikos von mittleren und starken Rauchern, die nicht täglich bzw. weniger als einmal pro Woche Alkohol zu sich nehmen.

In Tabelle 3 sind die Risiken für 17 von 31 Berufsgruppen dargestellt, in denen jeweils mehr als insgesamt 8 Personen beschäftigt waren. Für Textil- und Lederberufe ergibt sich nach Adjustierung für Alter, Rauchen und Alkoholkonsum ein signifikant erhöhtes OR von 8,19 (KI 1,49–45,03). Das adjustierte Risiko für Lager- und Transportarbeiter beträgt 1,83 (KI 0,94–3,56), für Hilfsarbeiter ohne nähere Tätigkeitsbezeichnung 1,72 (KI 0,46–6,43). Unter den Transportarbeitern konzentriert sich das Risiko v. a. auf die Seeverkehrsberufe (721–725) mit 13 Fällen zu 4 Kontrollen. Deutlich erniedrigte Risiken (unter 0,5) weisen die Berufsgruppen Bergleute (OR 0,41; KI 0,10–1,70), Zimmerer und Maurer (OR 0,47; KI 0,17–1,28), Techniker und Ingenieure (OR 0,32; KI 0,08–1,26) sowie die Friseur-, Gaststätten- und Reinigungsberufe (OR 0,41; KI 0,12–1,42) auf.

Da die Fallzahlen dieser Studie relativ klein sind, wurden sämtliche Berufe, die nach einer Literaturübersicht von Simonato u. Saracci (1983) mit einem vermuteten Larynxkarzinomrisiko behaftet sind, zu einer Gruppe „Risikoberufe" zusammengefaßt, um die Auswirkungen von Dauer und Latenz beruflicher Exposition betrachten zu können und einen Vergleich unserer Studienergebnisse mit dem bisherigen Forschungsstand zu ermöglichen (s. Tabelle 4). Hierzu zählen

Tabelle 3. Anzahl von Fällen und Kontrollen, die jemals in einer oder mehreren von 31 ausgewählten Berufsgruppen beschäftigt waren und resultierende Odds ratios

Berufsgruppe[a] (Schlüsselnummer)[d]	Fälle (n–100)		Kontrollen (n–85)		Odds ratio[b]		95% KI[c]
	n	%	n	%	adjust. 1	adjust. 2	
Landwirt (011 041-043)	21	24,7	24	24,0	1,04	1,08	0,53– 2,19
Bergmann (071-091)	3	3,5	7	7,0	0,49	0,41	0,10– 1,70
Tischler, Holzaufbereiter (181-184 501-504)	8	9,4	9	9,0	1,06	1,18	0,41– 3,42
Metallerzeuger u. -bearbeiter (191-252)	12	14,1	15	15,0	0,92	0,80	0,33– 1,92
Mechaniker, Schlosser, Klempner (261-306)	15	17,6	19	19,0	0,91	0,79	0,36– 1,74
Textil- u. Lederberufe (331-378)	8	9,4	2	2,0	5,17	8,19	1,49– 45,03
Ernährungsberufe (391-433)	7	8,2	8	8,0	1,02	0,84	0,28– 2,55
Zimmerer, Maurer (441-453)	8	9,4	14	14,0	0,64	0,47	0,17– 1,28
Straßen-, Tiefbau- u. Bauhilfsarbeiter (461-472)	14	16,5	13	13,0	1,33	1,13	0,48– 2,69
Maler, Lackierer (511-514)	3	3,5	7	7,0	0,47	0,52	0,12– 2,17
Hilfsarbeiter (531)	6	7,1	5	5,0	1,51	1,72	0,46– 6,43
Techniker, Ingenieur (601-635)	3	3,5	11	11,0	0,30	0,32	0,08– 1,26
Waren- u. Versicherungskaufmann (681-706)	17	20,0	28	28,0	0,64	0,67	0,33– 1,38
Lager- u. Transportarbeiter (711-744)	32	37,6	24	24,0	1,91	1,83	0,94– 3,56
Organisations- u. verwandte Berufe (751-784)	11	12,9	16	16,0	0,78	1,00	0,41– 2,42
Ordnungs- u. Sicherheitsberufe (791-805)	8	9,4	14	14,0	0,63	0,68	0,26– 1,78
Friseur-, Gaststätten- und Reinigungsberufe (901-937)	4	4,7	10	10,0	0,44	0,41	0,12– 1,42

[a] Alle Berufsgruppen in denen mindestens 10 Probanden für mindestens 6 Monate beschäftigt waren. Referenzkategorie sind jeweils alle Personen, die nie in der entsprechenden Berufsgruppe tätig waren.
[b] Odds ratios adjustiert nach Alter (adjust. 1) bzw. nach Alter, Rauchen (0–5, 6–19, 20 und mehr Packungsjahre) und Alkoholkonsum (weniger als 1mal/Woche, 1- bis 6mal/Woche, täglich) (adjust. 2).
[c] Konfidenzintervall für OR adjust. 2.
[d] Schlüsselnummer gemäß Klassifizierung der Berufe. Statistisches Bundesamt 1975.

die folgenden eingestuften Berufe mit der dazugehörigen Anzahl von Fällen und Kontrollen (Schlüsselnummern gemäß Statistisches Bundesamt (1975)): Dachdecker und Asphaltarbeiter 8 : 7 (452, 461, 546, 623), Asbestverarbeitung 6 : 1 (101, 112, 331, 342), Isolierer 1 : 1 (482), Schiffbau 4 : 2 (275), Hütten, Stahlerzeugung und Nickelproduktion 7 : 0 (191, 323, 625), sowie Lederarbeiter 2 : 0 (371–378). 28% der Fälle gegenüber nur 10% der Kontrollen waren jemals in einem oder mehreren dieser Berufe beschäftigt. Adjustiert für Alter, Rauchen und Alkoholkonsum ergibt dieses Verhältnis ein signifikant erhöhtes OR von 2,74 (KI 1,23–6,09). Dieser Wert liegt nur geringfügig unter dem, der sich bei aus-

Tabelle 4. Odds ratios für die Beschäftigung in Berufen mit vermutetem Larynxkarzinomrisiko (Risikoberufe) nach Dauer und erstem Jahr der Beschäftigung

Dauer (Jahre)	Beginn der Beschäftigung im Risikoberuf[a] (Anzahl von Fällen/Kontrollen)		OR (adjust. 2)[b]	95% KI
	vor 1955	nach 1955		
0,5–9	8/4	4/3	2,11	0,76–5,85
≧10	7/3	5/2	2,95	0,95–9,15
OR (adjust. 2)	2,98	2,06		
95% KI	1,10–8,10	0,60–7,08		
OR für jemals in Risikoberufen Beschäftigte			2,74	1,23–6,09

[a] Risikoberufe definiert nach Simonato u. Saracci (1983) (s. Text), Referenzgruppe sind alle Personen, die nie in einem dieser Berufe gearbeitet haben.
[b] Odds Ratio adjustiert nach Alter, Rauchen (3 Strata) und Alkohol (3 Strata).

Tabelle 5. Risiko für die Erkrankung an Kehlkopfkrebs fur ausgewahlte Arbeitsstoffe nach Angaben der Probanden (Stoffliste)

Arbeitsstoff	Anzahl exponierter[a]		OR[b] (adj. 1)	OR[c] (adj. 2)	95% KI[d]
	Fälle (n = 85)	Kontrollen (n = 100)			
Schweißen/Brennen	12	19	0,7	0,6	0,3–1,4
Hitze	30	40	0,8	0,7	0,4–1,3
Staub, allgemein	52	70	0,7	0,5	0,3–1,1
Holzstaub	6	10	0,7	0,7	0,2–2,2
Kohlenstaub	5	11	0,5	0,4	0,1–1,3
Pflanzenstaub	6	6	1,2	1,0	0,3–3,4
Rauch	18	22	0,9	0,7	0,3–1,4
Dampf	10	24	0,4	0,3	0,1–0,8
Asbest	18	18	1,2	1,1	0,5–2,4
Fasern (nicht Asbest)	5	6	1,0	1,1	0,3–4,1
Metallstaub	13	9	1,8	1,6	0,6–4,2
Chrom/Nickel	6	8	0,9	0,8	0,2–2,5
Metall nicht (Chrom oder Nickel)	7	10	0,8	0,9	0,3–2,7
Mineralöl	18	10	2,4	2,2	0,9–5,3
Benzin	15	6	3,4	2,8	1,0–7,7
Diesel	27	17	2,3	1,7	0,8–3,5
Teer/Bitumen	7	9	0,9	0,6	0,2–1,9
Farben/Lacke	25	29	1,6	1,5	0,8–3,0
Lösungsmittel	27	27	1,3	1,3	0,7–2,5

[a] Stoffliste: nach eigenen Angaben jemals exponiert.
[b] OR nur nach Alter adjustiert.
[c] OR nach Alter. Rauchen (0–5, 6–29, ≧30 Packungsjahre) und Alkoholkonsum (weniger als 1mal/Woche, 1- bis 6mal/Woche, täglich) adjustiert.
[d] Konfidenzintervall für OR (adj. 2).

schließlicher Adjustierung nach Alter ergibt (OR 2,88; KI 1,34–6,20). Die nach Adjustierung höchsten Risiken weisen unsere Daten für die Personen aus, die mindestens 10 Jahre in diesen Berufen beschäftigt waren (OR 2,95; KI 0,95–9,15) oder deren Beschäftigungsbeginn in einem dieser Berufe vor 1955 lag und damit mindestens 30 Jahre zurückreichte (OR 2,98; KI 1,10–8,10).

Tabelle 5 gibt die abgefragte Stoffliste wieder, mit der jeweiligen Anzahl der nach eigener Angabe exponierten Fälle und Kontrollen und den entsprechenden Risiken. Personen, die für eine gegebene Stoffgruppe mit „weiß nicht" geantwortet haben, wurden für den entsprechenden Stoff als nicht exponiert gewertet. Besonders auffällig ist der große Unterschied zwischen Fällen und Kontrollen, die gegenüber Mineralöl, Benzin oder Diesel exponiert waren. Die Adjustierung für Rauchen und Alkoholkonsum bewirkt zwar eine deutliche Absenkung für Benzin- und für Dieselexposition, jedoch bleibt das OR für Benzin mit 2,8 grenzwertig signifikant (KI 1,0–7,7). Für Metallstaub und Farben oder Lacke beträgt das OR nach Adjustierung 1,6 (KI 0,6–4,2) bzw. 1,5 (KI 0,8–3,0). Für die Exposition gegenüber den vermuteten Lungenkarzinogenen Asbest (OR 1,1; KI 0,5–2,4), Chrom oder Nickel (OR 0,8; KI 0,2–2,5) und Teer oder Bitumen (OR 0,6; KI 0,2–1,9) ergeben unsere Daten kein erhöhtes Risiko. Auch die Risiken für Schweißen oder Schneidbrennen (OR 0,6; KI 0,3–1,4) und für Lösungsmittel (OR 1,3; KI 0,7–2,5) sind im Sinne einer Risikoerhöhung unauffällig.

Diskussion

Die Ergebnisse dieser Studie können nur vor dem Hintergrund ihrer methodischen Limitationen diskutiert werden. Wegen der geringen für diese Studie zur Verfügung stehenden Personal- und Sachmittel wurden zur Erreichung eines kurzen Erhebungszeitraumes prävalente Fälle befragt. Inwiefern durch den Ausschluß von 15 Fällen, deren erste Diagnose im Befragungszeitraum älter als 2 Jahre war, eine mögliche Verzerrung der Fallgruppe tatsächlich ausgeschlossen ist, kann nicht mit Sicherheit entschieden werden. Jedenfalls besteht zwischen den 55 inzidenten Fällen und den 30 Fällen, die 1984 und 1985 erstmalig diagnostiziert wurden kein Unterschied hinsichtlich Alter, Tumorlokalisation oder Einzugsbereich. Auch die relativ gute Prognose für glottische Lokalisation, die die Mehrheit der Tumoren ausmacht, spricht gegen eine relevante Verzerrung der 85 in diese Analyse eingeschlossenen Fälle durch eine expositionsabhängige Überlebenszeit. Nach Becker et al. (1984) beträgt die Einjahresüberlebensrate 85%.

Response

Leider liegen weder für Kontrollen noch für die Fälle exakte Zahlen über alle im Erhebungszeitraum einbeziehbaren Probanden vor, die exakte Aussagen über die Responserate zulassen würden. Für die in der HNO-Klinik befragten Probanden (sämtliche Fälle und ca. 60% der Kontrollen) beträgt die Verweigerungsquote nach Schätzung des befragenden Arztes jedoch deutlich weniger als 10%, da die Befragung dort im Rahmen der üblichen Anamnese erfolgen konnte.

In der Augenklinik und in der Urologie haben insgesamt 8 Patienten ein Interview verweigert. Damit lag die Verweigerungsquote dort höher als in der HNO-Klinik, sie lag jedoch für die Kontrollen insgesamt unter 15%.

Daher können insbesondere die Fälle als repräsentativ für die Klinik angesehen werden, die aufgrund ihres Zentrumcharakters für Bremen und das Bremer Umland einen hohen Anteil der in dieser Region auftretenden Larynxkarzinome erfaßt.

Bekanntheit des Fallstatus

Eine wichtige Einschränkung der Studienergebnisse liegt in der Tatsache, daß der Fallstatus dem Interviewer bekannt war. Dies birgt insbesondere für „weiche" Expositionsvariablen die Gefahr, daß das Vorwissen und die Hypothesen die Fragetechnik und die Aufzeichnungen beeinflussen und zu falsch-positiven Ergebnissen führen. Als „weiche" Variablen in diesem Sinne sind insbesondere die Fragen nach stofflichen Expositionen anhand der Stoffliste und nach der Menge des Tabak- und Alkoholkonsums zu werten.

Alkohol und Rauchen

Da sich das primäre Ziel dieser Studie nicht auf die bereits bekannten Risikofaktoren richtete, wurden Rauchen und Alkoholkonsum relativ grob erfragt. Sie wurden primär erfaßt, um eine mögliche Verzerrung beruflicher Risiken durch diese Faktoren ausschließen zu können.

Das in dieser Studie beobachtete OR für täglichen Alkoholkonsum liegt mit 3,6 bzw. 3,2 (adjustiert für Rauchen) in einer Größenordnung, die sowohl in mehreren amerikanischen Fall-Kontrollstudien (Blot et al. 1980; Soskolne et al. 1984; Zagraniski et al. 1986; Byers et al. 1988; Falk et al. 1989) als auch aus einer multizentrischen Studie in Südeuropa (Tuyns et al. 1988) berichtet wurde. Im Gegensatz hierzu steht eine französische Studie mit deutlich höheren Risiken für die oberste Alkoholkategorie. Guenel et al. (1988) beobachteten für starke Trinker, deren gegenwärtiger Alkoholkonsum der Menge von 11 Gläsern Alkohol oder mehr (≥ 160 g Alkohol) täglich betrug, ein OR von 14,9 für glottische und von 35,7 für supraglottische Tumoren. In dieser französischen Studie gaben 60% der Fälle einen täglichen Alkoholkonsum von 7 und mehr Gläsern (≥ 100 g Alkohol) pro Tag an. Demgegenüber nimmt sich die Definition von Trinkern in den zitierten amerikanischen Studien, die zwischen 1 und 3 Gläsern Alkohol täglich liegt (Zagraniski 1986; Falk et al. 1989; Blot et al. 1980), sehr bescheiden aus. Möglicherweise ist der Alkoholkonsum unserer Studienpopulation eher mit amerikanischen Verhältnissen vergleichbar, so daß sich der Unterschied zur Studie von Guenel et al. (1988) also durch das unterschiedliche Spektrum in der konsumierten Alkoholmenge erklären läßt.

Unterschiede in der Befragung zwischen Fällen und Kontrollen in der französischen Studie – die Kontrollen wurden anläßlich eines nationalen Gesundheitssurveys befragt, die Fälle wurden mit einem anderen Fragebogen in einem Pariser Tumorzentrum befragt – und Unterschiede in der Genauigkeit der Erfassung des Alkoholkonsums zwischen den Studien sind in diesem Zusammenhang jedoch gleichfalls in Betracht zu ziehen. Darüber hinaus ist auch der unterschiedliche Kontext der Studie zu berücksichtigen. Da starkes Trinken in unserem Kulturkreis tabuisiert wird, können Schamgefühle gegenüber dem befragenden Arzt insbesondere bei starken Trinkern zu einem Underreporting führen, das eine Unterschätzung der entsprechenden Risiken zur Folge hätte. In diesem Zusammenhang sei auch auf die Beeinflussung des Antwortverhaltens durch die Wahl des in der Frage vorgegebenen Häufigkeitsspektrums hingewiesen, das die Selbsteinstufung der Probanden zur Mitte der vorgegebenen Häufigkeitskategorien verzerrt (Schwarz et al. 1988).

Blot et al. (1980) und Soskolne (1984) fanden einen ähnlich starken Zusammenhang zwischen Larynxtumoren und dem Zigarettenrauchen wie die vorgelegte Studie. Dabei wurde in allen 3 Studien das Rauchverhalten nur grob erfaßt. Die höheren Risiken in den übrigen Studien (Falk et al. 1989; Guenel et al. 1988; Tuyns et al. 1988) sind neben einer genaueren Erhebung der Rauchbiographie u. a. auch auf eine engere Definition von „Nichtrauchern" zurückzuführen, die in unserer Studie wegen der kleinen Fallzahl relativ breit gewählt werden mußte. Falk et al. (1989) beobachteten für gegenwärtige Raucher ein OR von 9,0, für das Rauchen von mehr als 40 Zigaretten täglich ein OR von 10,4. Die Risiken waren für supraglottische Tumoren etwas höher als für glottische, der Anteil der glottischen Tumoren am Gesamtkollektiv betrug wie in unserer Studie 61%. Tuyns et al. (1988) fanden Risiken zwischen 6,4 für das Rauchen von 8–15 Zigarettenäquivalenten und 16,0 für 26 und mehr Zigarettenäquivalenten täglich. In dieser Studie waren 50% der Tumoren supraglottisch. Die höchsten Risiken wurden von Guenel et al. (1988) beobachtet, mit Risiken zwischen 2,3 und 22,2 für glottische und zwischen 7,3 und 80,5 für supraglottische Tumoren, für das Rauchen von 10–19 bzw. 30 und mehr Zigarettenäquivalenten täglich. Zu den hohen OR in dieser Studie hat die Tatsache beigetragen, daß Exraucher ausgeschlossen waren und nur das gegenwärtige Rauchverhalten berücksichtigt wurde. Das Verhältnis von glottischen zu subglottischen Tumoren betrug 1 : 1.

In Übereinstimmung mit Falk et al. (1989); Guenel et al. (1988); Tuyns et al. (1988) beobachteten wir ein Absinken des Risikos für Exraucher.

Die neueren Studien von Guenel et al. (1988); Tuyns et al. (1988) und Byers et al. (1988) bestätigen die Ergebnisse älterer Studien, die von Saracci (1987) und Rothman et al. (1980) zusammengefaßt wurden, in bezug auf ein multiplikatives Zusammenwirken von Alkohol und Rauchen. Unsere Ergebnisse lassen aufgrund der kleinen Fallzahlen hierzu nur vorsichtige Aussagen zu. Der in Tabelle 2 dargestellte Zusammenhang zwischen Alkohol und Rauchen deutet ebenfalls darauf hin, daß das gemeinsame Risiko höher ist als die Summe aus beiden Einzelrisiken, es erreicht jedoch für die oberste Gruppe keinen multiplikativen Effekt, vgl. Falk et al. (1989).

Berufe

Berufs- und Branchenangaben sind in unserer Studie als die verläßlichsten Expositionsvariablen anzusehen, da diese Angaben am geringsten durch einen Recall- oder Interviewerbias beeinflußt werden. Die Angaben wurden nachträglich ohne Kenntnis des Fall- oder Kontrollstatus verschlüsselt. Auffälligstes Ergebnis ist die starke und signifikante Risikoerhöhung für Leder- und Textilarbeiter. Von den 8 Fällen in dieser Gruppe waren 3 als Spinner oder Weber beschäftigt, 2 waren Takler und je einer Lederhersteller und Schuhmacher. Die Kontrollen waren als Strickmaschineneinrichter bzw. als Schneider beschäftigt. DeCoufle (1979) beobachtete ein signifikant erhöhtes Larynxkarzinomrisiko bei Beschäftigten in der lederherstellenden und -verarbeitenden Industrie wobei die Rauchgewohnheiten berücksichtigt wurden. Das Risiko war insbesondere für längere Beschäftigung erhöht. Eine Reihe von Studien belegen ein erhöhtes Risiko für andere Krebsformen insbesondere Nasenkrebs, Blasenkrebs und Leukämien in dieser Industrie (Alderson 1980). In einer kanadischen Fall-Kontrollstudie gaben 5 Fälle und keine der Kontrollen eine Exposition gegenüber Textilstaub an (p < 0,05) (Burch et al. 1981). Olsen u. Sabroe (1984) konnten nach Probandenangaben eine (nicht signifikante) 40- bis 50%ige Risikoerhöhung für Woll- und Baumwollstaubexpositionen beobachten, nicht für Exposition gegenüber Textilfasern. Auch in einer britischen Studie ergaben die Probandenangaben keine signifikanten Unterschiede bezüglich Textilstaubexposition (Elwood et al. 1984). In einer amerikanischen Fall-Kontrollstudie lag das adjustierte OR für Beschäftigte in der Textilindustrie unter 1 (Zagranski et al. 1986). Flanders et al. (1984) beobachteten dagegen in einer nach Alter Geschlecht Wohnort Rauch- und Trinkverhalten gematchten Fall-Kontrollstudie ein signifikant erhöhtes Risiko in der Textilindustrie. Insbesondere für Tätigkeiten, die als Filtern, Trennen und Trocknen von Textilfasern beschrieben wurden, stieg das OR für Beschäftigungszeiten von 5 und mehr Jahren, die mindestens 5 Jahre zurücklagen, auf 5,6 (KI 1,4–29,1) an.

Die Identifikation möglicher karzinogener Noxen, die diese Befunde erklären können, war in den vorliegenden Studien nicht möglich. In der Lederindustrie ist der Kontakt mit einer Vielzahl von karzinogenen Färbemitteln, Nitrosaminen, Arsenverbindungen, Chromaten und Säuren in Betracht zu ziehen (IARC-Monographie 1981). In der Textilindustrie werden Maschinenöl, Acrylnitril und Chrom-, Nickel- und Kadmiumverbindungen diskutiert (Flanders et al. 1984). In unserem Fall müssen aufgrund der heterogenen Zusammensetzung dieser Berufsgruppe auch Asbestexpositionen (Asbesttextilien, Takler im Schiffbau) zu den möglichen Noxen gerechnet werden.

Zahlreiche Studien weisen auf erhöhte Risiken bei Kraftfahrern und Transportarbeitern hin. Dubrow u. Wegmann (1983) analysierten zahlreiche Querschnittstudien und beobachteten konsistent erhöhte Risiken für LKW- und Traktorfahrer, für Kraftfahrzeugführer und für Seeleute. Rauch- und Trinkgewohnheiten blieben hierbei unberücksichtigt. Eine nicht signifikante Risikoerhöhung für Kraftfahrer wurde von Wynder et al. (1976) und Flanders et al. (1984) berichtet. Olsen u. Sabroe (1984) fanden in einer dänischen Studie nach Adjustierung für Alkohol und Rauchen signifikante Risiken sowohl für die Berufsgruppe Kraftfahrer (exclusive Busfahrer), als auch für die Branchen Straßengütertransport, Taxi und sonstiger Transport. Im Bereich Hafendienste fand sich die ausgeprägteste Risikoerhöhung (OR 4,8 KI 1,3–17,7). In der Branche Transport, Nachrichtenübermittlung und Reinigungsdienste beobachteten Morris Brown et al. (1988) unter Berücksichtigung von Alkohol und Rauchen eine signifikante Risikoerhöhung, die am ausgeprägtesten den Bereich der Seeschiffahrt betraf. Für die Berufsgruppe Kraftfahrer ergab sich ein OR von 1,6 (KI 0,8–3,47). Unsere Daten stützen die Ergebnisse dieser Studien. Obwohl die Risikoerhöhung für Lager- und Transportarbeiter nach Adjustierung nicht signifikant ist, haben insbesondere in der Subgruppe Wasserverkehrsberufe überproportional viele Fälle gearbeitet. Über die Ursachen dieser Risikoerhöhung sind nur Spekulationen möglich, da eine Vielzahl von Stoffen umgeschlagen oder transportiert werden. Ein residuelles Confounding durch andere Rauch- und Trinkgewohnheiten ist eher unwahrscheinlich, da das OR nach Adjustierung für Rauchen und Alkohol nur geringfügig absinkt (s. Tabelle 3).

Für Bauarbeiter allgemein werden signifikant erhöhte Risiken berichtet (Dubrow u. Wegmann 1983; Morris Brown et al. 1988). Nicht signifikant waren die erhöhten Risiken für einzelne Subgruppen wie Zimmerleute (Morris Brown et al. 1988), Rohrinstallateure (Burch et al. 1981; Morris Brown et al. 1988) oder Maurer (Zagraniski et al. 1986). Eine schwedische Kohortenstudie ergab jedoch ein signifikantes Risiko unter Klempnern (Englund 1979). Für keine dieser Berufsgruppen ergeben unsere Daten einen Hinweis auf Risikoerhöhungen.

Wolf (1978) berichtet von einer überzufälligen Häufung von Holzberufen insbesondere Tischlern in seinem Untersuchungskollektiv. Auch Zagraniski et al. (1986) und Morris Brown et al. (1988) fanden eine auffällige Häufung von Holzverarbeitern, letztere insbesondere bei Möbelherstellern. Die Fallzahlen reichten jedoch in den letztgenannten Studien für eine statistische Absicherung der Befunde nicht aus. Eine schwedische Kohortenstudie ergab für Möbelhersteller ein deutlich erhöhtes Nasenkrebsrisiko, das Larynxkarzinomrisiko war mit 5 beobachteten zu 7 erwarteten Todesfällen jedoch erniedrigt (Gerhardsson 1985). Ohne positive Befunde in bezug auf Holzberufe oder Holzstoffexposition bleibt auch die Arbeit von Elwood et al. (1984).

Abgesehen von der Nickelproduktion werden Risikoerhöhungen auch für Metallarbeiter allgemein berichtet (Wolf 1978; Zagraniski et al. 1986; Burch et al. 1981; Morris Brown et al. 1988). Letztere beobachteten auch für Betriebsschlosser ("maintenance") erhöhte Risiken – ein Befund, der durch Zagraniski et al. (1986) für Maschinisten bestätigt wird. Für den Bereich Maschinenbau fand eine finnische Kohortenstudie (Tola et al. 1988) jedoch keine Auffälligkeiten. Wir fanden in keiner dieser Gruppen eine Häufung von Larynxkarzinompatienten im Vergleich zu den Kontrollen.

Weitere Berufsgruppen, für die signifikant erhöhte Larynxkarzinomrisiken beobachtet wurden, sind Beschäftigte in Bars oder Restaurants (Dubrow u. Wegmann 1983; Rothman et al. 1980; Olsen u. Sabroe 1984), Brauereiarbeiter (Jensen 1979), Baumwoll- und Getreidefarmer (Flanders et al. 1984), ungelernte Arbeiter (Olsen u. Sabroe 1984; Flanders et al. 1984) und Chemiearbeiter mit Exposition gegenüber Naphthalin, Säuren, Uran oder Senfgas (Wolf 1978; Soskolne et al. 1984; Dupree et al. 1987; Easton et al. 1988). Mit Ausnahme des nicht signifikant erhöhten Risikos für ungelernte Arbeiter fanden sich in unserer Studie keine vergleichbaren Hinweise; für Chemiearbeiter und Brauereiarbeiter sind auch die Fallzahlen zu klein um Aussagen zuzulassen. Bei Gaststättenpersonal ist v. a. an ein Confounding durch abweichende Rauch- und Trinkgewohnheiten als Erklärung für die in anderen Studien beobachteten Risikoerhöhungen zu denken.

In bezug auf Landwirte deckt sich der negative Befund unserer Studie mit 3 weiteren Fall-Kontroll-Studien (Wolf 1978; Elwood et al. 1984; Morris Brown et al. 1988) und einer Kohortenstudie (Wiklund u. Holm 1986), in bezug auf Gästeberufe deckt er sich mit 2 der Studien in denen Rauch- und Trinkgewohnheiten berücksichtigt werden konnten (Elwood et al. 1984; Morris Brown et al. 1988).

Stoffe

Staubexpositionen sind ganz allgemein mit einem Larynxkarzinomrisiko in Verbindung gebracht worden (Neuberger u. Kundi 1985; Olsen u. Sabroe 1984). Die Angaben der Befragten weisen jedoch weder für die Kategorie „Staub allgemein" noch für einzelne Unterklassen wie Pflanzen- oder Holzstaub auf ein Risiko hin. In den anderen Studien waren Holzstaubexpositionen überhaupt nicht (Soskolne et al. 1984; Elwood et al. 1984) oder nur mäßig aber nicht signifikant (Morris Brown et al. 1988; Wynder et al. 1976) mit dem Larynxkarzinom assoziiert.

Die Literatur bezüglich Metallstaubexpositionen, insbesondere gegenüber Chrom- und Nickelverbindungen ist widersprüchlich. Kohortenstudien belegen ein Risiko, das mit dem Abbau, der Verarbeitung und der Raffinierung von sulfidischen Nickelerzen verbunden ist (Shannon et al. 1984; Pedersen et al. 1973). Dies scheint jedoch nicht für silikathaltige Erze zuzutreffen (Goldberg et al. 1987). Probandenangaben bezüglich Nickel- und Chromstaubexpositionen waren in je drei Fallkontrollstudien unauffällig (Burch et al. 1981; Hinds et al. 1979; Soskolne et al. 1984; Olsen u. Sabroe 1984; Zagraniski et al. 1986). Jedoch fanden Olsen u. Sabroe (1984) bei Zusammenfassung unterschiedlicher Nickelexpositionen durch Metallegierungen, Batteriechemikalien und nickelhaltige Zusätze bei der Kunststoffherstellung eine signifikante Risikoerhöhung. Eine neuere Kohortenstudie weist auch auf ein erhöhtes Risiko durch Kobaltverbindungen hin (Mur et al. 1987). Die Angaben der in unserer Studie Befragten ergeben zwar eine mäßige Risikoerhöhung für Metallstaubexpositionen insgesamt, jedoch ergibt sich weder für Schweißen noch für Chrom- oder Nickelkontakt eine Auffälligkeit. Die geringe Häufigkeit dieser Nennung bedingt allerdings ein großes Konfidenzintervall, das ein mögliches Risiko durch Chrom- oder Nickelstaub nicht ausschließt.

Asbestexposition war in unserer Studie mit einem minimal erhöhten, statistisch signifikanten Risiko verbunden. Ob Asbestexposition ein ursächlicher Faktor für den Larynxkrebs ist, ist umstritten. In jüngster Zeit sind 2 Übersichtsartikel dieser Frage nachgegangen (Chan u. Gee 1988; Edelman 1989). Bei beträchtlicher Überlappung der analysierten Studien kommen beide Arbeiten zu dem Ergebnis, daß die positiven Befunde einiger Studien v. a. auf fehlende bzw. unzureichende Adjustierung der Rauch- und Trinkgewohnheiten zurückzuführen sind. Jedoch liegen die Schätzungen aller Fall-Kontrollstudien, die diese beiden Confounder berücksichtigt haben mit einer Ausnahme oberhalb von 1. Bei dieser Ausnahme handelt es sich um eine kleine Studie, die auch sog. Dysplasien in die Fallgruppe einschloß (Newhouse et al. 1980). Die „Kontrollgruppe" war wesentlich jünger als die Fallgruppe (55% unter 45 Jahre vs. 4%), so daß die von Edelman (1989) selbst durchgeführte Risikoberechnung, die weder die Altersunterschiede noch Rauchen und Alkoholkonsum berücksichtigte, äußerst problematisch ist. Nur in einer der übrigen Studien führt die Adjustierung für Alkohol zu einer Absenkung der OR von 1,75 auf 1,33 (Hinds et al. 1979), in drei der Studien ergibt sich nach Adjustierung ein OR zwischen 1,46 und 2,3 mit jeweils unteren Konfidenzschranken über 0,9 (Burch et al. 1981; Olsen u. Sabroe 1984; Morris Brown et al. 1988). Kohortenstudien haben gegenüber Fall-Kontrollstudien nicht nur den Nachteil, daß Rauch- und Trinkgewohnheiten in der Regel unberücksichtigt bleiben müssen, sondern auch für relativ seltene Erkrankungen wie das Larynxkarzinom nur niedrige Erwartungswerte haben. Daher hatte nur eine der berücksichtigten Kohortenstudien eine ausreichende statistische Macht, um eine zweifache Erhöhung eines möglichen Larynxkarzinomrisikos zu entdecken (Edelmann 1989). Darüber hinaus stellt sich angesichts der hohen Diskrepanz zwischen Mortalität und Inzidenz der Erkrankung die Frage nach konkurrierenden Todesursachen, da die meisten Kohortenstudien nur die Mortalität als Endpunkt untersuchen. Dies kann eine Unterschätzung möglicher Risiken zur Folge haben. Der Vorteil von Kohortenstudien liegt in der relativ guten Expositionsabschätzung auf der Grundlage von Betriebsmessungen. Hier liegt auch der Nachteil, den unsere Studie mit den meisten Fall-Kontrollstudien gemeinsam hat, denn die Expositionseinstufung beruht in der Regel nur auf Probandenangaben, die nicht durch externe Kriterien validiert werden können und daher anfällig für einen Recallbias sind. Risikoschätzungen von Fall-Kontrollstudien, deren Probanden ohne Kenntnis des Fallstatus durch einen "industrial hygienist" eingestuft wurden (Burch et al. 1981; Morris Brown et al. 1988), sind für eine solche Verzerrung vermutlich weniger anfällig. In diesem Zusammenhang scheint erwähnenswert, daß unsere Fälle häufiger in Berufen mit möglicher Asbesteinwirkung wie Dachdecker oder Schiffbauer tätig waren als die Kontrollen.

Im Hinblick auf stoffliche Expositionen auffälligstes Ergebnis dieser Studie ist die Assoziation mit Diesel-, Benzin- und Mineralölexposition, die in bezug auf Benzin grenzwertig signifikant ist. Auch Wynder et al. (1976) und Olsen u. Sabroe (1984) berichten von einer Risikoerhöhung für Öl- und Schmiermittelexpositionen – ein Befund, der von Morris Brown et al. (1988) nicht bestätigt werden konnte. Letztere berichten jedoch für Diesel- und Benzindämpfe oder -abgase von einer signifikanten Assoziation (OR 1,5, KI 1,0–2,3). Mineralölexposition wurde häufig von metallverarbeitenden Berufen angegeben. Dies könnte als Hinweis auf Ölaerosolexposition an Drehbänken gewertet werden, jedoch ist bisher nur ein negativer Befund bezüglich der Assoziation zwischen Kühlschmiermittelexposition und Larynxkarzinom festgestellt worden (Zagraniski et al. 1986).

Farben- und Lackexposition wurde in zwei Studien als signifikanter Risikofaktor identifiziert (Morris Brown et al. 1988; Englund 1979), Exposition gegenüber (potentiell chromathaltigen) Korrosionsschutzmitteln war in einer zweiten Studie grenzwertig signifikant (Olsen u. Sabroe 1984), Lösemittelexposition jedoch nicht. Unter Spritzlackierern in der Automobilindustrie wurde keine Risikoerhöhung beobachtet (Chiazze et al. 1980). Unsere Risikoschätzungen weisen für Maler und Lackierer in die entgegengesetzte Richtung wie für Farben- und Lackexposition, jedoch ist die Anzahl in dieser Berufsgruppe sehr klein.

Ein Risikopotential durch Exposition gegenüber Säuredämpfen, das erstmals in einer Kohorte von Metalloberflächenbearbeitern als möglicher Risikofaktor identifiziert wurde (Ahlborg et al. 1981), konnte durch Soskolne et al. (1984), Steenland et al. (1988), Olsen u. Sabroe (1984), nicht jedoch durch Morris Brown et al. (1988) bestätigt werden. In zwei neueren Kohortenstudien mit erhöhten Larynxkarzinomrisiken wurden neben Uranprodukten (Dupree et al. 1987) und Mineral- und Nickelexpositionen in der Seifenproduktion (Forastiere et al. 1987) ebenfalls relevante Schwefelsäureexpositionen als mögliche Ursachen diskutiert. Expositionen gegenüber Säuren wurden in unserer Studie nicht erfragt. Diese Exposition verdient in zukünftigen Studien zu beruflichen Einflußfaktoren verstärkte Aufmerksamkeit.

Die vorliegenden Daten sind im Hinblick auf ihre Aussagefähigkeit begrenzt. Die Berechnung einer Vielzahl von OR erhöht die Gefahr von zufällig signifikanten Ergebnissen. Daher ist bei ihrer Interpretation auf Plausibilität und Konsistenz mit den Ergebnissen anderer Studien zu achten. Unsere Daten bestätigen sowohl in bezug auf die bekannten Risikofaktoren Rauchen und Alkohol als auch im Hinblick auf ein Risiko für Berufe, die a priori auf der Grundlage der vorliegenden epidemiologischen Evidenz eingestuft wurden (Tabelle 4), den bisherigen Kenntnisstand.

Das Beispiel der Exposition gegenüber Säuredämpfen macht deutlich, daß in dieser Studie auch die Möglichkeit gegeben ist, relevante Expositionen zu übersehen. Insbesondere der Entdeckung relativ seltener Einwirkungen sind hier enge Grenzen gesetzt. Die geringen Fallzahlen in einzelnen Expositionsgruppen haben weite Konfidenzintervalle zur Folge und setzen tiefergehenden Analysen der Daten deutliche Grenzen. Die Bestätigung eines möglichen Risikopotentials durch Schmieröl- und/oder Treibstoffexpositionen und die Identifikationen karzinogener Agenzien, die für eine mögliche Risikoerhöhung von Textilarbeitern bzw. von Seeleuten verantwortlich gemacht werden können, bleibt daher zukünftigen Studien vorbehalten. Bezüglich eines möglichen Risikos durch Asbestexposition lassen unsere Daten keine eindeutige Aussage zu und spiegeln damit den augenblicklichen Forschungsstand wider. Gerade an dieser Frage wird die Begrenztheit eines Fall-Kontroll-Ansatzes deutlich, bei dem eine Expositionseinstufung ausschließlich auf der Grundlage einer Expositionscheckliste im Fragebogen erfolgt. Zur Vermeidung eines möglichen Recallbias, sollten in zukünftigen Studien vermehrt Anstrengungen unternommen werden, um potentiell karzinogene Stoffe besser identifizieren zu können. Dabei ist sowohl die Hinzuziehung von "industrial hygienists", die erhobene Berufsbiographien einzelfallbezogen bezüglich ihrer stofflichen Exposition einstufen, in Betracht zu ziehen (Gerin et al. 1985), als auch eine Verbesserung der Datenerhebung, die mit Hilfe von Zusatzbögen gezielter auf fragliche Expositionen eingeht (Bolm-Audorff et al. 1988).

Literatur

Ahlborg G jr, Hogstedt C, Sundell L, Aman CG (1981) Laryngeal cancer and pickling house vapors. Scand J Work Environ Health 7:241–251

Alderson M (1980) Cancer mortality in male hairdressers. J Epidemiol Comm Health 34:182–185

Becker N, Frenzel-Beyme R, Wagner G (1984) Krebsatlas der Bundesrepublik Deutschland. Springer, Berlin Heidelberg New York Tokyo

Blot WJ, Morris LE, Stroube R, Tagnon I, Fraumeni JF (1980) Lung and laryngeal cancers in relation to shipyard employment in Coastal Virginia. J Natl Cancer Inst 65(3):571–575

Bolm-Audorff U, Ahrens W, Jöckel K-H et al. (1988) Experience with supplementary questionnaires in a lung cancer case-referent study. Beitrag zum EC Workshop Methodology of assessment of occupational exposure to carcinogens in the context of epidemiological detection of cancer risk. Institut National de la Santé et de la Recherche Médicale, Paris

Burch JD, Howe GR, Miller AB, Semenciw R (1981) Tobacco, alcohol, asbestos, and nickel in the etiology of cancer of the larynx: A case-control study. J Natl Cancer Inst 67/6:1219–1224

Byers T, Swanson M, Marshall J, Vena J, Graham S (1988) Diet, alcohol, and tobacco in the etiology of laryngeal cancer SER 21st Annual Meeting. Toronto

Chan CK, Gee BL (1988) Asbestos exposure and laryngeal cancer: an analysis of the epidemiologic evidence. J Occup Med 30/1:23–27

Chiazze L jr, Ference LD, Wolf PH (1980) Mortality among automobile assembly workers. J Occup Med 22/8:520–526

Comprehensive Cancer Center South (IKZ), SOOZ-Cancer Registration (1985) Cancer incidence in the Netherlands, South eastern part 1978–1982, IKZ, Eindhoven

DeCoufle P (1979) Cancer risks associated with employment in the leather and leather products industry. Arch Environ Health 1:33–37

Dubrow R, Wegmann DH (1983) Setting priorities for occupational cancer research and control: synthesis of results of occupational disease surveillance studies. J Natl Cancer Inst 71/6:1123–1142

Dupree EA, Cragle DL, McLain RW, Crawford-Brown DJ, Teta MJ (1987) Mortality among workers at a uranium processing facility, the Linde Air Products Company ceramic plant, 1943–1949. Scand J Work Environ Health 13:100–107

Easton DF, Peto J, Doll R (1988) Cancers of the respiratory tract in mustard gas workers. Br J Ind Med 45:652–659

Edelman DA (1989) Laryngeal cancer and occupational exposure to asbestos. Int Arch Occup Environ Health 61:223–227

Elwood JM, Pearson JCG, Skippen DH, Jackson SM (1984) Alcohol, smoking, social and occupational factors in the aetiology of cancer of the oral cavity, pharynx and larynx. Int J Cancer 349:603–612

Englund A (1979) Cancer incidence among painters and some allied trades. In: Vainio H, Sorsa M, Hemminki K (eds) Occupational cancer and carcinogenesis. Proceedings of a conference. Hemisphere, Helsinki, pp 347–353

Falk RT, Williams Pickle L, Morris Brown L, Mason TJ, Buffler PA, Fraumeni JF Jr (1989) The effect of smoking and alcohol consumption on laryngeal cancer risk in coastal Texas. Cancer Res 49(14):4024–4029

Flanders WD, Cann CI, Rothman KJ, Fried MP (1984) Work-related risk factors for laryngeal cancer. Am J Epidemiol 119/1:23–32

Forastiere F, Valesini S, Salimei E, Magliola E, Perucci CA (1987) Respiratory cancer among soap production workers. Scand J Work Environ Health 13:258–260

Gerhardsson MR, Norell SE, Kiviranta HJ, Ahlbom A (1985) Respiratory cancers in furniture workers. Br J Ind Med 42:403–405

Gerin M, Siemiatycki J, Kemper H, Begin DB (1985) Obtaining occupational exposure histories in epidemiologic case-control studies. J Occup Med 27/6:420–427

Goldberg M, Goldberg P, Leclerc A et al. (1987) Epidemiology of respiratory cancers related to nickel mining and refining in New Caledonia (1978–1984). Int J Cancer 40:300–304

Guénel P, Chastang JF, Luce D, Leclerc A, Brugère J (1988) A study of the interaction of alcohol drinking and tobacco smoking among French cases of laryngeal cancer. J Epidemiol Comm Health 42:350–354

Hinds MW, Thomas DB, O'Reilly HP (1979) Asbestos, dental x-rays, tobacco, and alcohol in the epidemiology of laryngeal cancer. Cancer 44:1114–1120

International Agency for Research on Cancer (1981) Wood, leather and associated industries. IARC (Monographs vol 25), Lyon

Jensen OM (1979) Cancer morbidity and causes of death among Danish brewery workers. Int J Cancer 23:454–463

Maher KV, DeFonso LR (1987) Respiratory cancer among chloromethyl ether workers. J Natl Cancer Inst 78:839–843

Morris Brown L, Mason TJ, Williams Pickle L et al. (1988) Occupational risk factors for laryngeal cancer in the Texas gulf coast. Cancer Res 48:1960–1964

Mur JM, Moulin JJ, Charruyer-Seinerra MP, Lafitte J (1987) A cohort mortality study among cobalt and sodium workers in an electrochemical plant. Am J Ind Med 11:75–81

Neuberger M, Kundi M (1985) Gesundheitsrisiken beruflicher Staubbelastung. Staub Reinhalt Luft 45/3:131–135

Newhouse ML, Gregory MM, Shannon H (1980) Etiology of carcinoma of the larynx. In: Wagner JC (ed) Biological effects of mineral fibres, vol 2. International Agency for Research on Cancer, Lyon, pp 687·695

Olsen J, Sabroe S (1984) Occupational causes of laryngeal cancer. J Epidemiol Comm Health 38:117–121

Pedersen E, Hogetveit AC, Andersen A (1973) Cancer of respiratory organs among workers at a nickel refinery in Norway. Int J Cancer 12:32–41

Rothman KJ (1986) Modern epidemiology. Little Brown, Boston Toronto

Rothman KJ, Cann CI, Flanders D, Fried MP (1980) Epidemiology of laryngeal cancer. Epidemiol Rev 2:195–209

Saracci R (1987) The interactions of tobacco smoking and other agents in cancer etiology. Epidemiol Rev 9:175–193

Schwarz N, Bless H, Bohner G, Harlacher U, Kellenbenz M (1988) Response scales as a frame of reference: The impact of frequency range on diagnostic judgements. Zentrum für Umfragen, Methoden und Analysen e. V. (ZUMA) – Arbeitsbericht No 6, Mannheim

Shannon HS, Julian JA, Muir DCF, Roberts RS, Cecutti AC (1984) A mortality study of Falconbridge workers. In: Sundermann FW (ed) Nickel in the human environment IARC, Lyon, pp 117–124

Simonato L, Saracci R (1983) Occupational carcinogens. In: Encyclopedia of occupational safety and health. International Labour Office (ILO), Geneva

Soskolne CL, Zeighami EA, Hanis NM et al. (1984) Laryngeal cancer and occupational exposure to sulfuric acid. Am J Epidemiol 120/3:358–369

Statistisches Bundesamt (1975) Klassifizierung der Berufe. Statistisches Bundesamt, Wiesbaden

Statistisches Bundesamt (1979) Systematik der Wirtschaftszweige. Statistisches Bundesamt, Wiesbaden

Steenland K, Schnorr T, Beaumont J, Halperin W, Bloom T (1988) Incidence of laryngeal cancer and exposure to acid mists. Br J Ind Med 45:766–776

Tola S, Kalliomäki PL, Pukkala E, Asp S, Korkala ML (1988) Incidence of cancer among welders, platers, machinists, and pipe fitters in shipyards and machine shops. Br J Ind Med 45:209–218

Tuyns AJ, Estève J, Raymond L et al. (1988) Cancer of the larynx/hypopharynx, tobacco and alcohol: IARC international case-control study in Turin and Varese (Italy) Zaragoza and Navarra (Spain), Geneva (Switzerland) and Calvados (France) Int J Cancer 41:483–491

Waterhouse J, Calum M, Shammugaratnam K, Powell J, Peackam D, Whelan S, Davis W (1982) Cancer incidence in five continents vol IV IARC, Lyon

Wiklund K, Holm LE (1986) Trends in cancer risks among Swedish agricultural workers. J Natl Cancer Inst 77/3:657–664

Wolf O (1978) Berufliche und außerberufliche Faktoren beim Kehlkopfkrebs. Z Ges Hyg Grenz 24:174–177

Wynder EL, Covey LS, Mabuchi K, Mushinski M (1976) Environmental factors in cancer of the larynx. A second look. Cancer 38:1591–1601

Zagranski RT, Kelsey JL, Walter SD (1986) Occupational risk factors for laryngeal carcinoma: Connecticut, 1975–1980. Am J Epidemiol 124/1:67–76

Lung Cancer Mortality of Workers Employed
in Chromate Pigment Factories:
A Multicentric European Epidemiological Study *

R. Frentzel-Beyme

Introduction

This survey of mortality among men employed for more than 6 months in any one of five factories producing chromate pigments was started in 1976. The objective was to determine whether or not the mortality of exposed workers differed from that of comparable groups without this occupational exposure. The main aim of the study was to investigate the mortality from cancer of the respiratory tract, but all other causes of death were also evaluated. An increased risk of cancer of the upper respiratory tract from exposure to zinc and lead chromate pigments has been described in earlier clinical reports and in epidemiological studies done by Langard and Norseth in Norway (1975), Gaffey in the USA (Equitable Environmental Health Inc. 1976), and Davies in Great Britain (1978, 1979). This study was designed to investigate the health effects of exposure to lead chromate pigment, but the prevalent „mixed" production made it impossible to distinguish between persons exposed solely to lead chromate pigment and those subjected in mixed zinc and lead exposures.

Materials and Methods

As in other cohort studies in occupational epidemiology, the source of the study population was the personnel listings of the factories since the beginning of production. Table 1 depicts the size of the workforce over different time periods. Table 2 shows that, although production often commenced early in this century and mostly before 1930, complete personnel records were only available from 1945 or later. Concerning information about exposure, a rough classifcation was obtained by a joint evaluation of exposure categories by factory representatives. Table 3 gives the typical job titles and activities and the exposure class to which they were assigned.

Originally in this study, seven factories in four countries participated in the data collection phase. Only five factories in two countries have so far provided sufficient basic material for a differential mortality analysis including a complete follow-up, with documents on the causes of death. A standardized procedure was used to carry out the investigation in all factories. This included common data

---

* First published in *Journal of Cancer Research and Clinical Oncology* (1983) 105:183–188.

Table 1. Numbers in factory cohorts and the completeness of follow-up

Factory	Nationality of staff	Numbers		LTFU[a]		Other nationalities		LTFU	
		Before 1960[a]	After 1960	Before 1960	After 1960	Before 1960	After 1960	Before 1960	After 1960
1	German	271	136	28	18	13	76	5	41
2	German	116	111	26	21	0	153	0	116
3	German	88	55	0	0	1	22	0	2
4	Dutch	71	96	12	8	1	11	0	0
5	Dutch	230	222	10	13	54	194	4	27

[a] Lost to follow-up.
[b] Approximate time of major changes in technology and industrial hygiene, and the addition of foreign workers to staff on a large scale.

Table 2. Significant dates as to the chromate pigment production and characteristics of cohorts by factory

First recorded manufacture	Factory number				
	1	2	3	4	5
Lead chromate pigment	1921	1911	1925	1913	1916
Zinc chromate pigment	1921	1913	1925	1951	1916
Termination of zinc chromate	1970	1974	1969	1971	1970
Personal records as of	1945	1949	1945	1965	1944
Records contain type of job since	1945	1952	1945	1965	1944
Size of work force[a]	69	151	26	48	125
Average year of entry of the cohort members	1958	1963	1958	1960	1960
Average age at entry of a cohort member (years)	31,7	31,7	32,4	30,8	31,5
Average observation period (years)	14,6	8	15,8	13,8	14,0

[a] The number needed to operate the production process.

Table 3. Rating of exposure by type of job

Kind of work	Category of exposure
Drying of the filtered pigment paste	High exposure
Milling of the filtered pigment paste	
Wet processes	Medium exposure
Precipitation of the pigment	
Filtering	
Maintenance, craftsmen, cleaning[a]	
Storage, dispatch	Low or trivial exposure
Laboratory personnel	
Supervising	

[a] Decision based on the idea that workers of certain crafts (coopers, saddlers, fitters) or in repair jobs may be particularly exposed, if only for a short time.

Table 4. Sources of information as to the cause of death

	Factory number				
	1	2	3	4	5
Total deaths	89	23	27	23	104
Causes of deaths unknown	7	6	–	–	9
Causes of deaths known	82	17	27	23	95
Information from death certificate	57	3	18	–	60
Information from other sources	11	2	8	23	28
Information from death certificate and other sources	14	12	1	–	7

sheets and tracing procedures for all persons who left employment. The mortality study was carried out according to the standard method as a historical prospective cohort study. The follow-up was achieved by taking the last known residence and discovering all subsequent residences with the help of the official registration scheme in every community (Einwohnermeldeamt or Standesamt), which is well organized and usually permits complete tracing of every national and also of registered foreigners. The follow-up began in 1976 and was completed in the same year.

The causes of death were obtained from the death certificates wherever possible. When the need for data protection prohibited access to the death certificate, other sources of information had to be used (such as general practitioners and, in some cases, dependents, friends, and colleagues). Table 4 shows the proportion of cases based on other sources of information than the death certificate. It is assumed, however, that any diagnosis such as lung cancer would also have appeared on the death certificate as the underlying cause, even if the diagnosis was obtained through inquiries from other sources. This would be confirmed by validation of death certificates, which will be evaluated in more detail in a later publication.

The basic principle of the investigation is a comparison of deaths observed in the chromate-pigment exposed cohort with the number of deaths expected for these cohorts were they under a presumptive age-specific mortality prevailing for the total regional male population. Problems inherent in this assumption are discussed at large in the pertinent literature (Enterline 1976). Data from the administrative districts (Kreise) in the Federal Republic of Germany and from provinces of the Netherlands were used to establish the data base for the calculation of expected numbers. This approach was utilized in order to provide the best use of specific mortality within the general catchment area of employees of a factory. The comparison between observed and expected number of deaths was done within the same program. Evaluation of the total expected deaths is based on mortality rates for the period 1970–1975 on 5-year age increments and for lung cancer the rates for the years 1952–1970 could be obtained to calculate the specific numbers expected. This was necessary in order to correct to otherwise exaggerated expected values resulting from increased rates of the late period, which becomes evident from the trend observed in the last three decades (Fig. 1). The statistical test for the difference of both values is based on the Poisson distribu-

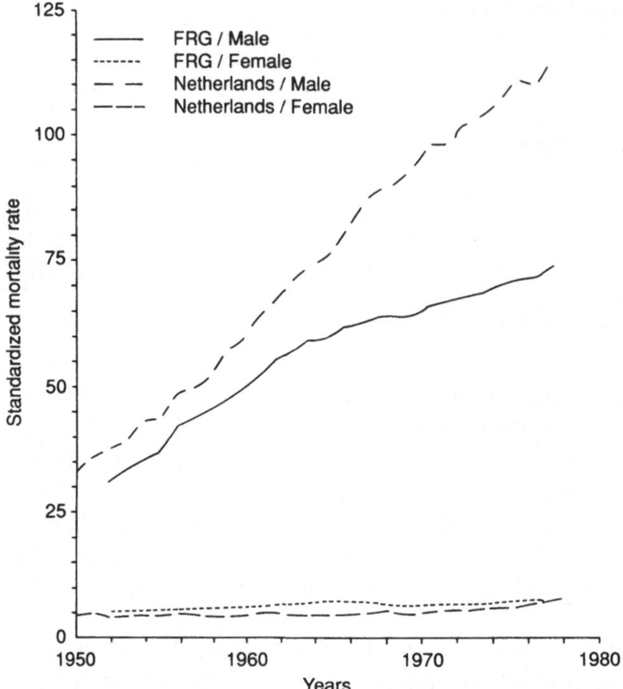

Fig. 1. Trends of lung cancer mortality in the Federal Republic of Germany and in the Netherlands (Becker et al. 1979)

tion, but p values were only given if the observed number was greater than expected. Persons lost to follow-up were included in the evaluation by counting those age-time-specific person years which they contributed to the observed period.

Further analysis concerns the comparison of observed and expected deaths of the „relevant cohort". This is defined by three criteria to achieve the best possible use of this data: minimum observation period of 10 years elapsed since employment started, which means beginning of exposure before 1965; complete records for the entire staff are available, which means omission of all persons from former times, who entered the cohort on their survivor status; exclusion of all foreign nationals because of difficulties in tracing and problems in assessing their mortality.

Results

The overall mortality showed no gross deviation from expectation. As compared with numerous other studies in the field of occupational health, however, no „healthy worker effect" was discernible, i.e., these cohorts did not show the favourable difference from general population mortality frequently observed in selected working populations. Summary results selected from more than a dozen

Table 5. Epidemiologic cohort studies in the chemical industry (BASF Ludwigshafen): selected results of observed and expected deaths in different cohorts

Study (reference)	Number of employees	Completeness of follow-up (percentage)	Person years	Deaths			
				Total		Cancer	
				Observed	Expected	Observed	Expected
Auramine (Kirsch et al. 1978)	191	G[a] 97/F[b] 44	3.423	45	40.46	10	8.07
Vinylchloride (Frentzel-Beyme et al. 1978a)	1,618	G 96/F 60	19.767	79	90.81	18	16.04
Vinylidene chloride (Thiess et al. 1977)	629	G 97/F 24	6.821	39	57.10	8	7.67
Styrene (Frentzel-Beyme 1978b)	1,960	G 97/F 58	20.138	73	96.46	12	19.80
Di-2-ethylhexylphthalate (Thiess et al. 1978)	221	G 100/F 55	2.538	8	16.97	1	3.33
o-Phthalodinitrile (Frentzel-Beyme et al. 1979)	221	G 97/F 23	2.034	13	11.92	4	2.29

[a] German   [b] Foreign

Table 6. Total number of persons, deaths, and lung-cancer deaths by factory and comparison cohorts in the five factories

	Factory					Vinyl chloride[a]	Styrene[b]
	1	2	3	4	5		
Number of persons	496	380	166	179	691	1,618	1,960
Total deaths	89	23	27	23	104	82	74
Cancer death	26	6	7	6	20	18	11
Lung cancer	14	4	3[c]	4	12	5	3
Lung cancer							
Percent age of all deaths	14.6	17.4	11.6	17.4	11.5	6	4
Average age of death	59.5	59.5	59.5	65.5	60.5		
Average year of death	1968	1970	1966	1969	1965		

[a] From Equitable Environmental Health Inc. (1976).
[b] From Frentzel-Beyme et al. (1978a).
[c] One death not definitely confirmed as primary lung-cancer.

                                                      R. Frentzel-Beyme

Table 7. Observed and expected number of deaths (from all causes and from lung cancer)

Factory	„Relevant"[b] cohort	Person years	Total deaths		Lung-cancer deaths	
			Observed	Expected[a]	Observed	Expected[a]
1	319	5.117	39	44.357	5	2.196
2	141	1.245	9	9.963	2	0.789
3	97	1.809	17	15.134	3[c]	0.778
4	174	2.388	16	15.360	2	1.270
5	248	4.517	36	36.944	7	4.310

[a] Expected deaths are calculated on the basis of the mortality rate of the *Kreis* (district or province).

[b] „Relevant:" a minimum observation period of 10 years has elapsed since employment; foreign nationals are excluded; complete records are available for the entire staff.

[c] $p < 0.05$.

similarly conducted studies in the chemical industry at Ludwigshafen (FRG), are presented for comparison in Table 5, where, in general, more deaths were expected than observed. Table 6 reveals the lung-cancer deaths in relation to total deaths for the five factories together with average ages at death and years of death and compares the results of two other cohort studies in the chemical industry. It is obvious that there is a considerably higher proportion of lung-cancer deaths among the pigment workers than among the employees in other branches of the chemical industry. Table 7 shows the total mortality observed in the five relevant cohorts, which closely corresponds to the total mortality expected (i.e., no healthy-worker effect) and also shows lung-cancer mortality above expectation. The observed lung cancer deaths are in excess of those expected in every instance, although owing to the small group sizes involved, only in one cohort was the increased incidence of lung cancer statistically significant.

Comparisons were made for cohorts classified according to the duration of employment and to the approximate exposure intensity and according to exposure group. The lung-cancer mortality pattern by duration of exposure (Table 8) indicates that the risk associated with the exposure does not show a clear dose-response effect with time. Risk ratios, the number of observed cases related to the calculated figure of expected deaths, range from about 1.6 up to about 8.5 if subcohorts are classified by type of job or exposure category, respectively (as shown in Table 3).

Other features of the analyses are: (a) In a control group exposed to ceramic dye and lead only, which consisted of 98 persons, no death from lung cancer was observed. (b) In only one factory was a case of death from lung cancer observed in the „low exposure" category compared with 0.9 expected (Table 9). (c) In the „high exposure" category there were consistently more deaths from lung cancer than would have been expected if the workers, as part of the total population, were subjected to a „normal" risk. This finding of a small to marked increase in the number of lung-cancer deaths is also found in the medium category to a certain extent. (d) Other tumor forms, such as stomach cancer, prostate cancer, cancer of the intestines or liver cancer, were observed rarely or not at all.

Table 8. Observed and expected[a] deaths from lung cancer by duration of exposure in the relevant cohorts

Factory	Duration of exposure								
	0–4 Years			5–10 Years			>10 Years		
	Observed	Expected	Persons	Observed	Expected	Persons	Observed	Expected	Persons
1	2	0.632	114	1	0.690	49	2	0.595	100
2	1	0.832	33	0	0.238	16	1	0.144	28
3	2[b]	0.287	51	1[c]	0.124	19	0	0.229	25
4	0	0.176	41	1	0.469	47	3	1.968	55
5	4	2.014	150	0	0.884	35	2	0.915	51

[a] Expected deaths are calculated on the basis of the mortality of the *Kreis* (district or province).
[b] $p < 0.01$.
[c] Not definitely confirmed as primary lung-cancer.
The „relevant cohort" considered in this table is that identified by selection criteria as being in unambiguously in the categories of exposure listed, i.e , (a) 1–4 years of (b) 5–10 years or (c) more than 10 years. It is not identical with the cohort considered in Tables 7 and 9.

A greater observed number of lung cancer deaths than that expected is found in the maintenance subcohort of the two factories, which specified rather large maintenance groups. This is shown in Table 9, where three subgroups with different levels of exposure are compared with the maintenance groups of those factories which gave the necessary information to allow a separate evaluation. The reason for the high risk of this particular group is as yet unknown but a case-control study is designed to investigate this issue in greater detail. As shown in Table 2, a mixed exposure to zinc and lead chromate prevailed in all factories for long periods of time. Furthermore, other possible exposure data and especially smoking histories were not available for the entire cohorts and only for a fraction of the cancer cases.

Table 9. Observed and expected[a] deaths from lung cancer by type of exposure in the relevant cohorts

Factory	Low			Medium			High			Uncertain (maintenance)		
	Observed	Expected	Persons	Observed	Expected	Persons	Observed	Expected	Persons	Observed	Expected	Persons
1	0	0.226	60	1	0 234	38	0	0.437	61	4[c]	1.241	171
2	0	0.036	7	2[b]	0.232	36	0	0.383	89			
3	0	0.032	15	0	0.227	31	2[c]	0.267	46			
4	0	0.467	65	2	0.761	38	2	1.267	39	0	0.421	35
5	1	0.864	94	0	0.988	41	3	1 766	70	3[b]	0.623	40

[a] Expected deaths are calculated on the basis of the mortality of the *Kreis* (district or province).
[b] $p < 0.05$.
[c] $p < 0.01$.
The „relevant cohort" considered in this table is that identified by selection criteria as being unambiguously in the categories of exposure listed, i.e., (a) low, (b) medium, (c) high, or (d) maintenance. It is not identical with the cohorts considered in Tables 7 and 8.

Discussion

The results of a trend within the five factories for an increased incidence of lung cancer are in keeping with previous reports. Owing to small numbers in the cohorts, only in one factory is the elevation above expectation statistically significant. The overall mortality was not different from that expected but there was no healthy worker effect. The summary results from more than a dozen similarly conducted studies in the chemical industry, as presented in Table 5, show that although such an effect is often observed, it is less likely to occur with increasing age of cohort members. The well appreciated fact that the healthy worker effect tends to disappear with increasing age of cohort members has been demonstrated in the Auramin study (Kirsch et al. 1978) and this probably applies also to this study. According to information from the factories involved, it was often difficult – in times of high employment – to attract and engage workers with excellent health as compared with other industries. Table 2 reveals that the average age at entry of the workers in all factories was about 32, whereas observed deaths had an average age of 60 (Table 6). Although a direct comparison of standardized mortality ratios is not permissible, the inspection of cohort size, numbers of observed and expected deaths from all causes and from cancer indicates the usual range of the differences. The relative proportions of cancer causes from the total number of deaths give a crude impression of the impact of cancer in a cohort, although this type of comparison is liable to bias because of differences in the age of compared cohorts. When either total cancer deaths or lung-cancer deaths are expressed as a percentage of total deaths, the figures of the five cohorts of this study are at least twice those obtained for other sizeable cohorts studied by similar methods, which are shown in Table 6 (vinyl chloride and styrene cohorts). The table reveals quite consistent rates of at least 50% lung-cancer deaths among cancer deaths and always more than 10% lung cancer among total deaths as compared with figures below 10% in the two chemical industry cohorts.

A far more reliable and valid comparison can be obtained with a comparable or even matched reference group, so every effort was made to establish „comparison" cohorts. Only one factory, however, could provide a suitable control group, which was characterized by its occupation in the ceramic dye department with exposure to lead, but never to chromate. Therefore, the expected deaths from all and from specific causes had to be calculated according to standard procedures on the basis of the population mortality by making use of person years of observation. Contrary to many studies using the national mortality rates as a reference, it was the principle of this study to consider the population of the small regional administrative unit available. This decision had been made on account of the well known fact that the mortality rate of individual regions of a country may show considerable deviations from the national average. This has been shown in particular as far as cancer and lung cancer are concerned. The differences by region have been demonstrated in the Cancer Atlas of the FRG and from the Netherlands (Frentzel-Beyme et al. 1980; Hayes et al. 1980). The results of this study suggesting carcinogenic effects associated with chromate pigment manufacture confirm findings from other studies, e.g., a British study (Davies 1978, 1979) carried out at roughly the same time in three factories. This study revealed an approximately two fold excess of lung cancer in workers exposed to zinc chromate pigment, but no excess mortality in a cohort exposed only to lead chromate pigment (Davies 1979). Results of this study have to be seen with particular caution concerning lead chromates in view of the impossibility of excluding mixed exposure. In the present study, it was impossible to confirm this apparent difference since a cohort without mixed exposure to lead and zinc chromate pigments could not be established with certainty.

Conclusion

It can be stated that, compared with the British study, the European survey suffered from serious disadvantages in that it has to deal, within the study, with different nationalities, different conditions of data acquisition, differences in the completeness of follow-up and basic medical information, and some obvious differences between the five factories, which made a pooled evaluation impracticable. It is virtually impossible, therefore, to say more concerning the causes of slightly increased risk than „that working in a chromate pigment factory either as production or maintenance staff is associated with an increased incidence of lung cancer and thus with a higher probability of dying from lung cancer compared to the general population." Nevertheless the fact that there is no increase in lung-cancer cases in the low exposure subgroup may indicate that a substantial reduction in the exposure to chromate pigment, which has been achieved in several factories during the last decade, is hoped to further reduce the risk of tumors of the respiratory system in persons employed in chromate pigment production.

Acknowledgements. For technical assistance in all matters of the follow-up I am indebted to the responsible persons at the factories. Without their invaluable cooperation this study would not have been possible. My thanks are also due to the physicians and heads of Departments of Public Health in those areas where investigations into the causes of deaths were necessary. The unlimited efforts of Mrs. R. Link, Mrs. U. Remle and Mr. R. Kattermann during the evaluations of the data are gratefully acknowledged.

Dedication. This contribution is dedicated to Prof. G. Wagner on his 65th birthday.

References

Becker N, Stenger HJ (1979) Monitor. Ein Programm-System zur Auswertung von Mortalitätsdaten. DKFZ, Heidelberg (Technical report, no 1/epidemiology)
Davies JM (1978) Lung cancer mortality of workers making chrome pigments. Lancet 1:384
Davies JM (1979) Lung cancer mortality of workers in chromate pigment manufacture: an epidemiological survey 62. J Oil Col Chem Assoc 5 157
Enterline PE (1976) Pitfalls in epidemiology research. J Occup Med 18:150–156

Equitable Environmental Health Inc (1976) An epidemiology study of lead chromate plants. Final report prepared for the Dry Color Manufacturer's Association. Equitable Environmental Health Inc, Berkley

Frentzel-Beyme R, Schmitz T, Thiess AM (1978a) Mortalitätsstudie bei VC/PVC-Arbeitern der BASF Aktiengesellschaft, Ludwigshafen am Rhein. Arbeitsmed Sozialmed Praeventivmed 10:218–228

Frentzel-Beyme R, Thiess AM, Wieland R (1978b) Survey of mortality among employees engaged in the manufacture of styrene und polystyrene at the BASF Ludwigshafen works. Scand J Work Environ Health [Suppl]4:231–239

Frentzel-Beyme R, Thiess AM, Wieland R (1979) Mortalitätssurvey bei Mitarbeitern aus der Ortho-Phthalodinitril-Produktion. Zentralbl Arbeitsmed 29:121–127

Frentzel-Beyme R, Leutner R, Wagner G, Wiebelt H (1980) Krebsatlas der Bundesrepublik Deutschland – Cancer atlas of the Federal Republic of Germany. Springer, Berlin Heidelberg New York

Hayes RB, de Guchteneire PFA, van der Knaap GA (1980) Geographic distribution of cancer mortality in the Netherlands. Studiecentrum Sociale Oncologie, Rotterdam

Kirsch P, Fleig I, Frentzel-Beyme R, Gebhardt C, Steinborn R, Thiess AM, Koch W, Seibert W, Wellenreuther G, Zeller H (1978) Auramin, toxikologische und arbeitsmedizinische Untersuchungen. Arbeitsmed Sozialmed Praeventivmed [Sonderh 2]13

Langård S, Norseth T (1975) A cohort study of bronchial carcinomas in workers producing chromate pigments. Br J Ind Hyg 32:62–65

Thiess AM, Frentzel-Beyme R, Penning E (1977) Mortality study of vinylidene chloride exposed persons in the BASF AG. 5th International Medichem Congress, Sept 5–11, San Francisco

Thiess AM, Frentzel-Beyme R, Wieland R (1978) Mortalitätsstudie bei Mitarbeitern mit Exposition gegenüber Di-2-athylhexylphthalat (DOP). Proceedings 18th Jahrestagung der Deutschen Gesellschaft für Arbeitsmedizin e.V, Frankfurt-Höchst, 24–27 May 1978

Unemployment, Health and Health Services in German-Speaking Countries *

D. Schwefel

For more than a decade, partly as a consequence of the economic crises since the early 1970s, social science research has increasingly tried to examine the links between unemployment and health. In the beginning, it was mainly research from the United States – such as the econometrical or epidemiological approaches of Brenner (in John et al. 1983, 27–80) and Kasl (in John et al. 1983, 338–370) – that helped to get research on this subject started in Europe. Gradually, however, various European regions developed their own approaches and research preferences in this area. Particularly in Britain, where the pressures of unemployment were felt strongly earlier on, research on unemployment had a head-start and, thanks to the widespread knowledge of English, it quickly received attention in many parts of Europe. In addition, there were several studies from Scandinavian and Iberian countries. Characteristic of this research is the very broad spectrum of approaches and methods it comprises. A host of academic disciplines participated in this collective endeavour: not only epidemiologists, sociologists but also economists, psychologists, psychiatrists, physicians and historians. Most studies examine the effects of unemployment on health, i.e. on physical, mental and social well-being. Topics such as the influence of health or illness on the occurrence and duration of unemployment or the fear of unemployed people to lose their jobs and its effects on their health status have so far been of minor interest only.

The purpose of this report is to review the recent research, conducted in German-speaking countries, on a large subject – unemployment and health – and the various methods to approach it.

Unemployment

In the Federal Republic of Germany, persons who are seeking work and are registered at the labour office, are officially classified as unemployed under the conditions that (a) they are not unable to work due to illness; (b) they are not working, or working only to a minor extent, as employees, homeworkers, family aids or self-employed; and (c) they are not trying to get only a minor job or a job at a specified enterprise or a job as homeworkers (except those receiving unemployment benefits), or that they seek a job for not more than three months (Frese and Mohr 1978).

---

* First published in *Social Science and Medicine* (1986) 22(4):409–430.

The concept of long-term unemployment is not clearly defined. In some studies, long-term unemployment is assumed in cases where an unemployed is (still or again) jobless one year after his/her first interview with the researcher; this concept may disguise 'hidden' long-term unemployment as several short-term jobs could well have been held in the meantime. For some unemployed, continuing and renewed phases of unemployment may add up to an extremely long duration of unemployment overall (Büchtemann 1983).

The official unemployment statistics do not include: young people not registered as unemployed at the labour office; women who have taken the role of housewives after having resigned from work; those who, after qualifying for unemployment benefits, were declared incapable to work and now receive social welfare; unemployed who work in schemes for job creation and rehabilitation measures; institutionalized people; and vagrant people (Kieselbach 1983).

'Disguised' unemployment is said to add up to an amount that equals about one-half of the official unemployment figure; so some sources estimate that in the Federal Republic of Germany today's actual unemployment rate is at about 15% (Bonss and Heinze 1984).

Major deviations from a traditional pattern of work – 8 hours a day, 5 days a week, regular vacations – and from a three-phase life pattern – education, work, retirement – as well as from a socially determined definition of potential labour force may be labelled as relative unemployment. This leads to highly relative definitions of unemployment. Seasonal work, underemployment, short-time work, long-term sick-leave, early disablement on the one hand, illicit work, additional (agricultural) activities and 'alternative' patterns of work, etc. on the other, demonstrate how unclear the limits between employment and unemployment are.

This often leads to an underestimation, sometimes to an overestimation, of the number of unemployed; in any case the real number is unknown. But there seems to be little doubt that since the employment crisis in 1974, and in spite of a reduction of foreign workers and the resulting relief of the German labour market (Kaiser and Westmüller 1978), 12.5 million Germans (or every third employed German) were hit by unemployment, and the total length of unemployment accumulated to about 1 year per unemployed, and each phase of unemployment lasted, on an average, for about 19 weeks (Karr 1983).

Thus, unemployment is no longer a problem of fringe groups. Estimates put the figure of the unemployed in the Federal Republic of Germany to about 3.6 million in 1985 (Bonss and Heinze 1984) and predict 6 million for the 1990s (Bonss et al. 1984).

Since the first oil crisis and the recession of 1974–1975, the traditional objective of full employment has apparently become utopian. There seems to be a crisis of the labour society (Bonss and Heinze 1984), a growing powerlessness of the labour force (Bonss et al. 1984) as well as a 'legitimation crisis' of the state (Kieselbach and Offe 1979a). Although clear differences between the unemployment in the 1930s and the 1980s well exist (Jahoda 1983b), some authors speak of a new poverty and of a considerable change in the social climate (Böhnisch and Schmitz 1978).

Although unemployment today is large-scale and obviously has a lot of causes beyond the control of individuals, it is still seen even by some unemployed themselves as the effect of insufficient individual adaptation and is labelled a psychological or even psychiatric problem (Bonss et al. 1984). It is often attributed to characteristics of problem groups, or to an individual inability to compromise, or to other traits of personality (Kieselbach and Offe 1979a). Unemployment is therefore not only an 'objective' societal problem but also a 'subjective' individual one that creates a host of secondary effects.

Research on Unemployment and Health

The following section presents the main characteristics of major empirical studies on unemployment and health in German-speaking countries, including the Federal Republic of Germany, Austria and Switzerland, but excluding the German Democratic Republic.

Studies

The first wave of German social science research on unemployment and health started in the 1930s, i.e. years after the peaks of unemployment during the Weimar Republic. A second wave followed in the years 1976–1977, again some time after the new economic crisis had begun. Unemployment research is, it seems, a belated product of slumps (Bonss and Heinze 1984).

One of the first large research projects was carried out around 1950 by Schelsky and dealt with unemployment and occupational problems of youth; a control group was not used (see Wilhelm-Reiss 1980).

Some of the most important cross-sectional research projects were the following:

- ISO Institute (Institute for the Study of Social Chances): survey of about 1300 unemployed and 1300 employed in North-Rhine Westfalia in 1976 (Fröhlich 1983a; Hentschel 1981; Hentschel et al. 1979)
- Henkel (1984; n.d.) survey of 243 unemployed and 267 employed alcohol-dependent patients, in 18 special clinics
- Bastiaan et al. (1980) survey of the care personnel for 33 psychiatric patients in inpatient and 44 in (semi-)outpatient care
- Vagt and Stavemann (1980) survey of 116 part-time, 509 short-time workers and 60 unemployed in 1978
- Bahnmüller (1981a, b) survey of 89 unemployed and 73 employed men during 1977, focusing on work, identity, social relations, time structure, (personal) assessment of the causes of the situation

Some cross-sectional research projects were extended to longitudinal studies:

- Infratest (1978a–e, 1980)
  1977: representative interviews with 1637 unemployed and 1236 reemployed

1978: 12–14 months after the first sampling, a second interview was carried out with 1125 and 823 persons of the respective groups
1978: representative study on the attitude of employed persons towards further training and mobility
1982: last interviews with all three samples (Büchtemann 1983, Infratest 1980)
– Institute for Labour Market and Occupational Research
1975: retrospective survey of a representative group of unemployed who had registered at the labour office the year before, including a survey of 1000 unemployed youth (Brinkmann 1977, 1981)
1981: survey of about 8000 unemployed in 25 representatively selected labour offices; personal interviews with about 2800, written interviews with about 2000 others as well as 2500 unemployed under the age of 25 (Brinkmann and Schober 1982)
1983: panel study on 1600 participants of the 1981 survey (Brinkmann 1984a); results were compared with a sample of employed people in cities (Brinkmann and Potthoff 1983)
– Wilhelm-Reiss (1980): surveys of 272 young people in 1976 and 252 in 1977; 29 unemployed youth participated in both surveys
– Frese (1979), Frese and Mohr (1977): surveys of unemployed workers over 45 years of age in 1975 and 1977

Heinemann (1978) combined several studies in order to assess the effects of youth unemployment: standardized personal interviews with 293 male German youths aged 15–20 as well as 277 employed young people; content analysis of records of delinquent youths in the years 1973–1976; semi-standardized interviews with employers; and expert meetings and group discussions.

Schwefel and coworkers are presently involved in research on unemployment and health at different levels: inventory of the most current international research and its publication in a newsletter (Schwefel and John 1982, 1983, 1984), application of the Medis health indicators to, for example, the longitudinal studies of the Institute for Labour Market and Occupational Research (Brinkmann and Potthoff 1983); time-series analyses of highly aggregated data on mortality and economic development (John 1982, 1983); and 'comparisons' between micro- and macrostudies (John et al. 1983; Brenner and Schwefel 1983; Schwefel 1983; Schwefel et al. 1984).

For research on unemployment (Brinkmann 1983) the following data were also used: routine investigations of the Federal Employment Office into the structure of unemployment (since 1973), routine data of the Statutory Sickness Funds including, for example, statistics on insured people, sick-leave, old age pensioners (Dennerlein and Schneider 1984; Halusa 1983; Preiser and Schräder 1983, 1984) as well as time series from other official statistics (John 1983).

Case studies were used either on an individual basis in a quasi-depth psychology manner (Demokratisches Gesundheitswesen 1983; Hertel and Holland 1984; Kieselbach 1984; Windolf and Klemm 1981) or as community-oriented case studies, e.g. to analyse consequences of plant closures (Bosch 1978, 1980).

A survey of privately practising physicians on the health effects of unemployment was undertaken by Thomann (1981, 1983c). Recently, Bosofo interviewed other experts on the same subject (Bochumer Sozialmedizinische Forschung 1984).

In Austria, Strotzka and Leitner (1969) were able to carry out a community study during an economic crisis in a small rural industrial town with about 5000 inhabitants. Action research was the core of the so-called Hamborn Project taking care of about 130 unemployed young people (Opaschowski 1976). Group discussions (see also Leithäuser 1984), and in-depth interviews with 311 youths were carried out by Burger et al. (1976).

Up to now, German research lacks monographic family studies, community studies, as well as studies on the relation between highly aggregated time series on economic development, unemployment, morbidity and mortality, as were carried out by Brenner (1979).

Concepts, Data and Methods

All these studies deal, directly or indirectly, with the subject of unemployment, illness and health; the concept of health used here includes physical as well as mental health and social well-being. Many different procedures to assess health status and health impairments are applied. Examples include:

- Questions as to whether a specific illness is officially acknowledged as a barrier to earning any income or practising any profession (Hentschel et al. 1979; Büchtemann and von Rosenbladt 1981; Preiser 1979)
- Registration of health problems at the Labour Office (Büchtemann and von Rosenbladt 1981)
- Sick-leave certificates issued by physicians (Wittig and Eberle 1984)
- Self-assessment of 'subjectively' experienced health status and of chronic impairments (Fröhlich 1983 a; Brinkmann 1984)
- Listing of complaints and diseases during the last 3 months (Büchtemann and von Rosenbladt 1981; Preiser 1979)
- Open questions on occupation-impeding diseases and handicaps (Hentschel et al. 1979)
- Medis scale of complaints (Brinkmann and Potthoff 1983; Brinkmann 1984 b)

Operationalizations of mental health and of personal characteristics, currently used, are manifold:

- Medis scale on emotional balance (Brinkmann and Potthoff 1983; Brinkmann 1984 b)
- Zung scale on depression (Balz 1984)
- Rosenberg scale on self-esteem (Balz 1984)
- Kaufmann scale on fatalism (Hentschel et al. 1979)
- Scales (of about 20 or more items) on nervousness, aggressivity, depression, irritation, sociability, relaxedness, domination, inhibition, openness, extraversion, emotional lability and masculinity (Wilhelm-Reiss 1980)
- Statements on the subjective experience of unemployment (Hentschel et al. 1979), achievement motivation, expectations of failure (Büchtemann and von Rosenbladt 1981) and anomia (Fröhlich 1983 a)

– Individual statements on anxiety in social situations (Preiser 1979), occupational orientation (Brinkmann and Potthoff 1983) and self-esteem (Brinkmann 1981)

With respect to operationalization of social well-being, single statements or questions regarding time budgets, frequency and quality of social contacts and social relations, are used (Fröhlich 1979).

Notwithstanding all the problems of registering unemployment correctly (Brinkmann 1980) and despite the misuse of the unemployed status (Hoppe 1981), unemployment is usually operationalized by its official registration and by the consequent self-assessment of the interviewee as an unemployed.

As a rule, results are analyzed descriptively; common are phenomenological approaches to interpretation. Items from lists or scales are, in the main, analyzed one by one. Multivariate statistics are as rare as scalographic procedures and time models (but see Wilhelm-Reiss 1980; Fröhlich 1983a; Brinkmann 1983; Schwefel and Schwefel 1973). Approaches at different levels – micro- versus macrostudies – are underrepresented (Schwefel 1983).

Frequent sources of error or bias in study designs and analyses are: confusion of long-term unemployed with temporarily short-time reemployed when comparing two points of time, underestimation of unemployment effects in the interview situation, and effects of anticipating unemployment during the first interview (in longitudinal research) or in the control group (Frese and Mohr 1978). When comparing a control group with the unemployed, the fact that unemployed people tend to be younger and proportionally more of female sex than the employed is often overlooked; this may lead to an underestimation of health problems caused by unemployment (Preiser 1979).

Health, Work and Society

Causes of Unemployment

Except when dealing with illness-induced unemployment, the wider causes of unemployment, and its changing meanings over time (Niess 1979), will not be dealt with in this report whose main subject are the effects of unemployment. In general, the causes of unemployment may be characterized as a complex problem related to population dynamics, economic crisis and to the transition towards intensive economic growth (Bonss and Heinze 1984; Bonss et al. 1984; Brandes 1977; Freiburghaus 1978; Goldberg et al. 1977).

Effects of Unemployment

When the more recent research on unemployment started off, it first tried to understand the present situation by going back to, and using, the results of former studies on the effects of unemployment. Looking back into history held the promise of helping to generate relevant hypotheses (Klönne 1984); so, among others, the Marienthal study, the Warsaw study and the Detroit study were reviewed (Wacker 1983).

In the beginning, results of foreign research were prominently adopted which, rather in a cookbook-like manner, emphasized effects of unemployment such as the following:

– Anticipatory fear, and the shock, of becoming unemployed
– Hopelessness, depression, general loss of control, helplessness, anomia, suicide, passivity, resignation, pessimism and reduced self-confidence
– Problems in the social sphere, social isolation and matrimonial difficulties
– Alcoholism
– Psychosomatic disorders: hypertension, high cholesterol level, high values of noradrenaline, or uric acid, and of creatinine in the serum, indisposition and days of reduced activity due to indisposition (Frese and Mohr 1978).

The work of Brenner and of Kasl and Cobb (in John et al. 1983) ranged high on the list of foreign studies that have been dealt with here. Some attempts to systematize the effects of (long-term) unemployment were made, resulting in classifications such as:

– Problem groups: directly affected unemployed, indirectly affected family members, people indirectly affected by their fear of job loss (von Berg 1977)
– Adaption of activities or attitudes to the situation of being unemployed: combining an 'intrinsic/extrinsic dimension' with an 'individualistic/collective dimension' to form four groups of reactions:
Intrinsic/individualistic: extreme reaction is suicide.
Extrinsic/individualistic: extreme reaction is criminality.
Intrinsic/collective: extreme reaction is illegal drug consumption.
Extrinsic/collective: extreme reaction is labour disputes (Wilhelm-Reiss 1980).
– Degree of effect intensity: selection according to health status, intensification of existing diseases, and development of new diseases, due to unemployment (Brinkmann and Potthoff 1983).

Theorems and Theories

Depending on the sort of problem stated, on professional socialization, academic discipline and theoretical orientation, some of the following constructs to investigate and understand the links between unemployment and health are preferably used.

Stress. Unemployment is considered a stressor; yet, there are arguments against approaches that are too much oriented towards individuals and pathologies as they tend to individualize problems (Bonss et al. 1984).

Life Event. Arguably, to think of unemployment only as a critical life-event, seems one-sided and too simple; rather, one should look into the processes of psychological adaptation and accomplishment, and thereby take into account two opposite hypotheses: the duration-of-exposition versus the initial-effect hypothesis (Frese 1984; Preiser 1983). Some results of life-event research are also criticized for being correlational only (Lauterbach 1984).

Labelling Approach. This approach, chosen to understand the negative consequences of unemployment, builds on the concept of stigma and the processes of stigmatization (Wilhelm-Reiss 1980).

Socialization. Some authors interpret unemployment as a learning process, an experience of socialization, etc. (Wacker 1976).

Strain Models. A coherent and operational concept of strain seems still missing (Brinkmann 1981). More attention should be given to the multi-factorial aetiology of diseases. Complex models of strain would be necessary in which, for instance, society could be conceived as a 'specific totality' (Bonss et al. 1984).

Course Models. A sociological analysis of the dynamic process of becoming and being unemployed is advocated for: entering an insecure segment of the labour market, becoming unemployed, situation during unemployment, ending of unemployment and consequences for professional careers (Büchtemann 1984).

Society. The point is also made that, increasingly, the labour market can no longer be considered the crucial mechanism to distribute opportunities for social participation and life (Büchtemann 1984), and that the meaning of work, social integration and working morale undergo rapid changes (Wacker 1983). Therefore, a comprehensive analysis of society is required.

Economics. Economic essays on unemployment often refer to trade-offs between inflation and unemployment, to problems of equilibrium assumptions and to the theory of voluntary unemployment (Rothschild 1978) as well as to theorems on the segmentation of labour markets (Heinze et al. 1981).

Psychology. Psychological and psychoanalytical interpretations stress the emotional meaning of job loss in terms of time perspectives and inability to act, of deprivation and *Trauerarbeit*, of identity crises and social stigmatization as well as of confidence and system loyalty (Wacker 1983).

Neomarxism. Some authors visualize unemployment in terms of capitalistic crises, mechanisms of competition, and of disposable alienated labour in highly developed capitalist systems where labour is not distinguished from work or activity. The distinction between labour as a value-in-use and an exchange value has been drawn (Bonss and Heinze 1984).

Relativity. As compared with the situation in developing countries or in Western Europe during the 1930s, the relative meaning of today's unemployment in this region is stressed and put against its absolute meaning in terms of poverty, catastrophic life-events, etc. (Schwefel and Schwefel 1973).

Chance. Unemployment is also considered to be a new chance of personal development (Wacker 1983), a 'creative unemployment' to open up alternative forms of living (Volpert 1979), one step in an individual and life-long development towards a change in life-style (Kaiser and Westmüller 1978; Beckmann and Hahn 1982).

In conclusion, a coherent theoretical conception that would help to grasp the topic unemployment and health intellectually is still not available.

The Role of Work

In order to understand the effects of unemployment, many authors refer to the positive functions of labour and work. Freud regarded work as the strongest link to reality, and the ability to work as a measure for the absence of neurotical disturbances (Jahoda 1983a). According to Jahoda (1983a) labour and work have five main functions: experience of time, social contacts, participation in collective objectives, status and identity and regular activity (Jahoda 1983b). According to 'Work in America', the importance of work lies in: social contacts, feeling of competence, sense of usefulness, social frame for self-esteem, individual concept of reality and personal identity (Kieselbach and Offe 1979a). Work and labour are therefore praised to guarantee income, acceptance, security and utility of life, although – as many polls show – professional roles have been considerably depreciated (Bonss and Heinze 1984), and wage labour seems to have lost a lot of its power (Bonss et al. 1984).

Various sources of strain, heavily destructive for body or mind, are still characteristic of many jobs, especially in the industrial sector (Jahoda 1983b). 'Learned helplessness' as a consequence of low control over strong stressors are still typical of the work situation of the underprivileged (Kieselbach and Offe 1979a). Increased rationalization and even more intensive labour may lead to further health problems (Heinze 1984). The high percentage of ill people among the unemployed is often indicative of the strains sustained during the last job (Büchtemann and von Rosenbladt 1981). As Büchtemann and von Rosenbladt conclude: "Unemployed with health problems suffered in their last jobs more than it is usual from strains such as uncomfortable and rigid posture, dull and uninteresting work, unfavourable weather conditions, increased risk of accidents, noise, polluted air, physically heavy labour as well as shifts and/or on-line production". The determination of the health status by the last occupation is shown in many studies (Preiser 1979). Psychosomatic complaints of unemployed are frequently caused by jobs held just before (Büchtemann and von Rosenbladt 1981).

In conclusion, it could well be expected that people, after having worked under very unfavourable conditions, might experience the loss of work as an improvement of their status of health (Fröhlich 1979). Classical authors, too (e.g. Hufeland), suggest that 'unhappy overwork', just like physical passivity and boredom, may reduce life expectancy (see also Thomann 1981).

Economic Recession and Health

In a period of mass unemployment and economic recession, both the suffering from work and the suffering from being jobless seem to increase (Bonss and Heinze 1984). Economic crises do not only hit the unemployed but all people (Wacker 1977) – a fact that makes unemployment research all the more difficult.

During the economic crisis with its mass unemployment, the rate of early disablement in the Federal Republic of Germany increased considerably; this was particularly true for psychiatric cases. At the same time, public rehabilitation services were cut down so that the chances of rehabilitation worsened (Bastiaan et al. 1980). Work (unhealthy working conditions, selection of the less healthy) seems to be the main factor for the increase in early disablement (Scharf 1980c). It is mainly the blue-collar female workers and the psychically disabled who are hit by early disability (Scharf 1980c; Bastiaan and Kaiser 1982; Henkel 1982). Cardio-vascular diseases, diseases of the musculo-skeleton system and the connective tissue as well as neoplasms are major causes (Scharf 1980c). While the rate of early disablement increases, the age of entry into early disablement decreases (Scharf 1980c).

Officially registered illnesses usually decrease in economic crises; insecurity of job seems to lower the number of sick-leaves (Böker 1971) – hence the argument that people tend to protract their illness out of fear to lose their job (Thomann 1983b). Yet, there is empirical evidence that, even in times of economic recession, the ill do go to see a doctor, only certificates of illness are not issued to the same extent as before; „recessions lower the number of sick persons, not the number of contacts with physicians" (Wittig and Eberle 1984).

Preiser and Schräder (1983) suggest that, during long-term economic crisis, employed people with health problems, and with an above average number of sick-leaves, are prominently forced out of the labour force. This is explained by: a reduction of the labour force quota of persons of 55–63 years of age, an increase in the number of early retirement due to disablement, an increase in unemployment due to health problems, and an increase in hospital cases and hospital days per retired.

This, however, must be considered a hypothesis as long as some inherent data problems and the influence of the jurisdiction on these interrelations are not satisfactorily coped with (Dennerlein and Schneider 1984; Preiser and Schräder 1984). Besides, the sick-leave frequency of the unemployed has the same procyclical variations as that of the employed (Dennerlein and Schneider 1984). Nevertheless, up to now, the relation between absenteeism, illness behaviour and unemployment has not been explored sufficiently (Orendi 1978).

Threatening unemployment – even if only assumed – changes health. Strotzka and Leitner (1969) report a marked increase in psychogenic diseases during economic crises: "The most interesting finding was that among 30 cases not one was directly hit by dismissal"; "an uncertain threat has stronger pathogenic consequences than the real strain." Wuggenig (1979) found a relationship between increased emotionality and anticipated unemployment. Pelzmann et al. (1984) conclude: "Among those employed who had reason to worry" about their jobs, we observed a significant increase in so-called dispositional diseases during the phase of their anticipating unemployment." Such findings highlight the danger of confounding objective unemployment and subjective handling of (threatening) unemployment in longitudinal studies on employed and unemployed people (Frese and Mohr 1978; Bonss et al. 1984).

In conclusion, complex interrelations exist between unemployment and health: (anticipated) unemployment interferes with health; health interferes with unemployment and employment; employment interferes with health; and health effects of (un-)employment may be buffered or increased by socio-economic conditions.

Thus, a review cannot only deal with the topic of unemployment-induced disease; it has to approach the much wider connections between society and economy on the one hand, and physical, mental and social well-being on the other. This is why in the following pages a distinction is to be made between the influence of health on unemployment, and the influence of unemployment on health.

The Influence of Health on Unemployment

In this section, the influence of (ill) health on unemployment, on its duration and its ending will be dealt with. Here, illness is regarded as one of the determinants, not as an effect of unemployment.

Illness and the Entry into Unemployment

Sick persons run a higher risk of becoming unemployed (Büchtemann and von Rosenbladt 1981). The risk of being sacked increases with the frequency and duration of illness (Dombois et al. 1982). In 1978, every fifth dismissal in private businesses, and every third in industry were due to illness (Büchtemann 1982a). One study showed that health problems accounted for 56% of all dismissals on personal grounds; 29% of all official explanations of dismissals referred to health problems (Bahnmüller 1981b). Several authors report on this link between ill health and dismissal (Preiser 1979; Aldinger-Mosseanu 1978; von Rosenbladt and Büchtemann 1980). Of those unemployed who had given up their job of their own will 11% mentioned health problems (von Rosenbladt and Büchtemann 1980).

Illness is one determinant of unemployment. Social selection processes are at work; people with health problems are pressured out of the labour market (Büchtemann 1982a, 1984). "In most cases, ill health was the main reason for terminating the last job" (Büchtemann 1982a). One-third of unemployed men – but only one-quarter of the women – indicated that their present illness was caused by their previous jobs (Hentschel et al. 1979).

Selection processes especially hit foreign workers, blue-collar workers in extremely strenuous jobs as well as women (Zimmermann 1983). In particular, elderly and disabled people run this risk (Heinze 1984). The unemployment rate of the heavily disabled was twice the total unemployment rate in September 1979

(Brinkmann 1982). Thomann (1983b) reports a „weeding of the weakest from the labour process".

Illness and the Duration of Unemployment

Persons with health problems run a very high risk of continued unemployment (Büchtemann and von Rosenbladt 1981); their unemployment lasts three times as long as that of the healthy unemployed (Preiser 1979). In addition, of all unemployed people the share of those who have health problems increases (Büchtemann and von Rosenbladt 1981).

A contrast group analysis to 'explain' the duration of unemployment by health impairments shows a variance reduction of 9.3% in the first analysis step; health problems rank as the first of the 27 variables to explain the duration of unemployment (Brinkmann 1978). Moreover, health status tends to deteriorate during unemployment (Brinkmann 1984c). Health problems play an even more important role during unemployment than at the beginning of it (Brinkmann and Potthoff 1983).

Illness and Reintegration of the Unemployed

According to employers, health problems are not the biggest obstacle to the reintegration of unemployed; more important were qualification, reliability, the number of previous jobs (Preiser 1979). By way of contrast, employment offices give health problems as the prime factor of the refusal of unemployed job applicants (Büchtemann and von Rosenbladt 1981; Büchtemann 1984). Routine data analyses of the Federal Employment Office show that every third unemployed suffered from health problems in September 1980, and that for every fifth person the chances of getting a job were considered low because of his/her health problems (Büchtemann 1982a). "The occupational reintegration of unemployed with health problems is primarily thwarted by the increasingly severe selection criteria applied by the enterprises" (Büchtemann 1982a). Nevertheless, the main determinant of occupational reintegration is the situation of the labour market (Brinkmann and Schober 1982).

According to an analysis of the determinants of continuing unemployment, health problems explained 3.19% of variance; civil status, sex, payment of financial benefits by the Federal Employment Office, occupational status of the spouse and duration of unemployment explained more of the variance (Brinkmann 1978). Next to age and duration of unemployment as explanatory variables for the reintegration into the work force, health problems rank third with a variance reduction of 1.64% (Brinkmann 1978). Because of strains at the new job, occupational reintegration does, however, not lead directly to a marked improvement of health status (Büchtemann and von Rosenbladt 1981).

"In most cases, occupational reintegration of unemployed with health problems leads to professional degradation and dequalification, but generally also to a diminished strain at the job as compared with the time before unemployment" (Büchtemann 1982a). "Unemployed with health problems ... have, more frequently than others, to accept changes in occupation, professional degradation and dequalification" (Büchtemann 1984); they have to accept jobs at a lower level, change of occupation and of industry, and a decreasing income (Preiser 1979). A typical result is the destabilization of the professional career (Büchtemann 1984).

"People with unstable reintegration patterns (show) a significant deterioration of health when compared with long-term unemployed" (Büchtemann and von Rosenbladt 1981). Such instability is not rare. Specific measures to increase job perspectives of the unemployed are often interrupted; 32% of people withdrawing from those programmes mention health problems (Hofbauer and Dadzio 1982).

Unemployment is often brought to an end by retreat into other social roles: the role of the ill, the retired, the housewife (Büchtemann 1982b, 1984; Frese and Mohr 1979).

The Influence of Unemployment on Health

This section will deal with the influences of unemployment on health. Although it is not contended that unemployment by itself causes illness, some evidence or plausibilities will be shown which suggest a sort of quasi-causality that exists in this relationship. At any rate, a lot of physical, mental and social effects of unemployment will be presented.

It is an indisputable fact that a high proportion of the unemployed is burdened with health problems. In 1979–1980 when about one-third of the male unemployed was affected by illness, this percentage was higher than in 1982 (21% only); yet, this figure is expected to increase in the future (Brinkmann and Potthoff 1983). The crucial question is whether those unemployed had been ill before, or fell ill during, unemployment.

Intervening Factors

There is no single form of unemployment nor of health. Individual attitudes and social conditions lead to a lot of different reactions towards unemployment.

Thomann (1981) gives the following list of factors which are assumed to increase illness connected with unemployment:

- Previous health status
- Financial situation of the unemployed
- Duration of unemployment
- Additional strains (e.g. family problems)
- Social or family support
- Position of the unemployed in society
- Values, ideals and social norms
- Socially accepted possibilities of conflict management
- Class-consciousness of the unemployed

- Importance of work in the life of the unemployed
- Age of the unemployed
- General level of education and occupational qualification of the unemployed
- Previous jobs
- Existence of a health insurance for the unemployed
- Psychic structure of the unemployed

In addition to this almost complete list of factors possibly influencing the state of health of the unemployed, other studies on unemployment and health mention the following factors alleviating or reinforcing illness connected with unemployment.

Long-term unemployment seems to have effects mostly on those people who spent their time inactively. Running a small-holding, moon-lighting and stop-gap activities – with or without payment – prove to be a protection against some effects of unemployment (Pelzmann et al. 1984).

The effects of unemployment are less negative when other roles can be adopted: the role of a housewife or a retired (Brinkmann 1981; Büchtemann and von Rosenbladt 1981). Persons who had to retire early did not show to be more depressive than employed people (Frese and Mohr 1979).

Status – whether as a (once more) unemployed or a housewife or a retired – is a more important predictor of psycho-social and psychosomatic strain than is duration of unemployment (Büchtemann and von Rosenbladt 1981). "The subjective health status of unemployment is less impaired by long-term unemployment and steady job-seeking than by their status and the behavioural requirements related with it" (Büchtemann 1982a).

Social support eases the psychological burden of unemployment on women (Gnegel and Mohr 1982). Support of the spouse alleviates the effects of unemployment (Fröhlich 1983b). A favourable family situation has a protective effect (Wilhelm-Reiss 1980). Social support is experienced as moderating the impact of unemployment (Wacker 1983).

"The public system of unemployment insurance and of social welfare (still) prevents unemployment from having a full impact on the individual existence" (Wacker 1981c). The same is true for health insurance.

The effects of unemployment are less incisive when unemployment is seen collectively as a widespread reality (as for example in the case of plant closures) or is experienced as a mass phenomenon in the neighbourhood (Heinemann 1978).

Depending on the general meaning of work, or on the specific importance of the last occupation, for the personal identity of the unemployed, the loss of job as a potential stressor varies considerably (Bonss and Heinze 1984; Bonss et al. 1984; Fröhlich 1983a, b).

Unemployment and anticipation of unemployment become greater problems when, after the loss of job, forced passivity is to be expected (Grundnig 1980).

Sociability, provided it is a stable trait of character, can act as a buffer against the immediate impacts of unemployment (Fröhlich 1983b; Hoppe 1981).

Many factors contribute to the interrelationship between unemployment and health; by no means is there a unilateral linkage. That is why highly differentiated research on unemployment is necessary.

Unemployment and Physical Health

The links between unemployment and physical health are relatively unknown. Research approaches are predominantly interpretative; ethiological models have hardly been developed at all (Thomann 1981).

From 1975 to 1978, the precentage of unemployed with health problems rose from 20 to 34% (Brinkmann 1983): early disablement and early retirement also increased during the 1970s (Heinze 1984). However, the overwhelming part of the unemployed cannot be classified as disabled (Preiser 1979). Likewise, in the 1930s, somatic impairments were less than was expected for the unemployed themselves, but had rather affected their children (Bonss et al. 1984).

When comparing the unemployed with employed people, twice as many unemployed are affected by health impairments; the rate is: 18% for male and 11% for female unemployed (Hentschel et al. 1979). In particular, the unemployed more often suffer from sleep disorders and circulatory ailments, whereas the employed mention headaches and fatigue more frequently (Preiser 1979). But the unemployed, too, often report nervousness, sleep disorders and tiredness (Büchtemann and von Rosenbladt 1981). Main complaints of unemployed males are: colds (21%), circulatory disorders (20%), headaches (18%), spinal disorders (16%), nervousness (15%) and flu (15%); women's complaints range from headaches (34%), circulatory disorders (28%), colds (21%), nervousness (20%), to flu (18%), cough (16%) and spinal disorders (16%) (Preiser 1979). Quite a few of these complaints are by no means specific to the unemployed. 21% of the interviewed unemployed were not suffering from any complaints or diseases during the previous 3 months; those who reported any complaints had about four complaints on an average; employed people reported more complaints than others (Preiser 1979). Predominantly, the health status of the unemployed remained the same as compared to when they were employed; for 21% of them, the health status even improved after becoming unemployed (especially when their previous work had been very strenuous), in the case of 24% it deteriorated (Fröhlich 1983a; see also Büchtemann 1983). Case studies on plant closures (no control group) report of nervousness, aggressivity, sleeplessness and gastric pains (Bosch 1980). At the level of highly aggregated health indicators such as general and infant mortality rate, significant relationships could only be shown between unemployment and the infant, but not with general, mortality rate (John 1983).

The interaction between sympatic and parasympatic leads Müller-Limmroth (1977) to assume that a reduction of activities by unemployment negatively affects the activity regulation through the vegetative nervous system. The result of unemployment could be that there are no marked phases of activity and recreation which, in turn, could lead to vegetative dystonia with symptoms like nervous heart complaints, circulatory instability, nervous gastric disorders, sleep disorders, cold sweat, etc. (Kieselbach and Offe 1979a). "By causing financial, social and occupational problems, unemployment works as a psychical and social stress-factor which, physiologically, produces an increased level of activation by means of hormonal control, with no change of simultaneous motoric release. If such a situation persists, increased arteriosclerosis, fatigue and digestive disorders might follow" (Kieselbach and Offe 1979a). Moreover, stress increases blood sugar, blood lipids and hyperacidity resulting in diabetes, arteriosclerosis, circulatory disorder and myocardial infarction as well as gastric and duodenal ulcers (Müller-Limmroth 1977). Pflanz also found a higher probability of ulcer incidence in the unemployed (in Thomann 1981). Effects of unemployment in terms of 'ACTH hormone' production are mentioned by Thomann (1983b) who, however, points out that unemployment is an unspecific burden; pathological effects are to be expected at the weakest point – "there is no specific unemployment disease" (Thomann 1981). A generally higher morbidity is much more probable than specific diseases of unemployed (Thomann 1981). Unemployment is only an external stimulus for the manifestation of disease or for the intensification of a previously existing but latent disease (Büchtemann and von Rosenbladt 1981).

During the first 3 months of unemployment, recovery outpaces effects of strain; the health status of the unemployed equals that of the employed, in special groups (e.g. young women) it is even better (Brinkmann and Potthoff 1983). Similar results are reported from Austria: "During the first four months of unemployment, diseases decreased and were about as frequent as in times of job security" (Pelzmann et al. 1984). A "recuperation and recovery factor of unemployment" is also reported by Brödel et al. (1976).

The effects on health of long-term unemployment are not totally clear. Brinkmann (1984b) reports a deterioration in all the indicators of the Medis complaint scale (with marked effects on mental health) in cases of long-term unemployment. His panel survey with unemployed quite strongly indicates that unemployment leads to a deterioration of health; 30%–40% of the diseases of long-term unemployed result from changes in health status during unemployment; the rest is said to be a structural effect of selection processes; so, long-term unemployment worsens existing diseases or causes new ones. Cross-sectional data of Fröhlich (1983a) also seem to indicate a deterioration of the health status due to long-term unemployment. An Austrian research project shows that long-term unemployed report a worse health status than the re-employed; 18.7% of the unemployed males, as compared to 2.6% of the employed, reported ill health (Bochumer Sozialmedizinische Forschung 1984). Psychosomatic and cardiovascular problems, in particular, seem to increase during long-term unemployment (Brinkmann 1984b). An Infratest study, however, found out that the health status of long-term unemployed, though worse than that of short-term unemployed and employed, had been similarly bad even before unemployment, implying that afterwards no deterioration took place (Preiser 1979). According to this source, long-term unemployment does not produce a bad health status. It is also said that persistent unemployment has no direct impact on the subjective health status (Büchtemann and von Rosenbladt 1981). These results strongly contradict the following statement: "In the long run, the burden of unemployment leads, for a considerable part of the affected, to the development or promotion or deterioration of a mental or physical disease" (Thomann 1983b).

A strong link can be found between age, health and unemployment (Heinze 1984). Occupational ability and health decrease with the age of the unemployed (Preiser 1979). In the case of unqualified blue-collar workers – despite their release from poor working conditions – health deteriorates very significantly during unemployment; their rate is at 29.1% as compared to an average of

24.3% for all unemployed men whose health status deteriorated during unemployment (Fröhlich 1979). The level of deterioration of physical health status increases with mounting economic deprivation (Fröhlich 1983a).

"Among patients in institutions for consultation, therapy and rehabilitation, a marked increase in dependence on alcohol can be found since massunemployment started in 1974. Today, about 50%–70% of all alcoholics in inpatient care are unemployed" (Henkel 1984). So far, very few studies deal with the relationship between unemployment and alcoholism, although unemployment may well be considered a psycho-social risk factor of alcoholism (Henkel 1984; Henkel et al. 1983). A study of Henkel (1984) shows that unemployment increases the risk of alcoholism and, in the case of addicts, reinforces their problem. According to the Trier Alcoholism Test, unemployed and employed differ quite significantly in the form and severity of alcoholism. Owing to financial problems, unemployed alcoholics tend to favour strong drinks; there is also an increase in the consumption of substitutional tranquilizers and sleeping drugs. As Henkel (1984) demonstrated, intensified and extended forms of alcoholism are rather a consequence of unemployment than a symptom of selective filter processes. Somatic secondary effects of alcoholism might as well increase (Henkel, n.d.). Given unemployment after discharge from a clinic, relapses into alcoholism increase dramatically and occur earlier in people who are not in a stable work situation (Henkel, n.d.). Unemployment seems to lead to a higher probability of relapses, but the empirical results are not totally convincing (Waldow and Börner 1984).

Unemployment and Mental Health

Research on mental health of the unemployed has used different constructs and produced divergent results (Bonss et al. 1984). In comparison with the situation of 1930s, the impact of unemployment today seems to be more of a psychological nature (Mohr and Frese 1981), a fact that apparently entails some problems for research (Maiers and Markard 1980).

A higher degree of nervousness and depressiveness and a lower degree of conviviality than in the population at large have been found among the unemployed by Wilhelm-Reiss (in Bochumer Sozialmedizinische Forschung 1984). The results of Gnengel and Mohr, admittedly achieved without using any controls, suggest a high share of depression, aggressivity and sleep disorders (in Bochumer Sozialmedizinische Forschung 1984). Henkel (1984) reports of psycho-social changes during unemployment in 30%–50% of the unemployed, especially in terms of growing worries about the future, nervousness, sleep disorders, depression and helplessness, and even suicidal tendencies among 30% of unemployed (alcoholic) patients as compared to 3% of employed ones. "None of the patients related their complaints, which were subjectively experienced as purely physical ones, to the economic crisis" (Strotzka and Leitner 1969).

For Müller, the self-esteem of unemployed is being imperiled by the underutilization of personal capabilities, causing long-term physiological reactions (in Kieselbach and Offe 1979 a). An awareness of general powerlessness has been shown by the work of Bahnmüller (1981 b). According to Fröhlich (1979), there is a correlational relationship between the state of health and the feeling of worthlessness.

Fröhlich (1983 a) also shows that 38 % of the unemployed have low anomia, 35 % middle anomia and 27 % a high degree of anomia. Bahnmüller (1981 b) links frustration and self-attribution of the blame with unemployment. But, according to Hentschel, employed and unemployed do not differ significantly on a fatalism scale (in Brinkmann 1981).

Wacker (1977) presupposes a relationship between unemployment and aggressivity, caused by emotional blocking, transfers into irrationality, self-hate and self-defence mechanisms.

Lauterbach (1984) points to the feeling of the unemployed not to be able to control negative life events. Self-stigmatization has also been reported as a personal way to deal with unemployment (Grau and Thomsen 1984; Kreehan 1978).

Comparing employed and unemployed, Infratest finds a lower achievement motivation and a higher expectation of failure among the latter. During unemployment, the achievement motivation increases smoothly (Büchtemann and von Rosenbladt 1988).

Most evidence has been gathered on the linkage between unemployment and depression. Based on the depression model of Seligmann and his concept of 'learned helplessness', Mohr and Frese (1981) are doing particular research on this relationship. Their hypotheses are: unemployment leads to depression; unemployment leads to a subjective feeling of non-control; and there is a relationship between non-control and depression.

After checking these hypotheses in the existing literature, a longitudinal study (with only a few interviewees, though) showed that unemployment evoked depressive states of health (Frese 1979; Frese and Mohr 1979; Mohr and Frese 1981), which are "characterized by passivity, resignation, planlessness, apathy, hopelessness, missing self-confidence, feeling of worthlessness and the like" (Frese and Mohr 1977). The average unemployed seems to be in a state of medium depression, which means that a considerable number of unemployed is very depressive and in need of clinical treatment (Frese and Mohr 1977; Thomann 1983 a). There is a strong relationship between the financial situation and depression (Frese and Mohr 1977). Long-term unemployment contributes to depression (Frese and Mohr 1977). "Long-term unemployment or renewed unemployment leads to heavy depression in the case of persons who still long to be able to control their future, whereas people who have lost this hope or desire are no longer heavily affected by long-term unemployment or new unemployment" (Frese 1979). Depression lessens when a new job is found or pension is granted (in Bochumer Sozialmedizinische Forschung 1984). Other studies have so far not revealed such trends (Bonss et al. 1984); Balz (1984) using the same Zung scale on depression, could not find significant differences between unemployed and employed.

As depression is one of the main causes of suicide (Frese and Mohr 1977), an increased suicide rate caused by unemployment should be expected. But John (1982) using macro-data, could not support this thesis. Friessem (1980) also

doubts that there is a linkage between suicide and unemployment, while others –
rather hypothetically – assume that occupational conflicts (i.e. also unemployment) play an important role, e.g. for male suicidals (Bauer et al. 1976).

A further deterioration, caused by unemployment, of the health status of
mentally ill people is reported by Bastiaan et al. (1980): for 37.2% the disease was
protracted, for 30.8% new psychic problems developed, and for 26.9% the treatment period had to be prolonged. Only in the case of 32.1% of the affected, no
additional effects could be found. Work can be a therapy for the mentally ill
(Bastiaan et al. 1980).

The emotional health of the unemployed is closely related to their financial
problems (Frese and Mohr 1977) as well as to their income-oriented attitude
towards work (Bochumer Sozialmedizinische Forschung 1984). In contrast to
that, Fröhlich (1983a) states that only work attitude is a significant factor of
psycho-social strain, but not so (as an indicator of economic deprivation) consumer behaviour. Personality variables such as individual strategies of management, ability to activate social support, openness and help-seeking behaviour,
help to moderate the effects (Kieselbach 1984a).

To understand the different phases of the emotional affection by unemployment, models are rarely used. However, in its initial phase – as was shown by
Brinkmann and Potthoff (1983) – unemployment is felt quite strongly as a mental
strain in terms of low morale, inner nervousness, and fear of the future. This is
particularly true for young unemployed males when compared to an employed
control group. According to Strotzka and Leitner (1969), flash-in-the-pan effects
can be seen in the case of emotionally unstable people. Later on, psycho-social
strain seems to lessen, yet this may be an artificial effect of statistics as
housewives and pensioners retreat from unemployment (Brinkmann 1981). In
the end, psycho-social burdens seem to increase again, though less for the long-
term unemployed than for those who lost their job several times (Büchtemann
1983). Due to the steadily diminishing chance of success for their own activities,
the long-term unemployed show clearly marked phases of reaction (Hentschel et
al. 1977). Wacker speaks of a special sequence: shock, optimism, pessimism,
fatalism (Deutsche Gesellschaft für Sozialpsychiatrie 1978).

As early as in the 1930s, some typologies of the unemployed were developed
distinguishing, for instance, between apathetic and stable personalities among
the unemployed (Bonss et al. 1984). WAL (1976) has not found any clear-cut
types of unemployed, whereas Heinemann (1978) has constructed the following
typology of activities of the young unemployed: instrumental-economical
oriented type of activity, interest oriented type of activity, self-value oriented type
of activity, social oriented type of activity, and leisure time oriented type of activity. In his action research with unemployed youths, Opaschowski (in Wacker
1981a) develops the following typology: the hopeful, about 10%; the apathical,
about 10%; the pragmatical, about 50%; the resigned, about 30%.

In 1978, the associations of German psychologists concluded: "Tendencies
towards 'giving up oneself' are strengthened (by unemployment), especially in the
area of addiction; attempts of suicide and depressive symptoms increase. A mul-
titude of other psychological strains and impairments are also worsened by the
effects of unemployment" (in Kieselbach and Offe 1979a). In contrast to this,

other research comes to somewhat milder results; it is unclear, however, whether this is only further evidence of the non-effect problem of evaluation research.

Unemployment and Social Well-Being

Usually, the employment of time, the degree of social isolation and of social prestige are the crucial criteria for assessing the social well-being of unemployed (Frese and Mohr 1977; Brenner and Schwefel 1983; Windolf and Klemm 1981; Fröhlich 1979). Again, a complex of psycho-social strains, rather than a series of individual social strains, has to be dealt with (Brinkmann 1976).

Fröhlich (1983a) has found that unemployed more often intensify social contacts (41%), instead of reducing them (17%). Brinkmann (1984c) points out that adult unemployed experience the social strains of unemployment – even those that affect other members of the household – as more pressing than the financial burden (see also Kieselbach and Offe 1979a). Additionally, a higher rate of trouble and conflict is found in the families of unemployed (Bonss et al. 1984). In contrast to that, Fröhlich (1983b) argues that unemployment actualizes problems of partnership, but does not create them.

Obviously, the time consumption pattern of unemployed changes during unemployment, but the results of research on this are contradictory (Fröhlich 1983b; Heinemann 1982).

Increasing financial constraints change the life style of unemployed. Sometimes, with no social net given they find themselves on the verge of starvation (Bonss and Heinze 1984; Beckmann and Hahn 1983).

Some studies deal with the question as to whether and how the unemployed organize themselves; so far, the results have been rather disappointing (Morgenroth 1982).

Bahnmüller (1981a) shows that unemployment more often leads to an aversion strategy than to a conflict strategy; apparently, the unemployed do not tend to politicize. Likewise, Bonss et al. (1984) see an inclination towards adaptation, resignation and apathy, i.e. a trend to 'depoliticization', in times of mass unemployment. Unemployment has no great impact on political awareness and attitudes (Kieselbach and Offe 1979a). A great potential of conflict does not seem to exist among the unemployed (Bahnmüller 1981b). Unemployment does not activate the electoral behaviour of the concerned (Bürklin and Wiegand 1984).

Contrary to frequent allegations that young unemployed tend to criminal behaviour, there is no evidence at all of an increase of criminality as an effect of unemployment (Kieselbach 1983; Wacker 1981b).

There is an argument between Brinkmann and Fröhlich as to whether the unemployed welcome their situation as giving them more leisure time. Brinkmann and Spitznagel (1984) criticize Fröhlich for his retrospective study design and a biased sample. The fact that 37% of long-term unemployed say to have more time for their families, and 33% to have more time for things they like, may well be attributed to rationalizations (Bonss et al. 1984). On the other hand, unemployment – provided a minimum of social security is given – might also be experienced as a liberation from labour and the routine of daily life (Bonss et al. 1984).

Financial Effects of Unemployment

There are quite a few intriguing studies on economic deprivation during unemployment (Hentschel et al. 1979), but occasionally the tendency is to play down the "actual processes of impoverishment" (Bonss et al. 1984). The financial problems of some unemployed are, despite a basic level of material security, astonishingly high (Brinkmann 1984a; Frese and Mohr 1977). As a maximum, the unemployed receive benefits which amount to about 62% of their last net income (singles about 7.5% less), and this is for a period of 12 months only (Kieselbach and Offe 1979a).

Fifty percent of the unemployed receive unemployment benefits, about 16% are only entitled to unemployment relief, and 34% get no subsidy at all (Bonss et al. 1984). According to Hentschel, 40% of the unemployed (according to Fröhlich 1979: 34%) have severe economic problems. Of long-term unemployed, 39% pay bills late or are indebted (Institut für Arbeitsmarkt- und Berufsforschung der Bundesanstalt für Arbeit 1984). Savings are used up (Brinkmann 1976). Attempts to cut down on expenditure are mostly made in the area of durable consumer goods and of high quality products. The longer unemployment lasts, the more areas of consumption are affected (Brinkmann and Spitznagel 1984). First, expenses for holidays, cars, etc. are reduced (Bahnmüller 1981b), then for clothing and, in 20% of the cases, even for food (Hillen 1971). As for the latter, most savings relate to the quality and diversity of food as well as to the frequency of eating out (Wacker 1983). Still, for most of the long-term unemployed, the risk not to subsist in terms of housing, nutrition and clothing seems actually not to be immediate and overwhelming (Bonss et al. 1984). "The financial burdens of long-term unemployment are generally not heavier than those of short-term unemployment, as is often alleged" (Brinkmann 1981). 30% of the unemployed have financial difficulties already in the initial phase of their unemployment (Brinkmann 1981).

The risk of impoverishment tends to increase with unemployment (Heinze et al. 1981). In German-speaking countries, only very few studies deal with the extent and impact of poverty on health (Brennecke 1980; Hauser et al. 1981). Brennecke (1980) shows that the spectrum of health complaints is different for poor and rich people. The poor suffer more from exhaustion, tiredness, sleeplessness, colds and kidney diseases, the rich more frequently have diabetes, digestive trouble, cardiovascular diseases and hypertension. There seems to be a U-shaped relationship between complaints and poverty/wealth (Brennecke 1980).

Problem Groups

As the results of unemployment research are generally too diverse to be consistent, it seems wise to develop typologies of the unemployed and to concentrate the investigations on specific 'problem groups' among them.

Social and Mental Problem Groups

Several studies speak of cumulative unemployment (Blanke et al. 1984) or of a "cumulative reinforcement of social inequality in terms of opportunities and risks at the labour market" (Büchtemann 1984). Apparently, unemployment is the burden of specific groups in society. The unequal distribution of labour market risks among different social groups is accompanied by unequal capabilities to manage without employment, constituting, for example, different mental groups (Büchtemann 1984; Heinze 1984).

In the main, these groups are composed of elderly and young, foreign, disabled and less qualified employed persons (Büchtemann 1984; Oehlke 1979). Health problems are more often found in blue-collar than in white-collar workers, more in single than married women, and more often among the elderly than the middle-aged unemployed (Büchtemann and von Rosenbladt 1981). Cumulative unemployment especially hits the sick (Büchtemann 1982c). 'One-sided cumulation of burdens' is characteristic of long-term unemployed (Büchtemann and von Rosenbladt 1981). Long-term unemployed weighs most heavily on men, individuals between 45–55 years of age, singles, and young people (Bonss et al. 1984).

According to Opaschowski (1976), some segments of the unemployed become problem groups as a consequence of their specific personality, e.g. the resigned and the apathical unemployed.

Unemployed Youth

About 10% of the unemployed are youth under 20 years of age (Wiemer 1981). There is no room here to report on the determinants, and the extent, of youth unemployment; only some effects will be mentioned.

According to Wilhelm-Reiss (in Bochumer Sozialmedizinische Forschung 1984), young unemployed are more aggressive and have more psychosomatic symptoms than young people in training courses. The Hamborn Project found a continued change from more positive to more negative attitudes in young unemployed; it also showed a tendency towards isolation, increased money instead of job orientation, and towards the family as a possible retreat (Wilhelm-Reiss 1980). Compared with young employed, unemployed youths "are more handicapped in somatic and psychosomatic terms, are more depressive and doubtful, more reactive, aggressive, less open to contacts and social affairs" (Wilhelm-Reiss 1980).

The impact of youth unemployment on physical health is rarely mentioned in the literature. Interestingly enough, more than 8% of school leavers have health impairments "which have to be regarded as factors that reduce their capacity of physical work"; postural disorders of the spine and various other anomalies of the skeletal system in addition to visual impairment and vegetative disablements (Aldinger-Mosseanu 1978).

There are parallel developments between increasing youth unemployment and an increased consumption of hazardous, illegal drugs by young people

(Bschor 1984). The empirical evidence of the proletarization of drug consumption as well as the theoretical assumption of a declining capability to consciously plan for the future lead Schneider and Weber (1982) to the conclusion that young unemployed become easily disoriented and are highly inclined to misuse drugs. Misuse of alcohol and drugs in the context of unemployment is often assumed (Engelland 1983; Prager 1977). Henkel (1984) finds the highest percentage of people who run the risk of becoming alcoholics in young unemployed. In contrast to this, the Hamborn Project did not find any escape into alcoholism, drug consumption or criminality (Opaschowski 1976).

"Spectacular forms of deviant behaviour such as organizing gangs, alcoholism and criminality" are frequently assumed (Wilhelm-Reiss 1980). Youth unemployment and criminality, however, are no cause-effect relationships but are parallel developments only (Heinemann 1978). The analysis of official statistics does not reveal any relationship between unemployment and criminality among young people (Prager 1977).

Youth unemployment changes self-esteem (Wilhelm-Reiss 1980) and leads to a somatization of conflict management (Engelland 1983).

Unemployed youth more often show boredom, helplessness, doubtfulness and hopelessness (Müller-Limmroth 1977; Börjes 1975). Boredom affects unemployed young women less than men (Opaschowski 1976).

In young age, unemployment is a permanent situation of high individual stress (Grundnig 1980). It blocks personal development (Bilden et al. 1981) and generates, at least for some, an irreversible retardation of the process of becoming socially mature (Opaschowski 1976).

Unemployed Women

Whether negative impacts of unemployment are particularly strong for women, is a moot point (Brinkmann and Potthoff 1983; Gnegel and Mohr 1982; Dobberthien 1977; Schoeps 1975; Westphal-Georgi 1983). After a phase of felt relief from the previous double burden, their sense of self-worth decreases markedly, and resignation grows in extrovert persons (Heinemann et al. 1983). Resignative moods are typical at the beginning of unemployment (Heinemann et al. 1983). Female singles are especially affected (Heinemann et al. 1983). Long-term unemployment furthers the acceptance of 'traditional role playing'; in the end, those women do no longer regard themselves as being unemployed (Heinemann et al. 1983). "Not unemployment itself but the ... intended professional and family activities constitute the identity and mental conditions of women" (Heinemann et al. 1983).

Unemployed White-Collar Workers

Uncertain are the effects of unemployment on highly qualified and white-collar workers. Wuggenig found more social problems and emotional stress with persons of higher qualifications. Fröhlich (1983 a) shows that people of this category suffer less when unemployed (see also Wuggenig 1984). There seems to be a strong tendency among unemployed white collar-workers to hold on to a world of illusion (Windolf et al. 1979). Results of special research projects are still awaited (Windolf and Klemm 1981).

Unemployed Elderly

For most of the elderly, unemployment is the preliminary (last) stage of a hard and relatively underprivileged occupational career (Infratest 1980; see also Bäcker 1978; Bäcker and Naegele 1981; Brinkmann 1979). For them, once dismissed, long-term unemployment is typical; they clearly show chronic diseases, caused by physical attrition (Infratest 1980). "Large differences between the unemployed and employed elderly can be shown as to health status and the deterioration of work capacity. Old employees with relatively poor health are highly likely to become unemployed. About two-thirds of the interviewed unemployed stated that they suffered from heavy chronic diseases – rheumatism, spinal, gastric, cardiac and circulatory disorders, etc. – during the last three months; these can be interpreted as a symptom of a continued deterioration of their individual working power" (Infratest 1980). "Older unemployed and/or unemployed having health problems who take over a new job after unemployment, are frequently forced to accept incisive professional losses for their reintegration into the work force. Especially for the older, not healthy unemployed, ... reemployment often coincides with a change of profession and branch of business, professional decline and dequalification" (Infratest 1980).

Children of the Unemployed

The impact of unemployment on family members, especially children, was dealt with much more intensively in the 1930s than today. Then it was found out that children of unemployed, as compared to employed parents "more often and more severely developed nervous symptoms, hyper-sensibility and functional impairments without clear organic causes" (Schneider 1932). The only topical research project of recent date revealed that 14–16 year-old school boys and girls of unemployed parents showed considerable differences in terms of psychologic symptoms, yet very low differences in their motivation to learn, and no differences as to the problem of professional orientation, when compared with children of employed parents (Schindler and Wetzels 1984). Another study shows that unemployment reduces the rate of participation in prevention programmes (Thiele 1983). It must be stated that the indirect effects of unemployment are underinvestigated. Results of macro-level studies on the link between unemployment and infant mortality suggest that research on this problem group should be much more intensive (John 1983; Schindler 1979; Zenke and Ludwig 1984).

Short-Time Workers

Short-time workers are not identical with part-time unemployment. "They do not differ much from the employed with a normal working time pattern. The tendency is rather a positive one: They seem to benefit from additional leisure time in contrast to the unemployed" (Vagt and Stavemann 1980). However, systematic and comprehensive analyses of the health effects of short-time work are still missing.

Diagnosis

Some of the main results can be summarized below.

Unemployment and overwork can induce similar psychosomatic impairments (Müller-Limmroth 1977); the obvious afflictions caused by unemployment should not lead to overlook those caused by employment. In both cases, the effects of stressors are considerably modified by personal capabilities to manage the situation.

More than 20% of the unemployed – in some groups up to 35% – regard unemployment as 'not so bad' (Brinkmann 1976). "Nevertheless, the manifold problems of the overwhelming part of the unemployed should not be disregarded even if some unemployed, including long-term unemployed, see some aspects of unemployment in a positive way" (Brinkmann 1984c).

Compared with the massive impoverishment in the 1930s, stress and distress seem to be much less for today's unemployed (Bonss et al. 1984); unemployment is rarely felt as a catastrophe or vital threat (Fröhlich 1979, 1983b; Niess 1979). Comparing the 1930s and the 1970s–1980s, Jahoda (1983b) speaks of a change from absolute physical deprivation to only relative damages. The unemployed suffer from fewer physical health problems than was expected by many (Preiser 1979). Present research results are quite modest in comparison with the most prominent health effects of unemployment stated by Moses in 1931 (in Thomann 1981).

Normally, unemployment causes more financial and psychological than physical burdens (Brinkmann and Spitznagel 1984). "Certainly, we cannot assume that unemployment always and necessarily leads to health disturbances. Financial constraints and psychosocial stress during unemployment play an important role, but vary depending on the individual case" (Brinkmann and Potthoff 1983).

Comparisons with the situation of the 1930s are misleading, as they disregard the process in social security that has taken place in Europe. At least in relative terms, there is a process of degradation and demoralization affecting the unemployed (Kieselbach 1984b; Wacker 1981a). However grave the health impacts may be, the unemployed have to carry their consequences individually, although they may not be personally blamed for their unemployment situation (Schwefel and Schwefel 1973). The right to work implies the right to physical and mental integrity (Frese and Mohr 1977). The latter might well be limited by the effects of both employment and unemployment.

Therapies

Proposals for a strategy to overcome unemployment or to smoothen its effects may look quite limited at present. There are too many open questions about the causes of unemployment and, therefore, about the right way to deal with it. Reform of a single institution or a single sector will certainly not help to overcome the problems cost-effectively.

Policies

Activities to combat unemployment or to soften its effects have to start on different levels: creation of new jobs, 'fair' distribution of work and working hours among the members of society, economic relief for the deprived and overburdened, minimization of physical and mental impairments caused by employment as well as unemployment. The need to change the organization of labour and to cut down the working hours seems to be inevitable (Kaiser and Westmüller 1978). Short-term employment schemes may rather lead to the construction of Keynesian pyramids than to a solution of the problem.

Case-oriented social policies are needed, as for example:

- Securing jobs for underprivileged groups (Heinemann 1978)
- Stop-gap relief in critical life situations for those members of problem groups who suffer most (Kieselbach 1983)
- Deployment of unemployed in social services which are labour intensive and need personnel (Blanke et al. 1984)
- Creation of, and support for, a second labour market (Blanke et al. 1984)
- Measures to facilitate the mobility of people (Siegrist and Wunderli 1982)
- Reform of the rules of 'reasonableness': when assessing the acceptability of professional degradation for re-employed people, the demands of the new job have to be taken into account, both in regard to the present state of health of the re-employed and to the long-term consequences on health and work performance
- Special programmes for the reintegration of the unemployed elderly to help them overcome their occupational isolation (Siegrist and Wunderli 1982)

Quite a number of organizations offer training programmes to improve job opportunities by requalification, further education and personality training (Beckmann and Hahn 1982; Hofbauer and Dadzio 1982; Siegrist and Wunderli 1982; Siegrist 1979, 1984). Most prominent are schemes of additional qualification as well as social-pedagogical and psychological training programmes to enhance self-management abilities on the cognitive, social, emotional and motivational level (Böhnisch and Schmitz 1978; Hockel and Kolb 1981). Such offers are used more frequently by unemployed middle-class people than by those in more urgent need of support (Kieselbach 1984 b).

In view of the labour market situation, such training programmes often lead to quite unrealistic hopes (Frese and Mohr 1978). West German associations of psychology therefore recommend political rather than psychological solutions (Kieselbach and Offe 1979 b).

Health Policies

In times of economic crisis and increasing unemployment, the need for advice as well as the number of contacts with physicians increase (Strotzka and Leitner 1969). Simultaneously, the supply of specialized social services diminishes (Kieselbach 1984b). There has been a considerable decrease of rehabilitation measures per retired person since 1974 (Henkel 1982). But the most important dilemma concerns the possibilities of medical rehabilitation and the low chances of reintegration due to high chronic unemployment (Thomann 1984). The small labour market implies that psychiatric and psychosocial therapy has no real perspective in cases where work is needed as a means of rehabilitation (Bastiaan et al. 1980). On the other hand, schemes to improve qualification or measures of social support or therapy may provoke unrealistic expectations (Frese and Mohr 1979). Increasing the supply of consultation may also add to the individualization of the problems and even reinforce the stigmatization by unemployment (Kieselbach 1984b; Rabatsch 1978).

Surveys of physicians about the link between unemployment and health show that only a few physicians are interested in this topic, and that the relationship between unemployment and illness is unclear to many of them (Thomann 1983c). A more 'clinical' perception of the problem creates new tasks and more work for the helping professions (Kleiber 1984). Yet, instead of pursuing a need- and employment-oriented budget policy in order to increase the number of medical staff, social workers and trainers, the present policy is to reduce personnel. While demand and need increase, the awareness of the problems is small, and so is effective supply.

It is proposed that the health services of Austria, Switzerland and West Germany may improve their curative and preventive functions in the following ways:

A prerequisite is the information and training of health personnel with regard to the results of psychological and medical research on unemployment (Kieselbach 1983, 1984b; Thomann 1983c). The training of general practitioners, internists and gynaecologists would be particularly important. Knowledge of the need for, and the supply of, advice as well as of the facilities available for the training of the unemployed should enrich the spectrum of therapies offered by physicians.

"The sick-leave problem is mainly a problem of morbidity; an adequate solution, therefore, requires intensified efforts to improve health care. Of special importance would be a higher emphasis on rehabilitative and prophylactic measures against cardiac and muscular-skeletal disorders as well as psychogenic diseases" (Halusa 1983). This concerns not only office-based physicians but also the services of confidential medical officers, who are to guarantee early rehabilitation in cases of relapses.

Psychological prevention is recommended mainly for young (unemployed) people. Essentially, this means an improvement of the medical and psychological measures of prevention and care in (pre-)school age as well as further education for physicians who are in charge of monitoring the youth protection laws concerning employment and working conditions. Usually, these physicians have little knowledge of the particulars of vocational training and of the special requirements for working places of youth. Improvements in this area may yield some results in terms of prevention (Aldinger-Mosseanu 1978).

Healthy working conditions can be an important protection against early disablement. If it is true that the link between unemployment and health is, to a large extent, conditioned by the effects of hazardous jobs, then a prevention-oriented occupational medicine and 'humanization of work' seem to be essential (Scharf 1980 a–c).

The unemployed are in great need of advice; they badly need help (Brinkmann 1984c; Brinkmann and Potthoff 1983). If, as is proven, unemployment leads to depression, the unemployed is entitled to therapies like any other patient (Frese and Mohr 1979). Because the personal problems caused by unemployment vary from person to person, individual forms of consultation and care are needed, as are offered, e.g. in the 'health park' of the Munich Volkshochschule (Hockel 1984). Counselling should help persons to stabilize and reduce the effects of their situation (Böhnisch and Schmitz 1978). But advisory boards exclusively for the unemployed are not be recommended; rather, it would be cost-effective to have agencies that comprehensively deal with all psychosocial problems which develop in the context of family, alcoholism, drug consumption, unemployment and life management. To establish such services may not primarily be the task of the health care system but of voluntary organizations; the latter, however, need professional support from the former. Prevention of unemployment and its consequences may preferably take on the form of 'empowerment strategies' (Kieselbach 1984a).

The unemployed, especially the most affected, tend to self-isolation, quite a few to self-disclosure (Kieselbach 1984b). Psychosocial advice is not only needed by those who look for help (Kieselbach 1984b). For problem groups, e.g. the mentally ill, outreach ambulatory services are necessary (Bastiaan et al. 1980).

In times of economic decline, the consolidation of the institutions of rehabilitation is important (Bastiaan et al. 1980), likewise the extension of psychosocial advice in existing organizations (Kieselbach 1984b).

Preventive and curative measures against alcoholism and depression, and special assistance for the unemployed young and elderly seem to be the most cost-effective services the health sector can provide to reduce or, at least, smooth the effects of unemployment. One other problem group deserves special attention: the children of unemployed.

Self-Help

Self-help activities of adult unemployed are still rare; the same applies to initiatives of young unemployed (Brinkmann 1984c; Blanke et al. 1984; von Bargen 1982; Grottian and Paasch 1984). To the extent that organizations of the unemployed exist, nearly all of them – as surveys show – were created from outside (von Kardoff 1984). Centres for the unemployed are offered mostly by social religious or trade-union related organizations. They often have advisory services for health problems (Möller-Lücking 1983). Help for self-help seems to be the one essential measure of personal prevention against unemployment although this would mean a boost for the shadow economy.

Research

Intensified and more diversified research (see "Additional Literature") could be helpful to design cost-effective therapies to reduce, and to offer relief from, the effects of unemployment. It will be most important to design scientific models on how to possibly minimize the strain of work and the stress of unemployment, and how to change the human organization of labour and the social distribution of working time.

Acknowledgements. Originally this report was submitted to the Council of Europe, I wish to express my thanks to Mr. Franco Marziale at the Council for assistance and support. I also would like to thank Ms. Melitta Kullmann and Mr. Walter Satzinger for revising the English version.

References

Aldinger-Mosseanu G (1978) Jugendarbeitslosigkeit – sozialmedizinische Aspekte und psychosoziale Probleme. Kinderarzt 9:1045–1047

Bäcker G (1978) Beschäftigungsprobleme älterer Arbeitnehmer in der Bundesrepublik Deutschland – Ausprägungen und Ursachen. In: Dieck M, Naegele G (eds) Sozialpolitik für ältere Menschen. Heidelberg

Bäcker G, Naegele G (1981) Arbeitsmarkt, Altersgrenze und die Ausgliederung älterer Arbeitnehmer. WSI Mitt 34:679

Bahnmüller R (1981 a) Arbeitslose als politisches Konfliktpotential? In: Wacker A (ed) Vom Schock zum Fatalismus? Soziale und psychische Auswirkungen der Arbeitslosigkeit. Campus, Frankfort, pp 107–133

Bahnmüller R (1981 b) Die ohnmächtige Wut. Soziale Lage und gesellschaftliches Bewußtsein von männlichen Arbeitslosen mit qualifiziertem Berufsabschluß. Campus, Frankfort

Balz H-J (1984) Psychische Auswirkungen von Arbeitslosigkeit und Handlungsperspektiven – Erste Ergebnisse einer Längsschnittstudie. In: Kieselbach T, Leithäuser T, Wacker A (eds) Arbeitslosigkeit – Psychologische Theorie und Praxis. Symposium, University of Bremen

Bastiaan P, Kaiser E (1982) Arbeitslosigkeit und psychische Erkrankung. Sozialpsychiatr Inf 12:81–91

Bastiaan P, Kaiser E, Kuhr A, Rockstroh D, Wernado M, Wulff E (1980) Arbeitslosigkeit und psychische Erkrankung. In: Jantzen J (ed) Arbeit und Arbeitslosigkeit als pädagogisches und therapeutisches Problem. Pahl-Rugenstein, Cologne, pp 75–93

Bauer M et al. (1976) Psychiatrie, Psychosomatik, Psychotherapie. Stuttgart

Baumann U, Becker U, Gerstenmaier J, Schickle O, Tippelt R (1979) Handlungsperspektiven und politische Einstellungen arbeitsloser Jugendlicher. Campus, Frankfort (Forschung, vol 108)

Beckmann N, Hahn K-D (1982) Arbeitslosigkeit und Veränderungen im Lebensstil. Mitt Arb Markt Berufsforsch 15:69–77

Beckmann N, Hahn K-D (1983) Unemployment and life-style changes. In: John J, Schwefel D, Zöllner H (eds) Influence of economic instability on health. Springer, Berlin Heidelberg New York, pp 321–337

Bilden H, Diezinger A, Marquardt R, Dahlke K (1981) Arbeitslose junge Mädchen. Berufseinstieg, Familiensituation und Beziehungen zu Gleichaltrigen. Z Padag 27:677–695

Blanke B, Heinelt H, Macke C-W (1984) Arbeitslosigkeit und kommunale Sozialpolitik. In: Bonss W, Heinze RG (eds) Arbeitslosigkeit in der Arbeitsgesellschaft. Suhrkamp, Frankfort, pp 299–330

Bochumer Sozialmedizinische Forschung (ed) (1984) Belastungen der Gesundheit und Veränderungen im Gesundheits- und Krankheitsverhalten als Folge der Arbeitslosigkeit. Diskussionspapier zur Expertenbefragung. Bosofo, Bochum

Böcker W, Olk T, Otto HU (1976) Jugendarbeitslosigkeit: Reaktionen und Perspektiven der Sozialarbeit – Aspekte der Lebens- und Arbeitssituation Jugendlicher in der Krise. Neue Prax 6:124–153

Böhnisch L, Schmitz E (1978) Jugendarbeitslosigkeit heute: sozialpolitisch verschoben? Betrifft Erziehung 11(9):46–50

Böker K (1971) Entwicklung und Ursachen des Krankenstandes der westdeutschen Arbeiter. Argument 69:901–927

Bonss W, Heinze RG (1984) Arbeit, Lohnarbeit, ohne Arbeit. Zur Soziologie der Arbeitslosigkeit. In: Bonss W, Heinze RG (eds) Arbeitslosigkeit in der Arbeitsgesellschaft. Suhrkamp, Frankfort, pp 7–49

Bonss W, Keupp H, Koenen E (1984) Das Ende des Belastungsdiskurses? Zur subjektiven und gesellschaftlichen Bedeutung von Arbeitslosigkeit. In: Bonss W, Heinze RG (eds) Arbeitslosigkeit in der Arbeitsgesellschaft. Suhrkamp, Frankfort, pp 143–188

Börjes I (1975) Sind sie alle Versager? Was es für Jugendliche bedeutet, arbeitslos zu sein. Gewerksch Monatsh 26:576–579

Bosch G (1978) Arbeitsplatzverlust. Die sozialen Folgen einer Betriebsstillegung. Campus, Frankfort

Bosch G (1980) Erleben und Erfahren von Arbeitsplatzunsicherheit. In: Maiers W, Markard M (eds) Lieber arbeitslos als ausgebeutet? Pahl-Rugenstein, Cologne, pp 71–80

Boseke H, Spitzner A (eds) (1983) Jugend ohne Arbeit. Lamuv, Bornheim-Merten

Brandes V (1977) Arbeitslosigkeit in der Bundesrepublik. Erscheinungsformen, Auswirkungen, Verarbeitungsweisen und Abwehrperspektiven. In: Backhaus F et al. (eds) Gesellschaft. Frankfort, pp 197–245 (Beiträge zur Marxschen Theorie, vol 10)

Braun F, Weidacher A (1976) Materialien zur Arbeitslosigkeit und Berufsnot Jugendlicher. Munich

Brennecke R (1980) Armut, Gesundheitsbeschwerden und Inanspruchnahme von Gesundheitsleistungen. Sonderforschungsbereich 3, Goethe University Frankfort (Arbeitspapier no 32)

Brenner MH (1979) Wirtschaftskrisen, Arbeitslosigkeit und psychische Erkrankungen. Urban and Schwarzenberg, Munich

Brenner MH, Schwefel D (1983) Study on the influence of economic development on health. Report on the WHO Planning Meeting. In: John J, Schwefel D, Zöllner H (eds) Influence of economic instability on health. Springer, Berlin Heidelberg New York, pp 492–522

Brinkmann C (1976) Finanzielle und psycho-soziale Belastungen während der Arbeitslosigkeit. Mitt Arb Markt Berufsforsch 9:397–413

Brinkmann C (1977) Arbeitslosigkeit und Mobilität. Aus der Untersuchung des IAB über Ursachen und Auswirkungen von Arbeitslosigkeit. Mitt Arb Markt Berufsforsch 2:201–223

Brinkmann C (1978) Strukturen und Determinanten der beruflichen Wiedereingliederung von Langfristarbeitslosen. Mitt Arb Markt Berufsforsch 11:178–197

Brinkmann C (1979) Arbeitslosigkeit und berufliche Ausgliederung älterer und leistungsgeminderter Arbeitnehmer. Mitt Arb Markt Berufsforsch 4:517–524

Brinkmann C (1980) Zum Unterschied in der Erfassung von Arbeitslosen durch die Bundesanstalt für Arbeit und von Erwerbslosen im Mikrozensus. Beitr Arb Markt Berufsforsch 14:172

Brinkmann C (1981) Finanzielle und psycho-soziale Belastungen während der Arbeitslosigkeit. In: Wacker A (ed) Vom Schock zum Fatalismus? Campus, Frankfort, pp 57–91

Brinkmann C (1982) Behinderte und Leistungsgeminderte auf dem Arbeitsmarkt: Arbeitslosigkeit, berufliche Ein- und Ausgliederung, arbeitsmarktpolitische Perspektiven. In: Heinze RG, Runde P (eds) Lebensbedingungen Behinderter im Sozialstaat. Opladen, p 113

Brinkmann C (1983) Health problems and psychosocial strains of unemployed. A summary of recent empirical research in the FRG. In: John J, Schwefel D, Zöllner H (eds) Influence of economic instability on health. Springer, Berlin Heidelberg New York, pp 263–285

Brinkmann C (1984a) Financial, psycho-social and health problems associated with unemployment. Empirical findings and measures for their alleviation. Symposium on "The Future of Work: Challenge and Opportunity", London

Brinkmann C (1984b) Physical health and mental well-being of unemployed – results of a longitudinal survey in the Federal Republic of Germany. In: van Eimeren W et al. (eds) Third international conference on system science in health care. Springer, Berlin Heidelberg New York, pp 168–171

Brinkmann C (1984c) Psychosoziale und gesundheitliche Folgen der Arbeitslosigkeit – Ergebnisse einer repräsentativen Längsschnittuntersuchung. In: Kieselbach T, Leithäuser T, Wacker A (eds) Arbeitslosigkeit – Psychologische Theorie und Praxis. Symposium, University of Bremen

Brinkmann C, Potthoff P (1983) Gesundheitliche Probleme in der Eingangsphase der Arbeitslosigkeit. Mitt Arb Markt Berufsforsch 16:378–389

Brinkmann C, Schober K (1982) Methoden und erste Ergebnisse aus der Verlaufsuntersuchung des IAB bei Arbeitslosen (Zugänge November 1981). Mitt Arb Markt Berufsforsch 15:408–425

Brinkmann C, Spitznagel E (1984) Haushalt und Beschäftigungskrise. Frühjahrstagung des Fachausschusses „Strukturwandel des Haushalts", Königstein

Brödel R, Müller H-F, Pelte K, Popp W, Schirner H, Stockhausen M (1976) Die soziale Situation von Arbeitslosen und ihr Verhältnis zur Weiterbildung – Zwischenergebnisse einer empirischen Untersuchung. Göttingen

Bschor F (1984) Recent trends in fatalities amongst young Berliners: suicides, drug addicts, traffic accidents. Medis-WHO-Meeting "Underlying Processes of Becoming Socially Vulnerable", Munich

Büchtemann CF (1982a) Arbeitsbelastungen, Arbeitsverschleiß und Arbeitslosigkeitsrisiko. In: Hauss F (ed) Arbeitsmedizin und präventive Gesundheitspolitik. Campus, Frankfort, pp 225–244

Büchtemann CF (1982b) Erwerbskarrieren im Anschluß an Arbeitslosigkeit. Ergebnisse einer Zwischenerhebung zum Verbleib der Arbeitslosen und Abgänger aus Arbeitslosigkeit vom Herbst 1977 drei Jahre später. Mitt Arb Markt Berufsforsch 15:120–130

Büchtemann CF (1982c) Gesundheitszustand und Arbeitslosigkeit: Zum Zusammenhang von Gesundheits- und Arbeitsmarktrisiken. In: Schmidt M et al. (eds) Arbeit und Gesundheitsgefährdung. Frankfort

Büchtemann CF (1983) Infratest Sozialforschung: Die Bewältigung von Arbeitslosigkeit im zeitlichen Verlauf 1978–1982. Bundesministerium für Arbeit und Sozialordnung, Bonn (Reihe Sozialforschung, vol 85)

Büchtemann CF (1984) Der Arbeitslosigkeitsprozeß. Theorie und Empirie strukturierter Arbeitslosigkeit in der BRD. In: Bonss W, Heinze RG (eds) Arbeitslosigkeit in der Arbeitsgesellschaft. Suhrkamp, Frankfort, pp 55–105

Büchtemann CF, von Rosenbladt B (1981) Arbeitslose 1978: die Situation in der Arbeitslosigkeit. Mitt Arb Markt Berufsforsch 14:22–28

Burger A, Seidenspinner G, Weidacher A (1976) Jugendarbeitslosigkeit im Spiegel der Betroffenen. WSI Mitt 29:115–122

Bürklin WP, Wiegand J (1984) Arbeitslosigkeit und Wahlverhalten. In: Bonss W, Heinze RG (eds) Arbeitslosigkeit in der Arbeitsgesellschaft. Suhrkamp, Frankfort, pp 273–297

Demokratisches Gesundheitswesen (1983) Arbeitslos. Demokrat Gesundheitswes 1:8–23

Dennerlein R, Schneider M (1984) Ist der Rückgang des Krankenstandes eine Folge von Entlassungen und Frühverrentung? Soz Fortschr 33:226–229

Deuermeir W, Sawalies D (1978) Psychische Auswirkungen der Jugendarbeitslosigkeit – der Einfluß der Kontrollerwartung und der Kausalattribuierung auf die individuelle Verarbeitung. Diploma thesis, University of Giessen

Deutsche Gesellschaft für Sozialpsychiatrie (1978) Stellungnahme zum Problem der Arbeitslosigkeit aus der Sicht von Organisationen der psychosozialen Versorgung. In: Forum kritische Psychologie, vol 3. Argument, Berlin, pp 205–208

Dobberthien M (1977) Probleme der Frauenarbeitslosigkeit, dargestellt am Beispiel Baden-Württembergs. WSI Mitt 8:519–538

Dombois R et al. (1982) Vom Heuern und Feuern zur stabilen Mindestbelegschaft – drei Jahrzehnte betrieblicher Beschäftigungspolitik eines Schiffsbauunternehmens. Mehrwert 23

Eichenhofer H (1979) Jugendarbeitslosigkeit im Saarland. Ursachen und Folgen. ArbSkam. Saarl 27:354–358

Eichenhofer H, Peter R, Treinen H (1980) Ursachen und Folgen der Jugendarbeitslosigkeit im Saarland. Arbeitskammer des Saarlandes, Saarbrücken

Engelland R (1983) „Jugendprobleme" und „Jugendpolitik" angesichts wachsender Jugendarbeitslosigkeit. Soz Fortschr 32:241–282

Freiburghaus D (1978) Dynamik der Arbeitslosigkeit. Hain, Meisenheim

Frese M (1979) Arbeitslosigkeit, Depressivität und Kontrolle: eine Studie mit Wiederholungsmessung. In: Kieselbach T, Offe H (eds) Arbeitslosigkeit. Individuelle Verarbeitung. Gesellschaftlicher Hintergrund. Steinkopff, Darmstadt, pp 222–257

Frese M (1984) Zur Verlaufsstruktur der psychischen Auswirkungen von Arbeitslosigkeit. In: Kieselbach T, Leithäuser T, Wacker A (eds) Arbeitslosigkeit – Psychologische Theorie und Praxis. Symposium, University of Bremen

Frese M, Mohr G (1977) Die psychischen Folgen von Arbeitslosigkeit: Depression bei älteren Arbeitslosen. WSI Mitt 11:674–679

Frese M, Mohr G (1978) Die psychopathologischen Folgen des Entzugs von Arbeit: der Fall Arbeitslosigkeit. In: Frese M, Greif S, Semmer N (eds) Industrielle Psychopathologie. Huber, Stuttgart, pp 282–320

Frese M, Mohr G (1979) Soziale Maßnahmen für Arbeitslose: Überlegungen im Rahmen einer psychologischen Untersuchung. Psychosozial 1:22–34

Friessem D (1980) Psychische Folgen von Arbeitslosigkeit unter besonderer Berucksichtigung psychiatrischer Erkankungen und des Suizids. In: Maiers W, Markard M (eds) Lieber arbeitslos als ausgebeutet? Pahl-Rugenstein, Cologne, pp 53–63

Fröhlich D (1979) Psycho-soziale Folgen der Arbeitslosigkeit. Eine empirische Untersuchung in Nordrhein-Westfalen. Verein zur Förderung des Instituts zur Erforschung sozialer Chancen, Cologne (Report no 23)

Fröhlich D (1983a) Economic deprivation, work orientation and health conceptual ideas and some empirical findings. In: John J, Schwefel D, Zöllner H (eds) Influence of economic instability on health. Springer, Berlin Heidelberg New York, pp 293–317

Fröhlich D (1983b) The use of time during unemployment. A case study carried out in West Germany. Van Gorcum, Assen

Gerstenmaier J (1979) Selbstakzeptanz, Autoritarismus und politische Handlungsbereitschaft arbeitsloser Jugendlicher. In: Baumann V et al. (eds) Handlungsperspektiven und politische Einstellungen arbeitsloser Jugendlicher. Campus, Frankfort, pp 49–78

Gnegel A, Mohr G (1982) Wenn Frauen ihren Arbeitsplatz verlieren. In: Mohr G, Rummel M, Rückert D (eds) Frauen. Psychologische Beiträge zur Arbeits- und Lebenssituation. Urban and Schwarzenberg, Munich, pp 88–102

Goldberg J, Günther B, Jung H (1977) Arbeitslosigkeit. Ursachen – Entwicklung – Alternativen. Frankfort

Gölter G (1977) Begleiter der Arbeitslosigkeit: Abstieg und Armut. Dokumentation zur wirtschaftlichen Lage der Arbeitslosen in der Bundesrepublik Deutschland. Ministerium für Soziales, Gesundheit und Sport, Rheinland-Pfalz, Mainz

Grau U, Thomsen K (1984) Zur Rolle des Arbeitslosen – Attribuierung des Vorwurfs der Arbeitsunwilligkeit. In: Kieselbach T, Leithäuser T, Wacker A (eds) Arbeitslosigkeit – Psychologische Theorie und Praxis. Symposium, University of Bremen

Grottian P, Paasch R (1984) Arbeitslose: Von der gesellschaftlichen Randgruppe zum politischen Faktor? In: Bonss W, Heinze RG (eds) Arbeitslosigkeit in der Arbeitsgesellschaft. Suhrkamp, Frankfort, pp 331–348

Grundnig J (1980) Jugendarbeitslosigkeit als permanente individuelle Überforderungssituation. In: Maiers W, Markard M (eds) Lieber arbeitslos als ausgebeutet? Pahl-Rugenstein, Cologne, pp 139–150

Halusa G (1983) Zur Regulation des Krankenstandes: Kontrolle und Gesundheitssicherung. Bundesministerium für Forschung und Technologie, Bonn (Forschungsbericht Teil II, GKV 06. Vorhaben: Berliner Krankenstand)

Harten H-C (1980) Jugendarbeitslosigkeit und politische Sozialisation. In: Claussen B (ed) Politische Sozialisation in Theorie und Praxis. Reinhardt, Munich, pp 201–223

Hauser R, Cremer-Schäfer H, Nouvertne U (1981) Armut, Niedrigeinkommen und Unterversorgung in der Bundesrepublik Deutschland. Bestandsaufnahme und sozialpolitische Perspektiven. Frankfort

Heinemann K (1978) Arbeitslose Jugendliche. Ursachen und individuelle Bewältigung eines sozialen Problems. Eine empirische Untersuchung. Luchterhand, Darmstadt

Heinemann K (1982) Arbeitslosigkeit und Zeitbewußtsein. Soz Welt 33:87–101

Heinemann K, Röhrig P, Stadie R (1983) Arbeitslose Frauen. Zwischen Erwerbstätigkeit und Hausfrauenrolle. Eine empirische Untersuchung. Beltz, Weinheim

Heinze RG (1984) Soziale Strukturierung der Arbeitslosigkeit: Auf dem Weg zu einer gespaltenen Gesellschaft? In: Bonss W, Heinze RG (eds) Arbeitslosigkeit in der Arbeitsgesellschaft. Suhrkamp, Frankfort, pp 106–142

Heinze RG, Hinrichs K, Hohn H-W, Olk T (1981) Armut und Arbeitsmarkt: Zum Zusammenhang von Klassenlagen und Verarmungsrisiken im Sozialstaat. Z Soz 10:219–243

Henkel D Arbeitslosigkeit und Alkoholismus: empirische Zusammenhänge und Analysen. Manuscript

Henkel D (1982) Frühinvalidität und Rehabilitation bei psychisch Kranken in der Rentenversicherung von 1968 bis 1979. Sozialpsychiatr Inf 12:92–104

Henkel D, Kleiber D, Roer D (1983) Arbeitslosigkeit und Alkoholismus aus epidemiologischer, ätiologischer und rehabilitativer Sicht. Suchtgefahren 29:233–245

Henkel D (1984) Arbeitslosigkeit als psychosozialer Risikofaktor von Alkoholgefährdung und Alkoholismus. In: Kieselbach T, Leithäuser R, Wacker A (eds) Arbeitslosigkeit – Psychologische Theorie und Praxis. Symposium, University of Bremen

Hentschel U (1981) Politische Einstellungen von Arbeitslosen. In: Wacker A (ed) Vom Schock zum Fatalismus? Campus, Frankfort, pp 92–106

Hentschel U, Möller C, Pintar R (eds) (1977) Zur Lage der Arbeitslosen in Nordrhein-Westfalen. Eine erste Darstellung. Cologne

Hentschel U, Möller C, Pintar R (1979) Zur Lage der Arbeitslosen in Nordrhein-Westfalen. Eine erste Darstellung und Interpretation von Befragungsergebnissen. Verein zur Förderung des Instituts zur Erforschung sozialer Chancen, Cologne (Report no 11)

Hertel G, Holland A (1984) Konkrete Probleme durch Arbeitslosigkeit im Zusammenhang mit stationärer Psychotherapie in einer psychosomatischen Klinik. In: Kieselbach T, Leithäuser R, Wacker A (eds) Arbeitslosigkeit – Psychologische Theorie und Praxis. Symposium, University of Bremen

Hillen KB (1971) Arbeitnehmer nach einem Arbeitsplatzverlust. Opladen

Hockel M (1984) Psychosoziale Betreuung Arbeitsloser in Institutionen der Erwachsenenbildung. In: Kieselbach T, Leithäuser R, Wacker A (eds) Arbeitslosigkeit – Psychologische Theorie und Praxis. Symposium, University of Bremen

Hockel M, Kolb W (1981) Prävention bei Risikozielgruppen: Das Beispiel langzeitig Arbeitsloser. In: Hockel M, Feldhege FJ (eds) Behandlung und Gesundheit. Munich, pp 1243–1264 (Handbuch der angewandten Psychologie, vol 2)

Hoelzle W (1977) Psychologische Probleme der Arbeitslosigkeit bei Jugendlichen. Ein empirisch-kasuistischer Beitrag zur Situation des arbeitslosen Jugendlichen unter besonderer Berücksichtigung der Veränderungen im Erleben und Verhalten. Naturwissenschaftliche Fakultät, University of Salzburg

Hofbauer H, Dadzio W (1982) Die Wirksamkeit von Maßnahmen zur Verbesserung der Vermittlungsaussichten für Arbeitslose nach § 41 a AFG. Mitt Arb Markt Berufsforsch 15:426–433

Hoppe W (1981) Statistik – richtig oder falsch? Zur Mißbrauchs-Diskussion um Arbeitslosmeldung und AFG-Leistungen. Soz Fortschr 30:97–103

Infratest Sozialforschung/Wirtschaftsforschung, Sögel W (1978a) Arbeitssuche, berufliche Mobilität, Arbeitsvermittlung und -beratung. Bundesministerium für Arbeit und Sozialordnung, Bonn (Reihe Sozialforschung, vol 5)

Infratest Sozialforschung (1978b) Teilprojekt 1: Repräsentativbefragung von Arbeitslosen und Abgängern aus Arbeitslosigkeit, Materialbd I/2. Infratest, Munich

Infratest Sozialforschung (1978c) Teilprojekt 2: Repräsentativbefragung zur Fortbildungs- und Mobilitätsbereitschaft beschäftigter Arbeitnehmer, Materialbd 5. Infratest, Munich

Infratest Wirtschaftsforschung (1978d) Teilprojekt 3: Repräsentativbefragung von Arbeitgebern, Materialbd 3. Infratest, Munich

Infratest Wirtschaftsforschung (1978e) Teilprojekt 4: Repräsentativbefragung von Vermittlern, Materialbd 4. Infratest, Munich

Infratest Sozialforschung (1980) Arbeitnehmer in der Spätphase ihrer Erwerbstätigkeit. Teilprojekt: Ältere Arbeitslose. Sekundäranalysen. Infratest, Munich

Institut für Arbeitsmarkt- und Berufsforschung der Bundesanstalt für Arbeit (1984) Zur finanziellen Situation von Langfristarbeitslosen: Arbeitslose gut 1 ½ Jahre nach dem Zugang. IAB-Kurzbericht. IAB, Nürnberg

Jahoda M (1983 a) Die sozialpsychologische Bedeutung von Arbeit und Arbeitslosigkeit. In: Jahoda M, Kieselbach T, Leithäuser T (eds) Arbeit, Arbeitslosigkeit und Persönlichkeitsentwicklung, Reihe A. Psychologische Forschungsberichte, University of Bremen (Bremer Beiträge zur Psychologie no 23)

Jahoda M (1983 b) Wieviel Arbeit braucht der Mensch? Arbeit und Arbeitslosigkeit im 20. Jahrhundert. Beltz, Weinheim

John J (1982) Health and economic instability: infant mortality and suicide reconsidered. WHO Workshop on Health Policy in Relation to Unemployment in the Community, Leeds

John J (1983) Economic instability and mortality in the Federal Republic of Germany. Problems of macroanalytical approach with special reference to migration. In: John J, Schwefel D, Zöllner H (eds) Influence of economic instability on health. Springer, Berlin Heidelberg New York, pp 113–138

John J, Schwefel D, Zöllner H (eds) (1983) Influence of economic instability on health. Springer, Berlin Heidelberg New York

Kaiser K, Westmüller H (1978) Probleme der Arbeitslosigkeit und das Ziel eines Neuen Lebensstils. In: Wenke KE, Zilleben H (eds) Neuer Lebensstil – Verzichten oder verändern? Wiesbaden, pp 220–247

Karr W (1983) Anmerkungen zur Arbeitslosigkeit in der nunmehr 10 Jahre dauernden Beschäftigungskrise. Mitt Arb Markt Berufsforsch 16:276–279

Kieselbach T (1983) Die individuellen und sozialen Kosten von Arbeitslosigkeit. In: Jahoda M, Kieselbach T, Leithäuser T (eds) Arbeit, Arbeitslosigkeit und Persönlichkeitsentwicklung, Reihe A. Psychologische Forschungsberichte, University of Bremen (Bremer Beiträge zur Psychologie no 23)

Kieselbach T (1984 a) Funktion und Perspektiven psychologischer Intervention und Forschung im Bereich Arbeitslosigkeit. In: Kieselbach T, Leithäuser T, Wacker A (eds) Arbeitslosigkeit – Psychologische Theorie und Praxis. Symposium, University of Bremen

Kieselbach T (1984 b) Self-disclosure and help-seeking behaviour as determinants of vulnerability. Medis-WHO-Meeting "Underlying Processes of Becoming Socially Vulnerable". Munich

Kieselbach T, Offe H (1979 a) Psychologische, gesundheitliche, soziale und politische Probleme als Folge von Arbeitslosigkeit – ein kritischer Überblick. In: Kieselbach T, Offe H (eds) Arbeitslosigkeit. Individuelle Verarbeitung. Gesellschaftlicher Hintergrund. Steinkopff, Darmstadt, pp 2–140

Kieselbach T, Offe H (1979 b) Stellungnahme zum Problem der Arbeitslosigkeit aus der Sicht von Organisation der psychosozialen Versorgung. In: Kieselbach T, Offe H (eds) Arbeitslosigkeit. Individuelle Verarbeitung. Gesellschaftlicher Hintergrund. Steinkopff, Darmstadt, pp 372–378

Kleiber D (1984) Arbeitslosigkeit und Handlungserfordernisse im psychosozialen Bereich. In: Kieselbach T, Leithäuser T, Wacker A (eds) Arbeitslosigkeit – Psychologische Theorie und Praxis. Symposium, University of Bremen

Klönne A (1984) Arbeitslosigkeit und politische Systemkrise. Ein Rückblick auf die Weimarer Republik. In: Bonss W, Heinze RG (eds) Arbeitslosigkeit in der Arbeitsgesellschaft. Suhrkamp, Frankfort, pp 191–213

Krehan G (1978) Arbeitslosigkeit als Stigma. In: Kutsch T, Wiswede G (eds) Arbeitslosigkeit II. Psychosoziale Belastungen. Hain, Meisenheim, pp 149–170

Leithäuser T (1984) Antizipation von Arbeitslosigkeit als psychosoziale Belastung im Betrieb. In: Kieselbach T, Leithäuser T, Wacker A (eds) Arbeitslosigkeit – Psychologische Theorie und Praxis. Symposium, University of Bremen

Laturner S, Schon B (eds) (1975) Jugendarbeitslosigkeit. Hamburg

Lauterbach W (1984) The psychological effects of unemployment: theory and assessment. Medis-WHO-Meeting "Underlying Processes of Becoming Socially Vulnerable", Munich

Maiers W, Markard M (1980) Probleme der individualwissenschaftlichen Perspektive auf die gesellschaftliche Massenerscheinung Arbeitslosigkeit. In: Maiers W, Markard M (eds) Lieber arbeitslos als ausgebeutet? Pahl-Rugenstein, Cologne, pp 93–108

Mohr G, Frese M (1981) Arbeitslosigkeit und Depression. Zur Langzeitarbeitslosigkeit älterer Arbeiter. In: Wacker A (ed) Vom Schock zum Fatalismus? Campus, Frankfort, pp 179–193

Möller-Lücking N (1983) Arbeitslose in die Gewerkschaftsarbeit einbeziehen. Quelle 34:178–180

Morgenroth C (1982) Ansätze zur Selbstorganisation von Arbeitslosen – Arbeitslosigkeit als Lernprovokation. In: Wacker A (ed) Vom Schock zum Fatalismus? Campus, Frankfort, pp 265–284

Müller-Limmroth W (1977) Die psychophysischen Auswirkungen der Arbeitslosigkeit. WSI Mitt 30:671–674

Nicolai H-P, Nicolai R (1977) Jugendarbeitslosigkeit und Persönlichkeitsentwicklung. Diploma thesis, University of Oldenburg

Niess F (1979) Geschichte der Arbeitslosigkeit. Pahl-Rugenstein, Cologne

Oehlke P (1979) Objektive Ursachen der Arbeitslosigkeit. In: Kieselbach T, Offe H (eds) Arbeitslosigkeit. Individuelle Verarbeitung. Gesellschaftlicher Hintergrund. Steinkopff, Darmstadt, pp 142–183

Opaschowski HW (1976) Zur Lebenssituation arbeitsloser Jugendlicher. Ergebnisse eines sozialpädagogischen Projekts. Politik Zeitgesch 39/40:24–47

Orendi B (1978) Fehlzeiten und Krankheitsverhalten. In: Frese M, Greif S, Semmer N (eds) Industrielle Psychopathologie. Huber, Stuttgart, pp 184–215

Pelzmann L, Winkler N, Zewell E (1984) Antizipation von Arbeitslosigkeit. In: Kieselbach T, Leithäuser T, Wacker A (eds) Arbeitslosigkeit – Psychologische Theorie und Praxis. Symposium, University of Bremen

Prager L (1977) Jugendarbeitslosigkeit und Kriminalität in Bayern. Arb Soz 32(4):7–14

Preiser K (1979) Gesundheitliche Beeinträchtigung und Arbeitslosigkeit. Befunde aus einer repräsentativen Längsschnittuntersuchung von Arbeitslosen und Abgängern aus Arbeitslosigkeit in der BRD. Infratest, Munich

Preiser K (1983) Methodological problems in the measurement of health consequences of unemployment in sample surveys. In: John J, Schwefel D, Zöllner H (eds) Influence of economic instability on health. Springer, Berlin Heidelberg New York, pp 371–385

Preiser K, Schräder W (1983) Der Rückgang des Krankenstandes in der ökonomischen Krise: eine Folge struktureller Veränderungen in der Erwerbsbevölkerung. Soz Fortschr 32:276–282

Preiser K, Schräder W (1984) Scheiden gesundheitlich eingeschränkte Arbeitnehmer in der ökonomischen Krise verstärkt aus dem Arbeitsleben aus? Soz Fortschr 33:234–236

Rabatsch M (1978) Beratung ist nutzlos, wenn man nicht helfen kann. Unterstützung für arbeitslose Jugendliche im Jugendamt. In: Balon KH, Dehler J, Schön B (eds) Arbeitslose: abgeschoben, diffamiert, verwaltet. Fischer, Frankfort, pp 11–35

Rothschild KW (1978) Arbeitslose: Gibt's die? Kyklos 31:21–35

Scharf B (1980a) Abbau psychischer Belastungen durch die Humanisierung der Arbeitswelt. Überlegungen zu einer Strategie gegen die psychische Verelendung in der Lohnarbeit. Soz Fortschr 29:130–136

Scharf B (1980b) Abbau psychischer Belastungen durch die Humanisierung der Arbeitswelt. Überlegungen zu einer Strategie gegen die psychische Verelendung in der Lohnarbeit. Soz Fortschr 29:176–179

Scharf B (1980c) Frühinvalidität – zur sozialpolitischen Bedeutung der beruflich-sozialen Ausgliederung leistungsgeminderter gesundheitlich Beeinträchtigter und Behinderter. WSI Mitt 33:550–563

Schindler H (1979) Familie und Arbeitslosigkeit. In: Kieselbach T, Offe H (eds) Arbeitslosigkeit. Individuelle Verarbeitung. Gesellschaftlicher Hintergrund. Steinkopff, Darmstadt, pp 258–286

Schindler H, Wetzels P (1984) Subjektive Bedeutung familiärer Arbeitslosigkeit bei Schülern in einem Bremer Arbeiterstadtteil. In: Kieselbach T, Leithäuser T, Wacker A (eds) Arbeitslosigkeit – Psychologische Theorie und Praxis. Symposium, University of Bremen

Schneider O (1932) Arbeitslosigkeit und Schulkind. Z Gesundheitsverwalt Gesundheitsfürs 3:409–418

Schneider W, Weber G (1982) Jugendlicher Drogenkonsum und Arbeitslosigkeit. Ein Beitrag zum Entstehungszusammenhang jugendlicher Desorientierung. Arch Wiss Prax Soz Arb 13:44–64

Schoen B (1979) Forschungen zur psychischen und sozialen Situation jugendlicher Arbeitsloser. Z Padag 25:795–798

Schoeps M (1975) Zeitbudgetvergleich zwischen erwerbstätigen und nicht-erwerbstätigen Hausfrauen. Gießen

Schwefel D (1983) Arbeitslosigkeit und Gesundheit. Ein europäisches (Forschungs-)Problem. Soz Fortschr 32:172–173

Schwefel D, John J (1982) Study on the influence of economic instability on health. Medis, Munich (Newsletter no 2)

Schwefel D, John J (1983) Study on the influence of economic instability on health. Medis, Munich (Newsletter no 3)

Schwefel D, John J (1984) Study on the influence of economic instability on health. Medis, Munich (Newsletter no 4)

Schwefel D, John J, Potthoff P, Hechler A (1984) Unemployment and mental health. Perspectives from the Federal Republic of Germany. Int J Ment Health 13:35–50

Schwefel E, Schwefel D (1973) The social meaning of unemployment. In: Wohlmuth K (ed) Employment creation in developing societies. The situation of labour in dependent economies. Praeger, New York, pp 249–280

Siegrist M (1979) Requalifizierung von Arbeitslosen. Psychosozial 1:35–50

Siegrist M (1984) Einsatzprogramme für Arbeitslose: Arbeit/persönlichkeitsorientierte Bildung/Betreuung. Erfahrungen des Arbeitsamtes Zürich 76–84. In: Kieselbach T, Leithäuser T, Wacker A (eds) Arbeitslosigkeit – Psychologische Theorie und Praxis. Symposium, University of Bremen

Siegrist M, Wunderli R (1982) Probleme psychologischer Betreuung von Arbeitslosen. In: Minsel W-R, Scheller R (eds) Brennpunkte der klinischen Psychologie, vol 4. Munich, pp 75–91

Strotzka H, Leitner I (1969) Sozialpsychiatrische Auswirkungen einer akuten ökonomischen Krise. Wien Med Wochenschr 10:196–199

Thiele W (1983) Die Auswirkungen der Arbeitslosigkeit auf die Nutzung von Kindervorsorgeuntersuchungen. Arb Gesundh Sozialpolit Mitt 3

Thomann K-D (1981) Die gesundheitlichen Auswirkungen der Arbeitslosigkeit. In: Wacker A (ed) Vom Schock zum Fatalismus? Campus, Frankfort, pp 194–240

Thomann K-D (1983a) Arbeitslosigkeit und Gesundheit. Demokrat Gesundheitswes 1:12–13

Thomann K-D (1983b) Die vergessene Krankheit: Arbeitslosigkeit. Prakt Arzt 20:2774–2783

Thomann K-D (1983c) The effects of unemployment on health and public awareness of this in the Federal Republic of Germany. In: John J, Schwefel D, Zöllner H (eds) Influence of economic instability on health. Springer, Berlin Heidelberg New York, pp 480–491

Thomann K-D (1984) Hohe Sockelarbeitslosigkeit: Perspektiven der medizinischen und beruflichen Rehabilitation. In: Kieselbach T, Leithäuser T, Wacker A (eds) Arbeitslosigkeit – Psychologische Theorie und Praxis. Symposium, University of Bremen

Tippelmann M (1931) Über die Auswirkungen der Arbeitslosigkeit auf Jugendliche. Freie Wohlfahrtspflege 303–321, 364–377

Vagt G, Stavemann HH (1980) Arbeitszeitverkürzung. Freizeitprobleme und Persönlichkeit. Eine psychologische Untersuchung an Kurzarbeitern, Arbeitslosen und Normalzeitbeschäftigten. Psychol Beitr 22:513–520

Volpert W (1979) Konvivale Produktionsstätten und schöpferische Arbeitslosigkeit – Die Suche nach alternativen Arbeitsformen. Psychosozial 1:51–76

Von Bargen H (1982) Junge Arbeitslose wehren sich. Marxist Bl 3:37–40

Von Berg V (1977) Jugendarbeitslosigkeit. Analysen und Einschätzungen zu einem Dauerthema. Soz Fortschr 26:217–224

Von Kardoff E, Koenen E (1984) Zur Rolle von Initiativen im Arbeitslosen- und Armutsbereich – Ergebnisse einer Befragung vom Arbeitsloseninitiativen. In: Kieselbach T, Leithäuser T, Wacker A (eds) Arbeitslosigkeit – Psychologische Theorie und Praxis. Symposium, University of Bremen

Von Rosenbladt B, Büchtemann CF (1980) Arbeitslosigkeit und berufliche Wiedereingliederung. Mitt Arb Markt Berufsforsch 13:552–572

Wacker A (1976) Arbeitslosigkeit als Sozialisierungserfahrung – Skizze eines Interpretationsansatzes. In: Leithäuser T, Heinz WR (eds) Produktion, Arbeit, Sozialisation. Suhrkamp, Frankfort, pp 171–189

Wacker A (1977) Arbeitslos und aggressiv? Soz Welt 28:364–381

Wacker A (1979) Jugendarbeitslosigkeit und Aggression. In: Furion M (ed) „Du tust mir weh …". Aggression im Leben der Kinder und Jugendlichen. Bonz, Fellbach, pp 163–179

Wacker A (1981 a) Ansätze, Probleme und Grenzen psychologischer Arbeitslosenforschung. In: Wacker A (ed) Vom Schock zum Fatalismus? Campus, Frankfort, pp 15–37
Wacker A (1981 b) Arbeitslos und aggressiv? – Zum Verhältnis von Arbeitslosigkeit, Aggression und Kriminalitätsentwicklung. In: Wacker A (ed) Vom Schock zum Fatalismus? Campus, Frankfort, pp 241–264
Wacker A (ed) (1981 c) Vom Schock zum Fatalismus? Soziale und psychische Auswirkungen der Arbeitslosigkeit. Campus, Frankfort
Wacker A (1983) Arbeitslosigkeit. Soziale und psychische Folgen. Europäische Verlagsanstalt, Frankfort
Wagenhals K (1980) Die Bedeutung der Arbeitslosigkeit für die politische Sozialisation Jugendlicher. In: Maiers W, Markard M (eds) Lieber arbeitslos als ausgebeutet? Pahl-Rugenstein, Cologne, pp 130–138
WAL (Sozialwissenschaftliche Arbeitsgruppe Göttingen) (eds) (1976) Die soziale Situation von Arbeitslosen und ihr Verhältnis zur Weiterbildung. Zwischenergebnisse einer empirischen Untersuchung. WAL, Göttingen
Waldow M, Börner A (1984) Berufliche Integration bei arbeitslosen Alkohol- und Medikamentenabhängigen. In: Kieselbach T, Leithäuser T, Wacker A (eds) Arbeitslosigkeit – Psychologische Theorie und Praxis. Symposium, University of Bremen
Westphal-Georgi U (1983) „Mutterarbeit" statt Arbeitslosigkeit. Demokrat Gesundheitswes 1. 83:14–15
Wiemer B (1981) Soziale und psychische Situationen arbeitsloser Jugendlicher. Theor Prax Soz Arb 32:375–379
Wilhelm-Reiss M (1980) Psychische Veränderungen bei Jugendlichen ohne Arbeit. Eine empirische Studie zu den Folgewirkungen der Arbeitslosigkeit. Beltz, Weinheim
Windolf P, Klemm S (1981) Zum Problem der arbeitslosen Angestellten. In: Wacker A (ed) Vom Schock zum Fatalismus? Campus, Frankfort, pp 134–178
Windolf P, Klemm S, Fischer H (1979) Arbeitslosigkeit, das Ende der Angestellten? In: Kieselbach T, Offe H (eds) Arbeitslosigkeit. Individuelle Verarbeitung. Gesellschaftlicher Hintergrund. Steinkopff, Darmstadt, pp 335–361
Wittig W, Eberle G (1984) Arztbesuche im Konjunkturzyklus. Zum Einfluß wirtschaftlicher Rezession auf Krankenstand und Inanspruchnahme ärztlicher Versorgung. Ortskrankenkasse 66:500–503
Wuggenig U (1979) Psychische Belastung und Krankheit als Bedingungen, Folgen und Antizipationseffekte von Arbeitslosigkeit bei Jugendlichen und Jungerwachsenen. Angew Soz 7:183–223
Wuggenig U (1984) Sozialer Rang und Arbeitslosigkeit: Unterschiede und Gemeinsamkeiten der Arbeitslosigkeitserfahrung von ungelernten Arbeitern und von Hochschulabsolventen. In: Kieselbach T, Leithäuser T, Wacker A (eds) Arbeitslosigkeit – Psychologische Theorie und Praxis. Symposium, University of Bremen
Zenke K, Ludwig G (1984) Projekt ‚Kinder arbeitsloser Eltern' – Zwischenergebnisse und Reflexionen über die organisatorischen, methodologischen und politischen Probleme bei der Aufklärung eines Massenphänomens. In: Kieselbach T, Leithäuser T, Wacker A (eds) Arbeitslosigkeit – Psychologische Theorie und Praxis. Symposium, University of Bremen
Zimmermann G (1983) Krankheitskündigung in der Praxis. In: Ellermann-With R et al. (eds) Kündigungspraxis, Kündigungsschutz und Probleme der Arbeitsgerichtsbarkeit. Opladen

Additional Literature

Abholz HE (1970) Die Rolle des industriellen Arbeitsplatzes für die Ätiologie psychischer Erkrankungen. Argument 60:141–151
Balon KH, Dehler J, Schön B (eds) (1978) Arbeitslose: abgeschoben, diffamiert, verwaltet. Fischer, Frankfort
Barnard K (1983) Influence of economic instability on health. Report of the symposium. In: John J, Schwefel D, Zöllner H (eds) Influence of economic instability on health. Springer, Berlin Heidelberg New York, pp 1–24

Beckmann D et al. (eds) (1979) Schwerpunktthema: Arbeit und Arbeitslosigkeit. Rowohlt, Reinbek (Psychosozial, vol 1)

Bonss W, Heinze RG (eds) (1984) Arbeitslosigkeit in der Arbeitsgesellschaft. Suhrkamp, Frankfort

Brinkmann C (1982) Arbeitslosigkeit und berufliche Ausgliederung älterer und leistungsgeminderter Arbeitnehmer. In: Dohse K, Jürgens U, Riessig H (eds) Ältere Arbeitnehmer zwischen Unternehmensinteressen und Sozialpolitik. Frankfort

Brinkmann C (1982) Health problems in the initial phase of unemployment – some research findings and policy implications

Brinkmann C, Schoeber-Gottwald K (1976) Zur beruflichen Wiedereingliederung von Arbeitslosen während der Rezession 1974/75. Mitt Arb Markt Berufsforsch 2

Büchtemann CF (1983) Gesundheitsverschleiß am Arbeitsplatz und Arbeitslosigkeit. Demokrat Gesundheitswes 1:IV–VIII

Bundesanstalt für Arbeit (1975) Zur Situation der Arbeitslosigkeit der Jugendlichen. Ergebnisse der Sonderuntersuchung von Ende Januar 1975. Amtl Nachr BFA 3:239–243

Cramer M (1981) Psychologenarbeitslosigkeit und psychosoziale Reform. In: von Kardoff E, Korenen E (eds) Psyche in schlechter Gesellschaft. Urban und Schwarzenberg, Munich, pp 75–100

Danckwerts D (1980) Anmerkungen zu einer Untersuchung über Deklassierungsprozesse bei Arbeitslosigkeit. In: Jantzen W (ed) Arbeit und Arbeitslosigkeit als pädagogisches und therapeutisches Problem. Pahl-Rugenstein, Cologne, pp 15–156

Dotterweich J, Hölzle C, Köster W (1979) Bewußtseinsstrukturen aktuell und potentiell arbeitsloser Jugendlicher. In: Kieselbach T, Offe H (eds) Arbeitslosigkeit. Individuelle Verarbeitung. Gesellschaftlicher Hintergrund. Steinkopff, Darmstadt, pp 287–333

Duda E (1979) Ein Jahr arbeitslos Eine Infratest-Untersuchung im Auftrage des BMA. Soz Sicherh 28:367–369

Frese M (1977) Psychische Störungen bei Arbeitern. Salzburg

Frese M (1980) Arbeitslosigkeit. In: Asanger A, Wenninger G (eds) Handwörterbuch der Psychologie. Beltz, Weinheim, pp 31–35

Frese M, Greif S, Semmer N (eds) (1978) Industrielle Psychopathologie. Huber, Stuttgart

Hartwich H-H, Laatsch-Nikitin N, Schaal M (1975) Arbeitslosigkeit. Analysen, Bd 16. Opladen

Hauss F et al. (1981) Betrieblicher Arbeitsschutz als gesundheitspolitische Strategie. In: Böhle F et al. (eds) Sozialpolitik und Produktionsprozeß. Cologne

Heinze RG, Hinrichs K, Olk T (1982) Produktion und Regulierung defizitärer Soziallagen. In: Heinze RG, Runde P (eds) Zur Situation von Behinderten und Leistungsgeminderten im Sozialstaat. Opladen, p 79

Hentschel U (1979) Politische Einstellungen und Interessenorientierung von Arbeitslosen. Institut zur Erforschung sozialer Chancen, Cologne (Report no 22)

Hentschel U (1980) Individuelle Auswirkungen der Arbeitslosigkeit – Ein Überblick über Ergebnisse einer Befragung. In: Maiers W, Markard M (eds) Lieber arbeitslos als ausgebeutet? Pahl-Rugenstein, Cologne, pp 64–70

Hufeland CW (1958) Makrobiontik oder die Kunst, das menschliche Leben zu verlängern, 8th edn. Stuttgart

Institut für Arbeitsmarkt- und Berufsforschung (IAB) (1982) Lebenssituation von Arbeitslosen, soziale und psychologische Auswirkungen von Arbeitslosigkeit. Literatur-/Forschungsdokumentation. IAB, Nürnberg (Profil L/F, vol 26)

Jahoda M (1981) Arbeitslose haben alles Recht der Welt, über ihre Lage unglücklich zu sein. Psychol Heute 8:71–76

Jahoda M, Lazarsfeld PF, Zeisel H (1960) Die Arbeitslosen von Marienthal. Demoskopie, Allensbach

Jahoda M, Kieselbach T, Leithäuser T (eds) (1983) Arbeit, Arbeitslosigkeit und Persönlichkeitsentwicklung, Reihe A. Psychologische Forschungsberichte. University of Bremen (Bremer Beiträge zur Psychologie no 23)

Jantzen W (ed) (1980) Arbeit und Arbeitslosigkeit als pädagogisches und therapeutisches Problem. Pahl-Rugenstein, Cologne

Keupp H (1980) Thesen zum Thema „Arbeitsfähigkeit als normative Kategorie im System der sozialen Sicherheit der BRD". In: Jantzen J (ed) Arbeit und Arbeitslosigkeit als pädagogisches und therapeutisches Problem. Pahl-Rugenstein, Cologne, pp 5–103

Kieselbach T, Offe H (eds) (1979) Arbeitslosigkeit. Individuelle Verarbeitung. Gesellschaftlicher Hintergrund. Steinkopff, Darmstadt

Kieselbach T, Offe H (1979) Bredaer Protokolle. Ausschnitte aus Interviews mit Arbeitern und Angestellten der von Schließung bedrohten ENKA-Werke (Breda). In: Kieselbach T, Offe H (eds) Arbeitslosigkeit. Individuelle Verarbeitung. Gesellschaftlicher Hintergrund. Steinkopff, Darmstadt, pp 363–371

Kieselbach T, Kleiber D, Schindler H (1979) Psychologenarbeitslosigkeit: Auswirkungen und Strategien ihrer Überwindung aus der Sicht von Betroffenen. Mitt Dtsch Ges Verhaltensther 11:742–763

Kieselbach T, Leithäuser T, Wacker A (eds) (1984) Arbeitslosigkeit – Psychologische Theorie und Praxis. Abstracts der Referate. Symposium, University of Bremen

Kreft I, Vattes H (1980) Theoretischer Rahmen zur Erfassung psychosozialer Probleme der Jugendarbeitslosigkeit und zur Entwicklung praktischer Konsequenzen, um eine dauernde gesellschaftliche Ausgrenzung von arbeitslosen Jugendlichen zu verhindern. In: Jantzen W (ed) Arbeit und Arbeitslosigkeit als pädagogisches und therapeutisches Problem. Pahl-Rugenstein, Cologne, pp 145–150

Kutsch T, Wiswede G (eds) (1978) Arbeitslosigkeit II: Psychosoziale Belastungen. Hain, Meisenheim

Leithäuser T (1983) Arbeitsbelastung und ihre Bewältigung in sozialpsychologischer Sicht. In: Jahoda M, Kieselbach T, Leithäuser T (eds) Arbeit, Arbeitslosigkeit und Persönlichkeitsentwicklung, Reihe A. Psychologische Forschungsberichte, University of Bremen (Bremer Beiträge zur Psychologie, no 23)

Leroy R (1965) Arbeitslosigkeit und Unterbeschäftigung. Verwirklichung einer Untersuchungsmethode. IESPO, Brussels, pp 3–107 (Reihe Sozialpolitik, no 9)

Levenstein A (1912) Die Arbeiterfrage. Mit besonderer Berücksichtigung der sozialpsychologischen Seite des modernen Großbetriebes und der psycho-physischen Einwirkungen auf die Arbeiter. Munich

Maiers W, Markard M (eds) (1980) Lieber arbeitslos als ausgebeutet? Pahl-Rugenstein, Cologne

Matthes J (ed) (1983) Krise der Arbeitsgesellschaft? Verhandlungen des 21. Deutschen Soziologentages in Bamberg 1982. Frankfort

Mohr G (1976) Zum Zusammenhang zwischen Arbeitslosigkeit und Depression bei älteren Arbeitern. Diploma thesis. Free University of Berlin

Möller-Lücking N (1982) Gewerkschaften und arbeitslose Arbeitnehmer. Soz Sicherh 31:33–43

Moses J (1931) Arbeitslosigkeit. Ein Problem der Volksgesundheit. Berlin

Mueller EF (1965) Selbst-Aktualisierung, Überlastung und Gesundheit: Ein theoretischer Bezugsrahmen. Köln Z Soz Psychol 17:855–878

Nathow R (1984) Auswirkungen der Arbeitslosigkeit auf die sozialpsychiatrischen Dienste. In: Kieselbach T, Leithäuser T, Wacker A (eds) Arbeitslosigkeit – Psychologische Theorie und Praxis. Symposium, University of Bremen

Offe C (ed) (1977) Opfer des Arbeitsmarktes. Zur Theorie der strukturierten Arbeitslosigkeit. Neuwied

Pflanz M (1962) Sozialer Wandel und Krankheit. Stuttgart

Pintar R (1978) Betroffenheit durch Arbeitslosigkeit. Überblick über die veränderte Situation und das Verhalten von Arbeitslosen. In: Kutsch T, Wiswede G (eds) Arbeitslosigkeit II. Psychosoziale Belastungen. Hain, Meisenheim, pp 14–95

Rattinger H (1979) Auswirkungen der Arbeitsmarktlage auf das Ergebnis der Bundestagswahl 1976. Polit Vierteljahresschr 20:51–70

Saterdag H (1975) Situationsmerkmale von Arbeitslosen Anfang 1975 und Voraussetzungen für die Aufnahme einer neuen Beschäftigung. Mitt Arb Markt Berufsforsch 8:136

Schienstock G (1979) Arbeitslosigkeit. Streß im Abseits der Gesellschaft. In: Karmaus W, Müller V, Schienstock G (eds) Streß in der Arbeitswelt. Cologne

Schindler H (1979) Politisches Bewußtsein und psychische Folgen der Arbeitslosigkeit. Ein Literaturbericht. Bl Dtsch Int Polit 24:599–609

Schmidt MG (1983) Arbeitslosigkeit und Vollbeschäftigung. Ein internationaler Vergleich. Leviathan 4:451–473

Schober K (1978) Arbeitslose Jugendliche: Belastungen und Reaktionen der Betroffenen. Mitt Arb Markt Berufsforsch 11:198–215

Schön B, Schott S (1978) Soziale Arbeit und Arbeitslosigkeit. Institutionelle Angebote und mögliche Alternativen. In: Balon KH, Dehler J, Schön B (eds) Arbeitslose: abgeschoben, diffamiert, verwaltet. Fischer, Frankfort, pp 95–112

Thomann K-D (1981) Arbeitslosigkeit macht krank! Demokrat Gesundheitswes 3:17–18

Thomann K-D (1982) Gedanken an einen moglichen Selbstmord kehren immer wieder Ergebnisse zweier Symposien der WHO über die gesundheitlichen Folgen von Arbeitslosigkeit. Frankfurter Rundschau

Thomann K-D (1983) Gesellschaftliche Funktion, Aufgaben und Probleme des Ärztlichen Dienstes der Arbeitsämter in der Krise. Med Soziol 3:83–102

Udris I (1984) Die Studie des Europarats zur Arbeitslosigkeit – Konzept und Zwischenergebnisse. In: Kieselbach T, Leithauser T, Wacker A (eds) Arbeitslosigkeit – Psychologische Theorie und Praxis. Symposium, University of Bremen

Unrein H (1978) Arbeitslosigkeit, Fakten, Aspekte, Wirkungen. Cologne

Wacker A (1976) Arbeitslosigkeit. Soziale und psychische Voraussetzungen und Folgen. Frankfort

Wacker A (1982) Psychologische Aspekte der Arbeitslosigkeit älterer Arbeitsloser und ihrer Ausgliederung aus dem Arbeitsprozeß. In: Dhose K, Jürgens U, Russig H (eds) Ältere Arbeitnehmer zwischen Unternehmensinteressen und Sozialpolitik. Campus, Frankfort, pp 157–184

Wacker A (1984) Arbeitslosigkeit als Krankheitsursache. In: Elsner G (ed) Was uns kaputt macht. VSA, Hamburg

Wacker A (1984) Gegenwärtiger Stand und zukunftige Perspektiven der psychologischen Arbeitslosenforschung. In: Kieselbach T, Leithäuser T, Wacker A (eds) Arbeitslosigkeit – Psychologische Theorie und Praxis. Symposium, University of Bremen

WAL (Sozialwissenschaftliche Arbeitsgruppe Göttingen) (1978) Die soziale und psychische Lage der Arbeitslosen – Ansatzpunkt für Weiterbildung. WAL, Göttingen

WAL (Sozialwissenschaftliche Arbeitsgruppe Göttingen) (1978) Die psychosoziale Lage von Arbeitslosen. WAL, Göttingen

Windolf P, Weirich H (1980) Die neue Arbeitslosigkeit und die Grenzen der Sozialpolitik. Internationales Institut für Management und Verwaltung, Berlin (IIM-papers 80-8)

Winter G (1984) Arbeitslosigkeit als kritisches Lebensereignis: Was leistet ein Forschungsparadigma für Beschreibung, Erklärung und Beratung? In: Kieselbach T, Leithäuser T, Wacker A (eds) Arbeitslosigkeit – Psychologische Theorie und Praxis. Symposium, University of Bremen

Wunderli R (1979) Alternative Formen der Arbeitszeitgestaltung. Psychosozial 1:77–79

Zoll R (ed) (1981) Arbeiterbewußtsein in der Wirtschaftskrise. Erster Bericht: Krisenbetroffenheit und Krisenwahrnehmung. Bund, Cologne

Weiterführende Literatur zum Thema „Arbeitswelt"

Heiber M (1983) Methodenentwicklung für die Expositionsabschätzung neuer Stoffe: Forschungsbericht Nr. 358. Bundesanstalt für Arbeitsschutz, Dortmund
Projektträger „Humanisierung des Arbeitslebens" (1989) Projektstatusbericht 1988/89: Bericht zu Fördermaßnahmen des BMFT im Rahmen des Programms der Bundesregierung „Forschung zur Humanisierung des Arbeitslebens"
WHO IARC monographs on the evaluation of the carcinogenic risk of chemicals to humans: Chemicals, industrial processes and industries associated with cancer in humans, vol 1–29

3 Gemeinde

Zur Weiterentwicklung des öffentlichen Gesundheitsdienstes: Wertung der gesundheitspolitischen und wissenschaftlichen Literatur

W. Müller, U. Laaser, E. Kröger, G. Murza

Vorbemerkung

Der Beitrag versucht, anhand eines Resümees der gesundheitspolitischen und wissenschaftlichen Literatur eine Bewertung für die Weiterentwicklung des öffentlichen Gesundheitswesens vorzunehmen. Es wird versucht, Entwicklungschancen für den öffentlichen Gesundheitsdienst (ÖGD) aufzuzeigen und Forderungen an das eigene Selbstverständnis des ÖGD zu formulieren. Als Prämisse wird unterstellt, daß der ÖGD ein integrativer Bestandteil des Gesundheitswesens ist und auch in Zukunft bleiben muß. Die Absicht des Beitrages ist daher keine detaillierte ausformulierte Einzelaufgabenbeschreibung des ÖGD, sondern das Aufzeigen verschiedener Strukturmodelle der dritten Säule des Gesundheitswesens, in dem Bewußtsein, daß innovatives Agieren und Handeln im öffentlichen Gesundheitsdienst nur durch gesundheitspolitische Prioritätensetzung und im Interessenausgleich der staatlichen und privaten Institutionen des Gesundheitswesens möglich sein wird.

Die rechtlichen Rahmenbedingungen

Der öffentliche Gesundheitsdienst – wie er durch das Gesetz über die Vereinheitlichung des Gesundheitswesens vom 3. Juni 1934 und seinen 3 Durchführungsverordnungen geschaffen wurde (Labisch u. Tennstedt 1985) – ist mit der Gründung der Bundesländer und der Bundesrepublik Deutschland sowohl von der Struktur als auch den rechtlichen Aufgaben her im wesentlichen fortgeführt worden. Bis heute gelten in den Ländern Bremen, Baden-Württemberg, Hamburg, Hessen, Niedersachsen, Nordrhein-Westfalen, Rheinland-Pfalz und Saarland in der jeweils geltenden Fassung des bereinigten Landesrechtes diese gesetzlichen Grundlagen fort, ohne daß eine wesentliche Weiterentwicklung stattgefunden hat (Federhen 1967; AÖG 1985; Hopf 1976). Im Gegensatz dazu hat es im gesamten Rechtsbereich des Gesundheitswesens – insbesondere im Zuständigkeitsbereich des Bundesministers für Arbeit und Sozialordnung als auch in den Bereichen des „Technischen Umweltschutzes" – eine Vielzahl auch für den ÖGD rechtlich relevanter Regelungen gegeben. Der Bundesgesetzgeber hat die in Artikel 74 des Grundgesetzes festgelegten, im Rahmen der konkurrierenden Gesetz-

---

Erstmals veröffentlicht in: Öff. Gesundheitswesen 50/1988:303–313.

gebung möglichen rechtlichen Handlungsspielräume insbesondere der Ziffern 11a, 12, 19, 19a, 20 sowie 24 ausgeschöpft.

Obwohl spätestens seit Ende der 40er Jahre die Diskussion nicht verstummt, wie das bestehende Vereinheitlichungsgesetz in den Ländern abgelöst werden kann und diese Diskussion 1972 zu dem „Entwurf eines Gesetzes über das Gesundheitswesen im Land … als Richtlinie für Ländergesetze zur Wahrung der Einheitlichkeit des öffentlichen Gesundheitsdienstes" leitete (Hopf 1975, 1976, 1978), führte der allseits vorgebrachte Handlungsbedarf bisher nur in den Ländern Schleswig-Holstein (vgl. GDG-Gesetz Schleswig-Holstein vom 14. März 1979), in Berlin (vgl. GDG-Gesetz vom 28. Juli 1980) und Bayern (vgl. GDG-Gesetz vom 12. Juli 1986) zu Landesgesundheitsdienstgesetzen. Vorentwürfe oder Entwürfe eines Landesgesundheitsdienstgesetzes sind in den meisten anderen Bundesländern in Diskussion, wobei die Landesgesetzgeber vor dem Problem stehen eine neue Standortfestlegung des ÖGD vorzunehmen, die gesetzlichen Aufgaben des ÖGD in den gesamten Rechtsbereich des Gesundheitswesens einzubetten und die unterschiedliche historische Entwicklung des ÖGD in den Kommunen (Städten und Landkreisen) seit der Kommunalisierung des Gesundheitswesens (in den meisten Bundesländern Ende der 40er Jahre) zu berücksichtigen. Die bisher verabschiedeten drei Gesundheitsdienstgesetze belegen, daß die Rahmenvorgabe nicht als Klammer der Weiterentwicklung der Landesgesundheitsdienstgesetze wirkt.

Trotzdem haben die verschiedenen Vorstellungen über den ÖGD gemeinsam, daß der ÖGD ein Teil des öffentlichen Gesundheitswesens ist, zu dem auch die ärztlichen Dienste der Sozialleistungsträger, versorgungsärztliche Dienste, Krankenversicherung, ärztliche Dienste der Rentenversicherung und der Arbeitsverwaltung, der gewerbeärztliche Dienst, das Sanitäts- und Gesundheitswesen der Bundeswehr und des Bundesgrenzschutzes, der polizeiärztliche Dienst sowie der ärztliche Dienst der Justizvollzugsanstalten hinzugezählt werden.

Gemäß dem bayerischen Gesundheitsdienstgesetz ist der veterinärärztliche Dienst Teil des ÖGD, in anderen Bundesländern ist die Veterinärfachverwaltung organisatorisch und inhaltlich vom ÖGD getrennt.

Die inhaltliche Umsetzung vieler Beschlüsse der Konferenz der Gesundheitsminister und Senatoren, die ein Steuerungsinstrument für ein bundesstaatlich möglichst einheitliches öffentliches Gesundheitswesen sein soll, wurde durch länderspezifische Weiterentwicklungen nur z. T. realisiert.

Standortbestimmung

Die Beibehaltung der Institution „Gesundheitsamt" als Träger staatlichen Handelns im Bereich des Gesundheitswesens zur Sicherung seiner Funktionsfähigkeit und Anpassung an neue Aufgabenschwerpunkte wird nur von wenigen grundsätzlich in Frage gestellt (Göpel 1986), dennoch müssen die Gestaltungsprinzipien des öffentlichen Gesundheitsdienstes vor dem Hintergrund beschränkter Ressourcen und Veränderungen in der Gesamtkonstellation der Partner im Gesundheitswesen neu überdacht werden. Insbesondere muß der öffentliche Gesundheitsdienst sich mit dem zunehmenden Druck aus dem Bereich anderer medizinischer Leistungsträger auseinandersetzen. Dabei hilft, wie Schmacke (1987) formuliert, das „larmoyante Festhalten am Vereinheitlichungsgesetz", welches im Selbstverständnis der Amtsärzte das Gesundheitsamt mit einer Allzuständigkeit in gesundheitlichen Fragen ausgestattet hatte, nicht weiter. Weiterhin führt Schmacke aus, daß die erhoffte Allzuständigkeit in medizinischen Fragen sich immer offensichtlicher zur Farce entwickelte, „da weder genügend fachliche Qualifikation in den Gesundheitsämtern vorgewiesen werden konnte, noch die Amtsärzte rechtlich wie politisch entscheidend in die Prozesse der Gesundheits-, Sozial- und Arbeitsverwaltung eingreifen konnten".

Die Standortbestimmung des ÖGD wird daher eher durch andere Sektoren des Gesundheitswesens bestimmt als durch den ÖGD selbst.

Generell besteht Einigung darüber, ein „leistungsfähiges" öffentliches Gesundheitswesen und ein „leistungsfähiges" Gesundheitsamt zu schaffen. Als leistungsfähig wird ein ÖGD verstanden, der „das System ambulanter und staatlicher Versorgung optimal ergänzt" (Bericht der Landesregierung 1983). Die deutsche Ärzteschaft fordert in ihrem Blauen Papier (GSVDÄ 1986) eine Zusammenarbeit mit „niedergelassenen Ärzten, Krankenhausärzten, Betriebsärzten, den Ärzten der Sozialversicherungsträger in kollegialer Partnerschaft". Objektive Kriterien, ob und inwieweit die Leistungsfähigkeit des ÖGD, insbesondere des Gesundheitsamtes, durch seine jetzige Struktur und Funktion erzielt werden, gibt es kaum. Auch sind Ansätze, das Gesundheitsamt auf Effektivität und Effizienz zu überprüfen, bisher kaum vorhanden. Nach welchen Kriterien die Leistungsfähigkeit abgeprüft werden soll, bzw. zu welcher Zielvorgabe diese Leistungsfähigkeit gefordert wird, bleibt offen, allenfalls wird in den diskutierten Positionen die gewünschte Stellung des Gesundheitsamtes innerhalb des Gesamtbereiches der Anbieter von Gesundheitsdiensten verdeutlicht (Gesetz über den Gesundheitsdienst 1980). Die Grünen möchten ein kommunales Gesundheitsamt, das mit allen anderen Einrichtungen der Regionen einen Verbund bildet und diesen Verbund koordiniert (Grüne 1984).

Reformüberlegungen im Rahmen der bestehenden Organisationsstrukturen wurden vom Bundesverband der Ärzte des ÖGD (Federhen 1967), Hopf (1984), der NRW-Landesregierung (Öffentliches Gesundheitswesen 1978) und Nittner (1976) angestellt. Bei Hopf wird als Koordinations-/Kooperationszentrale ein „Fachbeirat am Gesundheitsamt" vorgeschlagen, in dem alle Einrichtungen des Gesundheitswesens einer Region vertreten sind.

Letztlich ist es bis heute nicht gelungen, die sog. dritte Säule des Gesundheitswesens tatsächlich als integrativen Bestandteil darzustellen; dieses wird dadurch erschwert, daß von den insgesamt über 170000 aktiven Ärzten in der Bundesrepublik weniger als 3000 hauptamtlich im Gesundheitsamt und dessen Einrichtungen beschäftigt sind. Die Gesamtaufwendungen für den öffentlichen Gesundheitsdienst in der Bundesrepublik im Vergleich zu den Gesamtausgaben des Gesundheitswesens liegen unter 1% (Daten Gesundheitswesen 1985; Hoffmeister 1978; Labisch u. Ziesmann 1984). Es ist daher nicht verwunderlich, daß Versuche, die drei Systeme – ambulante Versorgung, stationäre Krankenhausversorgung und öffentlicher Gesundheitsdienst – in ein Gesamtsystem der gesundheitlichen Versorgung zur Kooperation und sinnvollen Arbeitsteilung zu bringen, gescheitert sind, nicht zuletzt aufgrund der unterschiedlichen Aufgabenstellung, des Selbstverständnisses und der Bedeutung der drei „Partner".

Neben dieser quantitativen Ungleichheit ist von Bedeutung, daß der öffentliche Gesundheitsdienst im allgemeinen Selbstverständnis, auch der Bundesländer, subsidiär zu handeln habe (vgl. bayerisches GDG, Bericht der rheinlandpfälzischen Landesregierung): Der ÖGD soll grundsätzlich nur Aufgaben übernehmen, die von privaten Trägern nicht gleichgut oder besser wahrgenommen werden können. Auch soll geprüft werden, ob „der Staat durch Rückübertragung bestimmter Aufgaben Freiraum für eine bessere Wahrnehmung wesentlicher Pflichten" gewinnen kann (Bericht Landesregierung 1983). Bei konsequenter Durchführung dieses Gedankens scheidet der ÖGD als aktiver, mitbestimmender und akzeptierter Partner aus. Ähnliche Präferenz bezüglich der Übertragung der Aufgaben des ÖGD auf private Leistungsanbieter äußert der Hartmann-Bund (Hartmann-Bund 1981). Auch von Manger-Koenig (1975) sieht den ÖGD auf die klassischen Aufgaben der öffentlichen Gesundheitspflege festgelegt. Wolters (1974) regt ein Geben und Nehmen an. Prinzipiell andere Vorstellungen entwickeln die SPD (Leitlinien öffentlicher Gesundheitsdienst 1986), die Grünen (1984), Labisch (1985), Schmacke (1987).

Hopf (1984) und Dewein (1981) bedauern den Fortfall von Aufgaben der Gesundheitsämter durch „Rechtsvorschriften aus dem Bereich des BMA". Hopf bezeichnet die mögliche Übertragung von ÖGD-Aufgaben auf Trägervereine (medizinischer Überwachungsverein „MÜV"), wie er in der Schrift der rheinlandpfälzischen Landesregierung diskutiert wird, als abwegig. Der Bundesverband warnt: „Privatisierung der Bevölkerungsmedizin wird die Sozialisierung unseres Gesundheitswesens" zwangsläufig nach sich ziehen. Steuer (1984) kritisiert die Bemühungen um neue Gesetze für den ÖGD; für die nordrhein-westfälische Landesregierung (Reuter 1982) ist eine dauernde Übertragung von Aufgaben des ÖGD auf private Leistungserbringer nicht denkbar, nicht vertretbar, da dadurch wesentliche Bevölkerungsgruppen der Beobachtung, Dokumentation und Beratung entzogen würden. Global meint Reuter (1982), daß ein öffentlicher Gesundheitsdienst in irgendeiner Form für jedes Staatswesen unverzichtbar ist, und es wird ihn immer geben, weil seine Probleme immer bestehen bleiben werden. Er sieht das neue Konzept für den ÖGD in großzügig eingerichteten und überörtlich ausgelegten Gesundheitszentren, die weniger Amts- vielmehr Institutionscharakter haben. Nach Reuter ist Hauptaufgabe, neben der Analyse der Standortbestimmung eine Prioritätsentscheidung für zukünftige Aufgaben zu treffen, diese haben elementare Auswirkungen auf die Organisationsstruktur, ein „Herumbasteln" am Vereinheitlichungsgesetz bzw. an den Durchführungsverordnungen zeigt keinen in die Zukunft weisenden Weg.

Dewein (1981) fordert einen neuen Ansatz, eine neue leistungsfähige und besonders bürgerfreundliche Struktur und Organisation, da der öffentliche Gesundheitsdienst im modernen Staat der Daseinsvorsorge ein Dienstleistungszweig ist, der mit dem Denken von Dienstleistungsunternehmern organisiert und gestützt werden muß.

Wesentlich für das zukünftige Selbstverständnis des ÖGD ist die Frage der „Gesundheit in Eigenverantwortung". Inwieweit soll Eigenverantwortlichkeit der Bürger für ihre Gesundheit bestehen oder sind – sozialstaatlichem Handeln gemäß – der Delegationsfähigkeit bevölkerungsmedizinischer Aufgaben Grenzen gesetzt und wo liegen diese?

Wird der sozialhygienische Auftrag vom Staat, der Gesundheitsfachverwaltung akzeptiert und ist sein Handeln auf Gemeindeebene in die konkrete Problemerfassung und Problembeseitigung im Sinne einer umfassenden Präventivmedizin eingebettet, dann sind die vielfältigen Diskussionen über Größe und Einzugsgebiet von Gesundheitsämtern hinfällig (vgl. Ziele der WHO – Regionalstrategie 1982, 1983).

Die bisherige Struktur, die Dienstbezirke der Gesundheitsämter grundsätzlich mit dem Gebiet eines Landkreises oder einer kreisfreien Stadt identisch zu gestalten, zur Schaffung der „Einräumigkeit der Verwaltung" sind primär aus pragmatischen, organisatorischen Grundüberlegungen entstanden (Bericht Landesregierung 1983). Dieses flächendeckende Netz führt zu einer Vielzahl von kleineren und. kleinsten Ämtern. Schmacke (1987) merkt hierzu richtig an, „daß in diesen Ämtern die Aufgabenvielfalt von wenigen Entscheidungsträgern unter der Leitung eines ‚allzuständigen' Amtsarztes wahrgenommen werden muß". Daß eine derartige Kumulation von Funktionen von Begutachtungen über Seuchenhygiene bis zur Umweltmedizin oftmals zum Verwalten von Problemen führen muß, ist evident.

Göpel (1986) will die Aufgaben des Gesundheitsamtes auf kommunaler Ebene abgetan wissen, will aber nicht unbedingt ein „Gesundheitsamt" weiter vorhalten, da die Aufgaben des Gesundheitsamtes von anderen Institutionen, z. B. den Sozialämtern und den Umweltverwaltungen, wahrgenommen werden könnten. Dewein (1981) und Nittner (1976) weisen darauf hin, daß ein Gesundheitsamt bei großem Einzugsbereich über Außenstellen verfügen muß. Auf die Nachteile der Anbindung der Gesundheitsämter an die Kommunen verweist von Manger-Koenig (1975). Den Ausbau von modernen, überregionalen und multidisziplinären Gesundheitsämtern fordert die FDP, mit der Übertragung von bisher von Ärzten wahrgenommenen Aufgaben im umwelthygienischen und sozialmedizinischen Bereich auf nichtärztliches Personal zur Entlastung der Ärzte für ihre eigentlichen Aufgaben, ohne diese Aufgaben näher zu präzisieren (Gesundheitspolitisches Programm FDP 1976).

Ganz den Rahmen der kommunalen Gebietskörperschaft zu verlassen schlägt Faerber (1972) vor, der eine Regionalinstitution oberhalb der Kreisebene mit einem Einzugsbereich von 500 000 Einwohnern vorsieht. Reuter (1982), der das bisher herkömmliche Gesundheitsamt ganz aufgeben will, fordert „großzügig eingerichtete überörtliche Gesundheitszentren".

Es bleibt bei der kommunalen Gliederung der Gesundheitsämter das Dilemma bestehen, daß die Kommunen und Kreise die Struktur, die personelle und die apparative Ausstattung der Gesundheitsämter aufgrund ihrer eigenen gesundheitspolitischen Vorstellungen und finanzpolitischen Verfügungsmasse bestimmen. Von daher ist die Möglichkeit intensiv zu prüfen, ob der Träger eines Gesundheitsamtes auch ein Zweckverband sein könnte, in dessen Rahmen unter Rationalisierungsgesichtspunkten Schwerpunktaufgaben durch Übereinkunft verschiedener Träger einem bestimmten Gesundheitsamt zugewiesen werden können. Diese Verzahnung der kommunalen und überkommunalen Aufgabenwahrnehmung würde die Möglichkeit geben, einen der Hauptkritikpunkte an dem allgemein beklagten schlechten Zustand des ÖGD und insbesondere des Gesundheitsamtes zu eliminieren, nämlich daß von jedem Gesundheitsamt alle gesetzlich vorgeschriebenen Aufgaben wahrgenommen werden müssen, unabhängig von der Größe des zu betreuenden Gebietes, der betroffenen Bevölkerungszahl, der Finanzkraft der Kommunen sowie den sächlichen und personellen Kapazitäten des Amtes.

Kennzeichnend für die Standortdiskussion ist die vorwiegend innerhalb des ÖGD geführte Auseinandersetzung. Eine den ÖGD einschließende Diskussion innerhalb der globalen gesamtgesundheitspolitischen Auseinandersetzung findet z. Z. noch nicht statt.

Aufgabenbereiche

Die Hauptfunktionen des Gesundheitsamtes – einerseits Gesundheitsüberwachung und -aufsicht sowie örtliche Beratungs- und Planungsinstitution in gesundheitsrelevanten Fragen sowie andererseits Fürsorgeinstitution schlechthin für alle benachteiligten, behinderten, psychisch und chronisch kranken Menschen – wurde im Vereinheitlichungsgesetz festgeschrieben. Der in manchen Bereichen kaum zu überbrückende Dualismus zwischen „Hoheitsträger/Seuchenpolizei" und „umfassende Fürsorgeinstitution" wirkt bis heute fort und findet sich auch in moderner Terminologie in den 5 Hauptbereichen der Richtlinie nach Hopf (1978):

– Medizinalaufsicht über Berufe und Einrichtungen des Gesundheitswesens,
– Aufgaben der Gesundheitshygiene und des Gesundheitsschutzes,
– Aufgaben der Gesundheitsförderung und -vorsorge sowie der Gesundheitshilfe,
– gutachterliche Aufgaben und
– Epidemiologie und Gesundheitsplanung.

Diese generellen Aufgaben wurden in einem umfänglichen Katalog von Femmer (1982) bis in kleinste Einzelaufgaben differenziert.

Medizinalaufsicht

Wesentliche Aufgaben der Medizinalaufsicht über die Gesundheitsfachberufe sind Selbstverwaltungskörperschaften wie z. B. den Ärztekammern übertragen worden. Andere Gesundheitsfachberufe verblieben im Zuständigkeitsbereich des ÖGD, wie z. B. Heilpraktiker. Bei anderen Berufsgruppen, die im Gesundheitswesen tätig sind, wie z. B. Diätberater etc., ist die Zuordnung als „Gesundheitsfachberuf" nicht gegeben. Es muß daher bezweifelt werden, ob die vielfältigen organisatorisch völlig getrennten Zuständigkeiten in der Medizinalaufsicht der Gesundheitsfachberufe eine effektive Qualitätskontrolle ermöglichen.

Eine weitere – grundsätzlich unbestrittene – Aufgabe des ÖGD in der Medizinalaufsicht ist die Überprüfung und Kontrolle von Hygienestandards. Es ist denkbar, diesen Bereich auf weitere Lebensbereiche auszudehnen, wobei in unverkennendem Maße der bisher vorwiegend bestehende ordnungspolitische Charakter der Medizinalaufsicht und Hygieneaufsicht als Hygieneberatung für öffentliche Einrichtungen und Privatpersonen erweitert werden sollte.

In den meisten Bundesländern obliegt die Apothekenaufsicht den Regierungspräsidenten (Gesundheitsdezernaten) und wird in erheblichem Umfang durch sog. Pharmazieräte wahrgenommen. Ob die Verlagerung der Apothekenaufsicht in den Zuständigkeitsbereich der Kommunen wie in NRW 1982 geschehen, eine bessere Qualitätskontrolle hervorbrachte, ist bisher nicht belegt worden, da diesbezügliche Untersuchungen noch nicht vorliegen.

Gesundheitsschutz (Verhütung und Bekämpfung übertragbarer Krankheiten und Lebensmittelüberwachung) und Umwelthygiene

Forderungen, den gesundheitlichen Umweltschutz als multidisziplinäre Aufgabenstellung zu sehen, die durch Hygieniker, Apotheker, Lebensmittelchemiker, Tierärzte etc. wahrgenommen werden soll, sind zwar sachlich nachvollziehbar, ihre inhaltliche und administrative Realisierung jedoch bisher kaum zu erkennen. Die in den letzten Jahren heftig geführte Diskussion, den öffentlichen Gesundheitsdienst durch vermehrte Aufgaben im gesundheitlichen Umweltschutz zu stärken (vgl. GMK-Position, Blaues Papier der Deutschen Ärzteschaft 1986; Steuer 1984; Moritzen u. Wodarg 1987) sind zu begrüßen. Jedoch muß der öffentliche Gesundheitsdienst sich hierbei selbstkritisch fragen, ob er in der Lage ist, dieser Problem- und Aufgabenstellung personell und apparativ gerecht zu werden. Darüber hinaus ist auffällig, daß bei den Obersten Landesbehörden und den Bundesbehörden der Umweltschutz und auch z. T. der gesundheitliche Umweltschutz nicht in den Sozialministerien bzw. in den Arbeitsministerien ressortieren, sondern eigene Umweltministerien geschaffen worden sind.

Durch die Einrichtung von „Gesundheits- und Umweltämtern" im Land Hamburg 1986 wurde dort diese gesundheitspolitische Frage eindeutig beantwortet. Es bleibt abzuwarten, ob die gestellte globale Forderung gesundheitspolitisch durchzusetzen ist, oder ob die bestehende meßtechnisch-apparative Minderausstattung der meisten Gesundheitsämter dazu führt, daß Umweltbehörden und andere Institutionen den öffentlichen Gesundheitsdienst überspielen und damit langfristig inhaltlich und fachlich in dieser Fragestellung bedeutungslos machen.

Ein öffentlicher Gesundheitsdienst, der selbst nicht in der Lage ist, Untersuchungen durchzuführen und bei allen umweltrelevanten Fragestellungen auf die Weitergabe bzw. Interpretation der Untersuchungsergebnisse von leistungsfähigen Drittinstituten angewiesen ist, wird von marginaler Bedeutung werden. Auch dürfte die rechtliche Weiterentwicklung z. B. des Bundesimmissionsschutzgesetzes die Kompetenz des öffentlichen Gesundheitsdienstes im Bereich dieser Rechtsmaterie noch weiter zurückdrängen. Auch in den bisher ausschließlich vom Gesundheitsamt wahrgenommenen Bereichen der Überwachung der Trinkwasserhygiene zeichnet sich regional eine Verlagerung in die Umweltämter ab (z. B. Wiesbaden, Lübeck). Eine zukünftige Arbeitsteilung mit „Meßinstitutionen" und den Gesundheitsämtern muß geschaffen werden, damit in enger Abstimmung die Ergebnisse von der Gesundheitsfachverwaltung epidemiologisch bewertet und interpretiert werden können. Solange sie dieses nicht leistet, wird sie im kommunalpolitischen Bereich nicht als der Sachwalter der Gesundheitsinteressen der Bevölkerung im gesundheitlichen Umweltschutz auftreten können. Somit ist der komplexen Aufgabenstellung des gesundheitlichen Umweltschutzes nur in einer engen Kooperation mit überregionalen Einrichtungen wie den Medizinaluntersuchungsämtern bzw. universitären Institutionen Rechnung zu tragen. Für Einzelaufgaben ist die Teilprivatisierung bzw. Übertragung an Einrichtungen nach dem Muster der technischen Überwachungsvereine denkbar.

Traditionell sind dem Gesundheitsamt die öffentlichen Aufgaben in der Seuchenhygiene zugeordnet. Die wesentliche Rechtsmaterie in diesem Gebiet wird durch das Bundes-Seuchengesetz geregelt. Die Anwendung des Bundes-Seuchengesetzes bzw. die Ergänzung des Bundes-Seuchengesetzes durch weitere Verordnungen nach § 11, wie auch die AIDS-Verordnung der bayerischen Landesregierung, haben unmittelbare Auswirkungen auf die gesundheitspolitische Stellung der Gesundheitsämter.

Die Aufgaben der Gesundheitsämter nicht nur in seuchenhygienischer Überwachung, sondern im Sinne einer seuchenhygienischen Präventionsarbeit, sind durch das Auftreten der Immunschwächekrankheit AIDS vor neue Dimensionen und neue Probleme gestellt worden. Seit mehreren Jahren sind in den Gesundheitsämtern, insbesondere in den Großstädten mit kommunalen Gesundheitsämtern (die meisten Gesundheitsämter in den Großstädten der Bundesrepublik Deutschland sind auch in den Ländern Baden-Württemberg und Bayern mit staatlichen öffentlichen Gesundheitsdiensten in kommunaler Trägerschaft), die sowohl in seuchenhygienischer Sicht, psychosozialer als auch pflegerischer Sicht gefordert waren, vielfältige kommunal gesteuerte, kommunal verantwortete und auch kommunal finanzierte Aktivitäten im Gange. Als Beispiel mögen die personalintensiven AIDS-Beratungsstellen der Gesundheitsämter in Düsseldorf und Köln gelten. Das Sofortprogramm der Bundesregierung zur Bekämpfung von AIDS, insbesondere das Großmodell „Gesundheitsämter", in dem für jedes Gesundheitsamt eine AIDS-Präventionskraft für die Dauer von 4 Jahren aus Bundesmitteln bezahlt werden sollte, gibt der zentralen Stellung des Gesundheitsamtes in der Seuchenprophylaxe und in der Seuchenabwehr eine zukunftsorientierte neue Aufgabe innerhalb des traditionellen Aufgabenkataloges. Das Problem AIDS wurde von den ärztlichen Standesorganisationen erst recht spät auch als ein Problem der niedergelassenen Ärzte gesehen (Flatten u. Allhoff 1987).

Es besteht eine zunehmende Tendenz mit dem Fortschreiten der Erkennungs- und Behandlungsmöglichkeiten, diesen Problembereich wiederum vollständig in den RVO-Bereich aufzunehmen und dem ÖGD allein die seuchenpolizeilichen Aufgaben zu überlassen.

Die Tuberkulose ist keine Volkskrankheit mehr, insofern stellt sich Tuberkulosefürsorge heute eher als Überwachungsmaßnahme der gesunden Befundträger und Diagnostikmethoden bei Ansteckungsverdächtigen dar (Bericht der Landesregierung 1983). Ziel der Tuberkulosefürsorge muß die Bekämpfung der Klein- und Kleinstepidemien sein. Das Gesundheitsamt ist aufgerufen, hier eine systematische Quellenermittlung wahrzunehmen (Bundesverband der Ärzte des öffentlichen Gesundheitsdienstes e. V. 1985).

Im Hinblick auf die Schutzimpfungen und die zu beobachtende Tendenz zu einer Verlagerung in den Bereich der niedergelassenen Ärzte (Vorreiter ist hier das Land Bayern gewesen) kommt dem Gesundheitsamt die besondere Bedeutung zu, etwa bestehende Impflücken aufzuspüren und durch ein ausreichendes Angebot von Schutzimpfungen zu schließen. Maier (1986) nennt „Impfungen, die alle Kinder erreichen müssen" als einen der 6 Schwerpunkte jugendärztlicher Arbeit. Auch wenn diese Forderung weitgehend unbestritten ist, ergibt sich doch auch hier das Problem, wie bestehende Impflücken aufgespürt und ein ausreichendes Angebot von Schutzimpfungen nicht nur bereitgestellt, sondern auch ein genügender Durchimpfungsgrad erreicht werden. Die bestehende Rechtslage bietet dem Gesundheitsamt hier nicht die Möglichkeit, dieser Aufgabe gerecht zu werden. Ob die lückenlose Erfassung der Kinder bzw. der Jugendlichen in betreffenden Altersgruppen durch Anschreiben bzw. gezielte Impfaufforderungen in den Schulen erreicht wird (Bundesverband der Ärzte des öffentlichen Gesundheitsdienstes e. V. 1985) ist fraglich. Ein Gesamtkonzept wird von Stürzbecher (1984) gefordert.

Die Aufgaben des ÖGD in der Krankenhaushygiene sind in den bestehenden Rechtsgrundlagen zu global und rechtlich nicht genügend abgesichert. Bei der Umsetzung der „Richtlinien" des BGA zur Verhütung und Bekämpfung von Krankenhausinfektionen werden die wissenschaftlichen Aufgaben Hygienekommissionen übertragen, wie dies auch das neue Landeskrankenhausgesetz NRW (1987) fordert. Die Aufsicht innerhalb der Krankenhäuser soll durch Schaffung verantwortlicher Hygienefachkräfte und Hygienekommissionen verstärkt werden.

Gesundheitspolitisch ist bisher die Frage, ob der Verbraucherschutz, d. h. der Bereich des Veterinärwesens, der Lebensmittelhygiene und -aufsicht ein substantieller Teil des ÖGD sein sollte nicht eindeutig beantwortet. Inhaltlich sind keine überzeugenden Argumente nach unserer Ansicht vorzutragen, diesen Bereich nicht als integrativen Bestandteil eines neuen GDG-Gesetzes aufzunehmen.

Gesundheitspflege
(Gesundheitsförderung und -vorsorge, Gesundheitshilfe)

Da die Leistungen im Bereich der Individualvorsorge und individuellen Gesundheitshilfe weitgehend durch die Reichsversicherungsordnung erfaßt sind, verbleibt dem öffentlichen Gesundheitsdienst die bevölkerungs- bzw. gruppenbezogene Gesundheitsfürsorge und -vorsorge als originäre Aufgabe. Diese Aufgabenbereiche hängen eng mit einer ausreichenden Infrastruktur für die epidemiologische Bewertung des Gesundheitszustandes und der präventivmedizinischen Versorgung (Health care research) der Bevölkerung zusammen. Nur bei Kenntnis des Gesundheits- und Versorgungszustandes können daraus aktuelle Schwerpunktaufgaben abgegrenzt, identifiziert und aufgegriffen werden. Die 50. GMK sieht für die Gesundheitsämter hier einen neuen Schwerpunkt im Bereich der Koordination und der federführenden Betreuung aller einschlägigen präventiven Aktivitäten. Diese müssen über die Programme der Aufklärung und Gesundheitserziehung im engeren Sinne hinausgehen und vor allem die Rahmenbedingungen für ein gesundheitsgerechtes Verhalten (Verbesserung der präventiven Angebote und ihrer Nutzung gerade auch bei sozial schwachen Gruppen) verbessern.

Für die der Primärprävention dienenden Aktivitäten und Maßnahmen ist ein Schwerpunkt beim Jugendärztlichen Dienst erforderlich, da Maßnahmen der Gesundheitsförderung im Wachstumsalter die größten Erfolgsmöglichkeiten bieten. Dagegen liegen Maßnahmen der sekundären (im Sinne der Früherkennung) und der tertiären (im Sinne der Rehabilitation) Prävention eher beim niedergelassenen Arzt bzw. im klinischen Bereich. Bei der Frage nach den Leistungsanforderungen an den jugendärztlichen Dienst ist zu berücksichtigen, daß in der Bundesrepublik Deutschland in den letzten 20 Jahren die Zahl der pro Jahr geborenen Kinder von ca. 1,2 Mio. auf ca. 600 000 gesunken ist, bei gleichzeitiger deutlicher Zunahme der niedergelassenen Kinderärzte, die in Zukunft die kassenärztlichen Möglichkeiten, wie sie das seit 1955 bestehende Kassenarztrecht bietet, nämlich die Verhütung von Krankheiten als kassenärztliche Aufgabe anzusehen, verstärkt wahrnehmen werden.

Vor diesem Hintergrund ist die Funktion und Bedeutung des schulärztlichen Dienstes zu diskutieren. Dieser kann nur als adäquater Partner zu den niedergelassenen Ärzten Stand haben, wenn der schulärztliche Dienst sich im Sinne eines sozialmedizinischen Anwalts des Schülers und Beraters der Schule versteht. Unterstützt wird dieses durch Artikel 71 des Grundgesetzes in dem es heißt, „das gesamte Schulwesen untersteht der Aufsicht des Staates", insofern sollte hier der jugendärztliche Dienst gefordert sein. Maier (1986) faßt diese Aufgaben des jugendärztlichen Dienstes in 6 Punkten zusammen:

1) ärztliche Hilfe für *alle* Kinder,
2) Impfungen, die alle Kinder erreichen,
3) ärztliche Hilfen für chronisch kranke und behinderte Kinder,[1]
4) ärztliche Einflußnahme auf Träger und Mitarbeiter der Schule, der Jugendhilfe und anderer Institutionen,
5) Gesundheitserziehung,
6) Epidemiologie im Säuglings-, Kindes- und Jugendalter.

Besonders die epidemiologischen Aufgaben sind über lange Jahre in den Hintergrund des Interesses und auch des Selbstverständnisses des ÖGD gerückt. Ein Beispiel dafür liefert die vielfach auf den Aspekt der medizinischen Schulfähigkeit reduzierte schulärztliche Untersuchung vor der Einschulung. Diese Untersuchung, die neben der Todesursachenstatistik die einzige Querschnitt- (und potentiell auch Längsschnitt-)Untersuchung der deutschen Bevölkerung darstellt, könnte bei entsprechender Standardisierung und Auswertung sowohl zur Qualitätsüberprüfung der Vorsorgeuntersuchungen (besonders U4–U8) wie auch zum vergleichenden epidemiologischen Monitoring der Entwicklung des kindlichen Gesundheitszustandes auf Bevölkerungsebene ausgebaut werden (Laaser et al., im Druck). Allerdings wäre dazu die Aufhebung widersinniger Einschränkungen durch den Datenschutz aufgrund der jetzigen Rechtslage erforderlich (Laaser u.

---

[1] Dazu gehört die Präsenz in sozialen Brennpunkten und Schwachstellen als auch die vermehrte Einrichtung sozialpädiatrischer und sozialpsychiatrischer Betreuungsangebote (Hopf 1984).

Wichmann 1985; Laaser et al., im Druck). Darüber hinaus sollten epidemiologische Begleiterhebungen und -analysen generell zu qualitätssichernden Maßnahmen für den kinder- und jugendärztlichen Dienst beitragen. Voraussetzung dafür ist die Sicherstellung einer entsprechenden epidemiologischen Methodenkenntnis in den Gesundheitsämtern. Hier haben auch die in der Bundesrepublik Deutschland insgesamt zur Verfügung stehenden Ausbildungsangebote noch erhebliche Lücken (Keil u. Laaser 1988; Laaser 1981).

Hervorgehoben werden muß die Bedeutung des jugendzahnärztlichen Dienstes für die Gesundheitsvorsorge und Gesundheitserziehung. Der Ausbau des jugendzahnärztlichen Dienstes zur Verbesserung der kindlichen Zahngesundheit, zur allgemeinen Gesundheitserziehung und zur Kostendämpfung im Gesundheitswesen bei intensiver Zusammenarbeit mit den RVO-Kassen ist eine wichtige und nicht verzichtbare gesundheitspolitische Maßnahme. Dies setzt jedoch voraus, daß der öffentliche Gesundheitsdienst freien Zugang zu allen kinderbetreuenden Einrichtungen auf kommunaler Ebene hat. Die Entwicklung der letzten Jahre deutet darauf hin, daß dieses zunehmend erschwert wird.

Eine besondere Frage, die am heftigsten umkämpfte Frage zwischen niedergelassenen und Klinikärzten auf der einen und dem ÖGD auf der anderen Seite, sind die Möglichkeiten und Zuständigkeiten des ÖGD in der „Therapie". Durch die Entschließungen der GMK, dort bezogen auf den sozialpsychiatrischen Dienst, wird grundsätzlich eine Behandlungsmöglichkeit für den ÖGD geschaffen. Die generelle Regelung des § 16 des Berliner GDG-Gesetzes erweitert diese Möglichkeit über den sozialpsychiatrischen Dienst hinaus. Hier öffnet sich eine Chance, dem hilfesuchenden und hilfebedürftigen Bürger durch den ÖGD die ärztliche Hilfeleistung zukommen zu lassen, deren Erbringung bei Ausklammerung der Behandlungsmöglichkeiten bzw. -erlaubnis aufgrund der Besonderheiten bestimmter persönlicher Bedingungen des Betroffenen und der Auswirkungen von Erkrankungen nicht möglich wäre.

Modellvorhaben – etwa im sozialpsychiatrischen Dienst – bestehen, hier sollte die Sachkompetenz und das im ÖGD vorhandene geeignete Personal (Ärzte, Psychologen, Sozialarbeiter, sozialmedizinische Assistenten) in multiprofessionellen Teams für die Bedürfnisse der psychisch Kranken in Behandlung und Betreuung bei fest umrissenen Indikationsgebieten genutzt werden.

Es ist unbestritten, daß die Gesundheitsämter in Zukunft stärker von den Landesvereinigungen für Gesundheitserziehung und der Bundeszentrale für gesundheitliche Aufklärung durch konkrete und verbesserte Arbeitshilfen unterstützt werden müssen.

Neben den z. Z. alle anderen Aktivitäten an den Rand drängenden Maßnahmen im Bereich der AIDS-Aufklärung dürften jedoch als gesundheitserzieherische Aufgaben die Probleme des Rauchens, des Alkoholismus, der Über- und Fehlernährung und des Bewegungsmangels in Verbindung mit der Kontrolle der Hypertonie und Hypercholesterinämie mit dem Ziel einer deutlichen Reduktion kardiovaskulärer Komplikationen in der Bevölkerung (Hoffmeister 1978) nicht vergessen werden.

Der ÖGD sollte sich der kollektiven Prävention ebenso wie der administrativen Prävention annehmen, Initiativen und fachliche Beratung bei Gesetzesvorhaben zur Gesundheitsvorsorge sind ebenso nötig wie anwendungsorientierte Feldforschungen und Interventionsprogramme. Das notwendige abgestimmte Handeln der verschiedenen medizinischen Versorgungsbereiche nebeneinander und miteinander als auch das in der regionalen Arbeit u. E. mangelhafte kooperative Zusammengehen mit den Sozialdiensten (Laaser et al., im Druck) bedarf der Verbesserung.

Hier liegt u. E. neben der Wiederbelebung einer epidemiologisch orientierten bevölkerungsmedizinischen Denkweise und Verantwortlichkeit (Laaser 1981) eines der für die weitere Entwicklung zentralen Aufgabenfelder (Murza u. Laaser 1988).

Begutachtungen

Eine weitere grundlegende Aufgabe des Gesundheitsamtes ist der Bereich des Gutachtenwesens, wobei zwar auch in Zukunft der durch Bundes- und Ländergesetze breite Katalog amtsärztlicher Individualgutachten einen großen Raum einnehmen wird, in Zukunft jedoch im Vordergrund der Aktivitäten die generelle Sachverständigentätigkeit zu gesundheitlichen Fragen stehen sollte.

Das Gesundheitsamt soll aufgrund seiner personellen und apparativen Ausstattung in der Lage sein, der unteren Verwaltungsbehörde sachlich fundierte Gutachten zu allen gesundheitlichen Bereichen zu erstellen, um lokale Entscheidungsträger in allen Fragen der „Volksgesundheit" gutachterlich beraten zu können. Es ist hierbei von ausschlaggebender Bedeutung, ob die erstellten Gutachten in ihrer Bewertung und Beweisführung als eine Meinungsäußerung eines „kommunalen Bediensteten" angesehen werden, oder ob Gutachten des Gesundheitsamtes eine Verbindlichkeit zukommt, die dem Grad externer Fachgutachten entspricht.

Bezüglich der amtsärztlichen Individualgutachten ist die Forderung des Hartmann-Bundes verständlich, alle diejenigen Gutachten an niedergelassene Ärzte oder Klinikärzte zu übertragen, die rechtlich übertragbar sind und die zur Erstellung eines solchen apparativen-technischen Aufwandes bedürfen, der nur in Spezialeinrichtungen vorhanden ist. Bezüglich der amtsärztlichen Gutachten merkt Schmacke (1987) kritisch an, daß empirische Untersuchungen zum amtsärztlichen Gutachtenwesen allenfalls in unzureichenden Ansätzen existieren, so daß in weiten Bereichen die Maßstäbe und Auswirkungen dieser Praxis nicht transparent sind.

Die bisher geübte Praxis, dem Amtsarzt die arbeitsmedizinischen Belange der Beschäftigten gemäß des Arbeitssicherheitsgesetzes von 1973 zu übertragen und keine eigenen arbeitsmedizinischen unabhängigen Dienste für den öffentlichen Dienst zu schaffen (mit wenigen Ausnahmen in Großstädten), führt zu einer „höchst unzureichenden Berücksichtigung" der arbeitsmedizinischen Belange der Beschäftigten (Schmacke 1987).

Hier bedarf es der Klarstellung zwischen den Aufgaben des ÖGD, des Amtsarztes und den Anforderungen, die das Arbeitssicherheitsgesetz vorschreibt.

Epidemiologie und kommunale Gesundheitsberichterstattung

Die bevölkerungsmedizinische – also in erster Linie an epidemiologischen Daten orientierte – Betrachtungsweise ist heute als Folge der Zurücknahme staatlicher Überwachungsfunktionen nach 1945 weitgehend verlorengegangen. Im Zuge seines immer wieder akzentuierten Subsidiärcharakters ist der ÖGD im allgemeinen Verständnis teilweise auf eine zweitklassige ärztliche Versorgung von sozialen Minoritäten geschrumpft.

Auszugehen wäre von den Formulierungen des § 1 der 2. Durchführungsverordnung, in der es heißt, „dem Gesundheitsamt obliegt es, die gesundheitlichen Verhältnisse des Bezirkes zu beobachten und sich auf Erfordern der zuständigen Behörde in Angelegenheiten des Gesundheitswesens gutachterlich zu äußern und ihnen Vorschläge zum Abstellen von Mängeln und zur Förderung der Volksgesundheit zu unterbreiten", fortgesetzt in den Bestimmungen des § 2 der 2. Durchführungsverordnung, aufgegriffen als § 6 des Schleswig-Holsteinischen GDG, als auch des § 1 Abs. 2 Ziffer 6 des Berliner GDG, obliegt es dem Gesundheitsamt „Daten zu sammeln" und diese zu epidemiologischen Zwecken auszuwerten und zu dokumentieren.

Ähnliche Formulierungen finden sich in der Länderrichtlinie (Hopf 1978). Allenthalben wird die Forderung erhoben, die Zuständigkeiten des Gesundheitsamtes im Bereich der regionalen Gesundheitsplanung und Gesundheitsberichterstattung zu erhöhen und Instrumentarien zu schaffen, die zur Klärung epidemiologischer Fragestellungen erforderlich sind.

Im Zuständigkeitsbereich des öffentlichen Gesundheitsdienstes bedarf es daher eindeutiger Regelungen von wem und wie die Daten für die notwendige sektorale Planung bereitgestellt werden müssen, wie diese Informationen umgesetzt werden sollen und wie die Koordinationsaufgaben des ÖGD bei der Ausarbeitung von Plänen für die ambulante und stationäre Versorgung und für die Prävention verbindlich geregelt werden können. Die Notwendigkeit der regionalen Gesundheitsberichterstattung ist gesundheitspolitisch unbestritten, Ziel und Methoden sind in Diskussion.

Ein besonderer Schwerpunkt der Gesundheitsberichterstattung soll auf die Beschreibung der gesundheitlichen Lage der Menschen und ihrer Determinanten gelegt werden. Einen Schwerpunkt bildet die Aufbereitung und Darstellung der Interdependenzen und Folgewirkungen zwischen Gesundheit/gesundheitlicher Lage/gesundheitlicher Versorgung und deren Finanzierung und den anderen menschlichen und gesellschaftlichen Lebensbereichen. Die Gesundheitsberichterstattung soll von den Gebietskörperschaften, wie Kommunen, Ländern und Bund sowie den Trägern der Selbstverwaltung in verschiedenen Berichtsformen entwickelt und getragen werden. Folgende Themenbereiche sind vorgesehen:

1) Gesundheitsprogramm,
2) Bevölkerung und bevölkerungsspezifische Rahmenbedingungen des Gesundheitswesens,
3) Gesundheitszustand,
4) gesundheitsrelevante Verhaltensweisen,
5) gesundheitsrelevante Bedingungen der natürlichen, technischen und sozialen Umwelt,

6) Leistungsinanspruchnahme der Gesundheitsversorgung,
7) Einrichtungen im Gesundheitswesen,
8) Beschäftigte im Gesundheitswesen,
9) Ausbildung und Forschung im Gesundheitswesen,
10) Ausgaben und Finanzierung,
11) Kosten und Nutzen und
12) Aufgabenplanungen.

Diese Konzeption der Gesundheitsberichterstattung (nach einem Arbeitspapier für Arbeitsgemeinschaft der leitenden Medizinalbeamten der Länder 1987) zielt also auf eine verdichtende Darstellung und beschreibende Bewertung von Gesundheits- und Medizinalstatistiken. Diese sollen nicht ersetzt, sondern breiter nutzbar und ergänzt werden (Schräder et al. 1986).

Eine Kompetenzsteigerung in diesem Bereich ist jedoch ohne Aufstockung der sachlichen und personellen Mittel sowie der Zusammenarbeit mit sonstigen Leistungsträgern des Gesundheitsdienstes nicht möglich. Im Bereich der Fortbildungsmaßnahmen sei auf die im Rahmen des deutschen akademischen Austauschdienstes zur epidemiologischen Weiterbildung geschaffenen Maßnahmen der Bundesregierung sowie auf die Epidemiology Summer School in Nordrhein-Westfalen (Keil u. Laaser 1988) hingewiesen.

Organisationsformen

Vielfältige Organisationsformen werden in dem Bericht der rheinland-pfälzischen Landesregierung (1983) vorgestellt. Eine diskussionswürdige These wird von Göpel (1986) vertreten, der vorschlägt, die Gesundheitsämter als Institution aufzulösen und die unbestreitbar vorhandenen gesundheitlichen Aufgaben in den Sozialverwaltungen oder den Umweltverwaltungen wahrzunehmen. Dies würde in der Konsequenz bedeuten, daß z. B. der schulärztliche Dienst in das Schulamt integriert wird und dort das ärztliche Fachwissen möglicherweise in einer multiprofessionellen Einheit eher den Belangen der Schüler Rechnung trägt als in der jetzigen Organisationsform, die häufig einer engen Zusammenarbeit von Ärzten und Pädagogen entgegensteht. Des weiteren wäre denkbar, daß der Gesamtbereich des gesundheitlichen Umweltschutzes von ärztlichem und sonstigem Fachpersonal der Umweltämter wahrgenommen wird.

Für die zukünftige Wahrnehmung der jetzigen Aufgaben der Gesundheitsfachverwaltungen lassen sich folgende sechs Hauptorganisationsformen diskutieren, unabhängig von rechtlichen Umsetzungsmöglichkeiten dieser Modelle und unabhängig von der „Effizienz" dieser Strukturen:

1) Wahrnehmung der Aufgaben durch eine überregionale staatliche oder kommunale Institution,
2) Wahrnehmung der Aufgaben durch städtische und kommunale Einrichtungen,
3) Wahrnehmung der Aufgaben durch die „bisherige Gesundheitsamtstruktur",
4) Wahrnehmung der Aufgaben durch noch zu schaffende Institutionen des öffentlichen Rechtes wie z. B. Medizinalüberwachungsvereine,

5) Wahrnehmung der Aufgaben durch freie Träger und
6) Durchführung der Aufgaben durch Privatpersonen und private Institutionen.

Perspektive

Bedingt durch die föderale Struktur der Bundesrepublik Deutschland und die unterschiedlichen politischen und gesundheitspolitischen Vorstellungen der Mehrheitsparteien in den Bundesländern und den bereits verabschiedeten Gesundheitsdienstgesetzen in den Ländern Bayern, Berlin und Schleswig-Holstein ist es eher unwahrscheinlich, daß es möglich sein wird, für den ÖGD eine allseits akzeptierte zukünftige Standortfestschreibung zu erreichen, da ein gesundheitspolitischer Bedarf für eine neue „Länderrichtlinie" z. Z. nicht gegeben ist. Gleichwohl bedarf es – in jedem Bundesland – letztlich grundlegender Entscheidungen bezüglich der Funktion und Struktur des ÖGD.

Grundsatzentscheidung

Die differenzierte Weiterentwicklung der Leistungserbringer im Gesundheitsdienst und außerhalb des Gesundheitsdienstes der letzten 30 Jahre führte dazu, daß die bisherige umfassende Zuständigkeit des ÖGD infolge des Vereinheitlichungsgesetzes für alle gesundheitsrelevanten Bereiche der Kommune letztlich eine Überforderung nach sich zog, die sich in einer auf vielen Bereichen diskutierten Kompetenzminderung niederschlug. Es ist daher erforderlich, eine Schwerpunktsetzung im ÖGD vorzunehmen, damit eine Eingrenzung der Aufgaben letztlich zu einer positiven Gesamtentwicklung führt. Folgende Schwerpunktaufgaben sind denkbar:

1) der ÖGD als staatliche/öffentlich-rechtliche Steuerungsfunktion für das Gesundheitswesen (über) kommunaler Ebene mit den Hauptaufgaben der epidemiologischen Datenerhebungsauswertung sowie umfassender Planungskompetenz in gesundheitlichen Fragestellungen,
2) der ÖGD als ärztliche bzw. kommunale Sachverständigenstelle für den Bürger und die Kommune mit den Hauptaufgaben der Beantwortung gesundheitsrelevanter Fragen das Verhältnis Umwelt, Bürger, Kommune betreffend,
3) der ÖGD als bürgerorientierte Beratungsinstitution für alle Fragen der Prävention mit den Hauptaufgaben der Allgemein- und Individualberatung in den Bereichen der Gesundheitserziehung und der Prävention sowie des Verbraucherschutzes als auch der Screeninguntersuchungen.
4) der ÖGD als komplementär tätiger umfassender sozialmedizinischer Dienst, der weit gefächert dezentral angelegt ist zur Betreuung aller Programmgruppen und Gefährdeten sowie Behinderten,
5) der ÖGD als staatliche Eingriffs-, Kontroll- und Beratungsinstitution im Gesundheitsbereich, dem umfassende gesundheitspolizeiliche Zuständigkeit, substantielle Medizinalaufsicht zukommt.

Dabei scheint es am realistischsten, einen organischen und allmählichen Umbau mit zunehmender Akzentuierung der Aufgabenfelder „epidemiologisches und ggf. Umweltmonitoring" (s. S. 343) und „Koordination einer kooperativen Prävention auf kommunaler Ebene" (s. S. 339) zu fordern.

Grundsatzaufgaben

Das bisher von den Gesundheitsämtern bzw. im Rahmen der Gesundheitsfachverwaltung des ÖGD wahrgenommene Aufgabenspektrum ist grundsätzlich zu überprüfen nach den Kriterien:

- Hoheitlichkeit der Aufgabe,
- Notwendigkeit der Aufgaben,
- Neutralitätserfordernis („anwaltliche" Rolle des Gesundheitsamtes) und
- Subsidiarität der Aufgabe.

Für die traditionellen Bereiche der Medizinalaufsicht, des Gesundheitsschutzes und der Gesundheitsfürsorge sowie für die in Zukunft zunehmend bedeutungsvolleren Bereiche der Gesundheitsvorsorge/Gesundheitsförderung und der epidemiologischen Überwachung des Gesundheitszustandes der Bevölkerung einschließlich der damit verbundenen Planungsaufgaben müssen Kriterien geschaffen werden. Es ist daher zu prüfen, ob das deckungsgleiche Agieren der Gesundheitsämter mit Kommunalverwaltungen und die damit verbundene Abhängigkeit der gesundheitspolitischen Aussagen des Gesundheitsamtes von den kommunalen Entscheidungsträgern eine auch in Zukunft bestehende Organisationsform sein soll. Falls die bisherige Struktur auch aus verfassungsrechtlichen Gründen nicht geändert werden kann, ist grundsätzlich die Frage nach der effizienten Fachaufsicht zu stellen, die ein zentrales Steuerungselement sein sollte, um einer durch die dezentrale Kommunalität der Gesundheitsämter gegebene Tendenz zur Aufsplitterung von Planungs- und Abstimmungsvorgängen entgegenzuwirken. Dies setzt jedoch eine drastische Erhöhung der personellen Ressourcen bei den Landesmittelbehörden bzw. bei den Obersten Landesgesundheitsbehörden voraus, die z. Z. kaum in der Lage sind, systematisch fachaufsichtlich und gleichzeitig innovativ tätig zu werden. Dabei muß die Verantwortlichkeit der Obersten Landesgesundheitsbehörden für das gesamte Gesundheitswesen erneut betont werden, auch wenn durch die Delegation der Aufgabenwahrnehmung die fachliche Zuständigkeit sowohl im ambulanten als auch stationären Bereich größtenteils außerhalb der direkten Einflußnahme der Ministerien liegt. Für den engeren Bereich des ÖGD ist zu überprüfen, ob die Aufgaben der Medizinalaufsicht tatsächlich der „staatlichen" Regelung bedürfen.

Die notwendige Prüfung der Einzelaufgaben hat neben dem hoheitlichen Aspekt bzw. den ordnungspolitischen Gesichtspunkten vor allem auch der „strukturellen Neutralität" des Gesundheitsamtes als einer letztlich vom demokratischen Konsens abhängigen Institution Rechnung zu tragen.

Die beim gesundheitlichen Umweltschutz (Umweltmedizin) anfallenden Aufgaben der gutachterlichen Stellungnahme zu den Problembereichen „Boden, Wasser, Luft" sollten – abgesehen von Einzelüberprüfungen und -kontrollen – wegen der Komplexität der Materie in überregionalen Institutionen angesiedelt sein, wobei diese Institutionen eine Meßkapazität benötigen, die zunehmend von bakteriologischen zu umwelttoxikologischen Bereichen einschließlich der Strahlenmessung verschoben werden muß.

Dies darf aber nicht dazu führen, auch die medizinisch-epidemiologische Bewertung von potentiell gefährlichen Expositionen bzw. deren Messungen aus den Gesundheitsämtern heraus zu verlagern. Nur dort kann und sollte aufgrund der Tradition des ÖGD, seiner strukturellen Einbindung und Aufgabenstellung und der Erfahrungs- und (zunehmend) der Ausbildungskompetenz seiner Fachkräfte eine solche abschließende und integrierende Bewertung angesiedelt und zugeordnet werden.

Für die vielfältigen Aufgaben im Rahmen der Gesundheitsvorsorge, -fürsorge und -hilfe ist das Festhalten an den Kriterien der absoluten Subsidiarität, gemessen an den Erfordernissen einer modernen Gesundheitsfachverwaltung, nicht hilfreich. Der große Vorteil des öffentlichen Gesundheitsdienstes in der strukturell vorhandenen großen Flexibilität sollte genutzt werden, um den Belangen der Bevölkerung Rechnung zu tragen, wobei verstärkt der Vorteil des ÖGD bezüglich der Effektivität und Effizienz gegenüber anderen Leistungserbringern jenseits ideologisierender Dogmen nachgeprüft und verdeutlicht werden muß.

Amtsärztliche Gutachten müssen im Individualbereich auf das vertretbare Minimum reduziert werden, der Bereich der Fachgutachten im Sinne des „Sachverständigenanwaltes" für gesundheitliche Belange der Bevölkerung sollte durch konsequente Schulung und Aufbau eines multiprofessionell agierenden Beratungsinstrumentariums wesentlich verstärkt werden.

Im Bereich der epidemiologischen Erfassung und Auswertung von relevanten Gesundheitsdaten zur regionalen Gesundheitsberichterstattung, die als Grundlage kommunaler gesundheitspolitischer Entscheidungen essentiell erforderlich ist, fehlt z. Z. noch das notwendige Instrumentarium der Umsetzung. Dem kann sich der ÖGD in Zukunft nicht entziehen, dieser Aufgaben sollte er sich nicht halbherzig widmen und im Zusammengehen mit den auf diesem Gebiete forschenden wissenschaftlichen Institutionen ein attraktives Konzept für die Gesundheitsberichterstattung zur Grundlage der Verbesserung der Lebensbedingungen und des Gesundheitszustandes der Bevölkerung entwickeln.

Die kaum geführte parlamentarische Diskussion bei der Verabschiedung der Landesgesundheitsdienstgesetze der Länder Schleswig-Holstein, Berlin und insbesondere Bayern hat gezeigt, daß der ÖGD nicht als Instrumentarium einer Gesundheits- und Sozialpolitik gesehen wird. Darin liegt eine Chance für eine parteipolitisch „neutrale" bürgerorientierte Fachbehörde. Darin dokumentiert sich jedoch auch die Gefahr, gesundheitspolitisch zur Bedeutungslosigkeit abzusinken, ausgestattet mit rudimentären ordnungspolitischen Aufgaben. Der einsetzende drastische Strukturwandel im Gesundheitswesen sollte vom ÖGD genutzt werden, um in den Aufgabenfeldern der Sozialhygiene und Prävention (Labisch 1985) und der kommunalen Gesundheitsförderung zum Vorreiter im Gesundheitswesen zu werden. Hierin bedarf es des Umdenkens, der inhaltlichen Gestaltung und der kommunalpolitischen Umsetzung. Ohne gesundheitspolitisches Engagement seitens der Handelnden im ÖGD – basierend auf dem Hintergrund einer fachkompetenten, multiprofessionellen Gesundheitsverwaltung – werden die Forderungen nicht mehrheitsfähig werden.

Schlußbetrachtung

Die Diskussion über die Zukunft des ÖGD hat sich bisher im wesentlichen auf das Umfeld des Berufsverbandes der Ärzte des öffentlichen Gesundheitswesens beschränkt und kaum den wissenschaftlichen (Sozialmedizin, Sozialhygiene, Medizinsoziologie, Gesundheitswissenschaften) oder gar gesundheitspolitischen Raum erreicht. Das Projekt zur Intensivierung der Gesundheitserziehung durch den öffentlichen Gesundheitsdienst der BZgA, gefördert vom BMFT und administriert von BZgA und WIAD, hat bisher nach mehr als fünfjähriger Laufzeit noch keinen Bericht, der für die allgemeine Öffentlichkeit zugänglich wäre, publiziert. Aus der Deutschen Herz-Kreislauf-Präventionsstudie (DHP) ist wenigstens ansatzweise über Erfahrungen mit der präventiven Koordination auf Gemeindeebene unter Federführung des ÖGD berichtet worden (Laaser 1986). Mit Ausnahme der historisierenden Betrachtung von Labisch u. Tennstedt (1985) ist von den einschlägigen universitären Instituten bzw. Lehrstühlen die Problematik zumindest nicht vertiefend aufgegriffen worden. Dies liegt sicher auch an dem oben schon angesprochenen Ausbildungsdefizit und den bisher geringen Karriereerwartungen.

Die aktuelle Diskussion über die Einrichtung von Graduiertenstudiengängen für Gesundheitswissenschaften oder den MPH (Master of Public health) vergleichbare Weiterbildungsmöglichkeiten an deutschen wissenschaftlichen Einrichtungen (Berlin, Bielefeld, Ulm etc.) eröffnet zumindest perspektivisch die Möglichkeit einer mittelfristigen Abhilfe. Die beiden Akademien für öffentliches Gesundheitswesen in Düsseldorf und München können mit der bisherigen Ausbildungsstruktur den Sachbedarf (vgl. dazu den Bestand von 21 Schools of Public health in den USA mit einer ca. 4mal so großen Bevölkerung) nicht abdecken (Kröger u. Müller 1987). Die Diskussion über die Zukunft des ÖGD und über die dafür notwendigen Voraussetzungen muß in eine breitere Öffentlichkeit getragen werden.

Literatur

Akademie für öffentliches Gesundheitswesen (Hrsg) (1985) Fünfzig Jahre Gesetz über die Vereinheitlichung des Gesundheitswesens. Tagung zur Geschichte und Zukunft des öffentlichen Gesundheitsdienstes am 18. und 19. Mai 1984 in Bremen. Bd 12 der Schriftenreihe der Akademie für öffentliches Gesundheitswesen in Düsseldorf. Selbstverlag, Düsseldorf
Arbeitsgemeinschaft der Leitenden Medizinalbeamten der Länder (1987) Rahmenplan für eine Gesundheitsberichterstattung in den Ländern. Berlin Bielefeld Hamburg Mainz Stuttgart
Bericht der Landesregierung über die Zukunft des öffentlichen Gesundheitsdienstes in Rheinland-Pfalz (1983) Landtag Rheinland-Pfalz, Drucksache 10/284 v. 6.11.1983
Bundesverband der Ärzte des öffentlichen Gesundheitsdienstes e.V. (1985) Die Aufgaben des öffentlichen Gesundheitsdienstes bei der Gesundheitssicherung in der Bundesrepublik Deutschland. Öff Gesundheitswes 47:235–239
Daten des Gesundheitswesens – Ausgabe 1985 – Band 154 der Schriftenreihe des BMJFG Stuttgart
Dewein P (1981) Die Zukunft des öffentlichen Gesundheitsdienstes. Öff Gesundheitswes 43:575–577
Faerber K-P (1972) Formen des öffentlichen Gesundheitsdienstes in der Zukunft. Öff Gesundheitswes 34:645–653

Federhen L (Hrsg) (1967) Der Arzt des öffentlichen Gesundheitsdienstes. Das Grüne Gehirn. Thieme, Stuttgart

Femmer H-J (1982) Zur Zukunft des öffentlichen Gesundheitsdienstes – Organisation und Aufgaben. Öff Gesundheitswes 44:805–814

Flatten W, Allhoff P (1987) AIDS als Problem in der kassenärztlichen Versorgung. Deutscher Ärzte-Verlag, Köln

Geissler H (1974) Was erwartet der Gesundheitspolitiker vom öffentlichen Gesundheitsdienst? Öff Gesundheitswes 36:97–103

Gesetz über den öffentlichen Gesundheitsdienst – Gesundheitsdienstgesetz (GDG) vom 28. Juli 1980. GVBl. Berlin 1495ff.

Gesetz über das öffentliche Gesundheitswesen – Gesundheitsdienstgesetz (GDG) vom 26. März 1979. GVOBl. Schleswig-Holstein 255ff.

Gesundheitspolitisches Programm der CDU, Bonn (1978)

Gesundheitspolitisches Programm der FDP, Bonn (1976)

Göpel E (1986) Kommunale Gesundheitspolitik und öffentlicher Gesundheitsdienst. In: Buckert H, Hoppe F, Schwandner G (Hrsg) Kritik des Gesundheitswesens und grüne Alternativen (Arbeitskreis Arbeit und Soziales der Grünen im Bundestag). Bonn, S 110–113

Göttsching C (1980) Die Zukunft des öffentlichen Gesundheitsdienstes. Öff Gesundheitswes 42:548–553

Grüne im Bundestag, Projektgruppe „Nationale Strategie Gesundheit 2000" (Hrsg) (1984) Gesund sein 2000. Wege und Vorschläge. Verlagsgesellschaft Gesundheit, Berlin, S 45ff., 53

GSVDÄ: Gesundheits- und sozialpolitische Vorstellungen der deutschen Ärzteschaft (1986). Das „Blaue Papier". Deutscher Ärzte-Verlag, Köln, 91ff.

Hartmann-Bund. Verband der Ärzte Deutschlands (Hrsg) (1981) Thesen zur Sozial- und Gesundheitspolitik. Selbstverlag, Bonn, S 56ff.

Hoffmeister H (1978) Die Kostenexplosion im Gesundheitswesen – Ein Anlaß zum Nachdenken über Auftrag und Chancen des öffentlichen Gesundheitsdienstes. Öff Gesundheitswes 40:408–417

Hopf E-J (1976) Das Gesundheitsamt heute und morgen. Öff Gesundheitswes 38:8–14

Hopf E-J (1978) Die Richtlinien für Ländergesetze über das Gesundheitswesen und ihre Umsetzung in Landesrecht. Öff Gesundheitswes 40:418–427

Hopf E-J (1975) Die Weiterentwicklung des öffentlichen Gesundheitsdienstes nach der Richtlinie für Ländergesetze. Eine Zwischenbilanz. Bundesgesundheitsblatt 18:333–344

Hopf E-J (1984) Zukünftige Aufgabenschwerpunkte des Gesundheitsamtes. Öff Gesundheitswes 46:347–351

Keil U, Laaser U (1988) The German American Epidemiology Summer School 1988 Universität Bochum und Institut für Dokumentation und Information, Sozialmedizin und öffentliches Gesundheitswesen, Bielefeld

Kröger E, Müller W (1987) Zur Situation der beruflichen und wissenschaftlichen Qualifizierungsmöglichkeiten in "Public Health" in der Bundesrepublik Deutschland. Akademie für öffentliches Gesundheitswesen, Düsseldorf

Labisch A (1985) Soziologische Grundlagenprobleme der primären Prävention und das Konzept der „gemeinschaftlichen Gesundheitssicherung" der Weltgesundheitsorganisation. In: Rosenbrock R, Hauß F (Hrsg) Krankenkassen und Prävention. Ed. Sigma, Berlin, S 51–75

Labisch A, Tennstedt F (1985) Der Weg zum „Gesetz über die Vereinheitlichung des Gesundheitswesens" vom 3. 7. 1934. Entwicklungslinien und -momente des staatlichen und kommunalen Gesundheitswesens in Deutschland. Bd 13. Schriftenreihe der Akademie für öffentliches Gesundheitswesen in Düsseldorf. Düsseldorf

Labisch A, Ziesmann U (1984) Zur Personalsituation (insbesondere der Ärzte) im ÖGD von 1951–1980 im Vergleich zur ambulanten und stationären Versorgung. Öff Gesundheitswes 46:63–67

Laaser U (1981) Epidemiologie: Wissenschaft, Methode oder Aufgabe? Med Klinik 76:407

Laaser U (1986) Die Deutsche Herz-Kreislauf-Präventionsstudie (DHP): Das Modell einer kooperativen Prävention. In: Halhuber C et al. (Hrsg) Die koronare Herzkrankheit – eine Herausforderung an Gesellschaft und Politik. Perimed, Erlangen, S 212–232 (Nachdruck in: Bundesvereinigung für Gesundheitserziehung (Hrsg) Gemeindenahe Gesundheitserziehung. Bonn, S 155–183

Laaser U, Wichmann H (f. d. AG Epidemiologie) (1985) Memorandum zur Verbesserung des Zugangs zu Sterbeunterlagen und Mortalitätsdaten in der Bundesrepublik Deutschland. Arbeitsmedizin, Sozialmedizin, Präventivmedizin 20:125–127 (Nachdruck in: Krasemann EO, Laaser U, Schach E (Hrsg) (1987) Sozialmedizin: Schwerpunkte Rheuma und Krebs. Springer, Berlin Heidelberg New York Tokyo

Laaser U, Gerdel W, Sassen G (1986) Gesundheitsentwicklung im Schulalter· Datenlage und Bewertung aus medizinischer und epidemiologischer Sicht. Prävention und Gesundheitserziehung: Kooperativer Ansatz, multidisziplinäre Aufgabe. Kongreß der Deutschen Gesellschaft für Sozialmedizin und der Zeitschrift Prävention, Bielefeld 23.–27. 9. 1986. Springer, Berlin Heidelberg New York Tokyo

Laaser U, Murza G, Gerdel W, Borgers D (1988) Strategien zur Prävention von Herz-Kreislauf-Krankheiten in der Bundesrepublik. SMP

Leitlinien für den öffentlichen Gesundheitsdienst (1986) Seminar der Landesarbeitsgemeinschaft Gesundheit der SPD Bremen in Bad Zwischenahn am 16.11.1985, Broschüre der SPD Bremen

Maier E (1986) Zukunft der Jugendgesundheitshilfe im öffentlichen Gesundheitsdienst. Öff Gesundheitswes 48:547–555

Manger-König L von (1975) Der öffentliche Gesundheitsdienst zwischen gestern und morgen. Öff Gesundheitswes 37:433–448

Moritzen P, Wodarg W (1987) Gesundheitlicher Umweltschutz – eine Aufgabe der Gesundheitsämter in Schleswig-Holstein. Öff Gesundheitswes 49:216–219

Murza G, Laaser U (1988) Kooperative Prävention auf dem Prüfstand der Praxis. Umfrage bei den Gesundheitsämtern in Nordrhein-Westfalen zur Existenz von Arbeitsgemeinschaften für Gesundheitsförderung. Prävention

Neuhaus R, Schräder WF (1986) Modellversuche zur kommunalen Planung im Gesundheitswesen. Öff Gesundheitswes 48:666–669

Nittner K-R (1976) Modellvorschläge zur Organisation zur kommunalen (und regionalen) Gesundheitsplanung. Öff Gesundheitswes 38:793–798

Öffentliches Gesundheitswesen (1978a) Antwort der Landesregierung NRW. Landtag NRW Drucksache 8/3889 v. 7.12.1978

Öffentliches Gesundheitswesen (1978b) Große Anfrage der SPD und FDP. Landtag NRW Drucksache 8/3050 v. 6.3.1978

Pfau E (1979) Muß es einen öffentlichen Gesundheitsdienst geben? Allgemeinmed 55:336–339

Reuter H (1982) Gibt es noch eine Alternative? Öff Gesundheitswes 44:805–814

Schmacke N (1987) Der Standort der Gesundheitsämter in der aktuellen gesundheitspolitischen Diskussion. Argument [Sonderband AS] 146:122–145

Schmidt G, Laaser U (1988) Gesundheitswissenschaft und öffentliche Gesundheitsförderung; aktuelle Modelle einer universitären Public-Health-Ausbildung. Fakultät für Soziologie der Universität Bielefeld und Institut für Dokumentation und Information, Sozialmedizin und öffentliches Gesundheitswesen, Bielefeld 5. u. 6.2.1988

Schräder WF et al. (1986) Kommunale Gesundheitsplanung. Birkhäuser, Basel

Steuer W (1984) Aufgabenwandlung des offentlichen Gesundheitsdienstes. Öff Gesundheitswes 46:68–70

Stürzbecher M (1984) Ein einheitlicher Jugendgesundheitsdienst vom Säugling bis zum Schulkind. Bundesgesundheitsblatt 27:151–154

Weltgesundheitsorganisation (WHO) (1982) Regionale Strategie zum Erreichen des Ziels „Gesundheit für alle bis zum Jahr 2000". EUR/RC 30/8 Rev 2

Weltgesundheitsorganisation (WHO) (1983) Einzelziele zur Unterstützung der Regionalstrategie für „Gesundheit 2000", EUR/RC 33/9

Wickenhauser K (1975) Aufgabenkatalog des Amtsärztlichen Dienstes. Öff Gesundheitswes 37:210–221

Wolters H-G (1974) Moderne Gesundheitspolitik im öffentlichen Gesundheitsdienst. Öff Gesundheitswes 35:727–737

Bürgerbefragungen als Beitrag gemeindebezogener Berichterstattung und Planung

J. von Troschke, K. Riemann

Seit ca. 15 Jahren werden weltweit mit Unterstützung der WHO gemeindebezogene Präventionsansätze erprobt. In epidemiologischen Modellstudien wurde die Bevölkerung von Wohngemeinden als Zielpopulation für Interventionsmaßnahmen genommen und mit entsprechenden Referenzgemeinden verglichen. Bei der Durchführung der Präventionsmaßnahmen stellte sich bald heraus, daß es notwendig war, sich mit den vorgefundenen lokalen, präventiv engagierten Personen und Organisationen zu arrangieren, wenn man die vorgesehenen Innovationen erfolgreich durchführen und stabil implementieren wollte. Die dabei angewandten Strategien zielen darauf, effektivere Maßnahmen zur Gesundheitserziehung, -aufklärung und -beratung in bestehende präventive Versorgungsstrukturen einzubringen, um damit bei der Wohnbevölkerung die Häufigkeit von Risikofakto-

Tabelle 1. Raucherverhalten im nationalen und regionalen Untersuchungssurvey (t_0: 1984–1985) (Alter: 25 bis 69 Jahre)

	Nationales Untersuchungssurvey	Region Berlin– Spandau	Region Bremen	Region Stuttgart	Region LK.Traunstein	Region Bruchsal/ Mosbach	Region Karlsruhe
Stichprobe (absolut)							
– Gesamt	4780	1832	1798	1788	1944	2144	1998
– Männer	2297	880	865	859	936	1025	962
– Frauen	2483	952	933	929	1008	1119	1036
Gesamt [%]							
– Raucher	34,0	44,0	42,6	35,6	26,1	29,9	30,6
– Ehemalige Raucher	24,7	23,3	24,1	25,7	22,3	24,6	24,9
– Nichtraucher	41,3	32,7	33,3	38,7	51,6	45,5	38,5
Männer [%]							
– Raucher	41,7	53,0	54,3	41,7	34,8	40,3	45,5
– Ehemalige Raucher	31,9	29,2	30,1	34,8	30,4	33,5	30,7
– Nichtraucher	26,4	17,8	15,6	23,5	34,8	26,2	23,8
Frauen [%]							
– Raucher	26,9	35,8	31,7	29,9	18,1	20,5	28,3
– Ehemalige Raucher	18,0	17,9	18,6	17,2	14,8	16,4	19,6
– Nichtraucher	55,1	46,3	49,7	52,9	67,1	63,1	52,1

ren (bzw. Morbiditäts- und Mortalitätsraten) statistisch signifikant zu reduzieren. In wissenschaftlich kontrollierten Evaluationsstudien wurde deshalb der Gesundheitszustand der Bevölkerung mit Befragungs- und Untersuchungssurveys erfaßt und zu mehreren Meßzeitpunkten miteinander verglichen. Ein Studienerfolg wurde dann konstatiert, wenn sich die Meßwerte der Studienpopulation statistisch signifikant in die erwünschte Richtung verändert hatten.

Die vergleichende Auswertung der Ergebnisse epidemiologischer Untersuchungen zeigt große Unterschiede, nicht nur zwischen verschiedenen Nationen, sondern auch im kleinräumigen regionalen Vergleich innerhalb einer Gesellschaft. So hat die Deutsche Herz-Kreislauf-Präventionsstudie gezeigt, daß sich in der Bundesrepublik Deutschland wesentliche Unterschiede in bezug auf gesundheitsrelevante Verhaltensweisen und somatische Befunde in der Wohnbevölkerung sowie auf präventive Versorgungsstrukturen zwischen den Gemeinden feststellen lassen. Exemplarisch können wir an dieser Stelle die Ergebnisse zum Rauchverhalten im nationalen und regionalen Untersuchungssurvey (t_0 1984/85) anführen (Kreuter et al. 1989; Tabelle 1). Die Raucherquoten bei den Männern schwanken zwischen 34,8 % im Landkreis Traunstein und 54,3 % in Bremen-West/Nord, bei den Frauen zwischen 18,1 % im Landkreis Traunstein und 35,8 % in Berlin-Spandau.

Auf der Basis derartiger Daten kann eine systematische Dokumentation gesundheitsrelevanter Verhaltensweisen in der Wohnbevölkerung von Gemeinden sowie der darauf bezogenen Gesundheitsdienste erstellt und als Basis für eine zielgerichtete Gesundheitsplanung genommen werden.

Gesundheitsberichte, wie sie in der Strategie der WHO für die europäische Region unter dem Titel „Gesundheit für alle bis zum Jahr 2000" gefordert werden, können zwei verschiedene Funktionen haben:

- die Dokumentation des Gesundheitsstatus einer Wohnbevölkerung und deren Veränderung im Zeitverlauf,
- die gesundheitspolitische Steuerung des Versorgungssystems mit Hilfe einer zielgerichteten Versorgungsplanung.

Für die Bundesrepublik Deutschland liegen bisher verschiedene Ansätze zur Gesundheitsberichterstattung vor, die sich auf das Bundesland Nordrhein-Westfalen (Idis 1987/88), den Landkreis Kronach (1985) und die kreisfreien Städte Osnabrück (1983), Köln (oJ) und Essen (1988) beziehen. Im Rahmen eines Modellprojekts des Bundesministeriums für Arbeit und Sozialordnung wurde das folgende Rahmenkonzept für eine kommunale Gesundheitsberichterstattung und einen kommunalen Gesundheitsplan erarbeitet (Schräder et al. 1986):

1) Ziele und Verfahren des Gesundheitsplans,
2) Gesundheitsprogramm,
3) Bevölkerung und Gesundheitszustand,
4) Gesundheitsschutz,
5) Gesundheitsversorgung,
6) Beschäftigte im Gesundheitswesen,
7) Aufgaben im Gesundheitswesen,
8) ausgewählte Aufgabenplanungen und bereichsübergreifende Programme.

Als Kriterien des Gesundheitszustandes einer Bevölkerung wurden die „Länge des Lebens, Morbidität und krankheitsbedingte Beeinträchtigungen der Mobilität und Arbeitsfähigkeit" (Neuhaus u. Schräder 1988) vorgeschlagen. Die Durchführung zeigte v. a. Schwierigkeiten in der Verfügbarkeit valider Daten sowie in der Interpretation der Ergebnisse. So konnten Heins und Stiens die „interregionale Mobilität als einen der wesentlichen ‚Störfaktoren' bei Untersuchungen der Zusammenhänge zwischen der Qualität der regionalen Lebensumwelt und den Strukturen regionaler Sterblichkeit" identifizieren (Heins u. Stiens 1984). Auch die Frage nach der Umsetzung der festgestellten Auffälligkeiten war oft schwer zu beantworten. So kam der Gesundheitsbericht des Landkreises Kronach vor dem Hintergrund einer hohen Sterblichkeit an Krankheiten der Atmungs- und Verdauungsorgane gegenüber dem Landesdurchschnitt lediglich zu dem Schluß: „Diese Entwicklung wird von dem Gesundheitsamt sorgfältig beachtet und geprüft, inwieweit mit dem Datenmaterial eine Eingrenzung der Problematik möglich ist" (Landkreis Kronach 1985).

Darüber hinaus vernachlässigen derartige Statistiken die Lebensrealitäten und die subjektiven Bedürfnisse der Bevölkerung. Die WHO hat ausdrücklich die Forderung aufgestellt, daß neben expertendefinierten Gesundheitsproblemen auch die Perspektive der sog. Laien bei der Planung präventiver Maßnahmen berücksichtigt werden soll. Zur Förderung der gesundheitlichen Fähigkeiten wurde vorgeschlagen, die „Messung des Gesundheitszustandes nach der subjektiven Einschätzung der Befragten" und eine „bessere Erforschung der Beziehung zwischen der subjektiven Wahrnehmung der Gesundheit, den Erwartungen und der ‚objektiven' Messung des Gesundheitszustandes" vorzunehmen (Einzelziel 2) (WHO 1985, S. 40). Für den Bereich des gesundheitlichen Umweltschutzes (Einzelziel 18) werden die Mitgliedsstaaten aufgefordert, Indikatoren zu entwickeln, z. B. „das Problembewußtsein der Öffentlichkeit" (WHO 1985, S. 214) betreffend.

Damit sind grundsätzlich neue Dimensionen gemeindebezogener Prävention angesprochen: Zum einen sollen die Bedürfnisse der Wohnbevölkerung selber erfragt und bei der Planung, Organisation und Durchführung präventiver Maßnahmen berücksichtigt werden, zum anderen werden neben die Individualprävention Maßnahmen zur Verhältnis- und Umweltprävention gestellt. Zur Umsetzung dieser Forderung bieten sich verschiedene Methoden an. In den meisten

Tabelle 2. Angaben (%) zum subjektiven Gesundheitszustand von Männern

Subjektiver Gesundheitszustand von Männern	Stuttgart	Berlin-Spandau	Bremen West/Nord	Karlsruhe	LK Traunstein
Sehr gut	5,5	5,6	6,0	7,8	7,9
Gut	38,4	35,4	33,7	41,1	38,7
Zufriedenstellend	39,4	44,0	45,3	37,0	40,7
Weniger gut	13,7	11,4	12,1	11,0	9,9
Sehr schlecht	2,8	3,2	2,2	2,8	2,3
Keine Antwort	0,3	0,4	0,7	0,0	0,5
n Gesamt	835	848	853	968	892

Bevölkerungsumfragen finden sich auch Fragen zur subjektiven Einschätzung des Gesundheitszustandes, die gemeindebezogen ausgewertet werden können. Im Gesundheitssurvey der Deutschen Herz-Kreislauf-Präventionsstudie (1984/85) zeigten sich wesentliche Unterschiede zwischen den Studiengemeinden (Tabelle 2).

Neben regionalen Aspekten wirken sich Alter, Geschlecht sowie Merkmale der sozialen Lage auf das subjektive Gesundheitserleben aus.

Ein anderer Ansatz zur Erfassung gemeindebezogener Informationen über gesundheitsbezogene Einstellungen der Wohnbevölkerung ist die Durchführung von weitgehend offenen Interviews. Zur Erprobung der Möglichkeiten von Straßenbefragungen wurden von uns mehrere Erhebungen durchgeführt (Tabelle 3).

Tabelle 3. Bürgerbefragungen zu Gesundheitsproblemen (Gesomed 1988/89)

Gemeinde	Erhebungsort -anlaß	Stichprobe	Alter
Saarbrücken	Veranstaltung: Altentag	n = 164	über 60 Jahre
Merchweiler	Veranstaltung: Gesundheitstag	n = 270	über 13 Jahre
Freiburg	Stadtteil Weingarten	n = 123	14–18 Jahre
Freiburg	Stadtteil Herdern	n = ca. 350 (läuft derzeit)	14–18 Jahre
Offenburg	Stadtgebiet	n = 1273	über 13 Jahre
Emmendingen	Stadtgebiet	n = ca. 1000	14–20 Jahre über 30 Jahre

Im Mittelpunkt der Untersuchungen stand die Frage nach den gesundheitsrelevanten Problemen, die nach Meinung der Befragten in ihrer Wohngemeinde gegeben sind. Bei den bisher durchgeführten Pilotstudien ging es v. a. um die Entwicklung eines angemessenen Ansatzes zur Durchführung von Straßenbefragungen zur Erfassung relevanter Daten für die Gesundheitsberichterstattung.

Anläßlich der Evaluation eines „Altentages" in Saarbrücken wurden den Teilnehmern lediglich zwei Fragen gestellt:

– „Was ist hier in Saarbrücken für Ihre Gesundheit und Ihr Wohlbefinden am besten?"
– „Was stört hier in Saarbrücken Ihre Gesundheit und Ihr Wohlbefinden am meisten?"

Es wurden keine Antwortvorgaben gegeben. Die Interviewer hatten die Anweisung, die Antworten ausführlich mitzuschreiben.

Die Kategorisierung der Ergebnisse erwies sich als außerordentlich schwierig, da die Nennungen ein breites Spektrum von Einzelangaben erhielten. Tabelle 4 zeigt das Spektrum der Angaben in bezug auf positive Einflußfaktoren für die Gesundheit.

Die Ergebnisse zeigen die besondere Wahrnehmung der Gemeinderealität aus der Perspektive alter Menschen (über 60 Jahre).

Tabelle 4. Positive Einflußfaktoren für die Gesundheit (aufgeschlüsselt; n = 164, Mehrfachnennungen)

	n	%
Umwelt		
Viel Wald, schöne Umgebung	42	26
Gute Luft	10	6
Ruhe	9	5
Saubere Stadt	3	5
Schöne Architektur	8	5
Lebensgefühl/soziale Kontakte		
Atmosphäre der Stadt	17	10
Viele Kontakte	3	2
Heimatgefühl	17	10
Nette Mitmenschen	10	6
Familie/Ehepartner	3	2
Kultur/Geselligkeit		
Kulturelle Angebote	12	7
Schöne Gaststätten + Cafes	6	4
Seniorentanz, -clubs etc.	26	16
Stadt- und Dorffeste	3	2
Freizeitmöglichkeiten		
Gute Wandermöglichkeiten	17	10
Grünanlagen	15	9
Schwimmbäder	8	5
Ökonomie/Wohnen		
Gute Wohnsituation	15	9
Genügend Geld	1	1
Infrastruktur (Verkehr, Einkaufen)		
Gute Verkehrsverbindungen	5	3
Gute Einkaufsmöglichkeiten	9	5
Indifferenz		
Nichts Besonderes	3	2
Zufrieden	5	3

Die gleiche Frage wurde den Besuchern eines „Gesundheitstages" in Merchweiler gestellt. Dabei zeigte sich, daß mit 51 % die Nennung von guten Sportmöglichkeiten an erster Stelle standen. Dem Befragungsanlaß entsprechend wurden von 13 % das Angebot von Gesundheitsvereinen und -verbänden als positiv bewertet.

Interessant ist der Vergleich der beiden Befragungen in bezug auf negative Einflußfaktoren für die Gesundheit (Tabelle 5).

Auffallend ist die Tatsache, daß 23 % der Befragten in Merchweiler sich durch die in dieser Region häufigen Tiefflieger belästigt fühlen. In Saarbrücken wird häufig Klage über schlechte Infrastrukturbedingungen geführt. Dieses Ergebnis charakterisiert eine „Orientierung an Vorhandenem" mit einer Tendenz zur steigenden Kritik bei höherem Versorgungsniveau. Die guten Einkaufs- und Verkehrsbedingungen der Großstadt werden kritischer betrachtet (insbesondere wenn kurz vor der Befragung ein Fahrplanwechsel stattfand), während die Einwohner der kleineren Gemeinde an ihren objektiv schlechteren Bedingungen keinen Anstoß nehmen. Hinter der Sammelkategorie „Umweltschäden" verbergen

Tabelle 5. Negative Einflußfaktoren für die Gesundheit
Frage: „Was stört in Ihrer Heimatgemeinde Ihre Gesundheit
und ihr Wohlbefinden am meisten?"

Einflußfaktor	Saar-brücken	Merch-weiler
Umweltschäden	64%	83%
Tiefflieger		23%
Infrastruktur (Einkauf, Verkehr)	24%	
Freizeitmöglichkeiten	15%	6%
Lebensgefühl sozialer Kontakte	15%	2%
Kultur, Geselligkeit	9%	
Ökonomie, Wohnen	8%	
Gesundheitsversorgung, Verbände, Vereine	2%	
nichts, indifferent	13%	12%
sonstiges	17%	7%

Saarbrücken: n = 164, Befragung „Altenburg".
Merchweiler: n = 270, Befragung „Gesundheitstag".

Tabelle 6. Negative Einflußfaktoren für die Gesundheit (Mehrfachnennungen; n = 123 Jugendliche in Freiburg-Weingarten)
Frage: „Was stört Dich hier, was findest Du schlecht?"

Einflußfaktor	n	%
Hochhäuser, Bauten	38	31
Ausländer, Asoziale	21	17
Dreck, Verkehr, Lärm	16	13
Kriminalität, Destruktivität	14	11
Soziale Kontakte	5	4
Verkehrsanknüpfung	7	6
Ghettobewußtsein	5	4
Kritik, Verbote der Alten	4	3
Kulturelle Angebote	4	3
Wohnen	2	2
Sonstiges	10	8
Nichts	11	9
Weiß nicht	26	21

sich in Merchweiler auch Aussagen über Grubenschäden (12 %) und industrielle
Lärmbelästigung (14 %).

Ein weiteres Problem zeigte sich bei der Befragung von Jugendlichen im Alter
von 14–18 Jahren in einem Problemstadtteil von Freiburg. Ein Pretest zeigte, daß
die Jugendlichen mit der Frage nach „Gesundheit" wenig anfangen konnten. Es
erwies sich als günstiger, die Frage allgemeiner zu stellen: „Was ist hier in Weingarten gut; was findest Du hier toll/prima?" und „Was stört Dich hier; was findest Du schlecht?" (s. Tabelle 6).

Auch nach der umformulierten Fragestellung zeigte sich, daß 30 % der Jugendlichen mit „weiß nicht" oder „nichts" antworteten. Die inhaltlichen Antwor-

Tabelle 7. „Wenn du an die Zukunft denkst – z. B. an das Jahr 2000 – was fällt dir dann ein?"

	n	[%]
Umweltprobleme allgemein	119	39,8
Ozonloch	18	6,0
Umweltkatastrophen	15	5,0
Bevölkerungs-/Ernährungsprobleme	14	4,7
Energie + Rohstoffprobleme	6	2,0
Weltuntergang, Krieg, Chaos, Angst, Schwarze Zeiten, Krankheiten	59	19,7
Schlechte Lebensqualität	31	10,4
Meine eigene Zukunft	22	7,4
Ausländerprobleme	9	3,0
Verkehrsprobleme	8	2,7
Ost-West Dialog, Frieden	18	6,0
Vereinigtes Europa	16	5,4
Fortschritte im Umweltschutz	12	4,0
Bessere Lebensqualität	6	2,0
Technischer Fortschritt	49	16,4
Keine großen Veränderungen	9	3,0
Sonstiges	47	15,7
Weiß nicht, keine Angaben	34	11,4
Gesamt	299	100,0

ten spiegeln die besonderen Probleme des Stadtteils wider: Hochhäuser, Ausländer, Verkehr, Lärm, Dreck und Kriminalität. In einer Vergleichsuntersuchung in einem der „besseren" Freiburger Wohngebiete soll der Stadtteileffekt genauer untersucht werden.

Die Auswertung einer Pilotstudie zur Befragung von Jugendlichen in der südbadischen Kleinstadt Emmendingen zeigte ein breites Spektrum von Angaben auf die Frage „Wenn du an die Zukunft denkst – z. B. an das Jahr 2000 – was fällt dir dann ein?" (s. Tabelle 7).

Auffallend ist die große Bedeutung, die von Jugendlichen inzwischen den Problemen der Umweltverschmutzung auch in einer Region mit eher geringen Belastungswerten beigemessen wird. Das Spektrum der assoziierten Themen ist relativ groß. Allerdings überwiegen die eindeutig negativen gegenüber den positiven Erwartungen.

Die derzeit laufende Auswertung in der Hauptuntersuchung wird zeigen, ob diese Ergebnisse repräsentativ für die Zukunftseinstellung von Jugendlichen in dieser Stadt (mit insgesamt 25 000 Einwohnern) sind.

Die Erhebungsbedingungen und Stichproben erlauben bisher noch keine Verallgemeinerungen der Ergebnisse. Interessant ist in diesem Zusammenhang eine von der Bundesforschungsanstalt für Landeskunde und Raumordnung durchgeführten Repräsentativerhebung zur Bewertung von Lebensbedingungen. Dort konnte festgestellt werden, daß die Bewohner „je nach Lebenslage unterschiedliche Aspekte ihrer Umwelt mehr oder weniger wahr(nehmen) und sie nach ihrer jeweiligen Lebenssituation (bewerten)." Entsprechend beziehen sich auch Handlungsorientierungen und Verhaltensweisen, z. B. Umzüge, nicht auf eine objektiv für alle Bewohner gleichermaßen gültige Stadt oder Stadtteilstruktur, sondern auf die nach Lebenslage relevanten Ausschnitte" (Böltken 1987). In den Befragungen wurde eine Liste verschiedener Aspekte zur Beschreibung der Lebensbedingungen vorgegeben, die von den Befragten gewichtet wurden. Abbildung 1 zeigt den Vergleich der Häufigkeiten, mit der diese Bedingungen in Großstädten und in kleinen Gemeinden als „sehr wichtig" bezeichnet wurden.

Diese Repräsentativdaten weisen Parallelen zu unseren Ergebnissen auf in bezug auf die besonders häufig genannten Kategorien saubere Luft, Parks/Grünanlagen, Einkaufsmöglichkeiten und öffentlicher Nahverkehr. Ein entscheidender Unterschied ergibt sich in bezug auf die gesundheitliche Versorgung. In der zitierten Repräsentativbefragung wurden auf einer Liste verschiedene Antwortkategorien vorgegeben. In unseren Interviews wurden die Fragen offen gestellt. Es ist anzunehmen, daß unstrukturierte Befragungen die Perzeption der Bevölkerung besser wiedergeben, wenn auch bei der Kategorisierung der vielen genannten Einzelaspekte Zuordnungsschwierigkeiten auftreten.

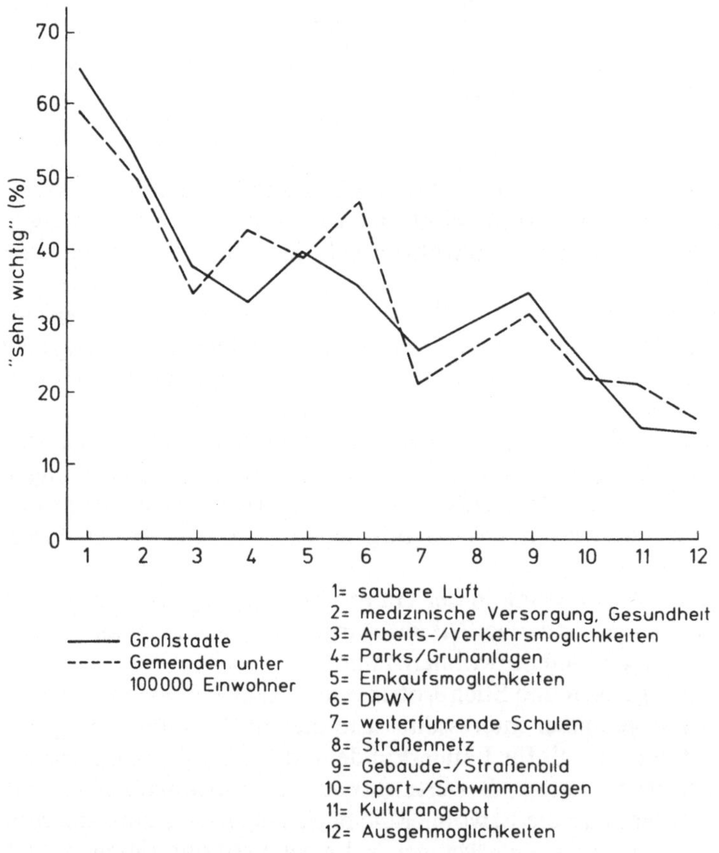

Abb. 1. Gewichtung von Lebensbedingungen in Großstädten und kleineren Gemeinden 1987

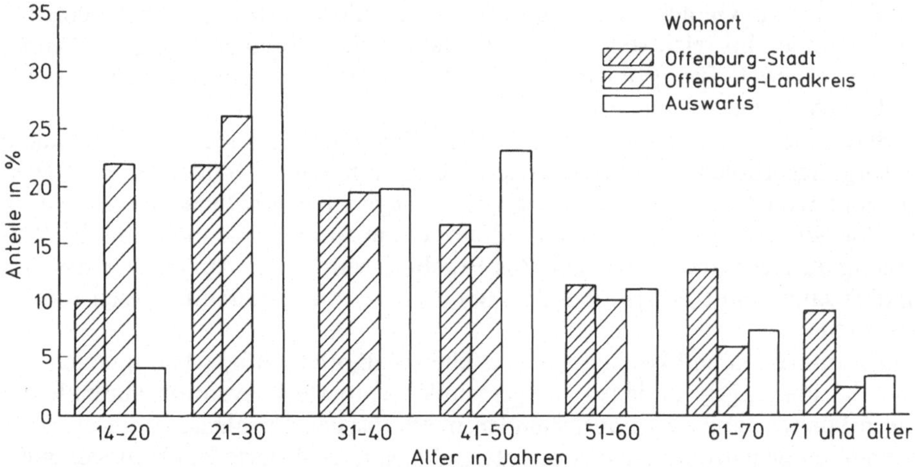

Abb. 2. Stichprobenbeschreibung: Wohnort nach Altersklassen

Die von uns durchgeführten Untersuchungen haben verschiedene methodische Probleme deutlich gemacht. Grundsätzlich ist davon auszugehen, daß mit Straßenbefragungen Selektionsphänomene verbunden sind. Als Beispiel soll die Stichprobenbeschreibung unserer Offenburger Befragung angeführt werden (Abb. 2).

Wie auch mit Erhebungen der maßnahmenbegleitenden Prozeßevaluation in der Deutschen Herz-Kreislauf-Präventionsstudie deutlich wurde, finden sich bei Veranstaltungs- und Straßenbefragungen immer hohe Prozentteile von Personen, die aus anderen Gemeinden oder Regionen kommen. Deshalb sollte jeweils möglichst präzise nach dem Wohnort gefragt werden. Verzerrungen in der Altersstruktur können möglicherweise durch gezielte Nacherhebungen ausgeglichen werden.

Bei Interviewernachbesprechungen und der Analyse von Videointerviews vermittelt sich der Eindruck, daß situative Aspekte das Antwortverhalten beeinflussen können. Fuhr während der Befragung ein Lastwagen lautstark vorbei oder fiel der Blick des Interviewten auf ein Hochhaus, so wurde mitunter der Verkehrslärm oder die Städteplanung der Gemeinde kritisiert. Derartige Effekte lassen sich ausgleichen, wenn die Befragungen an unterschiedlichen Standorten durchgeführt werden („Repräsentativität" der Erhebungspunkte für die Gemeinde).

Das methodische Hauptproblem stellt sich in der für statistische Auswertungen notwendigen Kategorisierung der qualitativen Antworten. Wir arbeiten derzeit an einem System, das die in Pretests ermittelten typischen Antwortkategorien grob vorgibt, in die der Interviewer dann die wörtlichen Aussagen des Befragten einträgt.

Die Ergebnisse derartiger Befragungen lassen sich in verschiedener Weise umsetzen. In aggregierter Form können sie für eine regelmäßige Gesundheitsberichterstattung nützlich sein, um die Problemwahrnehmung der Bevölkerung in angemessener Weise zu berücksichtigen. Für die kommunalpolitische Arbeit in den Parteien, im Gemeinderat und in der Gemeindeverwaltung können derartige Informationen hilfreich sein. Schließlich lassen sich Ergebnisse von Straßenbefragungen gezielt für problembezogene Veranstaltungen nutzen, z. B. mit Jugendlichen, Alten, Ausländern etc.

Stadtteilbezogene Erhebungen können Verwendung finden, um besondere Versorgungsprobleme politisch wirksam zu vertreten und Abhilfen einzufordern. So konnten die Ergebnisse von Bürgerbefragungen in einer Obdachlosensiedlung in München dazu genützt werden, um auf die unzureichende medizinische Versorgung aufmerksam zu machen. Als Ergebnis wurde eine Außenstelle des Gesundheitsamtes mit entsprechenden Beratungs- und Unterstützungsleistungen eingerichtet.

Zusammenfassend können wir feststellen, daß offene Bürgerbefragungen wesentliche Planungsgrundlagen für gemeindeorientierte Präventionsmaßnahmen liefern können. Die dabei auftretenden methodischen Probleme bedürfen einer besonderen Beachtung. Hier ist es notwendig, standardisierte Rahmenbedingungen vorzugeben, die gewährleisten, daß die gefundenen Ergebnisse aussagekräftig und hinreichend repräsentativ sind. Eine zukünftige umfassende Gesundheitsberichterstattung sollte nicht nur mit „Expertendaten" arbeiten, sondern auch die Problemwahrnehmungen der Bevölkerung in angemessener Weise berücksichtigen.

Literatur

Böltken F (1987) Wahrnehmung, Bewertung und Gewichtung von Lebensbedingungen aus Bürgersicht. Bundesforschungsanstalt für Landeskunde und Raumordnung: Informationen zu Raumentwicklung 11/12:756
Essen, Gesundheitsamt (1988) Gesundheitsbericht der Stadt Essen. Dezember
Heins F, Stiens G (1984) Regionale Unterschiede der Sterblichkeit. Untersuchung am Beispiel der Länder Nordrhein-Westfalen und Rheinland-Pfalz. In: Bundesforschungsanstalt für Landeskunde und Raumordnung (Hrsg) S 170 (Bonn)
Idis (Hrsg) (1987/88) Konzeption und statistische Materialien des Gesundheitsberichts Nordrhein-Westfalen. Gesundheitsberichterstattung Bd 1/1987, Bd 2/1988
Köln (Hrsg) (oJ) Das Gesundheitswesen in Köln. Aufgaben, Einrichtungen, Institutionen, Initiativen. Köln
Kreuter H, Zachcial M, Klaes L, Troschke J von (1989) Deutsche Herz-Kreislauf-Präventionsstudie: Programm-Report 1989. Design, Methoden, Ergebnisse zur Studienmitte. DHP-Forum Berichte Mitteilungen 1
Landkreis Kronach (Hrsg) (1985) Bereichsübergreifende Gesundheitsberichterstattung und kommunaler Gesundheitsplan Kronach. S 45
Neuhaus R, Schräder WF (1988) Möglichkeiten regionaler Gesundheitsberichterstattung. Gesundheitsdaten für kommunale Prävention. Prävention 1:7ff.
Osnabrück (Hrsg) (1983) Gesundheitsplan Osnabrück. Osnabrück
Schräder et al. (1986) Kommunale Gesundheitsplanung. Basel Boston Stuttgart, S 89ff.
WHO (Hrsg) (1985) Einzelziele für „Gesundheit 2000". Frankfurt am Main, S 40, 214

Weiterführende Literatur zum Thema „Gemeinde"

Evers A, Farrant W, Trojan A (eds) (1990) Healthy public policy at the local level. Campus/Westview, Frankfurt am Main

Hildebrandt H, Trojan A (Hrsg) (1987) Gesündere Städte – Kommunale Gesundheitsförderung. Sozialwissenschaften und Gesundheit e. V., Hamburg

Labisch A (Hrsg) (1989) Kommunale Gesundheitsförderung: aktuelle Entwicklungen, Konzepte, Perspektiven. Deutsche Zentrale für Volksgesundheitspflege e. V., Frankfurt am Main

Stark W (Hrsg) (1989) Lebensweltbezogene Prävention und Gesundheitsförderung: Konzepte und Strategien für die psychosoziale Praxis. Lambertus, Freiburg

Troschke J v, Klaes L, Maschewsky-Schneider U (Hrsg) (1991) Erfolge gemeindebezogener Präventions-Ergebnisse der Deutschen Herz-Kreislauf-Präventions-Studie (DHP). Asgard, Sankt Augustin

4 Gesundheitssystemforschung

Langfristige Entwicklungstrends im Gesundheitswesen: Strukturierung eines Forschungsschwerpunktes *

J.G. Brecht, E. Becker, A. Jenke, F. Beske

Vorbemerkung

Die Ergänzungsarbeiten zum Vorhaben „Langfristige Entwicklungstrends im Gesundheitswesen" sollen das Spektrum der anwendbaren Methoden zur Prognostik darstellen, die einzelnen Anwendungsbereichen Methoden zuordnen und eine konkrete, für die Etablierung eines Projekts geeignete Organisationsstruktur entwickeln, die interdisziplinäre und multizentrische Kooperation ermöglicht.

Die Ergänzungsarbeiten, deren Ergebnis im folgenden dargestellt wird, sollen sich an den Zielen des einzurichtenden Projekts ausrichten, die folgendermaßen beschrieben werden können:

1) Für die wichtigsten Bereiche des Gesundheitswesens sollen langfristige Entwicklungstrends erarbeitet werden.
2) Die Forschungsergebnisse des zukünftigen Projekts sollen für alle Entscheidungsträger in der Gesundheitspolitik Entscheidungshilfen darstellen.
3) Es sollen Strukturen etabliert werden, die die Umsetzung dieser Forschungsergebnisse in die Praxis der Gesundheitspolitik unterstützen.

Aus diesen Basiszielen lassen sich auf einer nächsten Ebene folgende Ziele ableiten:

4) Die Forschungsgegenstände, für die Langfristtrends entwickelt werden sollen, müssen ausgewählt werden. Daran sind Gesundheitspolitiker und wissenschaftliche Einrichtungen zu beteiligen.
5) Für jeden der ausgewählten Forschungsgegenstände ist mindestens ein Forschungsvorhaben im Rahmen des Projekts „Langfristige Entwicklungstrends im Gesundheitswesen" einzurichten. Ziel dieser Forschungsvorhaben ist die langfristige Prognose der zukünftigen Entwicklung des fraglichen Bereichs. Es sind Prognosemethoden zu wählen oder zu entwickeln, die entscheidungsorientierte Ergebnisse versprechen.
6) Wegen der thematischen und methodischen Verflechtungen zwischen den einzelnen Forschungsgegenständen sind die verschiedenen Forschungsvorhaben zu koordinieren.
7) Die Rahmenbedingungen und methodischen Annahmen, unter denen einzelne Projektionen zustande gekommen sind, sind detailliert darzustellen.

---

* Gekürzte Fassung einer Veröffentlichung des Instituts für Gesundheits-System-Forschung, Kiel, 1989.

8) In jedem Vorhaben sollen Vorschläge gemacht werden, welche Parameter und Annahmen über die eigentliche Vorhabenslaufzeit hinaus intensiv weiterverfolgt werden müssen, damit die Prognosen fortgeschrieben werden können.

Außerhalb des eigentlichen Projekts „Langfristige Entwicklungstrends im Gesundheitswesen" empfiehlt es sich, daß Entscheidungsträger im Gesundheitswesen Einrichtungen benennen oder schaffen, die die Forschungsergebnisse der Vorhaben in die Entscheidungsfelder ihrer eigenen Politik einbringen. Diese Einrichtungen sollen sich bei der Umsetzung der Forschungsergebnisse der Unterstützung durch wissenschaftliche Einrichtungen versichern können. Auch dies soll außerhalb des Projekts „Langfristige Entwicklungstrends im Gesundheitswesen" geschehen.

Methodische Ausgangslage

Prognosen als Entscheidungs- und Bewertungshilfen

Rationale Entscheidungen zielen auf die Wahl möglichst effektiver und effizienter Alternativen aus einem Bündel von möglichen Handlungen. Sie benötigen daher immer eine mehr oder weniger explizite Ex-ante-Evaluation ihrer Wirkungen. Die praktisch normative Entscheidungstheorie (Sieben u. Schildbach 1975) beschreibt diesen Zusammenhang in folgender Weise:

> Zu berücksichtigen sind zwei Kategorien von Informationen, nämlich Informationen über die vom Entscheidungsträger erstrebten Sachverhalte (*Ziel* oder *Zielsystem*) und Informationen über die ihm offenstehenden Handlungsmöglichkeiten, die Einflüsse von dritter Seite und die Konsequenzen der Entscheidungen (*Entscheidungsfeld*).
> Das Entscheidungsfeld wird hierbei untergliedert in
>
> - den *Aktionsraum*, der aus der Menge aller Aktionen besteht, die dem Entscheidungsträger offenstehen,
> - die *Umweltbedingungen*, die alles umfassen, was sich der Einflußnahme durch den Entscheidungsträger entzieht, aber die Handlungswirkungen beeinflussen kann,
> - eine *Bewertungsvorschrift*, die jeder Kombination von Umweltzuständen und Aktionen Werte auf der Zielebene zuordnet.

Da die Wirkungen von Entscheidungen erst in der Zukunft eintreten, sind sowohl für die entscheidungsspezifischen Wirkungen als auch für die bewertungsrelevanten Rahmenbedingungen, in die diese Wirkungen eingebettet sind, Prognosen erforderlich. In bezug auf eine Entscheidung oder ein Entscheidungsbündel kann die Zielebene dagegen als zeitlich konstant angenommen werden (Zielkonsistenz). Im allgemeinen trifft dies auch auf die Bewertungsvorschrift zu.[1]

Als erstes stellt sich die Frage nach dem Zweck von Prognosen im Gesundheitswesen. Gewöhnlich wird diese Frage mit dem Hinweis auf den Planungsbedarf im Gesundheitswesen beantwortet, wobei unterstellt wird, bei genügender Datenlage lasse sich der Bedarf an Gesundheitsleistungen in einer Weise progno-

---

[1] Es sei jedoch auf die Diskussion um die Diskontierung bei Kosten-Wirksamkeits-Untersuchungen hingewiesen (Drummond u. Stoddart 1985; HM Treasury 1982).

stizieren, welche die Bereitstellung der zur Deckung des festgestellten Bedarfs erforderlichen Ressourcen ermöglicht. Im Sinne der Entwicklung eines Projektvorschlags mit umsetzungsfähigen Ergebnissen liegt es daher nahe, von den tatsächlich gegebenen Planungs- und Entscheidungsstrukturen auszugehen. Diese sind zum einen weitgehend dezentral, zum anderen bisher eher an kurz- und mittelfristigen Entscheidungen orientiert.

Kurzfristige Entscheidungen sind dadurch gekennzeichnet, daß sich Rahmenbedingungen, die sich durch eigenes oder fremdes Handeln ergeben, nur in geringem Umfang verändern. Das Informationsfeld für solche Entscheidungen ist also einerseits gekennzeichnet durch größere Sicherheit der Erwartungen an die Entwicklung der relevanten Größen, andererseits durch eine geringere Zahl von Größen, die als veränderlich in Rechnung zu stellen sind. Je größer der Planungshorizont wird, desto mehr ist zu berücksichtigen, daß sich Rahmenbedingungen ändern können und daß unterstellte Entwicklungen von entscheidungsrelevanten Größen sehr viel unsicherer sind.

Prognosen sind nach ihren Zielgrößen zu unterscheiden in solche von Entwicklungen, die von Entscheidungen weitgehend unabhängig sind, und von Prognosen solcher Entwicklungen, die ihrerseits wieder von Entscheidungen (auch Dritter) bestimmt werden. Zusammen mit den Ausführungen im letzten Absatz folgt daraus, daß Prognosen um so *entscheidungssensitiver* sind, je langfristiger ihr Zielbereich ist. Dies ist eine erhebliche zusätzliche Komplikation bei der Voraussage von Langfristtrends.

Das niederländische Steering Committee on Future Health Scenarios hat daraus die Konsequenz gezogen, die rein rechnerische Ermittlung von langfristigen Prognosen nur punktuell einzusetzen, nämlich dort, wo Entscheidungssensitivität nicht oder nur in geringem Umfang zu befürchten war. Verwendet wurde hingegen die sogenannte Szenariotechnik (Kahn u. Wiener 1967), die schon allein wegen ihrer Entwicklungsgeschichte anhand militärischer Anwendungen für strategische Entscheidungen, bei denen die Handlungen anderer Entscheidungsträger in Rechnung gestellt werden müssen, besonders geeignet zu sein scheint. Selbst wenn unterstellt werden darf, daß die Schätzung einzelner Zeitreihen mit dieser Methode teilweise nur noch sehr ungenau möglich ist, z. B. durch Delphi-Verfahren, ist dieser Unschärfe der Vorzug vor einer vermeintlichen Präzision zu geben. Gerade der Rekurs auf die Befragung handelnder Personen in der Delphi-Technik kann die Erwartungen und zukünftigen Handlungen von Entscheidungsträgern auf einem allerdings eher qualitativen Niveau herausarbeiten.

Die bisherigen Ausführungen haben deutlich gemacht, daß Entscheidungen nicht einfach mechanistisch aus Prognosen resultieren, sondern im Idealfall bewußt auf die zukünftigen Gegebenheiten des Entscheidungsfeldes hin zu formulieren und zu treffen sind. Dazu bedarf es nicht nur einer genügenden Datenlage bei den Prognosegrößen, sondern vor allem eines für pragmatische Zwecke hinreichend gesicherten theoretischen Fundaments zur Auswahl der geeigneten Parameter des Entscheidungsfeldes und zur Beschreibung von Wirkzusammenhängen zwischen diesen Parametern, den Handlungsparametern und den Zielgrößen.

Eine bisher nur am Rande behandelte Komplikation tritt dann ein, wenn Entscheidungen nicht nur durch eine einzige Instanz getroffen werden sollen, sondern mehrere Entscheidungsträger betroffen sind. Ein derartiges System verteilter Entscheidungen kann hierarchisch organisiert sein in dem Sinn, daß eine Instanz für Grundsatzentscheidungen zuständig ist und weitere Entscheidungsträger für die Ausgestaltung vor Ort verantwortlich sind. Die Beteiligung mehrerer Entscheidungsträger ist – mit in der Regel unterschiedlichen Zielsetzungen – auch dann gegeben, wenn Entscheidungen als Folge von Verhandlungen entstehen. Im Gesundheitswesen sind wegen der föderativen Strukturen und der Selbstverwaltungskompetenzen beide Muster verteilter Entscheidungen zu beobachten, häufig in kombinierter Form (z. B. Honorarvereinbarungen auf regionaler Ebene nach zentralen Empfehlungsvereinbarungen).

Eine dieser Situation angemessene Differenzierung des Szenariobegriffs von Brenner (1986) unterscheidet explorative Szenarien, strategische Szenarien und Ressourcenallokationsszenarien. Hiernach sind explorative Szenarien der Beschreibung möglicher zukünftiger Entwicklungen, strategische Szenarien der Wahl bestimmter Optionen und Ressourcenallokationsszenarien der Ausgestaltung dieser Optionen gewidmet.

Nach Lagergren (1986) besteht der Hauptzweck von Szenarien in der Bewertung von langfristigen Konsequenzen politischer Entscheidungen. Dies rückt die Verwendung von Szenarien nahe an die Ebene der politischen Entscheidungsfindung. Sowohl strategische Szenarien als auch Ressourcenallokationsszenarien werden mithin nur in enger Anbindung an die Entscheidungsinstanzen entwickelt werden können. Für explorative Szenarien ist dies hingegen nicht notwendig. Es muß lediglich sichergestellt werden, daß entscheidungsrelevante Prognosegrößen gewählt werden. Explorative Szenarien können also auch der Vorbereitung von Entscheidungen in pluralistischen Systemen dienen.

Genauigkeit und Gültigkeit von Prognosen

Die wissenschaftstheoretische Untersuchung von Prognosen (Popper 1972) hat gezeigt, daß eine strukturelle Ähnlichkeit von Erklärung und Voraussage vorliegt. Beide basieren auf dem Eintreten eines Ereignisses E, das auf entsprechende Antezedensbedingungen und Gesetzmäßigkeiten zurückgeführt werden kann.

> Der pragmatische Unterschied zwischen den beiden Fällen äußert sich .. in folgendem: Wenn E in dem Sinn vorgegeben ist, daß man bereits weiß, der durch E beschriebene Sachverhalt habe stattgefunden, und wenn geeignete Antecedensbedingungen A_1, ..., A_n sowie Gesetze G_1, ..., G_r *nachträglich zur Verfügung gestellt* werden, aus denen zusammen E ableitbar ist, so sprechen wir von einer Erklärung. Sind hingegen die Antecedensbedingungen wie Gesetze *zunächst* gegeben und wird daraus E zu einem Zeitpunkt abgeleitet, *bevor* das durch E beschriebene Ereignis stattfindet, so handelt es sich um eine Voraussage. Die analoge Unterscheidung kann für den statistischen Fall gemacht werden (Stegmüller 1974).

Obwohl nun Prognosen nach ihrem logischen Aufbau nichts anderes sind als Erklärungen, besteht ein prinzipieller Unterschied zwischen ihnen insofern, als die Gültigkeit von Prognosen immer erst ex post facto überprüft werden kann. Im Falle von qualitativen Prognosen ist eine derartige Überprüfung nur mit Mitteln der entsprechenden Substanzwissenschaft möglich, während bei quantitativen Prognosen zusätzlich statistische Methoden verwendet werden können. Speziell für die Beurteilung der Gültigkeit von Prognosen ist das Standardrepertoire der

Fehlerrechnung erweitert worden um normierte Fehlermaße (z. B. Ungleichheitskoeffizient von Theil, 1966) und um qualitative Fehlermaße, die zur Beurteilung der korrekten Voraussage von Tendenzänderungen in einer Zeitreihe herangezogen werden können. Für eine umfassende Diskussion der verwendbaren Fehlermaße sei auf Schwarze (1980) verwiesen.

Während die *Gültigkeit* einer Prognose nur ex post überprüft werden kann, besteht bei statistischen Prognoseverfahren bereits ex ante die Möglichkeit, die *Genauigkeit* abzuschätzen soweit sie durch Zufallsfehler getroffen ist. Obwohl die mit Hilfe eines statistischen Modells gewonnene Prognose einer Zeitreihe und den dazu gehörenden Konfidenzintervallen einen erheblichen Vorteil gegenüber der einfachen Angabe von Punktschätzungen bietet, bleibt gerade bei langfristigen Prognosen die Frage offen, wie sehr zukünftige Einflüsse Antezedensbedingungen modifizieren, unterstellte Gesetzmäßigkeiten in Frage stellen und mithin zu systematischen Fehlern der Prognose führen können.

Im Gegensatz zu den Zufallsfehlern eines statistischen Prognosemodells sind systematische Fehler zum Prognosezeitpunkt in der Regel nicht abzusehen. Eine Möglichkeit, ihnen zu begegnen, besteht darin, nach einer expliziten Formulierung aller Prognosevoraussetzungen ein permanentes Monitoringsystem aufzubauen, das zur Fortschreibung der Antezedensbedingungen und zur Überprüfung der verwendeten Gesetzmäßigkeiten benutzt werden kann. Einschränkend wird angemerkt, daß dieser Aufwand nur für solche Prognosegrößen sinnvoll ist, die immer wieder für Entscheidungen benötigt werden.

Absichten und Rahmenbedingungen eines Projekts „Langfristige Entwicklungstrends im Gesundheitswesen"

Entscheidungsträger im Gesundheitswesen

Bei jeder Entscheidungsfindung ist im Grundsatz zwischen dem staatlichen Bereich und dem staatsfreien Raum zu unterscheiden. Das Verwaltungshandeln, entweder auf der Grundlage von Gesetzen wie bei Verordnungen, im Vollzug des Haushaltes oder in Einzelentscheidungen nach pflichtgemäßem Ermessen wird in aller Regel von einer intensiven Diskussion mit den Beteiligten, von fachgebundenen Publikationen und von Erörterungen in den Medien begleitet. Staatliche Entscheidungen auf allen Ebenen sind damit das Ergebnis eines umfangreichen Meinungsbildungsprozesses.

Die gesetzliche Krankenversicherung als ein wichtiger Bereich des deutschen Gesundheitswesens wird nach staatlichen Vorgaben und Rahmenbedingungen von der mittelbaren Staatsverwaltung im Rahmen der Selbstverwaltung gestaltet. Hierzu gehören in erster Linie Körperschaften des öffentlichen Rechts wie Krankenkassen und kassenärztliche/kassenzahnärztliche Vereinigungen. Aber auch die Kammern – Ärztekammern, Zahnärztekammern, Apothekerkammern – sind als berufsständische Organisationen Körperschaften des öffentlichen Rechts mit großen Befugnissen im Rahmen der Selbstverwaltung. In der gesetzlichen Krankenversicherung haben die zentralen Organe wie Ausschüsse der gemeinsamen Selbstverwaltung oder der Ärzte/Zahnärzte bzw. der Krankenkassen Fragen von grundsätzlicher Bedeutung zu regeln, während eine Vielzahl von Gremien im nachgeordneten Bereich mehr Einzelentscheidungen zu fällen haben, die wegen des dezentralen Charakters sehr unterschiedlich sein können. Dabei wirkt die dezentrale Ebene intensiv an den Entscheidungen der zentralen Ebene z. B. über Vertreterkammern oder Ausschüsse mit, ist jedoch andererseits an den Rahmen gebunden, der von der zentralen Ebene gesetzt wird.

Im staatsfreien Raum gibt es im Gesundheitswesen eine Vielzahl von Vereinen, Vereinigungen, Verbänden und losen Zusammenschlüssen, die in ihrer Entscheidungsfindung von ihren Mitgliedern getragen werden. Diese unterschiedlichen Gruppierungen können auf der Ebene, auf der sie tätig sind, über viel Einfluß verfügen, sei es über die Meinungsbildung bei ihren Mitgliedern, über die veröffentlichte Meinung oder durch ihre beratende Funktion für Parlamente und Verwaltung.

Diese knappe und stark vereinfachte Darstellung der Meinungs- und Entscheidungsbildung im Gesundheitswesen macht deutlich, daß wohl niemals Entscheidungen auf allen Ebenen und in sämtlichen Bereichen ohne einen intensiven und in der Regel breit angelegten Meinungs- und Entscheidungsbildungsprozeß getroffen werden können. Das hat zur Konsequenz, daß Entscheidungen zumindest von denjenigen mitgetragen oder respektiert werden, die an diesem Prozeß mitgewirkt haben, es sei denn, daß es aus politischen oder sachlichen Gründen weit von der Entscheidung abweichende Meinungen gibt. Dies bedeutet aber auch, daß Entscheidungsträger dann, wenn sie eine breite Zustimmung für ihre Entscheidungen wünschen, was ebenfalls die Regel sein dürfte, wissenschaftlich abgesicherte und von möglichst vielen Beteiligten miterarbeitete und mitgetragene Meinungen zur Grundlage ihrer Entscheidung machen sollten.

Forschungsgegenstände

Im Rahmen der Strukturierung des Forschungsschwerpunktes „Langfristige Entwicklungstrends im Gesundheitswesen" sollen vorzugsweise solche Themen behandelt werden, die eine hohe Relevanz für das jeweilige Problemfeld aufweisen und die aufgrund entsprechender Vorarbeiten – auch im Ausland – relativ leicht zugänglich sind. Deshalb stehen unter diesen Gesichtspunkten die im folgenden kurz aufgeführten Forschungsgegenstände im Vordergrund der Betrachtung.

Die *Altersstruktur der Bevölkerung* ist neben rein demographischen Voraussagen, die von einer Vielzahl von Interessenten für ihre Planungen benötigt werden, für darüber hinausgehende wirtschafts- und sozialpolitische Prognosen von erheblicher Bedeutung. Ein Erkenntnisgewinn gegenüber den bereits vorhandenen Bevölkerungsschätzungen ist durch die Beschreibung der zu erwartenden Konsequenzen auf weitere Änderungen des Morbiditätsspektrums und damit auch auf Bedarfsänderungen in der medizinischen und pflegerischen Versorgung sowie auf Änderung der sozioökonomischen Rahmenbedingungen zu erwarten. Die *Entwicklung der wirtschaftlichen Rahmenbedingungen* ist auf mehreren Ebenen mit dem Gesundheitswesen verknüpft. Zunächst ist der Sachverhalt zu berücksichtigen, daß die wirtschaftlichen Rahmendaten die Mittel bestimmen, die dem Gesundheitswesen zur Verfügung stehen. Eine weitere Verknüpfung mit dem Gesundheitswesen ergibt sich durch die direkte Wirkung sozioökonomischer Faktoren auf den Gesundheitszustand der Bevölkerung. Zu diskutieren sind in diesem Zusammenhang auch gesundheitsfördernde Wirkungen des „Wohlstandes" durch eine unspezifische Verbesserung der Lebensverhältnisse.

Grundsätzlich könnte die Einbeziehung von *Morbidität und Mortalität* von allen Krankheitsgruppen in langfristige Prognosen gefordert werden. Aus Gründen der Forschungsökonomie ist die Setzung von Prioritäten jedoch unerläßlich.

Im Bereich der *Herz- und Kreislauferkrankungen* wäre zu prüfen, inwieweit auf die Ergebnisse der niederländischen STG-Arbeitsgruppe (Steering Committee on Future Health Scenarios, 1986) zurückgegriffen werden kann. Ergänzungen dieser – wegen des Verzichts auf den Risikofaktorenansatz nicht unumstrittenen – Ergebnisse sind denkbar durch Morbiditäts- und Mortalitätsprognosen auf der Basis von Risikofaktorenmodellen sowie auf der Basis von Vergangenheitsdaten. Die Wichtigkeit von Prognosen der *Morbidität durch bösartige Neubildungen* begründet sich einerseits durch die Bindung erheblicher Teile der Versorgungsstrukturen durch die Versorgung von Krebskranken. Andererseits legt die Altersentwicklung der Bevölkerung eine steigende Morbidität an bösartigen Neubildungen nahe. Bedingung für Prognosen ist allerdings die Möglichkeit, genügend lange Zeitreihen herstellen zu können. Diese ist in der Bundesrepublik Deutschland gegenwärtig nur unzureichend erfüllt.

Der *Versorgungsbedarf durch Infektionskrankheiten* kann wegen der Möglichkeit des Entstehens neuer Krankheitsbilder ex ante kaum abgeschätzt werden. Die Prognose der Erkrankungshäufigkeit an einzelnen, abgrenzbaren Infektionskrankheiten kann dagegen mit dem methodischen Instrumentarium der Epidemiologie versucht werden. Verschiedene Szenarien zum Erfolg klinischer und pharmakologischer Forschung sowie ökonomische, soziale und psychologische Aspekte der Krankheitsausbreitung und der zu schaffenden Maßnahmen sind einzubeziehen. Eine weitere erhebliche Quelle von Morbidität und Mortalität stellen *Unfälle* dar, weil bei einer alternden Bevölkerung die Häufigkeit häuslicher Unfälle vermutlich zunehmen wird. Häufigkeit und Folgenschwere von Arbeits- und Verkehrsunfällen dürften in erster Linie mit sozioökonomischen und technischen Rahmenbedingungen zusammenhängen.

Vor dem Hintergrund ökonomischer, demographischer und kapazitätsbestimmter Entwicklungen ist damit zu rechnen, daß sich langfristig die *Versorgungsstrukturen im ambulanten und stationären Sektor* ändern werden. Obwohl anzunehmen ist, daß es – abhängig vom Selbstverständnis der Gesundheitsberufe – autonome Entwicklungen der Angebotsstruktur gibt, werden diese nur schwer von Antizipation einer sich verändernden Nachfragestruktur zu trennen sein. Entwicklungen der zukünftigen Versorgungsstruktur sind also in hohem Maße von der Erwartungshaltung der Gesundheitsberufe abhängig. Ein ähnliches Problem wie bei der Analyse der zukünftigen Versorgungsstrukturen zeigt sich bei Versuchen, den *technischen Fortschritt* zu prognostizieren. Da eine einzelne technische Neuentwicklung oft den technischen Fortschritt in völlig neue, vorher nicht absehbare Bahnen lenken kann, sind Langfristtrends über das gesamte Spektrum der technischen Entwicklung kaum abzuschätzen. Stattdessen wird vorgeschlagen, für einzelne technische Entwicklungen gezielte Technologiefolgeabschätzungen vorzunehmen. Dies bedeutet die bewußte Abkehr von Prognosen der technischen Entwicklung hin zu Ex-ante-Bewertungen der Auswirkung einzelner Technologien im Gesundheitswesen.

Verbindung mit anderen Bundesprojekten

Die thematische Breite eines möglichen zukünftigen Projekts „Langfristige Entwicklungstrends im Gesundheitswesen" läßt es in Verbindung zu nahezu jedem Vorhaben des Programms „Forschung und Entwicklung im Dienste der Gesundheit" treten. Soweit es hierbei nur um die langfristigen Konsequenzen geht, die aus den einzelnen anderen Vorhaben gezogen werden können, spielt das Projekt „Langfristige Entwicklungstrends im Gesundheitswesen" allerdings eine rein rezeptive Rolle. Abstimmungsvorgänge sind insoweit nicht erforderlich.

Anders ist die Verknüpfungsmöglichkeit mit zwei Projekten zu beurteilen, die zu dem hier entworfenen Projekt in engem Zusammenhang stehen, nämlich dem Projekt „Prioritäre Gesundheitsziele" und dem Projekt „Gesundheitsberichterstattung". Beide Projekte lassen sich zwanglos in die Kategorien der praktischnormativen Entscheidungstheorie[2] einordnen, wobei die prioritären Gesundheitsziele in natürlicher Weise die Rolle des Zielsystems übernehmen, während das Projekt „Gesundheitsberichterstattung" der Fundierung des Entscheidungsfeldes durch die kontinuierliche Beschreibung der Umweltzustände dient. Das zu strukturierende Projekt „Langfristige Entwicklungstrends im Gesundheitswesen" geht insofern über dieses auch von der Gesundheitsberichterstattung verfolgte Ziel hinaus, als die Methoden und Pilotanwendungen für langfristige Projektionen zu entwickeln sind. Wie weiter oben[3] dargestellt ist, wird als Konsequenz aus der Durchführung des Projekts jedoch die Fortschreibung einer Reihe von einzelnen Prognosen bzw. das Monitoring von einzelnen Szenarien als Daueraufgabe folgen. Diese Fortschreibung sollte, soweit nicht im Einzelfall grundlegend neue methodische Zugänge zu entwickeln sind, im Rahmen des Projekts „Gesundheitsberichterstattung" stattfinden.

Interdisziplinarität

Der auf S. 370 skizzierte Überblick über die im Projekt „Langfristige Entwicklungstrends im Gesundheitswesen" zu behandelnden Schwerpunkte zeigt, daß angesichts der thematischen Vielfalt die durchzuführenden Forschungsvorhaben in Einrichtungen mit unterschiedlichen fachlichen Schwerpunkten angesiedelt werden müssen. Bereits bei der Bearbeitung einzelner Forschungsvorhaben ist jedoch mit der Notwendigkeit interdisziplinärer Zusammenarbeit zu rechnen.

Als Beispiel soll der Themenbereich „Entwicklung der Altersstruktur der Bevölkerung" dienen. Dieser ist in erster Linie von Demographen zu bearbeiten. Bei

---

[2] Vgl. Abschn. „Prognosen als Entscheidungs- und Bewertungshilfen", S. 366.
[3] Vgl. Abschn. „Genauigkeit und Gültigkeit von Prognosen", S. 369.

der Weiterbearbeitung des Gegenstandes, die nach den Ausführungen auf S. 371 eine Vorausschau auf die Änderungen des Morbiditätsspektrums und die daraus folgenden Änderungen des Versorgungsbedarfs sowie eine Prognose der wirtschaftlichen und sozialen Konsequenzen umfassen soll, kann auf die Mitarbeit weiterer Disziplinen nicht verzichtet werden. Die exemplarisch gewählte Thematik verlangt somit die Bearbeitung mindestens durch die Disziplinen Demographie, Medizin, Epidemiologie, Versorgungsforschung, Pflegeforschung, Gesundheitsökonomie, Ökonometrie und Sozialforschung.

Ist bereits die Bearbeitung eines einzelnen Sachgebiets des Projekts „Langfristige Entwicklungstrends im Gesundheitswesen" nur mit einem interdisziplinären Ansatz möglich, so gilt dies erst recht für die Abwicklung des Gesamtprojekts. Da die einzelnen Forschungsvorhaben unter gemeinsamen Gesichtspunkten interpretierbar sein sollen, ist auf eine enge Koordination nicht zu verzichten. Diese sollte sich nicht nur auf thematische Abgrenzungen beziehen, sondern auch methodische Hilfestellungen geben.

Im Gesamtprojekt werden nach den auf S. 370 vorgestellten Forschungsgegenständen die Disziplinen Medizin (verschiedene Fachrichtungen), Epidemiologie und Sozialmedizin, Wirtschaftswissenschaften, Sozialwissenschaften, Psychologie, Biometrie und Operations research und Medizintechnik erforderlich sein. Diese Aufzählung ist nicht abschließend und im Interesse der Übersichtlichkeit bereits auf breit gefaßte Disziplinen bezogen.

Methodenpluralismus

Wie auf S. 369 angemerkt worden ist, ist das Ausmaß der Verzerrung von langfristigen Prognosen durch systematische Fehler zum Prognosezeitpunkt nur schwer abzuschätzen. Die dort aufgeführte Möglichkeit, mit Hilfe eines Monitoringsystems wenigstens entwicklungsbegleitend Prognosefehler zu korrigieren, hat zweifellos den Nachteil, möglicherweise erst nach Entscheidungen berichtigte Werte nachzuliefern. Von großem Nutzen wäre es deshalb, von vornherein zumindest Anhaltspunkte für das Ausmaß der Unsicherheit durch systematische Fehler zu haben.

Obwohl es zum Stand der Technik gerechnet werden kann, daß bei Vorliegen unsicherer Randbedingungen durch Sensitivitätsanalysen die Variationsbreite einzelner prognostischer Aussagen beschrieben wird, empfiehlt es sich, trotz der scheinbaren Gefahr von Doppelarbeiten die Entwicklung verschiedener Prognosemodelle für ein und denselben Sachverhalt zuzulassen. Dies ist insbesondere dann sinnvoll, wenn die Ansätze möglichst verschiedenen Fachrichtungen entstammen. Der Nutzen ähnlicher Prognosen bei verschiedenen Zugängen würde dann in einer erhöhten Sicherheit im Umgang mit den Vorhersagen liegen, während bei Diskrepanzen die wissenschaftliche Diskussion der Ursachen einen Gewinn für die jeweiligen Fachrichtungen und letzten Endes auch für die Nutzer ihrer Forschungsergebnisse verspricht.

Spektrum der anzuwendenden Methoden

Beim gegenwärtigen Stand der *Vorbereitung* eines Forschungsschwerpunkts ist es nicht möglich, zu einer detaillierten Zuteilung von Verfahren zu Fragestellungen gelangen zu wollen. Vielmehr bleibt die Wahl geeigneter Prognosemethoden für konkrete Fragestellungen den jeweiligen Substanzwissenschaften vorbehalten. Wenn im folgenden einzelne Prognoseverfahren diskutiert werden, geschieht dies mit der Zielsetzung, einen ersten Eindruck des voraussichtlichen Aufwandes zu vermitteln und bereits frühzeitig für die Voraussetzungen der technischen Kompatibilität der einzelnen Vorhaben des zukünftigen Forschungsschwerpunkts zu sorgen. Diese ist unerläßlich, um Einzelprognosen zusammenfassen zu können.

Für die zu wählenden Prognoseverfahren ist lediglich zu fordern, daß sie im Rahmen des gegebenen Gegenstandsbereichs zielführend sind und einer wissenschaftlichen Kritik standhalten können. Diese Minimalprämissen lassen einem Methodenpluralismus breiten Spielraum. Je nach dem Ausmaß theoretischer Vorarbeit soll die Verwendung von hochentwickelten ökonometrischen Modellen ebenso möglich sein wie etwa der Einsatz von Delphi-Befragungen. Die im folgenden gewählte Untergliederung von Prognoseverfahren in „quantitative" und „qualitative" Verfahren ist relativ willkürlich und in keiner Weise wertend. Insbesondere ist keine abschließende Aufzählung aller Prognoseverfahren beabsichtigt. Der Schwerpunkt der Aufzählung liegt bei statistischen Verfahren, von denen erwartet werden darf, daß die den weiter oben aufgeführten Forschungsgegenständen am ehesten angemessen sind. Soweit deterministische Verfahren angewendet werden können, werden sie sehr stark auf die entsprechende Substanzwissenschaft ausgerichtet sein, so daß sich ihre Besprechung hier erübrigt.

Das Postulat der Wissenschaftlichkeit verlangt bei der Anwendung aller Prognoseverfahren die Offenlegung sämtlicher Antezedensbedingungen und Gesetze, die in die Voraussage eingehen.

Quantitative Verfahren

Zeitreihenanalyse

Unter dem Oberbegriff der Zeitreihenanalyse werden Verfahren mit sehr unterschiedlichem methodischem Niveau zusammengefaßt. Allen diesen Verfahren ist gemeinsam, daß die Prognosewerte ausschließlich auf Vergangenheitswerten der Prognosevariablen beruhen. Wegen der fehlenden Berücksichtigung erklärender Variablen werden diese Prognoseverfahren i. allg. für langfristige Voraussagen als wenig geeignet angesehen. Als Ausnahmen gelten *Wachstums- und Sättigungsprognosemodelle* sowie *APC-Analysen*.

Wachstums- und Sättigungsmodelle:

Bei Wachstumsmodellen wird von der Grundannahme ausgegangen, daß das Wachstum Δx_t der Zeitreihe $\{x_t\}$ eine monotone Funktion $f(x_t)$ des im Zeitpunkt t erreichten Wertes x_t der Zeitreihe ist. Der einfachste Fall dieser Abhängigkeit ist mit der Funktion

$$\varDelta x_t = \text{konst}$$

gegeben, der zur linearen Trendextrapolation führt. Das exponentielle Wachstum wird durch die Funktion

$$\varDelta x_t = x_t \cdot \text{konst}$$

beschrieben. Kritisch angemerkt werden muß, daß die Grundannahme der Wachstumsmodelle oft nur schwer zu rechtfertigen ist. Da sie gegenüber Verletzungen dieser Annahme jedoch wenig robust sind, ist ihre Validität ex ante nur schwer abzuschätzen.

Sättigungsmodelle gehen von der Annahme aus, daß das Wachstum $\varDelta x_t$ der Zeitreihe $\{x_t\}$ eine in x_t und S monotone Funktion $f(x_t,S)$ des im Zeitpunkt t erreichten Wertes x_t der Zeitreihe und des Sättigungsniveaus S der Zeitreihe ist. Spezialfälle sind das logistische Modell mit

$$\varDelta x_t = x_t \cdot (S - x_t) \, \text{konst}$$

und das Gompertz-Modell mit

$$\varDelta x_t = x_t \cdot [\ln(S) - \ln(x_t)] \cdot \text{konst.}$$

Als nachteilig hat es sich erwiesen, die Schätzungen des Sättigungsniveaus S aus der Zeitreihe selber herzuleiten (Hansmann 1983). Statt dessen sollte das Sättigungsniveau aus Informationsquellen außerhalb der Zeitreihe geschätzt werden, womit ein erster Schritt zur Überwindung der reinen Zeitreihenanalyse getan wird. Beispielhaft für dieses Verfahren sind im Gesundheitswesen die Prognosen von Schäfer et al. (1984) zur Krankenhausverweildauer, die mit einem etwas modifizierten Sättigungsmodell arbeiten. In ihnen werden die Sättigungsniveaus aus einer Expertenbefragung erschlossen, die sich an das Delphi-Verfahren anlehnt, während die Zeitreiheneffekte selber aus der Krankenhausdiagnosestatistik Schleswig-Holstein (Heinemann 1986) ermittelt werden.

APC-Analysen:

Age-Period-Cohort-Analysen (APC-Analysen) wurden bisher in erster Linie auf Mortalitätsdaten angewendet, weil diese i. allg. aus der amtlichen Statistik verfügbar sind. Grundsätzlich steht einer Anwendung auf Inzidenzdaten jedoch nichts im Wege, wobei allerdings zu berücksichtigen ist, daß der Datenbedarf gewöhnlich nur mit Krankheitsregistern gedeckt werden kann.

Als eine Vorform dieser Methode kann die Age-Cohort-Analyse (AC-Analyse) betrachtet werden, die auch schon mit Daten der deutschen Todesursachenstatistik durchgeführt wurde (Robra u. Brecht 1984). Diese erlaubt einerseits eine Separierung des Alterseffektes, so daß die Altersabhängigkeit der Risiken dargestellt werden kann, ohne Verzerrungen durch unterschiedliche Risiken von i. allg. vermischt vorliegenden Geburtsjahrgängen in Kauf zu nehmen. Andererseits konnte der Kohorteneffekt unabhängig von Alterseinflüssen beschrieben werden, so daß eine vorsichtige Prognose der zukünftigen Krebssterblichkeit möglich ist.

Bei der Verwendung dieses multiplikativen Modells wird allerdings der Einfluß der (chronologischen) Zeit gänzlich den Faktoren Alter und Kohorte zugerechnet. Attribute, die dem Zeitabschnitt zugerechnet werden können, in dem die Sterbevorgänge tatsächlich stattgefunden haben, können in diesem Modell also nicht gesondert interpretiert werden. Als Attribute dieser Art sind alle Bedingungen anzusehen, die – anstatt über eine lange Latenzzeit zu wirken – die Mortalität kurzfristig beeinflussen. Zu denken ist hier beispielsweise an den „medizinischen Fortschritt" oder sonstige unmittelbar mortalitätswirksame Änderungen der Umweltbedingungen. Um diesen Effekt beschreiben zu können, ist ein Modell der Mortalitätsanalyse einzusetzen, das neben Alters- und Kohorteneffekten auch Zeiteffekte darzustellen vermag, ein sog. APC-Modell.

In der Literatur werden verschiedene APC-Modelle angeboten und geprüft. Allen diesen Modellen ist gemeinsam, daß – statistisch gesehen – der Kohorteneffekt nach Art eines Wechselwirkungsterms zusätzlich zu den Haupteffekten Alter und Sterbeperiode berücksichtigt wird. Dies kann in mathematisch unterschiedlicher Form geschehen. Eine systematische Übersicht über verschiedene Formulierungen der APC-Modelle geben Moolgavkar et al. (1979), die den Altersgang der Brustkrebsinzidenz in verschiedenen Populationen beschrieben haben.

Regressionsanalyse

Da für die Schätzung der Prognosewerte einer Zeitreihe in der (multiplen) Regressionsanalyse neben der Prognosevariablen andere, sog. *exogene Variablen* verwendet werden, insbesondere solche, denen man aufgrund theoretischer Erwägungen kausalen Charakter in bezug auf die Prognosevariable zuschreibt, wird die Regressionsanalyse gelegentlich auch als Kausalanalyse bezeichnet. Nach Ansicht der Verfasser sollte der Kausalitätsbegriff im statistischen Sprachgebrauch allerdings vermieden werden.

Der Vorteil des regressionsanalytischen Verfahrens besteht darin, daß theoretische Erkenntnisse über Zusammenhänge der Prognosegröße mit anderen in die Voraussage eingebracht werden können. Dieser Vorteil kann allerdings nur dann realisiert werden, wenn die exogenen Variablen entweder leichter zu prognostizieren sind als die Zielvariable oder die Prognosegröße von früheren Realisationen der exogenen Größen abhängen. Je nach der Länge dieses sog. time-lag kann dann die Prognosegröße sogar mit Gegenwarts- oder Vergangenheitsdaten geschätzt werden. Zu warnen ist vor der unkritischen Verwendung dieses Verfahrens bei Zusammenhängen, die nicht hinreichend theoretisch abgesichert sind. Gerade durch die Einflüsse der chronologischen Zeit werden oft Zusammenhänge vorgetäuscht, die eben nicht „kausal" sind.

Qualitative Verfahren

Delphi-Methode

Das Delphi-Verfahren stellt eine spezielle Form der Gruppenbefragung dar, wobei die Teilnehmer in der Regel schriftlich befragt werden. Durch die Rückkoppelung der Gruppenergebnisse an die einzelnen Teilnehmer mit einer oder mehreren anschließenden weiteren Befragungsrunden wird versucht, zu einem Konsens über zukünftige Entwicklungen zu gelangen. In der reinen Delphi-Technik wird in diesen Befragungsrunden der persönliche Kontakt zwischen den Befragten vermieden, um einem unerwünschten Gruppendruck entgegenzutreten.

Von dieser rein schriftlichen Vorgehensweise wird allerdings oft abgewichen, weil die Wartezeiten auf schriftliche Rückläufe unvertretbar lang sein können. Außerdem wird eine mehrfache Befragung von den Teilnehmern häufig als lästig empfunden, so daß Ausfälle entstehen. Neben diesen eher technischen Gründen für den Übergang zu mündlichen Gruppenbefragungen gibt es aber auch inhaltliche Gründe. Der wichtigste besteht darin, daß unterschiedliche Auffassungen über zukünftige Entwicklungen diskutiert werden können, wodurch sich für die Untersucher erhebliche Informationsgewinne einstellen.

Die Frage, ob mit der Delphi-Methode valide Voraussagen erzeugt werden können, läßt sich schwer beantworten. Eine Reihe von Delphi-Prognosen in Großbritannien zum Versorgungsbedarf in Krankenhäusern erreichte lediglich in etwa 50% der Voraussagen zufriedenstellende Ergebnisse (Taket, mündliche Mitteilung). Es liegt jedoch nahe, Delphi-Befragungen als ergänzende Kontrollmethode zu Prognosen zu verwenden, die auf andere Weise zustande gekommen sind. In der bereits oben aufgeführten Studie von Schäfer et al. (1984) wurde so vorgegangen.

Kritik an der Delphi-Methode wurde hauptsächlich aus 2 Gründen geübt: Erstens ist die Auswahl der zu befragenden Experten oft willkürlich, zweitens müßte bei der Erstellung eines gemeinsamen Urteils eine Gewichtung der einzelnen Beiträge erfolgen. Levine (1984) schlägt hierzu ein systematisiertes Vorgehen vor. Inwieweit dieses dazu geeignet ist, die beschriebenen Nachteile zu beheben, ist gegenwärtig allerdings noch offen.

Szenarien

Gegenüber den bisher besprochenen Verfahren der Prognose weisen die Szenarioverfahren einen Hauptunterschied auf: Es wird nicht nur auf die Beschreibung eines einzigen Verlaufs der zukünftigen möglichen Entwicklungen abgezielt, sondern es werden verschiedene Möglichkeiten der Zukunft aufgezeigt. Dieses Vorgehen ist deswegen besonders entscheidungsorientiert, weil die Konsequenzen von Entscheidungen unter Unsicherheit unter verschiedenen zukünftigen Umweltbedingungen bewertet werden können.

Nach Pannenborg (1986) hat die Szenarienanalyse folgende Eigenschaften:

- Sie beschreibt explizit und systematisch die Wahrscheinlichkeiten verschiedener möglicher Ereignisse in der Zukunft.
- Sie übernimmt Elemente sowohl aus den quantitativen als auch den qualitativen Prognoseverfahren.
- Sie macht die Voraussetzungen und Arbeitshypothesen des Modells und der Variablenauswahl explizit.

Er unterscheidet zwischen *explorativen* oder *prädiktiven Szenarien* und *normativen Szenarien*. Während explorative Szenarien dazu dienen, vom Prognosezeitpunkt aus die möglichen zukünftigen Verläufe zu beschreiben, besteht der Zweck von normativen Szenarien in der Ermittlung von Pfaden, die zu einem gesetzten Ziel führen. Normative Szenarien sollen hier nicht betrachtet werden.

Nach den bisherigen Aufführungen wird deutlich, daß sich ein Szenario viel stärker an seiner Thematik orientiert als an einer speziellen Prognosemethodik. Die Szenariotechnik kann als der Versuch bezeichnet werden, das zum Prognosezeitpunkt verfügbare Wissen zu einem Gegenstandsbereich zu einer Beschreibung von zukünftigen Entwicklungslinien zu verknüpfen. Hierzu gehört die Prognose – ersatzweise Annahmen über verschiedene Verläufe – von Einflußfaktoren auf die Zielgröße ebenso wie die Entwicklung von Theorien über ihr Zusammenwirken. Dies bedeutet, daß in einem Szenario – je nach Gegenstand und methodischem Vorwissen – alle Prognosemethoden Platz finden können. Dabei wird der Prognosecharakter um so deutlicher, je genauer einzelne Elemente des Szenarios vorhergesagt werden können und je stringenter der logische Zusammenhang zwischen den Einflußfaktoren und der Zielgröße ist.

Der Szenariotechnik wird gelegentlich vorgeworfen, daß sie sehr stark subjektiven Einschätzungen ihrer Anwender ausgesetzt sei. Dies kann kaum bestritten werden, ist jedoch nicht so sehr ein Kritikpunkt an der Technik selber als vielmehr an ihrer Ausgestaltung bei der Wahl und dem Einsatz ihrer einzelnen Methodenelemente.

Ein anderer Vorwurf bezieht sich auf die Auswahl der möglichen „Zukünfte". Ein Blick auf die möglichen Anwendungsfelder der Szenariotechnik im Gesundheitswesen – etwa auf dem Gebiet der Altersstruktur der Bevölkerung – zeigt, daß die Zahl der Einflußgrößen sehr groß ist und eine Vielzahl denkbarer Entwicklungen gestattet. Andererseits verlangt die beabsichtigte Verwendung von Szenarien bei Entscheidungen eine sinnvolle Beschränkung ihrer Zahl. Nach Ansicht von Anwendern in der Industrie (Boezeman 1986) ist eine Beschränkung auf maximal drei Alternativen angebracht. Die Auswahl von wenigen Alternativentwürfen aus einem Universum von Möglichkeiten ist zweifellos eine weitere Quelle subjektiver Verzerrungen. Andererseits reduziert sich die Zahl möglicher Alternativen dadurch erheblich, daß bestimmte Entwicklungslinien nicht miteinander verträglich sind. So zeigt beispielsweise Pannenborg, daß von 9 Entwicklungsalternativen zur Struktur der gesundheitlichen Versorgung Betagter von vornherein 3 als unerreichbar angesehen werden müssen.

Die beiden kritischen Anmerkungen bestätigen jedoch, daß die bereits weiter oben[4] geforderte Offenlegung der Voraussetzungen und Arbeitshypothesen die wissenschaftliche Qualität von Szenarien bestimmt.

Schlußfolgerungen und Empfehlungen

Vorschläge zur Methodik
bei der Behandlung einzelner Forschungsgegenstände

Im folgenden wird der Versuch unternommen, den auf S. 370 aufgeführten Forschungsgegenständen geeignete Prognoseverfahren zuzuweisen. Der endgültigen

---

[4] Vgl. Abschn. „Vorbemerkung", S. 365.

Gestaltung der einzelnen Forschungsvorhaben soll hiermit jedoch nicht vorgegriffen werden.

Altersstruktur der Bevölkerung

Die Abschätzung der Konsequenzen einer Veränderung im Altersaufbau der Bevölkerung auf die gesundheitliche Versorgung ist einerseits durch quantitative Verfahren möglich. Zum Einsatz kann hier bei Schaffung der entsprechenden Datenlage die APC-Analyse kommen, in einer vereinfachten Version könnten erste Hochrechnungen jedoch auch auf der Basis der heutigen altersspezifischen Inanspruchnahmeziffern des stationären und ambulanten Sektors vorgenommen werden. Ein Beispiel für eine derartige Studie für die Schweiz haben Minder u. Abelin (1986) veröffentlicht. Andererseits ist es erforderlich, diese Konsequenzen auch auf qualitativem Niveau zu diskutieren. Zu berücksichtigen ist hierbei insbesondere der Einfluß von Änderungen der heute üblichen pflegerischen Versorgung.

Neben dem Einsatz ökonometrischer Methoden zur Abschätzung der wirtschaftlichen Konsequenzen eines veränderten Altersaufbaus sind vor allem qualitative Verfahren zur Beschreibung der sozioökonomischen Entwicklungen einzusetzen.

Morbidität und Mortalität durch einzelne Krankheitsgruppen

Das vorrangige Interesse von Langfristprognosen liegt hier sicher nicht bei der Mortalität, sondern bei der Schätzung der *Morbidität*, insbesondere bei Prognosen der absoluten Krankheitshäufigkeiten. Auf der Grundlage von Daten aus dem finnischen Krebsregister geben Hakama et al. (1986) eine Prognose für die Inzidenz von Krebs insgesamt und 6 einzelnen Krebslokalisationen ab. Die Datenlage für vergleichbare Untersuchungen ist in der Bundesrepublik Deutschland allerdings schlecht.

Sofern nicht die Existenz von Krankheitsregistern wenigstens Hochrechnungen auf der Grundlage alters- und geschlechtsspezifischer Morbiditätsdaten erlaubt, können hilfsweise Inanspruchnahmedaten aus dem ambulanten und stationären Sektor verwendet werden. Für den stationären Sektor stehen mit der Krankenhausdiagnosestatistik Schleswig-Holstein und der Statistik der Krankenkassen längsschnittlich organisierte Datenkörper zur Verfügung, die eine diagnose- und altersspezifische Analyse gestatten. Die Analyse der Inanspruchnahme des ambulanten Sektors steht in der Bundesrepublik Deutschland dagegen erst am Anfang. Zwar hat das Zentralinstitut für die Kassenärztliche Versorgung in der Bundesrepublik Deutschland mit der EVaS-Studie eine entsprechende Untersuchung vorgelegt (Kerek-Bodden et al. 1984), diese bezieht sich jedoch nur auf einen einzelnen Zeitraum (1982/83). Im übrigen sei darauf hingewiesen, daß Inanspruchnahme für Morbiditätsschätzungen nur nach entsprechenden Korrekturen verwendet werden können.

Eine weitere Möglichkeit, Morbiditätsschätzungen mit bereits vorhandenen Daten durchzuführen, bietet sich bei Erkrankungen mit hoher Letalität durch den Rekurs auf die Todesursachenstatistik.

Eine Sonderrolle spielt die Gruppe der Verletzungen. Als ihre Hauptursache sind Verkehrsunfälle und häusliche Unfälle zu nennen. Zumindest bei Verkehrsunfällen sind langfristige Prognosen nur dann sinnvoll, wenn versucht wird, zukünftige technische Entwicklungen zu antizipieren. Der Einsatz der Delphi-Technik unter Einschluß von Experten aus dem Kreis der Automobilindustrie könnte dazu geeignet sein, grobe Eckdaten zu setzen.

Für Prognosen der *Mortalität* ist je nach Todesursache unterschiedlich vorzugehen. Bei Todesursachen, deren Häufigkeit mit der Zugehörigkeit zu verschiedenen Geburtsjahrgängen assoziiert ist, kann eine Prognose mit Mitteln der APC-Analyse vorgenommen werden. Hierzu sind vor allem chronische Erkrankungen mit langer Latenzzeit zu rechnen, so daß ein erheblicher Teil des Mortalitätsgeschehens in entwickelten Ländern einer vorsichtigen Prognose zugänglich ist.

Todesursachen, die mit der APC-Analyse nicht zu prognostizieren sind, sind in ihrer Häufigkeit in erster Linie durch Bedingungen des Sterbezeitraums charakterisiert. Beispiele sind die Mortalität durch Unfälle, Suizide oder Infektionskrankheiten. Voraussagen scheinen hier nur mit qualitativen Methoden möglich zu sein.

Wirtschaftliche und soziale Rahmenbedingungen, Versorgungsstruktur

Der Genauigkeitsgrad von langfristigen Prognosen im wirtschaftlichen Bereich ist gering. Es ist deshalb angebracht, auf verschiedene Szenarien zur Beschreibung des möglichen Verlaufs zukünftiger sozioökonomischer Entwicklungen zurückzugreifen. Die Entwicklung der Versorgungsstruktur kann nicht unabhängig von der zukünftigen Leistungsfähigkeit der Gesamtwirtschaft gedacht werden und unterliegt somit hinsichtlich ihrer Prognostizierbarkeit denselben Einschränkungen.

Die zu entwickelnden Szenarien sollten mindestens folgende Elemente enthalten:

- Entwicklung des Sozialprodukts,
- Entwicklung der Beschäftigtenzahl,
- Entwicklung der Einkommensverteilung,
- Personalentwicklung in den Gesundheitsberufen,
- Entwicklung besonderer Leistungsangebote zur geriatrischen Versorgung,
- Entwicklung präventiver Leistungsangebote,
- Entwicklung der Abgrenzung von stationären und ambulanten Leistungsangeboten.

Vorschlag einer Projektorganisation

Vorgaben für die Organisation

Die Organisation eines Projekts „Langfristige Entwicklungstrends im Gesundheitswesen" hat folgenden Gegebenheiten Rechnung zu tragen:

1) Die Auswahl der Forschungsgegenstände richtet sich nach dem gesundheitspolitischen Entscheidungsbedarf. Sie ist auch nach den ersten Vorschlägen in

dieser Studie nicht abgeschlossen. Sie wird in erheblichem Umfang von der Einschätzung ihrer Wichtigkeit durch Entscheidungsträger im Gesundheitswesen zu bestimmen sein.

2) Im Vorgriff auf genauere Schätzungen der Projektlaufzeit ist von einer mehrjährigen Dauer auszugehen. Die gesundheitspolitischen Prioritäten können sich im Lauf dieser Zeit ändern.

Die Punkte 1) und 2) verlangen die aktive Mitwirkung der interessierten Entscheidungsträger in der Gesundheitspolitik bei der Auswahl der zu bearbeitenden Gegenstände. Sie erzwingen weiterhin eine offene Struktur des Projekts in dem Sinne, daß neue Gegenstände während der Laufzeit an das Projekt angelagert werden können.

3) Die bisher skizzierten Forschungsgegenstände sind schwerpunktartig verschiedenen Disziplinen zuzuordnen.

Punkt 3) verlangt die Aufgliederung des Projekts in mindestens ein Forschungsvorhaben je Gegenstandsbereich. Damit die entscheidungsunterstützende Zielsetzung des Projekts trotzdem erhalten bleibt, müssen die Einzelvorhaben koordiniert werden. Diese Koordination bezieht sich zum einen auf die Beibehaltung der ursprünglichen Forschungsabsichten, zum anderen auf das methodische Vorgehen. Sie soll gewährleisten, daß die Einzelvorhaben gemeinschaftlich interpretierbar sind. Dies bezieht sich zunächst auf die Prognosezeiträume und auf die Prognosegegenstände, sodann aber auch auf die kompatible Definition einzelner Elemente wie Altersklassen, Diagnosegruppen usw.

4) Je nach Differenzierungsgrad der einzelnen Forschungsvorhaben werden diese auch selber entweder nur interdisziplinär oder mit einem erhöhten Koordinationsaufwand zu bearbeiten sein.

Bei niedrigem Differenzierungsgrad (im Extremfall ein Vorhaben je Gegenstand) kann ein großer Teil der Koordinationsaufgaben in das einzelne Vorhaben verlagert werden. Dies verlangt jedoch der durchführenden Einrichtung ein hohes Maß an Interdisziplinarität ab und bringt den Verlust von Steuerungsmöglichkeiten mit sich.

5) Für jeden Forschungsgegenstand ist Methodenpluralismus anzustreben, weil so die für Langfristprognosen typischen Unsicherheiten hinsichtlich der Validität der Ergebnisse kontrolliert werden können.

Dieses Vorgehen legt es nahe, die Anwendung verschiedener Methoden in unterschiedlichen Forschungseinrichtungen zu plazieren. Unerwünschte frühzeitige Abstimmungsprozesse über Ergebnisse können so vermieden werden. Es entsteht jedoch eine weitere Koordinationsaufgabe.

6) Aus Gründen der Arbeitsökonomie ist auf Vorarbeiten Dritter zurückzugreifen. Dies gilt auch für Vorarbeiten im internationalen Raum, wo v. a. auf Erfahrungen der niederländischen STG zurückgegriffen werden könnte.

Die Entwicklung von Prognosemethoden könnte dadurch arbeitsteilig gestaltet werden. Einzelne Prognosen oder Szenarien müssen jedoch vor Ort erstellt werden. Die STG hat gegenüber den Verfassern ihre Kooperationsbereitschaft geäußert.

7) Die Forschungsergebnisse müssen der gesundheitspolitischen Umsetzung zugeführt werden.

Dies erfordert die Aufnahme der Studienergebnisse in einer Einrichtung, der Gesundheitspolitiker angehören.

Organisationsentwurf

Die Projektaufgaben sind wie folgt zu gliedern:

1) Inhaltliche Kompetenzen

Hierzu gehören: Auswahl der Forschungsgegenstände und ihre Begründung, Aufbereitung der Forschungsergebnisse zu ihrer Umsetzung.

2) Durchführungskompetenzen

Bearbeitung der einzelnen Forschungsvorhaben.

3) Koordinationskompetenzen

Abstimmung zwischen den verschiedenen Einzelvorhaben hinsichtlich ihrer Ziele, Abstimmung zwischen den verschiedenen Einzelvorhaben hinsichtlich ihrer Methoden, Zusammenführung der Ergebnisse aus den einzelnen Vorhaben zu einheitlichen Darstellungen (bei niedrigem Differenzierungsgrad der Einzelvorhaben teilweise entbehrlich), Ergebnisabstimmung bei Einzelvorhaben zur gleichen Thematik mit unterschiedlichem methodischen Ansatz, Herstellung von Verbindungen zwischen verschiedenen Forschungsgruppen, insbesondere bei internationaler Kooperation.

4) Finanzielle Kompetenzen

Mittelbewilligung und Mittelzuteilung für die einzelnen Vorhaben.

Die Verteilung der aufgeführten Kompetenzen auf einzelne Einrichtungen sollten sich nach Ansicht der Verfasser aus organisatorischen Gründen eng am üblichen und bisher bewährten Verfahren der Forschungsförderung im Rahmen des Programms „Forschung und Entwicklung im Dienste der Gesundheit" ausrichten. Dieses verweist die finanziellen und auch einen Teil der inhaltlichen Zuständigkeiten an die Projektträgerorganisationen des Bundes. Die Durchführungskompetenzen wären wie üblich an Auftragnehmer bzw. Zuwendungsempfänger zu delegieren.

Die inhaltlichen Kompetenzen sollten von einem neu zu schaffenden Gremium (Lenkungsausschuß) wahrgenommen werden, dem Vertreter der mit Gesundheitspolitik befaßten Gebietskörperschaften, aber auch Vertreter sonstiger Entscheidungsträger der Gesundheitspolitik angehören. Zu nennen sind hier insbesondere die Selbstverwaltungseinrichtungen der „Anbieter von Gesundheitsleistungen" und der Krankenkassen. Weiterhin sollten einschlägig ausgewiesene Wissenschaftler diesem Gremium angehören.

Mit den Koordinationskompetenzen, die der Projektträger nicht selber übernehmen kann oder will, ist eine Einrichtung zu betrauen, die in enger Abstimmung mit dem Projektträger, den durchführenden Einrichtungen und dem Lenkungsausschuß zusammenarbeitet (Koordinationsinstitut).

Literatur

Boezeman JEM (1986) Scenarios by Royal Dutch Shell. Vortrag im STG/WHO-Workshop on Scenarios and Methods to Support Long Term Planning. Noordwijk aan Zee

Brenner H (1986) Review on scenarios as an instrument for health policy design. Vortrag im STG/WHO-Workshop on Scenarios and Methods to Support Long Term Planning. Noordwijk aan Zee

Drummond MF, Stoddart GL (1985) Principles of economic evaluation of health programmes. World Health Stat Q 38:355–367

Hakama M, Hakulinen T, Läärä E (1986) Predicting cancer incidence and prevalence. In: WHO Regional Office for Europe (ed) Health projections in Europe: methods and applications. WHO Regional Office for Europe, Kopenhagen, pp 25–39

Hansmann KW (1983) Kurzlehrbuch Prognoseverfahren. Gabler, Wiesbaden

Heinemann A (1986) Zur Diagnosestatistik des Landes Schleswig-Holstein. Stat Monatsh Schleswig-Holstein 38:4–17

HM Treasury (1982) Investment appraisal in the public sector. Her Majesty's Stationary Office, London

Holmes DR, Elveback LR, Frye RL, Kottke BA, Ellefson RD (1981) Association of risk factor variables and coronary artery disease documented with angiography. Circulation 63:293–299

Kahn H, Wiener AJ (1967) The year 2000: a framework for speculation on the next thirty-three years. Macmillan, New York

Kerek-Bodden HE, Schach E, Schach S, Schwartz FW, Wagner P (1984) EVaS-Study: Survey instruments. In: Eimeren W van, Engelbrecht R, Flagle CD (Hrsg) 3rd Int Conf on System Science in Health Care. Springer, Berlin Heidelberg New York Tokyo, pp 1352–1354

Lagergren M (1986) Methodological considerations in long-range planning. Vortrag im STG/WHO-Workshop on Scenarios and Methods to Support Long Term Planning. Noordwijk aan Zee

Levine A (1984) A model for health projections using knowledgeable informants. World Health Stat Q 37:306–317

Minder CE, Abelin T (1986) Projections of needs, impairments and morbidity of the elderly in Switzerland. In: WHO Regional Office for Europe (ed) Health projections in Europe: methods and applications. WHO Regional Office for Europe, Kopenhagen, pp 56–73

Moolgavkar SH, Stevens RG, Lee JAH (1979) Effect of age on incidence of breast cancer in females. J Natl Cancer Inst 62:493–501

Pannenborg CO (1986) Scenarios as a method of exploring the future of health care. In: WHO Regional Office for Europe (ed) Health projections in Europe: methods and applications. WHO Regional Office for Europe, Kopenhagen, pp 236–251

Popper KR (1972) Objective knowledge. An evolutionary approach. Clarendon, Oxford

Robra BP, Brecht JG (1984) Kohortenanalyse der Krebssterblichkeit in der Bundesrepublik Deutschland 1955 bis 1979. Lebensversicherungsmedizin 36:26–28

Schäfer T, Schmidt R, Wachtel HW (1984) Gutachten über die Entwicklung der Bedarfsdeterminanten für die Fortschreibung des Krankenhausbedarfsplans. Dornier System, Friedrichshafen

Schwarze J (1980) Statistische Kenngrößen zur Ex-post-Beurteilung von Prognosen. In: Schwarze J (Hrsg) Angewandte Prognoseverfahren. Verlag Neue Wirtschafts-Briefe, Herne, S 317–344

Sieben G, Schildbach T (1975) Betriebswirtschaftliche Entscheidungstheorie. Mohr, Tübingen
Steering Committee on Future Health Scenarios (oJ) Structure and terms of reference. Steering Committee on Future Health Scenarios, Rijswijk
Steering Committee on Future Health Scenarios (Hrsg) (1986) The heart of the future – the future of the heart. Scenarios on cardiovascular diseases 1985–2010. Steering Committee on Future Health Scenarios, Leidschendam
Stegmüller W (1974) Probleme und Resultate der Wissenschaftstheorie und Analytischen Philosophie. Bd 1: Wissenschaftliche Erklärung und Begründung. Springer, Berlin Heidelberg New York
Theil H (1966) Applied economic forecasting. North-Holland-Publishing Company, Amsterdam

Weiterführende Literatur zum Thema „Gesundheitssystemforschung"

Bundesministerium für Arbeit und Sozialordnung: Reihe Gesundheitsforschung: Forschungsberichte
Eimeren W van, Horisberger B (Hrsg): Reihe Gesundheitssystemforschung, Springer, Berlin Heidelberg New York Tokyo
Sachverständigenrat für die Konzertierte Aktion im Gesundheitswesen (1987) Medizinische und ökonomische Orientierung: Vorschläge für die Konzertierte Aktion im Gesundheitswesen, Jahresgutachten 1987. Nomos, Baden-Baden
Sachverständigenrat für die Konzertierte Aktion im Gesundheitswesen (1988) Medizinische und ökonomische Orientierung: Vorschläge für die Konzertierte Aktion im Gesundheitswesen, Jahresgutachten 1988. Nomos, Baden-Baden
Sachverständigenrat für die Konzertierte Aktion im Gesundheitswesen (1989) Qualität, Wirtschaftlichkeit und Perspektiven der Gesundheitsversorgung: Vorschläge für die Konzertierte Aktion im Gesundheitswesen, Jahresgutachten 1989. Nomos, Baden-Baden

5 Gesundheitsberichterstattung

Zum Aufbau einer Gesundheitsberichterstattung: Bestandsaufnahme und Konzeptvorschlag *

Redaktionskomitee der Forschungsgruppe „Gesundheitsberichterstattung"

Ansatz und Vorgehensweise

Im Rahmen des Programms „Forschung und Entwicklung im Dienste der Gesundheit" wurde die Forschungsgruppe Gesundheitsberichterstattung mit der Durchführung des Forschungsvorhabens „Aufbau einer Gesundheitsberichterstattung – Bestandsaufnahme und Konzeptvorschlag" beauftragt.

Gegenstand des Auftrags war im wesentlichen:

- Ermittlung und Strukturierung des Nutzungsbedarfs einer Gesundheitsberichterstattung,
- Bestandsaufnahme und Bewertung von Datenquellen hinsichtlich ihrer Eignung für eine Gesundheitsberichterstattung,
- Vorschlag für eine Basisgesundheitsberichterstattung,
- Skizzierung verschiedener Szenarien, in denen Voraussetzungen für den Aufbau und die dauerhafte Funktion einer Gesundheitsberichterstattung beschrieben werden.

Im Vorhaben wird zwischen einer *Basis-* und einer *Spezialberichterstattung* unterschieden. Berichtsthemen, die eine hohe Nutzervielfalt und Relevanz aufweisen, werden einer kontinuierlichen Basisberichterstattung zugewiesen. Für spezielle Themen, die nur für einzelne oder wenige Nutzer relevant sind, episodenhaften Charakter besitzen oder einen hohen, noch offenen Forschungsbedarf aufweisen, können Spezialberichte entwickelt werden.

Thematisch wurde die Gesundheitsberichterstattung in folgende Bereiche gegliedert:

- Soziodemographie,
- Gesundheitszustand der Bevölkerung,
- Ressourcen des Gesundheitswesens,
- Inanspruchnahme von Leistungen des Gesundheitswesens,
- Kosten und Finanzierung des Gesundheitswesens.

---

* Überarbeitung der Kurzfassung des Endberichts zum Vorhaben Aufbau einer Gesundheitsberichterstattung – Bestandsaufnahme und Konzeptvorschlag.

Grundfragen einer Gesundheitsberichterstattung

Es bestehen in der Bundesrepublik Deutschland – gemessen am Informationsbedarf, aber auch im internationalen Vergleich – offensichtliche Lücken in den bisher verfügbaren Daten und Analysen über Soziodemographie, Gesundheitszustand der Bevölkerung, Ressourcen, Kosten und Finanzierung des Gesundheitswesens. Diese sollen mit dem Aufbau einer Gesundheitsberichterstattung systematisch und gezielt geschlossen werden.

Darüber hinaus soll, wo immer möglich, die systemhafte Verflechtung der genannten Einzelbereiche hervorgehoben werden. Damit soll die bisher übliche Praxis, wonach einzelne Datenquellen für den Informationsbedarf einzelner Institutionen in unterschiedlicher Form erhoben worden sind, schrittweise an eine einheitliche Systematik herangeführt werden.

Ausgangslage und inhaltliche Zielsetzung einer Gesundheitsberichterstattung hat der Sachverständigenrat für die Konzertierte Aktion im Gesundheitswesen (SVR) wie folgt dargestellt:

> Um die längerfristige Entwicklung der gesundheitlichen Versorgung und ihre medizinischen, vor allem aber ihre wirtschaftlichen Auswirkungen analysieren zu können, muß der zugrundeliegende Versorgungsprozeß beschrieben, in die Zukunft projiziert und schließlich anhand von Zielsetzungen bewertet werden. Nur so kann beurteilt werden, ob bestimmte gegenwärtige oder für die Zukunft erwartete Entwicklungen im Hinblick auf bestimmte gesundheitspolitische Ziele als „positiv" oder „negativ" einzustufen sind, und nur so können längerfristige Prioritäten für den Abbau von Versorgungsdefiziten und bestehender Überversorgung auf rationaler Basis entwickelt werden.
>
> Angesichts dieser Ausgangslage ist eine sektorübergreifende, funktionale Bestandsaufnahme und -analyse sinnvoll. Bestimmte Entwicklungen – in der Bevölkerungsgröße und -struktur, in den Mortalitäts- und Morbiditätsmustern, in der gesundheitlichen Versorgung, in den finanziellen und wirtschaftlichen Rahmenbedingungen u.a.m. – können identifiziert und ihre Implikationen für die Zukunft aufgezeigt werden. Daraus lassen sich mittel- und langfristige Optionen für die Gesundheitspolitik ableiten (SVR 1987)[1].

Der SVR empfiehlt die Einrichtung eines Berichtswesens ähnlich der volkswirtschaftlichen Gesamtrechnung. Die Position des SVR wird nicht nur von seiten der Gesundheitsforschung allgemein geteilt. Vielmehr zeigt sich auch bei einzelnen Bundesländern Unbehagen über die im Jahr 1975 zuletzt aktualisierten Ländergesundheitsberichte. Die Arbeitsgemeinschaft der leitenden Medizinalbeamten der Länder hat deswegen im Jahr 1987 eine Arbeitsgruppe mit dem Auftrag eingesetzt, ein bedarfsgerechtes System der Gesundheitsberichterstattung einzurichten.

Die Notwendigkeit eines solchen Systems wurde bereits anläßlich der Großen Anfrage von Abgeordneten der Bundestagsfraktionen der CDU/CSU und der FDP im Jahr 1985 deutlich: Zwar war es möglich, die Fragen zur *personellen* und *institutionellen Struktur* des Gesundheitswesens auf der Grundlage der amtlichen Statistik eingehend zu beantworten, eine adäquate Stellungnahme zu den Fragen der Abgeordneten nach dem Gesundheitszustand der Bevölkerung konnte jedoch trotz intensiver Bemühungen nicht gegeben werden. Der Parlamentarische

---

[1] SVR (1987) Medizinische und ökonomische Orientierung: Vorschläge für die Konzertierte Aktion im Gesundheitswesen. Baden-Baden.

Staatssekretär beim MBJFG stellte dazu fest: „Die gegenwärtig in der Bundesrepublik Deutschland verfügbaren Datengrundlagen reichen für umfassende, gesicherte Aussagen über die gegenwärtige Situation und zukünftige Entwicklungen nicht aus" (BT-Drucksache 10/3374, 1985).

Lückenhaft sind insbesondere die Aussagen zur Krankheitshäufigkeit und zur Krankheitsdauer, für die lediglich auf Ergebnisse des Mikrozensus zurückgegriffen werden konnte. Zur Frage nach der Leistungsfähigkeit der gesundheitlichen Versorgung konnte nur auf den Anteil der Krankenversicherten an der Bevölkerung und die Ausgaben für das Gesundheitswesen und seine einzelnen Bereiche hingewiesen werden.

Das Grundproblem der Gesundheitspolitik besteht, wie weiter ausgeführt wird, „nicht darin, zu wenig Mittel zur Verfügung zu haben, sondern darin, die richtigen gesundheitspolitischen Prioritäten zu setzen und die Rahmenbedingungen in den einzelnen Leistungsbereichen so zu gestalten, daß die medizinischen Leistungen effektiv und effizient erbracht und sparsam nachgefragt werden" (BT-Drucksache 10/3374, 1985).

Die verteilten Kompetenzen im deutschen Gesundheitswesen verlangen darüber hinaus, daß die Wahl von Prioritäten von den jeweiligen Entscheidungsträgern mitgetragen wird. Orientierungsdaten im Gesundheitswesen haben somit nicht in erster Linie einen technokratischen Planungscharakter, sondern v. a. eine Informations- und Konsensbildungsfunktion. Das vorgeschlagene System einer Gesundheitsberichterstattung soll hierfür notwendige Informationsgrundlagen liefern.

Ergebnis der Nutzeranalyse

Für die einzelnen Themenbereiche ergeben sich nach der Nutzeranalyse v. a. folgende Anforderungen an Indikatoren zu Status, Entwicklung und Bewertung des Gesundheitswesens:

Soziodemographie

Es sind erforderlich
- Bevölkerungsaufbau und Bevölkerungsentwicklung nach
  - Alter,
  - Geschlecht,
  - Region (für Nutzung in einer kleinräumigen Berichterstattung auch kleine Gebietseinheiten),
  - sozioökonomischen Merkmalen wie Art des Krankenversicherungsschutzes, Beschäftigung, Ausbildung.

Nur für einzelne Nutzungsebenen wird als notwendig angesehen
- Risikostruktur der Bevölkerung nach Versicherungszweigen (Nutzungsebene Strukturreform der GKV).

Gesundheitszustand der Bevölkerung

1) Mortalitätsindikatoren:
   – Lebenserwartung von Neugeborenen und bestimmten Altersgruppen,
   – Müttersterblichkeit,
   – Kindersterblichkeit, Säuglingssterblichkeit, perinatale Mortalität, Anteil von Neugeborenen mit einem Mindestgeburtsgewicht von 2500 g nach Geschlecht,
   – für bestimmte auszuwählende Krankheiten Mortalität.

2) Morbiditätsindikatoren:
   – Für bestimmte auszuwählende Krankheiten Inzidenz, Prävalenz, Wiederherstellungsraten,
   – Trendunterschiede im Gesundheitszustand einzelner Bevölkerungsgruppen,
   – Karies-(DMF-T-)Index bei Kindern, Anteil von über- und untergewichtigen Kindern, Grad der Durchimpfung gegen bestimmte Krankheiten,
   – subjektiver Gesundheitszustand, gesundheitsrelevante Verhaltensweisen, Pflegebedürftigkeit, Activities-of-daily-living-(ADL-)Skalen.

3) Risikoindikatoren:
   – Konsum von Tabakwaren und Alkohol pro Kopf, Anteil von Nichtrauchern und starken Rauchern,
   – Pro-Kopf-Verbrauch von Proteinen, Lipiden und Kohlenhydraten.

4) Indikatoren der Krankheitsfolgen:
   – Verrentungshäufigkeiten, zeitweilige Behinderung, Anteil dauerhafter Behinderter,
   – Arbeitsunfähigkeit,
   – Berufskrankheiten.

Alle angegebenen Indikatoren sollen – soweit anwendbar – nach den weiter oben aufgeführten soziodemographischen Merkmalen gleichartig differenziert werden können. Für die Nutzung auf Bundesebene genügt dabei eine grobe Regionalisierung, etwa nach Ländern oder Regierungsbezirken. Für die Nutzung in einer kleinräumigen Berichterstattung wird darüber hinaus die Ermittlung von Schwerpunkten von Krankheit und Behinderung mit der Absicht des zeitlichen und regionalen Vergleichs gefordert. Dazu wird eine kleinräumige Erfassung von Mortalität, Morbidität, Gesundheitsrisiken und Krankheitsfolgen benötigt.

Ressourcen des Gesundheitswesens

– Angebot von Personal und ausgewählten Sachmitteln nach
  Sektoren (ambulant, stationär etc.),
  Einrichtungen,
  Leistungen,
  jeweils bezogen auf die Gesamtbevölkerung und Bevölkerungsgruppen,
– Beschäftigte im Gesundheitswesen,
– Angehörige von Gesundheitsberufen in Ausbildung,
– Beschäftigungs- und Ausbildungssituation und regionaler Arbeitsmarkt für Gesundheitsberufe (für eine kleinräumige Berichterstattung).

Inanspruchnahme

- Inanspruchnahme nach
  Diagnose und Krankheitsgruppen,
  Leistungen,
  Personal und Einrichtungen,
  Sektoren,
- Kombinationen dieser Merkmalsgruppen, z. B. nach Leistungen für Sektoren.

Alle angegebenen Indikatoren sollen – soweit anwendbar – nach den weiter oben aufgeführten soziodemographischen Merkmalen gleichartig differenziert werden können, also v. a. nach Alter, Geschlecht, Region, Art des Krankenversicherungsschutzes usw.

Kosten/Finanzierung

- Indikatoren der wirtschaftlichen Rahmenbedingungen,
- Anteil der Gesundheitsausgaben am Bruttosozialprodukt,
- Einnahmen und Ausgaben im Gesundheitswesen nach
  Art,
  Träger,
  Finanzierung,
  Sektor,
- soziale Lasten und Kosten einzelner Krankheiten,
- Kosten und Wirkungen einzelner Verrichtungen,
- Ausgaben für gesundheitsbezogene Forschung und Entwicklung,
- Preisindizes nach Sektoren,
- kleinräumige Differenzierung von Leistungs- und Ausgabenstatistiken (für eine kleinräumige Berichterstattung).

Soweit möglich sollen die Indikatoren aller Themenbereiche einer Gesundheitsberichterstattung nicht nur im Querschnitt dargestellt werden, sondern auch in ihrer zeitlichen Entwicklung.

Es ist ausdrücklich darauf hinzuweisen, daß auch eine Basisberichterstattung sich nicht in der tabellarischen Auflistung von Indikatoren und deren Kommentierung erschöpfen kann, sondern Zusammenhänge zwischen den genannten Themenbereichen aufzeigen soll. Von den Mitgliedern der Forschungsgruppe werden insbesondere genannt Zusammenhänge zwischen Gesundheitszustand und Inanspruchnahme von Leistungen des Gesundheitswesens, zwischen demographischer Lage und ökonomischen Konsequenzen sowie Konsequenzen für den Gesundheitszustand der Bevölkerung. Nutzungsbedarf wird auch hinsichtlich der Beurteilung von Effektivität und Effizienz einzelner Leistungen des Gesundheitswesens gesehen.

Ergebnis der Bestandsaufnahme

Übersicht

Insgesamt wurden 276 Datenquellen oder Datenquellengruppen aufgenommen und bewertet. In dieser Sammlung sind sowohl umfassende Datenquellen mit mehreren hundert Merkmalen enthalten (z. B. Daten der Gesetzlichen Krankenversicherung) als auch Datenquellen mit geringer Merkmalanzahl (z. B. Statistik der Schwangerschaftsabbrüche). Diese Bestandsaufnahme ist damit bisher die umfangreichste ihrer Art in der Bundesrepublik Deutschland. Sie ist dennoch nicht vollständig. So sind z. B. gesundheitsbezogene Daten nach dem Bundessozialhilfegesetz nicht bearbeitet worden, obwohl sie sozialmedizinisch bedeutsam sind.

Die Datenquellen wurden nach Herkunft und Thematik gruppiert und danach bewertet, ob sie grundsätzlich für eine Basisberichterstattung geeignet sind, ob ihre inhaltliche und methodische Qualität für eine Nutzung ausreicht, ob der Zugang zu den Datenquellen ausreichend ist und welche Bearbeitungskosten für die Verwendung in einer Gesundheitsberichterstattung entstünden.

Es zeigt sich, daß die bestehenden Datenquellen nur für den Themenbereich Sozialdemographie inhaltlich und methodisch ausreichend sind. Für die Mehrheit der vorhandenen Datenquellen gibt es erhebliche Zugangsschwierigkeiten. Die Nutzung im Rahmen einer Gesundheitsberichterstattung wird bei allen Berichtsthemen beträchtliche Zusatzkosten gegenüber der jetzigen Verwendung mit sich bringen, insbesondere bei Datenquellen zum Gesundheitszustand der Bevölkerung und zur Inanspruchnahme.

Datenquellen zur Soziodemographie

Die Datenquellen zur Soziodemographie stammen zum großen Teil aus der amtlichen Statistik. Sie sind für eine Gesundheitsberichterstattung von großer Bedeutung, da sie auch von nahezu allen anderen Themenbereichen als Nennerdaten benötigt werden. Die Daten liegen jedoch derzeit nicht so aufbereitet vor, daß sie für eine Basisberichterstattung einfach verfügbar wären. Vielmehr müßten für die meisten der etwa vom Sachverständigenrat für die Konzertierte Aktion im Gesundheitswesen genannten Teilthemen aus dem Gebiet der Soziodemographie gezielte Auswertungen durchgeführt werden.

Für folgende Teilbereiche liegen Datenquellen vor:

- kleinräumiger Bevölkerungsaufbau nach Alter, Geschlecht sowie Ausländer-/ Inländerstatus bzw. Familienstand und Anzahl von Haushaltsmitgliedern,
- Jugend-, Alten- und Gesamtlastquoten für In- und Ausländer,
- Geburtenrate nach Alter der Frauen im Alter zwischen 15 und 44 Jahren.

Soziodemographische Daten insbesondere auch über soziale Merkmale wie Versichertenstatus und Berufszugehörigkeit *liegen in hinreichender regionaler Differenzierung nicht vor.*

Datenquellen zum Gesundheitszustand der Bevölkerung

Zur Beschreibung des Gesundheitszustandes der Bevölkerung können in einer Gesundheitsberichterstattung folgende bestehende Datenquellen herangezogen werden, teilweise allerdings erst nach einer Verbesserung ihrer Aussagekraft:

- Todesursachenstatistik,
- Statistik der Schwangerschaftsabbrüche,
- Statistik der meldepflichtigen Krankheiten,
- Musterungsuntersuchungen,
- Krankheitsregister,
- Daten der Gesetzlichen und Privaten Krankenversicherung,
- Daten des vertrauensärztlichen Dienstes (VäD),
- Krankenhausstatistik,
- Statistik zur häuslichen Krankenpflege,
- Statistik der Rentenversicherung,
- Statistik der Arbeitslosenversicherung,
- Statistik der gesetzlichen Unfallversicherung,
- Diagnose und Therapieindex.

Die *Todesursachenstatistik* erfaßt für jeden Verstorbenen demographische Angaben und die nach der ICD verschlüsselte Todesursache. Die Validität der ärztlichen Angaben auf dem Leichenschauschein wird verschiedentlich in Zweifel gezogen. Die bisherige Auswertung der Todesursachenstatistik reicht für detaillierte Analysen nicht aus. Es fehlt vor allem an einer laufenden Darstellung nach regionalen Merkmalen und der Erfassung von sozioökonomischen Größen.

Mit dem 15. Strafrechtsänderungsgesetz von 1976 wurde eine *Bundesstatistik über Schwangerschaftsabbrüche* eingeführt bzw. neu geordnet. Erfaßt werden neben wenigen soziodemographischen Daten Angaben zu früheren Schwangerschaften und zum jetzigen Abbruch. Die Meldungen gelten als nicht annähernd vollständig. Ein Abgleich mit GKV-Abrechnungsdaten wird diskutiert.

Die *Statistik der meldepflichtigen Krankheiten* ist die einzige amtliche Morbiditätsstatistik in der Bundesrepublik. Seit 1969 besteht eine unveränderte Rechtsgrundlage für eine Bundesstatistik (Bundesseuchengesetz, Gesetz zur Bekämpfung der Geschlechtskrankheiten). Erhoben werden die Neuerkrankungen an ca. 40 infektiösen Erkrankungen. Eine Meldepflicht für AIDS besteht nicht. Es gibt Zweifel an der Notwendigkeit und der Vollständigkeit der Statistik.

Die *Musterungsuntersuchungen* eines jeweils nahezu geschlossenen Jahrgangs der jungen männlichen Bevölkerung stellen eine potentiell wertvolle Informationsquelle dar. Es wird eine umfangreiche Liste medizinischer Merkmale erhoben, diese werden jedoch nur für den administrativen Bedarf verschlüsselt und erfaßt. Für die Nutzung in einer Gesundheitsberichterstattung wären weitgehende Änderungen notwendig.

Bevölkerungsbezogene Krankheitsregister sind für wesentliche Fragen der gesundheitlichen Gefährdung und Versorgung der Bevölkerung entscheidende und durch Ad-hoc-Studien in der Regel nicht ersetzbare Hilfsmittel. Krebsregister sind in der Bundesrepublik Deutschland bis auf das saarländische Krebsregister und das kooperative Register für Malignome im Kindesalter in Mainz nicht voll funktionsfähig verwirklicht. Häufiger sind klinische Krebsregister als Dokumentationshilfsmittel klinischer Versorgungseinrichtungen vorhanden. Hier fehlt teilweise die notwendige personelle Infrastruktur für eine ausreichende wissenschaftliche Aufbereitung und Veröffentlichung. Befriedigend arbeitende, längerfristige Register im kardiovaskulären Bereich fehlen bzw. sind als befristete Register im Aufbau (Monica: Augsburg, Heidelberg, Bremen). Das *psychiatrische Fallregister in Mannheim* ist geschlossen. Für wesentliche Krankheitsgruppen fehlen Register.

Die Daten der *Gesetzlichen Krankenversicherung* (GKV) dokumentieren für mehr als 90 % der Bevölkerung der Bundesrepublik Deutschland versichertenbezogen und bezogen auf die jeweiligen Leistungserbringer die Anlässe der medizinischen Behandlung, in erheblichem Umfang auch deren Inhalte. Sie sind die einzige umfassende Datenquelle für den Gesundheitszustand der in Anspruch nehmenden Bevölkerung. Die Liste der erhobenen Merkmale ist umfangreich, aber nach Vollständigkeit, Qualität und Interpretierbarkeit im Sinne einer Gesundheitsberichterstattung sehr heterogen. Die bisherige Statistik ist fiskalisch, nicht epidemiologisch orientiert. Das Mitglied, nicht der Behandelte, ist die zentrale Bezugseinheit, der Beitragsaufkommen, Leistungsmengen und Ausgaben zugeordnet werden. Ansätze für Analysen unter sozialmedizinischen und gesundheitsökonomischen Fragestellungen aus dem gegenwärtigen Routinematerial heraus sind äußerst begrenzt. Mit geringfügigen Veränderungen der Bearbeitung wären die Daten für eine Gesundheitsberichterstattung erheblich nützlicher als heute.

Anders sind die *Sondererhebungen* aus den gleichen primären Datenquellen zu beurteilen, die im Rahmen von „Kassenmodellen" durchgeführt wurden, bisher jedoch zu kleinräumig, zu heterogen und unstetig für eine kontinuierliche Gesundheitsberichterstattung sind.

Die *privaten Krankenversicherer (PKV)* in der Bundesrepublik Deutschland erstellen über den Verband der privaten Krankenversicherung zur Abrechnungskontrolle und zur Kostendokumentation für ihre Vertragskrankenhäuser eine *Krankenhausdatei.* Sie ist nicht öffentlich verfügbar und unter Morbiditätsgesichtspunkten wenig ergiebig. Eine allgemeine diagnosebezogene Wagnisstatistik ist nicht zugänglich.

In der *Krankheitsartenstatistik (Wagnisstatistik)* der *privaten Krankenversicherer* werden die Leistungsausgaben für Krankenhauspflege nach 15 Diagnosegruppen gemäß ICD („Krankheitsarten") gegliedert. Die Daten sind über den Verband der privaten Krankenversicherung beschränkt verfügbar. Teilveröffentlichungen erfolgen unregelmäßig im Rechenschaftsbericht des PKV-Verbandes.

Mit der *neuen amtlichen Krankenhausstatistik* erfolgt ein Einstieg in eine bundeseinheitliche Morbiditätsstatistik für den stationären Versorgungssektor; zugleich entsteht eine der umfassendsten Datenquellen der amtlichen Statistik im Bereich des Gesundheitswesens. Neben den Grunddaten und Kosten werden Alter, Geschlecht, Hauptdiagnose und Wohnort der Patienten erhoben. Damit wird für Verwaltung und Wissenschaft ein Datenangebot geschaffen, das die Basis für weitreichende gesundheitspolitische Untersuchungen liefern kann. Die voraussichtliche Anwendung der 3stelligen Version der ICD zur Verschlüsselung der Diagnosen wird in bestimmten Fachgebieten jedoch zu einem begrenzten Informationsgehalt führen. Eine Sonderrolle spielt die *Krankenhausdiagnosestati-*

stik Schleswig-Holstein, die auf freiwilliger Basis (Erfassungsgrad knapp zwei Drittel der Krankenhäuser) im wesentlichen die Daten erhebt, die nach der Neuordnung der amtlichen Statistik bundesweit zu erwarten sind. Für aktuelle Morbiditätsschätzungen im Krankenhaussektor ist dies die derzeit am weitesten entwickelte öffentlich erstellte Datenquelle. Zu nennen ist ferner die *Dokumentation der Landeskrankenhäuser Schleswig-Holsteins*, die für die Beschreibung der psychiatrischen Morbidität im stationären Bereich von Bedeutung ist.

Der *Kosten- und Leistungsnachweis (KLN)* ist vorwiegend Informationsgrundlage für Pflegesatzverhandlungen. Seine Auswertung enthält nur wenige medizinisch verwertbare Angaben zur Patientenklientel.

Die bisherige Statistik des *vertrauensärztlichen Dienstes (VäD)* ist anonymisiert. Ihre hauptsächliche Funktion liegt in der Unterstützung interner administrativer Aufgaben. Für hochaggregierte Diagnosegruppen (ICD 3stellig) werden rudimentäre, aber nicht schlüssig zu interpretierende Auswertungen zu epidemiologischen sozialmedizinischen Fragestellungen veranlaßt.

Die bisherigen *Statistiken zur häuslichen Krankenpflege* weisen noch erhebliche Mängel auf. Dies betrifft sowohl den fehlenden Bezug auf Fälle und Personen als auch fehlende Angaben zur Diagnose, die den Grund der Pflegebedürftigkeit bildet.

Prozeßdaten der Rentenversicherung liegen nahezu vollständig in den Versicherungskonten der einzelnen Träger vor. Diese sind nach den Gesichtspunkten der Verwaltung und nicht nach denen wissenschaftlicher Untersuchungen aufgebaut. Die *Statistik* über abgeschlossene *Rehabilitationsmaßnahmen* berichtet über Reha-Behandlungsfälle und nicht über Reha-Gesamtverläufe. Die Versicherten, die eine Reha-Maßnahme in Anspruch nehmen, stellen wegen des Antragsprinzips eine Selektion dar, deren Mechanismus bis heute nur wenig erforscht ist. Analysen zur Beurteilung des Reha-Erfolgs sind nur eingeschränkt möglich. Die *Rentenzugangsstatistik* beschreibt Zugänge zur Frühberentung, sobald Rentenzahlungen einsetzen. Der Datensatz enthält sozioökonomische Angaben (einschließlich Einkommen und Berufsgruppe) sowie morbiditätsbezogene Angaben. Die Qualität der diagnostischen Angaben gilt wegen des ausführlichen Begutachtungsprozesses als valide, bei interregionalen Vergleichen können verfahrensabhängige Unterschiede bestehen. Die *Reha-Verlaufsstatistik* versucht, über die reine Ereignis-Querschnittsstatistik hinaus Verläufe darzustellen. Unter versorgungsepidemiologischen Gesichtspunkten sind zum Abschluß noch laufender Entwicklungsarbeiten Verbesserungen des bislang nicht befriedigenden Auswertungsverfahrens der RV-Prozeßdaten zu erwarten.

Die *Statistik der Arbeitsverwaltung* liefert als Sekundärstatistik Strukturinformationen über den Beschäftigungsstand in der Bevölkerung. Die Daten sind nach Wirtschaftszweigen, Berufsgruppen, Stellung im Beruf und sonstigen Personenmerkmalen aggregiert. Bei Lösung datenschutzrechtlicher Probleme liefern sie aktuelle Nennerinformationen zur Ermittlung berufsbezogener Risiken in der Bevölkerung in geeigneter Verknüpfung mit entsprechenden Zählerdaten. Gesundheitsbezogene Aussagen anhand der Routinestatistik sind begrenzt möglich, nicht jedoch für Arbeitslose.

Die gesundheitsbezogenen Aussagen der *Gesetzlichen Unfallversicherung* sind prima facie zuverlässig. Deskriptive epidemiologische Untersuchungen sind be-

Tabelle 1. Bestehende Datenquellen zu den Ressourcen des Gesundheitswesens nach Funktionsbereichen (Auswahl)

Funktionelle Gliederung des Gesundheitswesens	Personal	Einrichtungen	Verfahren	Intermediäre Güter
Prävention, Vorsorge, Gesundheitszustand	Statistik der Gesundheitsämter	Statistik der Gesundheitsämter		
Ambulante Versorgung	Statistik der Berufe des Gesundheitswesens, Arbeitsstättenzählung, Apothekenbestandsstatistik, EVaS-Studie, Arzt-/Zahnarztregister	Arbeitsstättenzählung, Kostenstrukturstatistik, Apothekenbestandsstatistik, EVaS-Studie, Kammerstatistiken	Patentanmeldungen, BGA, Statistik BPI, EVaS-Studie	Einzelhandels- und Großhandelsstatistiken, Produktionsstatistik
Stationäre Versorgung	Krankenhaus-, Hochschulstatistik	Krankenhausstatistik, PKV-Krankenhausdatei, Apothekenbestandsstatistik	Operationsstatistik	Kosten- und Leistungsnachweis
Pflege und Betreuung	Jugendhilfestatistik, Arbeitsstättenzählung	Jugendhilfestatistik, Arbeitsstättenzählung		
Rettungswesen	DRK-Statistiken, Unfallverhütungsbericht Straßenverkehr	Statistik der Gesundheitsämter	Dokumentarische Studien, Rettungsdienst und Krankentransport	
Rehabilitation	Krankenhausstatistik, Reha-Statistik	Krankenhausstatistik, Reha-Statistik	Reha-Statistik	Kosten- und Leistungnachweis, Reha-Statistik
Berufliche Ausbildung	Hochschulstatistik, Statistik der beruflichen Schulen	Hochschulstatistik, Statistik der beruflichen Schulen		
Forschung	Hochschulstatistik, Statistik des BPI	Hochschulstatistik, Statistik des BPI		
Verwaltung	Statistik der Sozialversicherungsträger	Statistik der Sozialversicherungsträger		

grenzt möglich. Die publizierten Statistiken wenden sich überwiegend an interne Nutzer. Einer intensiven externen Nutzung aus wissenschaftlicher Sicht stehen z. T. datenschutzrechtliche Probleme entgegen. Die *Berufskrankheitendokumentation* erlaubt die Beschreibung bereits erkannter Ursachen. Eine Ursachenforschung ist damit jedoch nicht möglich. In begrenztem Rahmen lassen sich Schwerpunkte arbeitsmedizinischer Gefährdung aufzeigen. Die *Daten der arbeitsmedizinischen Vorsorgeuntersuchungen* nach den berufsgenossenschaftlichen Grundsätzen stellen eine potentiell wertvolle, noch nicht genügend genützte Datenquelle dar. Die *Rehabilitationsstatistik der Unfallversicherungsträger* gibt einen Überblick über die medizinischen und beruflichen Merkmale der einzelnen Verläufe. Die Verknüpfung von Qualität und Erfolg einer Maßnahme ist noch nicht befriedigend gelöst.

Der *Diagnose- und Therapieindex (DTI)* von Infratest stellt seit ca. 10 Jahren fallbezogene Personen-, Diagnose-, Leistungs- und Strukturdaten der Akutkrankenhäuser zusammen. Die Morbiditätsangaben lassen sich mit den Leistungsvariablen verknüpfen. Die Erhebungsqualität, insbesondere die Gültigkeit der Diagnosen, ist schwer einschätzbar. Trotz der langfristigen Erhebung gibt es keine regelmäßigen Veröffentlichungen der Morbiditätstrends.

Datenquellen zu Ressourcen des Gesundheitswesens

Die amtliche Statistik verfügt hinsichtlich der Ressourcen „Personal", „Gesundheitseinrichtungen" und „Intermediäre Güter" bisher über kein geschlossenes Berichtssystem. Eine Fülle von Indikatoren läßt sich dennoch aus zahlreichen Einzelstatistiken entnehmen, die zusammen ein grobes Bild über die Ressourcen des Gesundheitswesens zeichnen. Umfang und Aussagefähigkeit der vorhandenen Daten in den einzelnen Aufgabenbereichen des Gesundheitswesens ist allerdings sehr unterschiedlich. Einen Überblick über verfügbare Datenquellen nach Funktionsbereichen gibt Tabelle 1.

Datenquellen zur Inanspruchnahme von Leistungen des Gesundheitswesens

Tabelle 2 zeigt verfügbare Datenquellen in der Bundesrepublik Deutschland zu einzelnen Themen der Inanspruchnahme von Leistungen des Gesundheitswesens.

Datenquellen zur Finanzierung und zu Kosten des Gesundheitswesens

Die Daten der *Gesetzlichen Krankenversicherung* sind unter versicherungsökonomischen Gesichtspunkten zwar konsistent, es fehlt jedoch die Möglichkeit, finanzielle Größen auf Behandlungen oder relevante Teilbevölkerungen zu beziehen. Analysen der Wirtschaftlichkeit und der Bedarfsgerechtheit sind somit nicht möglich.

Tabelle 2. Datenquellen zur Inanspruchnahme von Leistungen des Gesundheitswesens (+: Der so bezeichnete Datenkörper enthält relevante Daten)

Leistungs-bereiche	Datenquellen							
	GKV, PKV	Renten-versi-cherung	Unfall-versi-cherung	Krankenhausstatistik		Bevolke-rungser-hebungen	Spezielle Studien	Sonstige amtliche Statistik
				Statistische Ämter	Diagnose-statistik			
Ambulante Versorgung	+		+			+	+	
Stationäre Versorgung	+		+	+	+		+	
Versorgung mit Heil- und Hilfs-mitteln	+		+			+	+	
Kuren	+					+		
Fruh-erkennung	+				+			
Vorsorge	+						+	
Rehabilita-tionsmaß-nahmen	+	+	+					
Schwanger-schafts-abbruche								+
Laien- und Selbsthilfe							+	

Die Finanzierungsströme im Gesundheitswesen werden in der Statistik über *Ausgaben für Gesundheit nach Leistungsarten und Ausgabenträger* des Statistischen Bundesamtes dargestellt. Sie ist jedoch zu gering gegliedert, einige Merkmalsausprägungen fehlen. Die Ausgaben der privaten Haushalte für Gesundheitsgüter können nur mit Hilfe der Einkommens- und Verbrauchsstichprobe geschätzt werden. Auch für die Ausgaben der Arbeitgeber liegen keine exakt nachgewiesenen Zahlen vor. Die Verknüpfbarkeit der Statistik mit anderen Themenbereichen einer Gesundheitsberichterstattung ist gering.

Eine der Aufgaben in einer Gesundheitsberichterstattung wird darin gesehen, die Datenlage für die *Erstellung von Krankheitskostenstudien* zu verbessern. Hierzu sind in erster Linie die Ausgabendaten der gesetzlichen und privaten Krankenversicherung nach Diagnose, Alter und Geschlecht zu spezifizieren.

Konzeptvorschlag für eine Basisberichterstattung

Die Basisberichterstattung bezieht sich auf Themen oder Zusammenhänge, die von allgemeinem Interesse und für mehrere Nutzergruppen relevant und zugleich für die Volksgesundheit oder die Volkswirtschaft so bedeutend sind, daß regelmäßig über sie berichtet werden sollte. Es handelt sich dabei in der Regel um eine Berichterstattung mit hohem Verdichtungsgrad.

Ein Basisbericht in traditioneller Form soll aus Tabellen, Graphiken und kommentierenden Texten bestehen und eine Standortbeschreibung zur gesundheitlichen Lage der Bevölkerung und zum Gesundheitssystem des Landes darstellen.

Ergänzend zu einer derartigen Ausgabe in Papierform und als technische Voraussetzung hierfür soll ein System der informationellen Infrastruktur geschaffen werden, das für einen kontinuierlich zu pflegenden Informationssatz den Rückgriff auf DV-gespeicherte Tabellen mit niedrigerem Aggregationsgrad ermöglicht.

Themenbereich Soziodemographie

Die Bereitstellung von Datenquellen aus dem Bereich der Soziodemographie hat wegen ihrer Verwendung als Bezugsgröße gegenüber anderen Themenbereichen der Gesundheitsberichterstattung vor allem Vorleistungscharakter. Insofern ist in diesem Bereich die Schaffung der oben geforderten Informationsstruktur vordringlich.

Da die Gliederungstiefe der soziodemographischen Daten die Grenze jeder weiteren bevölkerungsbezogenen Aussage darstellt, sollte sie möglichst weit gehen. Insbesondere ist die Verknüpfung von Daten der GKV mit soziodemographischen Daten auf kleinräumiger Ebene erforderlich. Hier zeigt sich ein wesentlicher Entwicklungsbedarf der amtlichen Statistik, die gegenwärtig solche Nennerdaten für Auswertungen von GKV-Daten nicht ausreichend zur Verfügung stellt oder von der GKV bezieht.

Themenbereich Gesundheitszustand der Bevölkerung

Das Konzept einer Basisberichterstattung sollte im Themenbereich Gesundheitszustand der Bevölkerung ein differenziertes Indikatorensystem zu Mortalität, Morbidität, Funktionseinschränkung, Befindlichkeit und Risiko verwenden.

Datenquelle für *Mortalitätsindikatoren* ist die amtliche Statistik, wobei sich für die Todesursachenstatistik die Notwendigkeit ergibt, die Validität zu verbessern oder zumindest durch „nachgehende Stichproben" Fehlerspannen abschätzbar zu machen.

Morbiditätsindikatoren können die tatsächliche Morbidität der Bevölkerung abbilden oder die Morbidität, die sich durch Nachfrage nach Gesundheitsleistungen manifestiert. Es ist zu prüfen, ob Surveys wie der nationale Gesundheitssurvey der Deutschen Herz-Kreislauf-Präventionsstudie (DHP) für eine Gesundheitsberichterstattung stärker eingesetzt werden sollten. Für die Erfassung der Morbidität im stationären Bereich sollten Krankenhausdiagnosestatistiken auf der Grundlage der Bundespflegesatzverordnung oder ein weiterentwickelter Diagnose-Therapie-Index verwendet werden. Für die Morbidität im abulanten Bereich nach Inanspruchnahmegrund bzw. Diagnose ist in der Bundesrepublik Deutschland bisher keine repräsentative Statistik vorhanden, die einen längsschnittlichen Vergleich ermöglicht. Ansatzpunkte für eine höhere Transparenz sind in der Erhebung zur Versorgung im ambulanten Sektor (EVaS-Studie) gegeben, die periodisch wiederholt werden sollte. Ebenso ist eine verbesserte Analyse von Prozeßdaten der GKV v. a. in ausgewählten Referenzkassen oder anhand von Stichproben denkbar. Morbitätsindikatoren sollten zusätzlich zu Diagnosedaten auch Angaben zum Schweregrad von Krankheiten und zu ihrem Verlauf aufweisen.

Indikatoren der *Funktionseinschränkung* sind mit der Statistik der Rentenversicherung, der Schwerbehindertenstatistik und der Arbeitsunfähigkeitsstatistik im Ansatz für Teilgesamtheiten gegeben. Hier müssen Maßnahmen für eine Validitätsverbesserung getroffen werden. Kenntnisse über Funktionseinschränkungen bei Aktivitäten des täglichen Lebens (ADL-Skalen) fehlen in der Bundesrepublik Deutschland weitgehend. Entsprechende Erhebungen im Mikrozensus oder in Surveys sind beim Aufbau einer Gesundheitsberichterstattung unverzichtbar.

Indikatoren des *subjektiven Gesundheitszustands* und des *Gesundheitsverhaltens* können in Mikrozensusform oder in Surveys erhoben werden und sollten Bestandteil einer regelmäßigen Gesundheitsberichterstattung sein.

Themenbereich Ressourcen des Gesundheitswesens

Zu unterscheiden sind
- Personal des Gesundheitswesens,
- Einrichtungen des Gesundheitswesens,
- diagnostische und therapeutische Verfahren,
- intermediäre Güter (Arzneimittel, Heil- und Hilfsmittel).

Bisher gibt es für die Ressourcen kein geschlossenes Berichtssystem, jedoch läßt sich aus zahlreichen Einzelstatistiken eine Fülle von Indikatoren entnehmen.

Eingang in eine Gesundheitsberichterstattung sollten Daten aus den Registern der Kassenärztlichen und Kassenzahnärztlichen Vereinigungen und den Ärzte- und Zahnärztekammern finden, ebenso Daten aus der derzeit überarbeiteten Krankenhausstatistik des Bundes.

Wenig bekannt ist über Kapazitäten von stationären und ambulanten Einrichtungen zur Pflege von Behinderten und Alten. Wegen der zunehmenden Wichtigkeit dieses Versorgungsangebots sollte in der Aufbauphase der Gesundheitsberichterstattung eine detailliertere Erhebung erreicht werden.

Themenbereich Inanspruchnahme von Leistungen des Gesundheitswesens

Für eine Gesundheitsberichterstattung werden folgende Arbeitsschritte für erforderlich gehalten:

- Darstellung des Umfangs der Inanspruchnahme nach Leistungsarten. Bei regelmäßiger Berichterstattung läßt sich so die Entwicklung des Ausmaßes der Inanspruchnahme und der Wandel in der Inanspruchnahmestruktur nach Leistungsarten ablesen.

- Durch eine Gegenüberstellung der in Anspruch genommenen Leistungsarten mit der Entwicklung des Angebots von Gesundheitseinrichtungen und -leistungen läßt sich das Verhältnis zwischen Angebot und Inanspruchnahme aufzeigen.
- Von besonderem Interesse ist die Frage, wie sich die Inanspruchnahme innerhalb der Bevölkerung verteilt und inwieweit sich diese Verteilung mit dem Gesundheitszustand verschiedener Bevölkerungsgruppen deckt. Die Beantwortung dieser auch mit dem Begriff der Bedarfsgerechtigkeit der Gesundheitsversorgung zu umschreibenden Frage erfordert eine Darstellung des Umfangs der Inanspruchnahme, bei der nach sozialen Gruppen differenziert wird.
- Ebenfalls im Zusammenhang mit der Bedarfsgerechtigkeit kann die Inanspruchnahme nach Krankheitsgruppen(arten) untersucht und dem Morbiditätsspektrum gegenübergestellt werden. Ebenso abzugleichen ist der Bedarf an präventiven Leistungen und Betreuungsleistungen.
- Im Rahmen des Ziels der Schaffung und Erhaltung vergleichbarer Lebensverhältnisse in der gesamten Bundesrepublik kann die regionale Verteilung der Inanspruchnahme dargestellt werden.
- Durch Vergleiche der Inanspruchnahmemuster der Bundesrepublik Deutschland mit denen des Auslandes können Hinweise auf Einflüsse gesundheitssystembedingter Unterschiede auf die Inanspruchnahme gewonnen werden.

Die erforderlichen Daten können im Rahmen der Aufbauphase einer Gesundheitsberichterstattung schrittweise aus einer Vielzahl von Quellen ermittelt werden. Hierbei spielen besonders die Daten der Kranken- und Sozialversicherung eine große Rolle, die jedoch für eine Gesundheitsberichterstattung sowohl eines gezielten Zuschnitts (kassenübergreifende Stichprobe) als auch gezielter Auswertungen (Versichertenbezug) bedürfen.

Themenbereich Kosten und Finanzierung des Gesundheitswesens

Die Kenntnis der finanziellen Situation im Gesundheitswesen und der Bestimmungsfaktoren von Einnahmen und Ausgaben insbesondere der GKV ist sowohl für die Beurteilung der gesundheitlichen Versorgung der Bevölkerung als auch für den Aufbau einer Basisberichterstattung erforderlich.

Im Kontext der Weiterentwicklung des Gesundheitswesens und der dabei auftretenden Probleme sind nicht nur GKV-spezifische Informationen, sondern auch übergreifende Angaben erforderlich, um die Interdependenzen struktureller Anpassungsprozesse in der Gesundheitsversorgung aufzuzeigen. Zu den Grunddaten, die bereits vorhanden sind, zählen:

- Gesundheitsausgaben nach Ausgabenträgern, Ausgabearten und Leistungsarten,
- Angaben zur Finanzierungsverflechtung,
- Gesundheitsquoten (Anteil der Gesundheitsausgaben am Sozialprodukt) auf der Grundlage unterschiedlich abgegrenzter Gesundheitsausgaben (Statistisches Bundesamt, Sozialbudget, GKV-Statistik),
- Einnahmen und Ausgaben der GKV.

Innerhalb dieser Bereiche können jeweils einige Basisstatistiken in den Vordergrund gestellt und zur ersten Beurteilung der finanziellen Situation im Gesundheitswesen herangezogen werden.

Folgende zusätzliche Angaben und veränderte Schwerpunkte in der statistischen Analyse wären wünschenswert und teilweise in Spezialberichten abzuhandeln:

- Angaben zu finanziellen Beziehungen der GKV mit den anderen Zweigen der Sozialversicherung (GRV, GUV, ALV) und dem Bundeshaushalt;
- Angaben zu direkten und indirekten Kosten von Krankheiten nach ausgewählten ICD- und Ursachengruppen;
- Behandlungskosten pro Fall für ausgewählte Behandlungsverläufe (z. B. bei AIDS, Dialysebehandlung etc.);
- Strengere funktionale Erfassung der Gesundheitsausgaben innerhalb und zwischen den Sektoren (z. B. Zuordnung der Arzneimittelausgaben der Krankenhausapotheken);
- Stärkere gruppen- und damit risikoorientierte, insbesondere alters- und regionsbezogene Erfassung von Leistungen und Kosten in der GKV und im Gesundheitswesen insgesamt;
- Differenziertere Erfassung der finanziellen Situation unter Einbeziehung von Steuervergünstigungen im Gesundheitswesen;
- Bessere Erfassung der Selbstbeteiligung in der GKV (nach Höhe und sozioökonomischen Gruppen) und in Form direkter Konsumausgaben für Gesundheitsleistungen;
- Bestandsaufnahme zur Finanzlage von öffentlichen und privaten Pflegeeinrichtungen und Pflegeleistungen;
- Berücksichtigung weiterer Ausgabenträger: private Krankenversicherung, karitative Organisationen, betriebsärztliche Versorgung, öffentlicher Gesundheitsdienst, Heilpraktiker und andere nichtmedizinische Leistungserbringer, laienmedizinische Einrichtungen etc.;
- Einkommen im Gesundheitswesen beschäftigter Personengruppen;
- Erfassung von Arbeitszeiten der Beschäftigten im Gesundheitswesen als auch der jeweiligen Arbeitslosenzahlen, um die Einkommen auf Arbeitszeiten und Beschäftigungsrisiken beziehen zu können.

Auch für diese Bereiche wäre es wünschenswert, Basisstatistiken zu entwickeln, die der Beurteilung der unterschiedlichen finanziellen Entwicklung in der Gesundheitsversorgung dienen können.

Vorschlag für die Organisation einer Gesundheitsberichterstattung

Den Organisationsvorschlägen für die Aufbau- und Arbeitsphase einer Gesundheitsberichterstattung liegen folgende Randbedingungen zugrunde:

Randbedingung 1:

Es sollte eine möglichst weitgehende Trennung folgender Funktionen angestrebt werden:

- Datenerheber, -hersteller, -sammler und -verarbeiter auf der Ebene primärer Daten,
- Datensammler und -aufbereiter auf der Ebene aggregierter Daten im Format der Gesundheitsberichterstattung,
- anregende oder beauftragende Stellen für Berichtsthemen der Gesundheitsberichterstattung,
- themenbezogene Analyse und Interpretation, Ausarbeitung von Berichten der Gesundheitsberichterstattung,
- Nutzer der Gesundheitsberichterstattung, berichtsempfangende Stellen, Stellen der politischen praktischen Umsetzung.

Randbedingung 2:

Die Organisationsform einer Gesundheitsberichterstattung sollte auf Dauer angelegt sein und auf einem Grundkonsens der Beteiligten beruhen.

Für die Organisation einer Gesundheitsberichterstattung wurden 8 Optionen auf ihre Praktikabilität und die Verträglichkeit mit diesen Randbedingungen überprüft. Darunter waren folgende Optionen mit *zentraler* Organisationsstruktur, die z. T. Änderungen des geltenden Rechts verlangen:

- interministerielle Arbeitsgruppe als Leit- oder Entscheidungsgremium,
- Zuweisung der Gesundheitsberichterstattung an das Bundesgesundheitsamt als Dienstaufgabe,
- Zuweisung der Gesundheitsberichterstattung an das Statistische Bundesamt als Dienstaufgabe,
- Übertragung der Gesundheitsberichterstattung als Stiftungsaufgabe,
- Zuordnung der Gesundheitsberichterstattung zu einem gesetzlich verankerten Rat oder Beauftragten mit Berichtsvorlage an den Bundestag.

Als Optionen einer dezentralen Organisation wurden diskutiert:

- Fortführung des jetzigen Zustandes,
- Ringstruktur: Zuständigkeitsvieleck mit gemeinsamem wissenschaftlichem Sekretariat,
- reduzierte Ringstruktur mit zentralem Sekretariat mit wissenschaftlicher Dienstleistungsfunktion, Beraterkreisen und Konsultationsdiensten durch vertraglich eingebundene wissenschaftliche Institute.

Die Erfahrungen der Konzeptphase zeigen, daß es in der Bundesrepublik Deutschland kein Institut gibt, in dem das für die Einschätzung aller einzelnen Datenquellen erforderliche spezialisierte Erfahrungswissen an einem Platz vorhanden ist. Dies gilt erst recht für die Aufbauphase einer Gesundheitsberichterstattung. Diese Aufbauphase wird daher notwendigerweise wie die Konzeptphase arbeitsteilig geleistet werden müssen, so daß sie aus einer koordinierten Durchführung einzelner Forschungsvorhaben mit dem Ziel der Verbesserung bestehender und der Schaffung neuer Datenquellen bestehen wird.

Wenn derartige Forschungsvorhaben Pilotfunktion für eine Gesundheitsberichterstattung haben oder im Hinblick auf die politische Entscheidung für eine bestimmte Organisationsform neutral sind, könnten sie unabhängig von der Wahl bestimmter Organisationsoptionen bereits vorher mit den derzeit bestehenden Forschungsstrukturen eingeleitet werden. Dies würde einen organischen Übergang von Konzeptphase zur Aufbauphase und danach zur endgültigen Routinephase erlauben. Eine Aufstellung von geeigneten Forschungsvorhaben ist Bestandteil dieses Berichts. Besonders berücksichtigt wurden Vorhaben zur ambulanten ärztlichen und zahnärztlichen Versorgung, die unter methodischen Gesichtspunkten eine Brücke zwischen Analysen der bereits bestehenden Prozeßdaten und von Erhebungen bilden.

Wenn jedoch bereits für die Aufbauphase der Gesundheitsberichterstattung eine Option mit zentraler Organisationsstruktur gewählt werden sollte, müssen schon nach Abschluß der gegenwärtigen Konzeptphase an einer Stelle Personal und Sachmittelstrukturen geschaffen werden, die es erlauben, die zur Datenverbesserung erforderlichen Forschungsvorhaben durchzuführen. Das gleiche gilt dann, wenn eine zentrale Organisationsstruktur erst nach Abschluß der Aufbauphase etabliert werden soll, jedoch bereits während der Aufbauphase solche Forschungsvorhaben begonnen werden sollen, deren Umstellung von einer dezentralen auf eine zentrale Organisation nur schwer möglich wäre.

Der Aufbau einer zentralen Organisationsstruktur wird unter den gegebenen Verhältnissen vermutlich bei der Beschaffung der erforderlichen personellen Ressourcen scheitern. Die Forschungsgruppe ist weiterhin der Ansicht, daß sowohl unter sachlichen (Randbedingung 1) als auch politischen Gesichtspunkten (Randbedingung 2) eine zentrale Organisation der Gesundheitsberichterstattung zumindest für die Aufbauphase erhebliche Hindernisse mit sich bringen würde.

Die Forschungsgruppe gibt daher der dezentralen Organisation einer Gesundheitsberichterstattung den Vorzug. Die effektivste dieser Organisationsformen dürfte die reduzierte Ringstruktur um ein Zentrales Sekretariat mit wissenschaftlicher Dienstleistungsfunktion, Beraterkreisen und Konsultationsdiensten durch vertraglich eingebundene wissenschaftliche Institute sein.

Entsprechend dem Ergebnis der Bestandsaufnahme werden Einzelvorhaben vorgeschlagen, die während der Aufbauphase einer Gesundheitsberichterstattung verfolgt werden sollten. Hohe Priorität haben dabei Vorhaben mit dem Ziel:

- verbesserte Zugänglichkeit von Ergebnissen der amtlichen Statistik,
- Erhebung zuverlässiger Morbiditätsstatistiken durch verbesserten Mikrozensus und Surveys,
- Aufbau einer repräsentativen Stichprobe von Daten der GKV,
- periodische Erhebungen bei niedergelassenen Ärzten und Zahnärzten zur diagnosebezogenen Erfassung von Inanspruchnahme und Ausgaben.

Die Federführung bei diesen Aufgaben soll für Vorhaben aus der amtlichen Statistik beim Statistischen Bundesamt liegen, für die GKV-Vorhaben bei den Instituten der Selbstverwaltung. Diese Einrichtungen sollen sich der Mitarbeit vertraglich eingebundener wissenschaftlicher Institute versichern. Die Ergebnisse der Einzelvorhaben sollen zu einem offiziellen Gesundheitsbericht integriert werden, dessen Federführung beim Bundesgesundheitsamt oder bei einer Großforschungseinrichtung liegen soll.

Weiterführende Literatur zum Thema „Gesundheitsberichterstattung"

Ausschuß Gesundheitsberichterstattung, Arbeitsgemeinschaft der leitenden Medizinalbeamten der Länder (AGLMB) (1989) Gesundheitsberichterstattung der Länder: Konzepte, Themen, Pilotbericht. Behörde für Arbeit, Gesundheit und Soziales der Freien und Hansestadt Hamburg, Hamburg
Forschungsgruppe Gesundheitsberichterstattung (1990) Aufbau einer Gesundheitsberichterstattung: Bestandsaufnahme und Konzeptvorschlag, Endbericht, 3 Bde. Asgard, St. Augustin
Schäfer T, Wachtel H-W (1989) Umweltbezogene Gesundheitsberichterstattung: eine Planungsstudie. Asgard, St. Augustin

6 Evaluationsforschung, Qualitätssicherung und Technologiebewertung

Qualitätssicherung in der Medizin:
Ziele und Forschungsbedarf*

H. K. Selbmann

Einleitung

Die Qualitätssicherung in der Medizin ist sicher kein eigenständiges, in sich abgeschlossenes Forschungsgebiet. Lediglich die Probleme und ihr gedanklicher Lösungsansatz lassen sie als Einheit erscheinen. Dieser aber ist fächerübergreifend und bedient sich u.a. der Methoden der Informationsverarbeitung, Biometrie, Epidemiologie und Gesundheitssystemforschung. Überall dort, wo sich das ärztliche Handeln auf gesichertes medizinisches Wissen stützen kann, läßt sich die Qualität beurteilen und können Maßnahmen zu ihrer Sicherung und – wenn notwendig – Verbesserungen entwickelt und in den ärztlichen Alltag eingeführt werden. Damit sind 2 der Hauptschwierigkeiten ärztlicher Qualitätssicherung aufgezählt: die Definition gesicherten Wissens – benötigt zur Auswahl der Anwendungsfelder und der Messung der Qualität – und die Kontrolle bzw. Intervention eines laufenden Prozesses. Insbesondere im zweiten Punkt unterscheidet sich die Qualitätssicherung von der medizinischen Forschung im üblichen Sinn.

Man wird im folgenden zwischen Qualitätssicherungsprogrammen und qualitätssichernden Maßnahmen zu unterscheiden haben. Qualitätssichernde Maßnahmen tragen nachweislich entweder – präventiv – zur Verhinderung medizinischer Qualitätsprobleme bei oder helfen – kurativ –, Qualitätsprobleme zu beseitigen. Die Qualitätsprobleme spiegeln dabei den Gesundheitszustand der medizinischen Versorgung wider. Qualitätssicherungsprogramme beinhalten i. allg. neben der möglichst zeitigen Erkennung von Qualitätsproblemen auch meist längerfristige Kontrollen der eingesetzten qualitätssichernden Maßnahmen. Die Einführung von Qualifikationsnachweisen oder erweiterten klinischen Dokumentationen ist erst dann eine qualitätssichernde Maßnahme, wenn ihre Wirkung auf die Qualität der medizinischen Versorgung nachgewiesen wurde, für sich genommen aber noch kein Qualitätssicherungsprogramm.

Zur Strukturierung der folgenden Diskussion des Forschungsbedarfs im Bereich der Qualitätssicherung soll das aus 5 Schritten bestehende Paradigma eines Qualitätssicherungsprogramms herangezogen werden (Selbmann 1983):
1. Beobachtung der Qualität der medizinischen Versorgung,
2. Problemerkennung und Setzen von Prioritäten,
3. Analyse des ausgewählten Problems und Erarbeitung von Lösungsvorschlägen,

---

* Erstmals veröffentlicht in: Gross RWJ (Hrsg) (1986) Wege der Gesundheitsforschung. Springer, Berlin Heidelberg New York Tokyo, S. 251–259.

4. Auswahl des geeigneten Lösungsvorschlags und Umsetzung in die Praxis,
5. Kontrolle, ob durch die neuen Maßnahmen das Problem auch tatsächlich beseitigt wurde.

Beobachtungstechniken im Rahmen von Qualitätssicherungsprogrammen

Ausgangspunkt jedes Qualitätssicherungsprogramms ist die geeignete Beobachtung der medizinischen Versorgung. Diese Beobachtung sollte dort erfolgen, wo Qualitätsmängel häufig auftreten können bzw. wo sie schwerwiegende Folgen hinterlassen. Sowohl die Problemfelder als auch die Beobachtungsinstrumente variieren zwischen den medizinischen Fachgebieten und müssen daher für jedes Fachgebiet neu überprüft bzw. erarbeitet werden.

Es sind 3 Maßnahmen zur Erzielung geeigneter Beobachtungen für Qualitätssicherungsprogramme zu unterscheiden:

- die Standardisierung der routinemäßig anfallenden Beobachtungen,
- die Sammlung zerstreut anfallender Beobachtungen an geeigneter Stelle und
- die Erzeugung spezieller qualitätsrelevanter Informationen.

Standardisierung von Beobachtungen

Die Standardisierung der routinemäßig anfallenden Beobachtungen erfolgt mit dem Ziel, eine Vollständigkeit, Gültigkeit und Vergleichbarkeit der Beobachtungen im zeitlichen Verlauf und zwischen ähnlichen Versorgungseinrichtungen herzustellen. Hierzu gehören insbesondere die bewußte Beobachtung und Registrierung durchgeführter diagnostischer und therapeutischer Maßnahmen einschließlich ihrer Indikationen und Ergebnisse. Die Erhebungen in der Perinatologie, Gynäkologie und Chirurgie sind Beispiele dafür. Die Erarbeitung des Prototyps eines die Qualitätssicherung unterstützenden fachgebietsspezifischen Krankenblatts – evtl. mit Hilfestellung der EDV – ist eine besondere Herausforderung.

Sammlung von Beobachtungen an den qualitätssichernden Stellen

Viele Beobachtungen fallen derzeit routinemäßig an, ohne daß sie immer die sich um die Qualitätssicherung bemühenden Stellen – i. allg. die Leistungserbringer – erreichen. Es sei nur an die Sterblichkeit von Säuglingen oder die Spätergebnisse von Operationen erinnert. Zwei der Hauptgründe für die verwinkelten und unvollkommenen Kommunikationswege sind die Zweiteilung der Gesundheitsversorgung in einen ambulanten und einen stationären Teil und der Datenschutz. Wenn aber ein Operateur z. B. nicht erfährt, daß die von ihm operierten Leistenhernien häufig rezidivieren, schätzt er seine Qualität falsch ein. Die Suche nach gangbaren Kommunikationswegen muß ein Hauptanliegen zukünftiger Forschung im Bereich der Qualitätssicherung sein. Es erscheint dabei naheliegend, an den Patienten als Träger der meisten Informationen zu denken und ihn bei Rückmeldungen (z. B. Mutterpaß oder onkologischer Nachsorgepaß) einzuschalten.

Inwiefern die *Zufriedenheit der Patienten* bei der Messung der Qualität ärztlichen Handelns eine Rolle spielt, wird derzeit kontrovers diskutiert. Eine Übersicht über vorhandene Studien zur Zufriedenheit der Patienten ergab u. a., daß

1. die Zufriedenheit mehrere Dimensionen – zufrieden mit den „technischen Fähigkeiten des Arztes, dem Arzt-Patienten-Verhältnis und dem Zugang zur ärztlichen Versorgung – besitzt,
2. die Zufriedenheit mit dem rein ärztlichen Handeln i. allg. höher ist als mit dem Arzt-Patienten-Verhältnis oder dem Zugang,
3. die Erwartungshaltung eine große Rolle spielt, die ihrerseits etwa mit der Schulbildung der Patienten korreliert ist, und
4. die Zufriedenheit positiv, aber mit großer Streubreite mit anderen Qualitätsmaßen korreliert ist (Lebow 1982).

Da die Beurteilung der Qualität ärztlichen Handelns durch den Patienten immer mehr an Bedeutung gewinnt, sind methodisch gute Studien zur Zufriedenheit unbedingt notwendig. Wegen der zu erwartenden großen Probleme – unscharfe Antworten, veränderliches Antwortverhalten, ungeeignete Befragungszeitpunkte und -instrumente, mangelnde Fähigkeit der Patienten, das ärztliche Handeln beurteilen zu können usw. – dürfte die Zufriedenheit aber immer nur in Verbindung mit anderen Maßen der Qualität gesehen werden.

Gerade in der ambulanten Versorgung, wo die Patienten oft von sich aus die Behandlung abbrechen, ist das Verständnis des Patienten für die Qualitätssicherungsbemühungen des Arztes vonnöten. Mushlin u. Appel (1980) haben für Symptome akuter Erkrankungen einen *Problemstatusindex* entwickelt, der per Post nach Ablauf einer gewissen Zeit beim Patienten erhoben wird und Rückschlüsse auf die Qualität der ärztlichen Versorgung erlaubt. Auf diese Weise lassen sich Spätergebnisse – auch bezüglich der diagnostischen Qualität – ermitteln. Es erscheint lohnend, diesen Ansatz auf andere Krankheitsbilder zu übertragen und dem deutschen Gesundheitswesen anzupassen.

Die Qualität der *Versorgungsstruktur* (apparative und personelle Ausstattung, Zugang, Ausbildungsstand des Personals usw.) wird oft nicht bewußt wahrgenommen. Zu ihrer Messung eignen sich u. a. Checklisten und Visitationen, wie sie u. a. von der Joint Commission on Accreditation of Hospitals (Roberts et al. 1984), dem Concilium Chirurgicum in den Niederlanden (den Otter 1982) oder bei uns im Bereich des Verletzungsartenverfahrens vorgenommen werden. Auch hier ist eine Übertragung auf andere Fachgebiete (Zahnarztpraxis usw.) denkbar und erscheint erfolgversprechend.

Erzeugung spezieller qualitätsrelevanter Beobachtungen

Die Erzeugung spezieller den Zwecken der Qualitätssicherung dienenden Informationen hat – nicht zuletzt wegen der damit erzielten Erfolge – in der letzten Zeit an Bedeutung gewonnen. Es sei nur an die Ringversuche in der Laboratoriumsmedizin, den Einsatz von Testkörpern in der Röntgenologie oder das Einholen von Expertenwissen in der Pathologie (Referenzzentren) oder Chirurgie (Zweitbeurteilungsprogramme) erinnert.

Einer Systematik von Eißner u. Selbmann (1984) zufolge lassen sich diese speziell erzeugten Informationen wie folgt klassifizieren:

1) Synthetischer Ursprung des Untersuchungsgegenstandes (Präzisions- und Richtigkeitskontrollen im Labor, Testkörper in der Röntgenologie, Patientensimulationen auf dem Rechner, hypothetische Tracerfragebögen usw.
2) Natürlicher Ursprung des Untersuchungsgegenstandes
   a) patientenfern
   – Gewebeproben (Slideseminare, pathologische Referenzzentren usw.),
   – Körperflüssigkeiten (Ringversuche in der Laboratoriumsmedizin und Mikrobiologie usw.),
   – Biosignale (Bildqualität und Informationsgehalt von Mammographien und Röntgenaufnahmen, Kardiotokogramm [CTG], EEG, EKG usw.),
   – Daten (Fallbesprechungen anhand von Krankengeschichten, Gutachten usw.);
   b) patientennah
   – (Zweitbeurteilungen von Operationsindikationen usw.).

Die meisten dieser Informationen betreffen nur Detailbereiche ärztlichen Handelns und hier fast ausschließlich die Diagnostik. Dadurch ist man in der Lage, Zwischenschritte der medizinischen Versorgung in ihrer Qualität zu überprüfen. Wie innovativ und kreativ derzeit in diesem Bereich geforscht wird und werden kann, zeigt die jüngste Entwicklung eines Silikonmammaphantoms für die Krebsvorsorge (Fletcher et al. 1985).

Potentielle Problemfelder

Jeder Leistungserbringer sollte sich ständig seiner potentiellen Schwachstellen bewußt sein und sie besonders genau beobachten. Da ein Großteil dieser Vorsorgeprobleme in allen Kliniken und Praxen dieselben sein werden, wirkt eine extern zusammengestellte Liste von Problemen – zu den neben den medizinischen auch organisatorische (z. B. zu lange Wartezeiten) und finanzielle gehören können – für die einzelne Klinik oder Praxis stimulierend. Die Niederländische Organisation für Qualitätssicherung in Krankenhäusern (CBO) verfügt über eine Liste mit mehr als 250 Problemfeldern (Tabelle 1) aus allen Bereichen der stationären Versorgung, beginnend bei den ärztlichen Entscheidungen bis hin zu den Kommunikationsproblemen (Reerink 1984). Auch in der ambulanten Versorgung sind solche Listen denkbar, wenn man etwa das Handbuch Teaching in General Practice des Departments Community Health der Universität Nottingham betrachtet (Sheldon et al. 1981).

Die Suche nach potentiellen Schwachstellen ist ein sensibles Unterfangen und muß fächerspezifisch, neutral und unter Beteiligung der Ärzte durchgeführt werden. Aktivitäten zur Aufdeckung von Versorgungsproblemen sind allenfalls

Tabelle 1. Problemliste für Qualitätssicherungsprogramme in allgemeinen Krankenhäusern (Reerink 1984)

Ärztliche Entscheidungen	
Onkologie	Diagnostische Strategien in der urologischen Onkologie
Diagnostik	Angiographie beim Diabetes mellitus, Komplikationen nach zerebraler Arteriographie
Therapie	Vorübergehende ischämische Anfälle, Ergebnisse bei Totalendoprothesen
Vorbeugung	Wundliegen
Nachtkontrolle	Patienten mit Selbstmordabsichten
Allgemein	Sepsis, Anorexie
Ärztliche Maßnahmen	
Intravenös	Postoperative Therapien
Katheterisierung	Verhütung von Infektionen
Laboruntersuchungen	Notfalluntersuchung, zu viele Untersuchungen
Invasiv	Zu viele Verfahren bei Kindern
Wiederbelebung	Verbessern der Methoden
Präoperative Maßnahmen	Anzahl und Indikationen
Hygiene	Chirurgische Infektionen
Strahlenschutz	Verbessern des Schutzes
Autopsien	Erhöhung der Autopsiezahlen
Medikamente	
Antibiotika	Effektiverer Einsatz (Ampicillin, Aminoglykoside)
Antikoagulantien	Zunahme der prophylaktischen Gabe, Therapie durch Ärzte und Pflegepersonal
Blut	Einsatz von Blutderivaten, Indikationen
Organisation und Management der medizinischen Versorgung	
Abteilungen	Wartezeit der Patienten, Liegezeit, Aufnahmevoraussetzungen, einheitliche Pflege
Registrierung/Dokumentation und Informationsaustausch	
Krankengeschichten	Einsicht und Benutzung durch Ärzte
Kommunikation	
Zwischen Ärzten	Konsultationen
Zwischen Angehörigen verschiedener Berufsgruppen	Kontakte zwischen Ärzten und Pflegepersonal
Information/Aufklärung der Patienten	
Im Zusammenhang mit Operationen	Prä- und postoperative Aufklärung
Im Zusammenhang mit ärztlichen Verordnungen	Anweisung der Patienten

Qualitätssicherungsmaßnahmen, aber noch keine Qualitätssicherungsprogramme.

Methoden der Problemerkennung

Zur Erkennung von Qualitätsproblemen bedarf es nach der Beobachtung der Beurteilung der Qualität. Im allgemeinen versucht man, die erzielte Qualität mit den Ergebnissen anderer Leistungserbringer oder mit vorformulierten Erwartungen zu vergleichen. Vergleiche mit den Ergebnissen anderer Kliniken oder Praxen wurden in den vergangenen 10 Jahren bzw. werden derzeit u. a. in der Perinatologie, Neonatologie, Pädiatrie, Gynäkologie, Allgemein-, Gefäß-, Herz-, Neuro-, Kinder- und Unfallchirurgie, Urologie, Pathologie, Röntgenologie, Laboratoriumsdiagnostik, Mikrobiologie, Krankenhauspflege, Hypertonie und Diabetologie durchgeführt. Auffällig ist, daß in dieser Liste die nichtoperativen Fächer wenig vertreten sind. Hier scheint, wie auch in der Allgemein- und Zahnmedizin, noch Entwicklungs- und Forschungsbedarf zu bestehen.

Viele der oben aufgeführten Erhebungen bzw. Studien versuchen, über die interkollegialen Vergleichsmöglichkeiten hinaus den beteiligten Einrichtungen in Ansätzen auch Orientierungshilfen zur absoluten Beurteilung ihrer Prozeß- und Ergebnisqualität zu geben. Bei großen Abweichungen von diesen Orientierungshilfen oder Standards – in ihrer einfachsten Form z. B. zu hohe Komplikationsraten oder zu häufiger Einsatz einer bestimmten Operationstechnik – sollen sich die betroffenen Kliniken oder Praxen auf die Suche nach den Ursachen machen. Entscheidungsbäume, wie sie u. a. von Greenfield et al. (1975) für 50 internistische Krankheitsbilder oder Symptome erstellt wurden, sind sicher eine geeignete Form für komplexere Versorgungsstrategien. Oft fehlt jedoch die explizite und damit einem größeren Personenkreis vermittelbare Ausformulierung der Standards, obwohl mittlerweile neuere Lehrbücher in zunehmendem Maße solche Entscheidungsbäume enthalten.

Die Erarbeitung von Orientierungshilfen – bei speziell erzeugten Informationen allerdings oft von vornherein bekannt – ist eines der Hauptanliegen und wohl die größte Herausforderung der Qualitätssicherung (zur Systematik s. Selbmann 1984). Die Festlegung ihrer Indikationsstellung (was ist eine Standardsituation?) und ihre Konstruktion gehören mit zu den Aufgaben der medizinischen Fachgesellschaften und können mit Hilfe von Konsensusmeetings, Delphi-Methoden oder nominalen Gruppenprozessen erfolgen. Nicht vergessen sei die praktische Erprobung und die laufende Überwachung ihrer Gültigkeit.

Auch die Entwickler wissensbasierender Expertensysteme, die in Teilbereichen eine Algorithmisierung der Medizin versuchen, leisten ihren Beitrag zur Formulierung von Standards. Überhaupt sollte in Zukunft dem "knowledge engineering" vermehrt Bedeutung beigemessen werden. Es wird die Zeit kommen, wo größere Mengen medizinisches Wissen aus EDV-gestützten Wissensbanken abrufbar sein werden.

Problemanalyse, -lösung und Umsetzung

Dort, wo die Problemerkennung durch Vergleich mit einem Prozeßstandard (z. B. keine intraoperative Cholangiographien bei Gallenoperationen) erfolgte, liegt die Problemlösung oft sehr nahe. In den anderen Fällen, wie etwa den outcome-orientierten Ansätzen, wird man zunächst versuchen, durch *statistische Analysen* der vorhandenen Daten nach den Ursachen zu forschen. Diese Analysen sind allerdings oft von 2 Handicaps begleitet: Zum einen können sie nur statistische und keine kausalen Zusammenhänge aufzeigen, und zum anderen ist der Datenumfang meist beschränkt. Während das erste Handicap allen Beobachtungsstudien zu eigen ist, läßt sich das zweite meist durch eine gezielte prospektive Studie mit erweitertem Beobachtungsumfang in der Klinik oder Praxis beseitigen. Solche Intensivstudien – im englischen Sprachraum als "medical care evaluation studies" bezeichnet – besitzen methodische Gemeinsamkeiten, die in Manualen niedergelegt werden können. Bei kleinen Patientenzahlen oder offensichtlichen Grenzen der Datenanalyse sind *Einzelfallanalysen* in interdisziplinären Qualitätszirkeln oder -kommissionen ("peer review committees") angezeigt. Studien haben gezeigt, daß dieses Vorgehen durch die Gesamtbetrachtung der Patienten und ihrer medizinischen Versorgung eine höhere Sensitivität bei der Erkennung tatsächlicher Probleme und ihrer Lösungen besitzt als das explizite, statistische Vorgehen. Auch für die Planung und Durchführung solcher Einzelfallanalysen, die sich durch ihr retrospektives Vorgehen auf gute Dokumentationen stützen müssen, lassen sich Prozeduren entwickeln.

Die Auswahl der geeignetsten Problemlösung muß jede Klinik oder Praxis für sich selbst vornehmen, es sei denn, die Auswahl wird ihnen durch die Kostenträger, kassenärztlichen Vereinigungen, Fachgesellschaften oder Regierungen abgenommen. Hierbei spielen mit Sicherheit bekannte Ergebnisse klinischer Studien eine große Rolle (s. Victor 1986). Die Entwicklung einer am Bedarf des einzelnen orientierten *Fortbildung* unter Zuhilfenahme der neuesten Beobachtungs- und Kommunikationsmedien ist eine weitere Herausforderung an die Forschung im Bereich der Qualitätssicherung. Nicht nur aus juristischen Gründen sind Studien wünschenswert, die die Wege der Wissensverbreitung – vom Feststellen gesicherten Wissens bis zum routinemäßigen Einsatz – und die benötigte Zeit angeben können.

Viele Studien haben gezeigt, daß zwischen Wissen (d. h. Kenntnis der Orientierungshilfen) und Tun ein Unterschied besteht. Selbst die Ersteller der Orientierungshilfen halten sich nur zu 60–70 % daran (s. z. B. Hulka 1979). Daraus ist zunächst zu schließen, daß ein Qualitätssicherungsprogramm sich nicht nur auf die Überprüfung des Wissens verlassen darf, sondern die Beobachtung der Praxis miteinschließen muß. Die bei der Mehrzahl der Studien offengelassene Ursachenforschung für diese *Umsetzungslücken* ließe Erkenntnisse über die Gültigkeit der Orientierungshilfen, die Mängel der Fortbildung und die Motivierbarkeit der Ärzte erwarten.

Evaluationstechniken

Jede neue Richtlinie und jede neue diagnostische oder therapeutische Maßnahme sollte in der ersten Zeit nach ihrer Einführung einer genauen Beobachtung unterworfen werden, um ihre Effektivität unter Routinebedingungen beurteilen zu können. Dies gilt insbesondere für Arzneimittel in der Phase IV, aber auch für medizinische Großgeräte oder Operationstechniken. Das Fachgebiet der medizinischen Biometrie und Informationsverarbeitung bietet dafür eine Reihe von Methoden an, beginnend bei Registern, Interventionsstudien bis hin zu den kontrollierten klinischen Studien. Die besondere Problematik besteht bei diesen Evaluationsstudien z. T. darin, daß die Beobachtung den routinemäßigen Ablauf der medizinischen Versorgung nicht beeinflussen darf und man daher oft vorhandene

Datenquellen (Gutachterstellen, Arzneimittelkommissionen, KV-Daten usw.)
mit heranziehen muß. Die Erarbeitung von Evaluationstechniken und ihre Vermittlung ist ein lohnendes Ziel.

In einem Qualitätssicherungsprogramm stellt jede Änderung oder Einführung einer neuen Orientierungshilfe eine Intervention dar, die i. allg. in einem
Vorher-nachher-Vergleich zu evaluieren ist. Auch ein Qualitätssicherungsprogramm muß evaluiert werden, eine Forderung, die nur von wenigen Qualitätssicherungsprogrammen derzeit erfüllt wird.

Übergeordnete Aspekte

Der Weg von einer Idee für die Qualitätssicherung zu ihrem Routineeinsatz ist
weit, und nicht jede Idee wird ihr Ziel erreichen. Ähnlich wie ein Arzneimittel
durchläuft auch ein Qualitätssicherungsmodell mehrere Phasen (Selbmann
1981):

- Phase I: Wissenschaftliche Studie, bei der die Idee von motivierten Ärzten in
  ausgewählten Problemfeldern realisiert, operationalisiert und ihre Wirksamkeit beobachtet wird.
- Phase II: Breitenstudie mit multizentrischem Ansatz und reduzierter, auf das
  Machbare beschränkter Methodik und organisatorischen Vorbereitungen für
  Phase III.
- Phase III: Routineeinsatz, in dem u. a. die Fragen nach der Effektivität und
  der Motivierbarkeit der beteiligten Personen ständig neu zu beantworten
  sind.

Bei den Phasen I und II existiert jedoch in der Bundesrepublik Deutschland ein
Nachholbedarf, während allzuoft versucht wird, direkt in die Phase III zu sprin-
gen. Dies ist nur ein Symptom dafür, wie wenig das Gedankengut der Qualitätssicherung bei uns bekannt ist. Auch die Tatsache, daß bei der Diskussion der Mit-
telverteilung im Gesundheitswesen (z. B. Bundespflegesatzverordnung) die Qualität keine Rolle spielt, müßte zu denken geben. Das Verhältnis zwischen Qualität
und Kosten der medizinischen Versorgung wurde in den vorausgegangenen Abschnitten bewußt ausgeklammert, da erfahrungsgemäß Kostengesichtspunkte die
Entwicklung von Qualitätssicherungsprogrammen in den Phasen I und II behindern. Dieses Verhältnis jedoch in anderem Zusammenhang zu analysieren und zu
verbessern ist sicher eine wichtige zukünftige Aufgabe.

Eine Anregung der WHO (1985) aufnehmend, empfiehlt sich die Einrichtung
einer Zentralstelle für Qualitätssicherung, die u. a.

- die interessierten Forscher bzw. Forschergruppen bei der Planung, Finanzierung und Durchführung von Qualitätssicherungsprojekten aus neutraler
  Sicht berät,
- eigene Initiativen für Qualitätssicherungsmodelle entwickelt und ggf. mit medizinischen Partnern realisiert,
- als Auskunftsstelle über Programme, Methoden, Standards, Problemlisten
  usw. für alle medizinischen Disziplinen und Hilfsdisziplinen agiert,

– Weiter- und Fortbildungsprogramme für Ärzte und andere heilberuflich Tätige erstellt und einrichtet und
– die Qualitätssicherungsprogramme evaluiert.

Schlußbemerkungen

Die Frage nach dem Forschungsbedarf läßt ein Gebiet oft im falschen Licht erscheinen, weil die in der Vergangenheit erzielten Erfolge dabei oft unter den Scheffel gestellt werden. In der Tat hat sich in den vergangenen 20 Jahren in der Qualitätssicherung der medizinischen Versorgung einiges zum Guten verändert. Dies aufzulisten, war jedoch nicht die Aufgabe dieses Beitrags.

Das systematische Durchgehen der Stufen eines Qualitätssicherungsprogramms hat m. E. eine Reihe von Anregungen für Forschungsvorhaben zutage gebracht, die von den verschiedenen medizinischen Disziplinen in konkrete Forschungsprojekte umgesetzt werden könnten. Die Auflistung mußte allerdings unvollkommen bleiben, weil

1. der Autor die Qualitätssicherung sicher etwas durch die Brille seines Fachgebiets – der medizinischen Informationsverarbeitung – sieht und
2. der Bereich der Qualitätssicherung, deren Grundgedanken Reerink (1984) für eine Innovation hält, immer wieder für weitere Innovationen gut ist.

Literatur

Eißner HJ, Selbmann HK (1984) Zur Bedeutung externer Vergleiche in der Qualitätssicherung. In: Selbmann HK (Hrsg) Qualitätssicherung ärztlichen Handelns. Bleicher, Gerlingen, S 169–176
Fletcher SW et al. (1985) Physicians' ability to detect lumps in Silicone breast models. JAMA 15:2224–2228
Greenfield S et al. (1975) Peer review by criteria mapping: criteria for diabetes mellitus. Ann Intern Med 83:761–770
Hulka B (1979) Peer review in ambulatory care: use of explicit criteria and implicit judgements. Med Care [Suppl] 17:1–73
Lebow J (1982) Consumer satisfaction with medical care. Bleicher, Gerlingen, pp 153–164
Mushlin AI, Appel FA (1980) Testing an outcome-based quality assurance strategy in primary care. Med Care [Suppl] 18:1–100
Otter G den (1982) The Dutch Concilium Chirurgicum as an instrument of quality assessment in surgical training. In: Selbmann HK, Überla KK (eds) Quality assessment of medical care. Bleicher, Gerlingen, pp 41–47
Reerink E (1984) Qualitätssicherung in den Niederlanden – Erfahrungen mit der interkollegialen Qualitätssicherung im Krankenhaus. In: Selbmann HK (Hrsg) Qualitätssicherung ärztlichen Handels. Bleicher, Gerlingen
Roberts JS, Walczak R, Widmann DE (1984) Das Qualitätssicherungsprogramm der Gemeinsamen Kommission zur Akkreditierung von Krankenhäusern. In: Selbmann HK (Hrsg) Qualitätssicherung ärztlichen Handelns. Bleicher, Gerlingen
Selbmann HK (1981) Quo vadis, Qualitätssicherung? MMW 123:1099–1100
Selbmann HK (1983) Die Rolle der medizinischen Informationsverarbeitung in der Qualitätssicherung geburtshilflichen Handelns. Geburtsh Frauenheilkd [Sonderheft] 43:82–86

Selbmann HK (1984) Standards ärztlichen Handelns. In: Selbmann HK (Hrsg) Qualitätssiche-
rung ärztlichen Handelns. Bleicher, Gerlingen, S 161–168
Sheldon MG et al. (1981) Teaching in General Practice. Department of Community Health,
Nottingham University
Victor N (1986) Die Begleitung von Projekten der Therapieforschung durch die medizinische
Biometrie. In: Gross RWJ (Hrsg) Wege der Gesundheitsforschung. Springer, Berlin Heidel-
berg New York Tokyo, S 237–250
WHO (1985) The principles of quality assurance. Euro Reports and Studies 94. WHO, Copen-
hagen, pp 1–37

Überlegungen zu Diffusion und Kosten medizinischer Technik *

S. Kirchberger

Einleitung: Was heißt „Medizintechnik"?

Der Begriff „Medizintechnik" ist vieldeutig. Die in der internationalen Diskussion übliche Bezeichnung "health care technology" oder "medical technology" umfaßt alle Verfahren und Techniken der Versorgungspraxis wie auch deren Substrat: Organisationsstrukturen und Medikamente ebenso wie Instrumente und Apparate.[1] Nur von den letzteren soll hier die Rede sein. Was diese „Technik" bedeutet, interessiert nach überaus divergenten Gesichtspunkten. Der Patient kennt Röntgen-, EKG- und Ultraschallgerät, vielleicht auch Inhalationsapparat, Hörgerät oder Herzschrittmacher. Was ein Perimeter oder Spirograph ist, weiß er i. allg. nicht, obgleich Gesichtsfeldmessung und Atemvolumenbestimmung wichtige, durchaus gängige Untersuchungen sind. Der Patient fragt gewöhnlich nicht nach. Er bekommt ohnehin nur einen Teil der Geräte zu sehen, die sich in Klinik und Praxis versammeln. Die Analyse von Körperflüssigkeiten und Gewebeproben etwa findet ohne ihn statt. Daraus resultiert eine definitorisch nützliche Unterscheidung zwischen

- Geräten, Apparaturen, Instrumenten, mit denen der Patient unmittelbar in Berührung kommt, denen er zu diagnostischen oder therapeutischen Zwecken ausgesetzt wird, und
- solchen, mit denen Arzt oder MTA arbeiten, der Patient jedoch nicht konfrontiert ist.

Die Geräte, mit denen der Patient in Kontakt tritt, bezeichne ich als „Medizintechnik". Diejenigen, die gleichsam hinter den Kulissen und nur vom Arzt und dessen Mitarbeitern angewandt werden, bezeichne ich als „Technik in der Medizin".

Die Unterscheidung trägt der Tatsache Rechnung, daß im zweitgenannten Technikbereich die *Geräte* nicht medizinspezifisch sind, sie finden sich ebenso in anderen Praxisbereichen.[2] Elektronenmikroskop, Präzisionswaage, Elektropho-

---

* Erstmals veröffentlicht in: Gäfgen G, Oberender P (Hrsg) (1988) Technologischer Wandel.

[1] "The term 'medical technology' is a very general one which has many meanings depending on the user ... it can encompass anything from sterilized bandages to open-heart surgery". Vgl. Altman u. Blendon 1979, S. 3; Gordon u. Fisher 1975; McNeill u. Cravalcho 1982; Anderson u. Jay 1985, S. 49–64.

[2] Soweit es um Verfahren und nicht um Geräte geht, gilt dies auch für einen Teil der „Medizintechnik". Röntgen- und Ultraschallverfahren werden z. B. zur Materialprüfung angewandt, allerdings handelt es sich dabei um andere Geräte.

resegerät, Photometer und Filmentwickler sind so wenig spezifisch medizinische
Geräte wie die Hardware, die die Basis zur Verarbeitung organisatorischer oder
auch diagnostischer Probleme liefert. Zudem entspricht die Unterscheidung der
Industriestatistik, insofern diese keine Differenzierungen nach Käufergruppen
kennt.

Allerdings entspricht sie nicht der Kostendiskussion, jedenfalls insoweit, als
das diagnostische Labor – Paradefall einer „Technik in der Medizin" – immer
wieder als ein wesentlicher Kostenfaktor diskutiert wird. Die in diesem Zusammenhang erörterten Kostenprobleme betreffen jedoch in erster Linie Mengenef-
fekte, die durch Rationalisierungs- und Automatisierungstechniken induziert
sind.

Unbeschadet dieser Abgrenzung, bleibt das Feld der Medizintechnik höchst
heterogen, reicht vom Nierenlithotripter bis zum chirurgischen Besteck. Dennoch ist jede weitere Klassifikation unergiebig, insbesondere die zwischen diagnostischen und therapeutischen Geräten. Die Technik, mit der der Patient unmittelbar in Berührung kommt, kann der Diagnostik oder der Therapie, aber
auch beidem dienen.

Röntgenstrahlen dienen der Diagnostik wie der Behandlung Krebskranker.
Die Endoskopie hat die nichtinvasive Diagnostik von Körperinnenräumen beträchtlich erweitert – flexible Endoskope sind mit Biopsiekanälen ausgerüstet,
mit deren Hilfe ein Sekret abgesaugt oder mit einer kleinen Zange Gewebe zur hi-
stologischen Untersuchung entnommen werden kann. Zugleich können durch
den Kanal therapeutische Eingriffe vorgenommen werden, z. B. das Abtragen
von Polypen mittels einer Drahtschlinge oder die Zertrümmerung von Gallen-
steinen.

Die Grenzen zwischen diagnostischer und therapeutischer Technologie sind
also fließend. Von all dem abgesehen, würde eine systematische Trennung von
diagnostischer und therapeutischer Technik den medizinischen Handlungszu-
sammenhang zerreißen, der für eine Erörterung der Kosten, soll sie nicht unter
betriebswirtschaftlichen, sondern gesundheitsökonomischen Aspekten erfolgen,
konstitutiv ist.

Was kostet „Medizintechnik?"

Auf einem Symposium, organisiert durch das "Sun Valley Forum on National
Health" zum Thema: "Medical Technology the Culprit behind Health Care
Costs" rivalisierten zwei Thesen miteinander:

– Ein Teil der anwesenden Experten vertrat die Ansicht: "Adopting new health
  care technology is a major cause of the large yearly increases in national
  health expenditures."
– Die anderen meinten: "We find at least for the period 1930–1975 that biomedical research on balance reduces outlays rather than increases them."[3,4]

Die Kontrastierung zeigt, wie schwer die Bedeutung des technischen Fortschritts
für die Gesundheitskosten abzuschätzen ist. Über eine Korrelation von Kosten-

---

[3,4] Altman u. Wallack 1979, S. 24.

entwicklung und Verbreitung technischer Innovationen lassen sich Hypothesen aufstellen, die sich am Anstieg der Personal- und Kapitalkosten, der technischen Ausstattung in Klinik und Praxis, der Zahl der Arztbesuche, der erhobenen Laborparameter, sonstiger diagnostisch-technischer Maßnahmen usw. orientieren, die Auslastungsgesichtspunkte oder Ausweichstrategien in den Mittelpunkt rükken – aber, wie jede Fragestellung, so sind auch diese Hypothesen durch das jeweilige Erkenntnisinteresse organisiert. Die Kostendimensionen der Medizintechnik lassen sich mit den Begriffen

- Forschungs- und Entwicklungskosten,
- Investitionskosten,
- Betriebs- und Folgekosten,
- Sensitivitäts- und Spezifitätskosten

bezeichnen. Doch ihr quantitatives Ausmaß scheint kaum eruierbar, weil

- erstens Daten fehlen und
- zweitens vielfältige Interdependenzen Globaldaten als zu pauschal, spezifizierte Daten als zu selektiv erscheinen lassen.

Forschungs- und Entwicklungskosten

Wie alle angewandten Wissenschaften bezieht die Medizin ihre Technologie aus allen möglichen Lebensbereichen und modifiziert sie für ihre Zwecke. Wesentliche Fortschritte in der Endoskopie verdankt sie der HiFi-Technik, der berühmte Scribner-Shunt, der die Dauerdialyse terminal nierengeschädigter Personen ermöglichte, der Entwicklung des „Teflon" für Zwecke der Raumfahrt.[5] Die Abgrenzung von Forschungs- und Entwicklungskosten bliebe in jedem Falle willkürlich. Das EKG ist 100 Jahre alt,[6] das Endoskop – oder Kystoskop, wie es ursprünglich hieß – noch älter,[7] F + E-Kosten für so entscheidende Veränderungen wie die Koppelung des EKG mit Mikroprozessoren zur Kurvenauswertung oder den Übergang zum wesentlich leistungsfähigeren Glasfiberendoskop angeben zu wollen, ist aussichts- und sinnlos.

Investitionskosten

Ebenso fragwürdig sind alle Angaben über die Höhe der Investitionskosten. Die verfügbaren Daten sind völlig unzulänglich. Vielmehr kursieren einmal in die Welt gesetzte und repetierte Zahlen. 1980 führte die Diskussion über den Einsatz moderner Medizintechnik in der ärztlichen Standespresse – gleichsam als Beitrag zur Rechtfertigung der steigenden Gesundheitskosten – zu einigen – seitdem oft wiederholten – Angaben über den Umfang der medizintechnischen Investitionen der niedergelassenen Ärzte.

---

[5] Vgl. Rettig 1978, S. 156.
[6] Vgl. Burch u. Pasquale 1964.
[7] Vgl. Graf 1968, S. 50ff.; Lux u. Demling 1983, S. 107ff.

Nach „vorsichtigen" Schätzungen belaufe sich das gesamte Anlagevolumen medizintechnischer Geräte in der BRD auf 25 Mrd. DM, wovon 10 Mrd. DM auf ärztliche und zahnärztliche Praxen entfielen.[8] Eine etwas weniger „vorsichtige" Schätzung des gleichen Jahres (1980) spricht von 35 Mrd. DM, von denen 60%, also 21 Mrd. DM, dem ambulanten, die restlichen 40% dem stationären Sektor zuzurechnen seien.[9] Für medizinisch-technische Geräte wird in der Literatur üblicherweise eine durchschnittliche Nutzungsdauer von 10 Jahren angegeben. Demnach betrug, um den Stand der Technik zu erhalten, der Bedarf an Ersatzinvestitionen allein in der ambulanten Versorgung 1 bzw. 2 Mrd. DM jährlich. Dabei ist anzunehmen, daß der Umfang der jährlichen Investitionen in den vergangenen Jahren gestiegen ist.[10] (Sofern die genannten Zahlenangaben realistische Größen darstellen sollten, beruht die Divergenz der Schätzungen auf der Unzulänglichkeit der Kenntnisse sowie der Unklarheit, was mit dem Begriff „Medizintechnik" erfaßt werden soll.) Allerdings fragt sich, welche gesundheitsökonomische Relevanz solchen Zahlen beizumessen ist, solange eine Produktivitätsmessung nicht möglich scheint.

Betriebs- und Folgekosten

Was ist mit den „Betriebs- und Folgekosten" gemeint? Hierzu eine qualifizierende Überlegung.

In einem Referat „Gewinnt die Technik ein Übergewicht in der kurativen Medizin?" meint Günter Reiff, Abteilungsleiter beim Bundesverband der landwirtschaftlichen Krankenkassen, daß die Technik die kurative Medizin in der Bundesrepublik Deutschland weitgehend beherrsche.[11] Er fährt fort: „Damit soll die Technik ... soweit sie beispielsweise einer gezielten und genaueren Diagnosestellung dient, keineswegs abqualifiziert oder gar verteufelt werden. Aber nicht alles, was technisch machbar ist, muß sinnvoll und finanzierbar sein." Reiff spricht von einem Übergewicht der Technikanwendung im Verhältnis zur Anwendung anderer Mittel. Ich stelle umgekehrt die Frage: Was eigentlich ist nicht Technikanwendung in der medizinischen Versorgung?

Vor 2 Jahren hat Siegfried Häussler ein Buch mit dem Titel *Diagnose ohne technische Hilfsmittel* herausgegeben.[12] Ein spannendes Buch, weil es dem Nichtmediziner beeindruckend deutlich macht, was alles aufgrund der sozialen und persönlichen Biographie, der vom Kranken an sich selbst beobachteten Symptome, ihrer Heftigkeit und ihrem zeitlichen Verlauf, was durch den „klinischen Blick" des Arztes mit fünf geschulten Sinnen wahrgenommen werden kann – wie sich aus einer Fülle kleiner Beobachtungen und anamnestischer Bausteine, vom Körperbau, der Beschaffenheit und Farbe der Hautoberfläche, dem Rede- und

---

[8] Vgl. Clade 1980, S. 2264.
[9] Vgl. Hartung 1980, S. 2293.
[10] Durch eine wachsende Zahl an Praxisneugründungen, durch gestiegene Wiederbeschaffungspreise, durch weitere Verbreitung der sogenannten „Großgeräte", aber auch durch neue aufwendigere Gerätegenerationen dürfte der Kapitalstock nicht unerheblich gestiegen sein.
[11] Vgl. Reiff 1986.
[12] Vgl. Häussler 1985.

Bewegungsverhalten bis zu den mitgeteilten Symptomen langsam eine Diagnose aufbaut. „Diagnose ohne technische Hilfsmittel" ist ein Lehrbuch der Semiotik, der Zeichendeutung der älteren Medizin, die in ihrer Funktion der juristischen Topik gleichzusetzen ist.[13] Teilweise sind diese Informationen sehr exakt, in vielen Fällen ist eine über das unmittelbar Beobacht- und Erfahrbare hinausgehende Diagnostik unnötig – insbesondere dann, wenn die therapeutischen Konsequenzen kein Risiko für den Patienten darstellen.

„Nichttechnik" heißt also zunächst einmal, daß der Arzt seine 5 Sinne einsetzt, um eine Verdachtsdiagnose zu stellen. Jede Diagnose ist Verdacht, ist eine Vermutung. Sofern sie hinreichend begründet erscheint, um daraus therapeutische Konsequenzen zu ziehen, erfolgt wiederum eine nichttechnische Handlung, die „Verordnung". Auch sie kann einen nichttechnischen Inhalt haben, z. B. die Verschreibung eines Medikaments, eine Empfehlung zur Bettruhe, zu weiteren Gesprächen, etwa in Form einer Psychotherapie. Anamneseerhebung, körperliche Untersuchung und die Verordnung nichttechnischen Inhalts – das sind die Mittel, die der Arzt jenseits von „Medizintechnik" zur Verfügung hat. Im Krankenhaus kommt noch die Pflege hinzu. Die gesamte übrige Praxis ist Anwendung von Medizintechnik. Was heißt – so gesehen – „Übergewicht" an Technik? Ist sie der gesamte Rest, wird jede Diskussion über Betriebs- und Folgekosten medizintechnischer Geräte absurd. Die Gebührenordnung unterscheidet nicht zwischen den Kosten der Erstellung eines Röntgenbildes und denen seiner Interpretation. Die Kunstfertigkeit des Umgangs mit dem Gerät ist genauso wenig kalkulierbar wie die Probleme, die sich aus der Physis des Patienten (z. B. Fettleibigkeit) für die Technikanwendung ergeben. Darum gestattet beispielsweise die Ermittlung „der" Kosten der Sonographie keinerlei Aussagen, die die Qualität der Versorgung, d. h. den Nutzen der Anwendung der Untersuchungsmethode betreffen. Ebensowenig besagen sie über institutionelle und professionelle Konsequenzen, die sich kostenträchtig bemerkbar machen. Auf Medizintechnik bezogen stellen sich „Betriebs- und Folgekosten" als Problem erst in einem Gesamtzusammenhang, der sich über die einzelnen Krankheiten bzw. Krankheitsgruppen und die Infrastruktur, in der sie nach dem jeweils gegebenen Stand des Wissens verarbeitet werden, konstituiert.

Sensitivitäts- und Spezifitätskosten

Dieser Sachverhalt ist nicht unbekannt. Bezeichnenderweise wird er vorwiegend gesellschaftspolitisch-sozialphilosophisch diskutiert. So wird einer technisch möglichen, iterativen Diagnostik, wenn aus ihr nach dem Stand des Wissens keine therapeutischen Folgen resultieren können, das Recht des Patienten auf „Nicht-Wissen" entgegengesetzt.[14] Therapeutische Technik wiederum – die regelmäßig der Verbesserung der Lebensqualität oder der Lebensverlängerung zu dienen bestimmt ist – wird unter dem Gesichtspunkt überflüssigen Komforts oder mangelnder Humanität in Frage gestellt: überflüssigen Komforts in der Dis-

---

[13] Vgl. Kırchberger 1986a, S. 100.
[14] Vgl. Jonas 1984, S. 75ff.

kussion um eine stärkere Selbstbeteiligung bei den Heil- und Hilfsmitteln, mangelnder Humanität in der Diskussion um die Sterbehilfe. Nur repräsentiert all dies lediglich die Grenzfälle der Problematik, die Sensation. Unspektakulärer sind die gleichsinnig strukturierten Regelfälle, die sich im Bereich der Sensitivitäts- und Spezifitätskosten medizintechnischer Entwicklungen niederschlagen.

Die Leistungsfähigkeit moderner Medizintechnik wird vielfach in ihrer hohen Sensitivität, also darin gesehen, daß sie es beispielsweise gestattet, selbst kleinste morphologische Veränderungen zu registrieren. Deshalb wird auch der semiotisch orientierte Arzt von Fall zu Fall auf technische Diagnostikhilfen rekurrieren; je risikoreicher nämlich die therapeutischen Konsequenzen einer Diagnose sind, desto abgesicherter muß sie sein. Umgekehrt ergibt sich aus der hohen Sensitivität die Möglichkeit des diagnostischen Zugriffs, ehe sich die Krankheit überhaupt manifestiert, d. h. in Symptomen sichtbar, semiotisch deutbar wird. Auf dieses Faktum spekulieren alle Diagnosezentren mit ihrem Screeningangebot (s. Tabelle 1).

Ein solcher "Check-up" (der von einigen Firmen für Führungskräfte sogar zur Pflicht gemacht wird) ist nicht nur medizinisch sinnlos, sondern hat für die Krankenkassen nicht unerhebliche Kosten zur Folge.

- Der Test ist medizinisch sinnlos, weil er nur in seltenen Ausnahmefällen zur frühzeitigen Aufdeckung einer Krankheit und entsprechenden therapeutischen Maßnahmen führen kann, weshalb die Testkosten selbst von der GKV zu Recht nicht getragen werden.
- Er ist kostspielig, weil die Krankenkassen die Folgen, nämlich die Notwendigkeit der weiteren Abklärung positiver Befunde – und seien es nur Normabweichungen ohne Krankheitswert – zu finanzieren haben, vor allem: die Kosten einer durch ein derartiges, medizinisch irreales Sicherheitsdenken provozierten Hypochondrie.

Normabweichungen ohne Krankheitswert werden zu vermeintlichen Risiken, die Risikosuche selbst zur Gesundheitsbedrohung. Ein gesunder Mensch ist, wie der englische Arzt E. A. Murphy zynisch bemerkt, ein jemand, der nicht hinreichend untersucht wurde.

Mit einem vergleichbaren, wenn auch anders gelagerten Problem – in Form des sog. Zufallsbefundes – haben alle Kliniker zu rechnen: er wird „bei Gelegenheit" entdeckt, nämlich im Zusammenhang mit einer auf Anderes zielenden Fragestellung, ohne daß ein Symptom auf ihn hingewiesen hätte. Die „Risikofaktorenmedizin"[15] schließlich vernachlässigt bewußt das Symptomkonzept. Sie ersetzt es durch das Risikokonzept: Anlaß für eine Untersuchung ist die Zugehörigkeit zu einer Risikogruppe.

In allen genannten Fällen tritt folgende Situation auf: Technische Diagnostik bedarf der interpretativen Absicherung auf dem Hintergrund von Anamnese und klinischem Bild; fehlen diese Informationen, weil keine Symptome vorliegen, die eine Interpretation gestatten, stellt sich die Frage, wie mit den Befunden zu verfahren ist. Verweisen sie doch lediglich auf das mögliche (!) Vorliegen einer

---

[15] Abholz et al. 1982.

Tabelle 1. Diese Institutionen testen Ihre Gesundheit (Aus: *Capital* 3/1987, S. 240)

Einrichtung	Zeitaufwand	Kosten	Vorteile	Nachteile
Hausarzt, falls er über ein Labor und die nötigen medizinischen Geräte verfügt	Einige Stunden	300–1100 DM	Billig und schnell, Reisen unnötig	Effizienz hängt von der Diagnostik-Erfahrung des Arztes und seiner apparativen Ausstattung ab
Facharzt für innere Medizin, Praxis oder Klinik	Einige Stunden	300–1100 DM	Wie Hausarzt	Wie Hausarzt
Institut für Arbeits- + Sozialhygiene (IAS), Siegfried-Kühn-Straße 1, 7500 Karlsruhe 1, (0721/811005)	8.30 bis 16.30 Uhr	1231 DM	Große Testerfahrung, gute apparative Ausstattung, persönlicher Arzt für jeden, viel Zeit für die Untersuchung	Nicht ganz billig; in der Regel Anreise am Vortag erforderlich, daher zeitaufwendig
Deutsche Klinik für Diagnostik (DKD), Aukammallee 33, 6200 Wiesbaden 1, (06121/577481-484)	1 bis 3 Tage	Zirka 1750–2450 DM	Wie IAS; zusätzlich: In Zweifelsfällen kann sofort ein Spezialist aus der DKD hinzugezogen werden	Noch teurer als IAS: unter Umständen auch zeitaufwendiger
Mayo Clinic, Rochester MN 55905, USA, (001/5072842546)	2 bis 4 Tage	600 bis 800 $	Wie DKD, aber größere Erfahrung als DKD	Noch zeitaufwendiger zu den Kosten des Checks kommen die Reisekosten

Krankheit, jedoch nicht mehr. Grundsätzlich kann jeder Befund falsch-positiv sein, auf einem Artefakt, einer Normabweichung, einer Fehlbeurteilung beruhen. Ein Dilemma erwächst nun daraus, daß es zwar häufig weitere diagnostische Mittel zur Absicherung eines Befundes gibt, sie im allgemeinen jedoch weitaus invasiver, für den Patienten risikoträchtiger sind – so etwa könnte ein computertomographisch gewonnener Tumorverdacht bei fehlender Symptomatik durch eine Biopsie erhärtet werden. Bedeutet eine weitere diagnostische Absicherung ein Risiko, sollte es – gemäß der Hippokratischen Maxime des „nihil nocere" – nur dort eingegangen werden, wo tatsächlich eine Krankheit vorliegt. Ob dies der Fall ist, soll aber gerade ermittelt werden.[16]

Andererseits wäre es unverantwortlich, einen einmal erhobenen Befund ohne Konsequenzen bestehen zu lassen, d.h. dem Betreffenden mitzuteilen: Bislang sind keine Symptome ersichtlich, aber möglicherweise haben Sie Krebs.[17] Mithin fragt sich nicht nur, ob der Aufwand der systematischen Untersuchung einer Risikopopulation und die weitere Abklärung der Befunde in einem sinnvollen Verhältnis zueinander stehen – das Problem aller Früherkennungsuntersuchungen – sondern auch, ob nicht letztlich mehr Schaden als Nutzen, mehr Angst als Hilfe das Resultat ist.

Fazit aus der Kostendiskussion

Die Überlegungen sollten deutlich machen,

- daß es – außer unter engen, betriebswirtschaftlichen Gesichtspunkten – unsinnig ist, einzelnen Geräten einzelne Kosten zuzurechnen,
- daß interessant die Kostenketten sind, die durch die Inbetriebnahme eines Gerätes bzw. einer Gerätegruppe entstehen und
- daß solche Kostenketten nur über die thematische Vernetzung von Versorgungskontexten in ihrer Bedeutung erkannt und als Fragestellung formuliert werden können.

Damit habe ich die derzeitige Kostendiskussion um Medizintechnik bagatellisiert und problematisiert zugleich, nicht nur, weil es an validen Daten fehlt, sondern auch deshalb, weil im Zuge der Diskussion um eine „Strukturreform des Gesundheitswesens" das Kostenargument so aufgebläht erscheint, daß zentrale Fragen nach der längerfristigen Strukturentwicklung der medizinischen Versorgung ganz in den Hintergrund zu rücken drohen – Entwicklungen, die teilweise ohne empirischen Aufwand eingeschätzt werden können.

Paradigmatisch hierfür steht die Verbreitung des Nierenlithotripters.[17a] Fraglos bedeutet er eine Verbesserung der Versorgungsqualität. Aber niemals hätte er sich derart rasch durchgesetzt, wenn nicht die Krankenkassen dem Argument, daß mit seiner Hilfe erhebliche Einsparungen erzielt werden könnten, auf-

---

[16] Hierzu Abholz 1986, S. 29ff., sowie Borgers 1986, S. 49ff.
[17] Dieses Problem stellt sich verschärft bei diagnostischen Befunden, denen keine therapeutischen Maßnahmen entsprechen, wie bei dem genetic screening oder bei Aids. Zu letzterem Problem cf. Rosenbrock 1986, S. 104–115 et passim.
[17a] Hierzu Kirchberger 1988 und 1991.

gesessen wären.[18] Hier wurde die Kostenfixierung der Reformdiskussion selbst zum Promotor einer Gerätediffusion mit enormen Folgekosten.

Entscheidendes Argument für die rasche, flächendeckende Versorgung in der Bundesrepublik Deutschland mit Nierenlithotriptern war die Behauptung, der Einsatz des Gerätes bewirke eine nicht unerhebliche Kostensenkung der Nierensteintherapie: Je nach Rechenweise wurden zwischen 40 und 140 Mio. DM pro Jahr veranschlagt.[19] Die Einsparungseffekte sollten durch

- Verkürzung der Verweildauer,
- Verkürzung der Arbeitsunfähigkeitsdauer,
- Verringerung der durch Nierensteinleiden verursachten Dialysefälle

entstehen. Nachdem ich bereits 1986 darauf hingewiesen hatte, daß diese Annahmen über mögliche Kostensenkungen auf abstrakten Modellrechnungen beruhten, denen realiter eher Kostensteigerungen gegenüberstehen dürften,[20] hat nun E. Bruckenberger die Kosteneffekte der ESWL erstmals empirisch untersucht[21] und diese These bestätigt.

- Ausgangspunkt der Modellrechnungen zur Aufwandsenkung war eine geschätzte Zahl von jährlich ca. 50 000 offenen Steinoperationen im Jahr 1982. Bruckenberger erhebt die Zahl der Operationen für Niedersachsen und rechnet sie hoch auf das Bundesgebiet. Er kommt auf ca. 33 000 offene Steinoperationen – immerhin rund 35 % weniger.
- Zweifellos hat die ESWL-Therapie eine kürzere Verweildauer zur Folge als die offene Steinoperation. Bruckenberger verweist aber auf den Fehlschluß, eine Reduzierung der Verweildauer – und damit der Pflegetage – führe automatisch zu Ausgabensenkungen bei den Krankenkassen. Der Fehlschluß beruht darauf, daß im Modell die Gesamtheit aller einsparbaren Pflegetage über alle Krankenhäuser der Bundesrepublik Deutschland hinweg zugrundegelegt wurde, obwohl konkrete Ausgabesenkungen nur dort möglich sind, wo in der urologischen Abteilung eines einzelnen Krankenhauses so viele Operationen entfallen, daß Betten eingespart, bzw. eine OP-Schwester, eine Pflegekraft freigesetzt werden könnte. Die Überlegung hätte also erst ab einer gewissen Abteilungsgröße mit entsprechender Zahl an Nieren- bzw. Harnleitersteinoperationen greifen können. Demgegenüber weist Bruckenberger nach, daß

---

[18] So meinte der geschäftsführende Direktor des „Landesverbandes der Ortskrankenkassen in Bayern" gemäß einem Bericht der *Ärzte Zeitung*, daß „bei der Entscheidung der gesetzlichen Krankenkassen in Bayern für die Einführung des Lithotripsieverfahrens in Münchens außerhalb des Krankenhausfinanzierungsgesetzes alle Kosten einschließlich der Investitionen zu tragen, der humane Aspekt aber auch gleichzeitig der der Ökonomie" von Bedeutung war. Nach Berechnungen des Landesverbandes werden bei 1000 Anwendungen des Lithotripters rund 2 Mio. DM weniger aufzuwenden sein, da die Operationskosten und Geldleistungen wegen Arbeitsunfähigkeit der Patienten entfielen. Somit sei Sparen und Gestalten verbunden, meinte Sitzmann." (*Ärzte Zeitung*, 21. 3. 1984). Ähnlich berichtet der *Münchner Merkur* am 10. 4. 1985. Im September 1985 berichtet „Die Ortskrankenkasse" von den gleichen Einsparungserwartungen (S. 382).
[19] Vgl. z. B. Rassweiler et al. 1985; vgl. Chaussy 1985.
[20] Vgl. Kirchberger 1986, S. 287.
[21] Vgl. Bruckenberger 1987; sowie Kirchberger 1988.

keine Personaleinsparungen erfolgten, es im Gegenteil zu Kapazitätsausweitungen kam.
- Die behauptete Kostenersparnis durch eine Verkürzung der Arbeitsunfähigkeitsdauer betrifft keine Einsparungen auf seiten der Krankenkassen. Brukkenberger verweist zu Recht auf das Fehlen jeglicher Kostenuntersuchung, die die Mehrfachbehandlung bzw. die zusätzliche Arbeitsunfähigkeit aufgrund vom Komplikationen als Folge der ESWL-Behandlung in Rechnung stellt.
- Was die Kostenersparnis als Folge der nierensteinbedingten Dialysefälle betrifft, verweist Bruckenberger darauf, daß es sich um spekulativ ermittelte Kosten handelt, da nachprüfbare Daten über den betroffenen Personenkreis nicht vorliegen. Wenn im übrigen den Berechnungen ein mittlerer Dialysezeitraum von 15 Jahren zugrundegelegt werde – so würde beispielsweise „ein Ersatz dieser fiktiven Dialyse durch eine fiktive Nierentransplantation ... die geschätzten Kostenersparnisse sofort auf ein Fünfzehntel reduzieren. Ebenso ist es nicht unproblematisch, für die Dauer von fünfzehn Jahren eine Stagnation des medizinischen Fortschritts zu unterstellen.

So kommt die Untersuchung zu dem Resultat, daß die Nieren-ESWL statt behaupteter Einsparungen allein für 1986 zusätzliche Kosten in Höhe von etwa 42 Mio. DM verursacht haben. Ohne hier spezifische Kausalzusammenhänge herstellen zu wollen: der Betrag entspricht etwa der Höhe der Kosten für ESWL desselben Jahres. Im Sinne meiner Feststellung zur Notwendigkeit einer thematischen Vernetzung der Versorgungskontexte gelangt Bruckenberger zu dem forschungsstrategischen Ergebnis: „Die medizinischen und wirtschaftlichen Auswirkungen der extrakorporalen Stoßwellen-Lithotripsie können nicht durch Analysen der Nachfrage- bzw. Leistungsentwicklung einzelner der derzeit vorgehaltenen 21 ESWL-Zentren ermittelt werden – wie das bisher geschah –, sondern müssen das Verhalten aller urologischen Abteilungen umfassend berücksichtigen.“[22]
Die Untersuchung, die erstmals in der Bundesrepublik eine empirische Ermittlung der sozioökonomischen Folgen der Verbreitung einer neuen Technologie unternimmt, wirft eine Reihe von Fragen auf:
Die Mehrzahl der Überlegungen von Bruckenberger hätte auch schon vor 5 Jahren erfolgen können und fraglos zu realistischeren Einschätzungen geführt.[23] Es hätte keines großen Aufwandes bedurft, um die tatsächliche Zahl der Operationen in der Bundesrepublik Deutschland zu erheben. Ebenso offensichtlich war, daß der Rückgang der Pflegetage in den urologischen Abteilungen sich in Dimensionen bewegen würde, die keine Personalfreisetzung gestatteten, sondern die Mindereinnahmen der urologischen Abteilungen durch die Erhöhung des allgemeinen Pflegesatzes für alle Abteilungen der betreffenden Krankenhäuser finanziert werden mußten. Und vor allem hätte jede vernünftige Prognose zu der Überlegung geführt, daß – insoweit Überweisungen zur ESWL erfolgten – die

---

[22] Bruckenberger 1987, S. 303.
[23] Vollends unverständlich ist es, wenn nunmehr W Heitzer in einem Vortrag vom 23.5.86 von „theoretischen Kosteneinsparungen von 120 Mio. DM" spricht, und den Mediziner Prof. Chaussy als Zeugen für Wirtschaftlichkeitsuntersuchungen heranzieht. Jeder Ökonom im Hause des AOK-Bundesverbandes hätte diese Theorie unschwer falsifizieren können.

einzelnen Abteilungen kompensatorische Aktivitäten ergreifen würden. Es wäre verfehlt, die Notwendigkeit solcher Aktivitäten pauschal in Frage zu stellen – aber ihre Struktur ist untersuchenswert.

Realistischer scheint hier die Politik der Niederlande, die nicht von Einsparungen ausgeht, sondern davon, daß die Nierenlithotripsie zumindest keine zusätzlichen Kosten verursacht. Sofern dies zutrifft, müßte es möglich sein, die ESWL-Investitions- und Folgekosten ohne zusätzliche Mittel allein über einen Finanzausgleich zu finanzieren. In diesem Sinne erhalten die Krankenhäuser keine zusätzlichen Mittel, vielmehr wird davon ausgegangen, daß sich die urologischen Abteilungen verschiedener Krankenhäuser zusammentun und Investition und Nutzung der Technologie aus dem laufenden Etat finanzieren.[23a]

Es ist deshalb unverständlich, daß die These der Kostensenkung von den gesetzlichen Krankenkassen kritiklos übernommen wurde. Nur auf diesem Hintergrund ließ sich die Durchsetzung einer derart kurzfristigen, flächendeckenden Versorgung rechtfertigen – mit dem Ergebnis des heute schon akuten Problems der Durchsetzung neuer, billigerer und ggf. auch besserer Geräte anderer Firmen[24] bzw. ihrer Durchsetzung nur unter Inkaufnahme einer erheblichen Überversorgung.[24a] Damit komme ich zum zweiten Teil meines Referates, zur Diffusionsproblematik.

Wie und warum verbreitet sich „Medizintechnik"?

Mit dem Diffusionsbegriff fasse ich nicht nur die Verbreitung, sondern auch die Nutzung von Medizintechnik. Was sollen Untersuchungen über die Verbreitung eines Gerätes, wenn seine Nutzung das eigentliche Problem darstellt? Bedarfsplanung bezieht sich allerdings durchweg auf die Verbreitung von Geräten – und ist insoweit als politisches Instrument ineffektiv.[25] So zeigt eine Untersuchung von 1978, daß CT-Untersuchungen keine Änderung der Therapieplanung bei Schlaganfallpatienten zur Folge haben. Diese Erkenntnis hat aber bis heute keinen Einfluß auf die bei solchen Patienten angewandte Diagnostik. Ferner belegen einige Erhebungen, daß sich ca. 20 % aller CT-Untersuchungen auf Kopfschmerzen beziehen. Andererseits gibt es genügend Erkenntnisse, aus denen klar hervorgeht, daß Patienten mit einem normalen neurologischen Befund, wie er über eine gründliche körperliche Untersuchung erhoben wird, auch keinen Befund im Computertomogramm erkennen lassen. Die CT-Untersuchung wäre demnach überflüssig.

Freilich: an den bis heute international vorliegenden Forschungsergebnissen gemessen ist die Verbreitung und Nutzung medizinischer Technik terra incognita. Welche Faktoren Umfang und Standard der Verbreitung technischer Innovatio-

---

[23a] Hierzu Kirchberger 1991.

[24] Neun weitere Firmen haben mittlerweile Lithotripter entwickelt. Vgl. Biomedical Business International Vol. X, No. 10/11, S. 94.

[24a] Während offiziell von einem Bedarf für etwa 21 Geräte die Rede ist, werden Ende 1990 mindestens 85 Geräte in der Bundesrepublik in Betrieb sein.

[25] So gibt es z. B. in Frankreich erheblich weniger Computertomographen als in der Bundesrepublik, ihre durchschnittliche Nutzung liegt mit ca. 6200 Untersuchungen jährlich jedoch erheblich höher als bei uns. Vgl. Fagnani et al. 1987.

nen in der medizinischen Versorgung bestimmt haben und bestimmen, welche
Einflüsse behindernd oder fördernd auf die Anwendung einzelner Geräte einwirkten, wie der Technisierungsprozeß über die letzten 80 Jahre in der Praxis der
medizinischen Versorgung verlaufen ist – darüber existieren kaum einschlägige
Studien.[26]

Geläufige Thesen zur Verbreitung und Nutzung medizinischer Technik

Fehlt die Kenntnis struktureller Determinanten, liegt der Rückgriff auf
individualisierend-psychologisierende Handlungsparameter nahe. An ihnen
richten sich die geläufigen Thesen zur Diffusion von Medizintechnik weitgehend
aus.[27] Ihnen zufolge erklärt sich die Diffusionsdynamik v. a. durch

– eine allgemeine Wissenschafts- und Technikgläubigkeit,
– Prestige- (und Konkurrenz-) Gesichtspunkte der Anwender,
– das Inanspruchnahmebewußtsein der Abnehmer,
– den Spielraum des Arztes und sein Absicherungsverhalten.

An die Stelle struktureller Determinanten treten Motivationen des Umgangs mit
der Apparatur. Zweifellos sind sie existent. Nur erklären sie nicht den bewußtseinsprägenden, spezifische Formen medizinischen Wissens generierenden und
Versorgungsabläufe determinierenden Einfluß, den die Medizintechnik als diagnostisches und therapeutisches Potential ausübt. Sie erklären auch nicht, inwiefern bestimmte Problemkonstellationen der medizinischen Versorgung im ambulanten oder stationären Sektor diffusionsbefördernd wirken. Und sie lassen keine
Aussagen über systemimmanente Grenzen des Einsatzes medizinischer Technik
zu.
    Die reduzierte Betrachtungsweise hat strategisch-politische Konsequenzen.
Als Modus der Intervention verbleibt die Bewußtseinsänderung. Verknappte
man die Mittel, würde sich aus dieser Sicht das Problem von alleine erledigen: mit
der geringeren Manövriermasse korrelierte der allseits reduzierte Anspruch, daraus wieder resultierte eine Konzentration auf die „wirklich wesentlichen" Fälle,
auf das „medizinisch Erforderliche".
    Paradigmatisch für solche Fehleinschätzungen ist die Diskussion um die
Höherbewertung kommunikativer Leistungen, wie sie sich in der neuen Gebührenordnung niedergeschlagen hat. Allein die Tatsache, daß so etwas wie „Schrotschußdiagnostik" konstatiert werden kann,[28] belegt, daß das Motiv für die Diagnostik nicht bloß die bisherige Höherbewertung der apparativ vermittelten Leistungen war, sondern das ausbildungs- und zeitökonomisch bedingte Unvermö

---

[26] Einen – wenn auch kursorischen – Überblick gibt Reiser 1978. Die Probleme der konventionellen Röntgenologie und die Arbeitsplatzentwicklung des diagnostischen Labors werden
dargestellt bei Kirchberger 1986 a. Die Geschwindigkeit, mit der sich die Röntgenologie von
1896–1906 weltweit verbreitete, ist ein Phänomen, das vermutlich einige Aufschlüsse über aktuelle Diffusionsprozesse in der Medizin bieten kann. Bislang liegt hierzu keine Untersuchung
vor.
[27] Vgl. z. B. Gordon u. Fisher 1975.
[28] Vgl. Vilmar 1980, S. 1249ff.

gen des Arztes zum Gespräch.[29] Und nicht nur dies. Die technische Leistung läßt sich dem Einzelleistungsdenken besser adaptieren als eine kommunikative, nach allgemeinem Verständnis ganzheitlich zu bewertende, nicht teilbare Leistung. Darum muß auch sie, die Kommunikation, der Technik angeglichen werden. Das wird z. B. deutlich an dem Leserbrief eines Arztes, veröffentlicht in der "Medical Tribune", der die Frage stellt, ob er ein Gespräch mit der doppelten Gebühr abrechnen dürfe, wenn es eine Minute länger dauere als nach der entsprechenden Gebührenposition vorgesehen.

Hier wird Technik nicht nur zum Substitut, sondern zugleich zum auslösenden Faktor des professionellen Verlernens einer Fähigkeit, die sich gegen diese Technik erst wieder durchzusetzen hätte. Umgekehrt folgte die professionelle Konzentration auf die apparative Leistung einem immer stärker sich durchsetzenden, Versorgung scheinbar objektivierenden Interaktionskonzept.

Die wesentliche Intention des neuen EBM dürfte es in diesem Punkte denn auch gewesen sein, interne Einkommensausgleiche zwischen den verschiedenen Fachrichtungen herzustellen. Den Kinderärzten und Allgemeinpraktikern zum Beispiel, aber auch technisch weniger ausgestatteten Internisten sollten Einkommensverbesserungen verschafft und so die Schere zwischen ihnen und den technischen Facharztgruppen nicht weiter vergrößert werden. Angesichts der wachsenden Zahl niedergelassener Ärzte erscheint dies dringlich, um die Homogenität der Interessen zu wahren.

Gesundheitspolitik und Technologiepolitik

Vergleichbare Fehleinschätzungen bestehen über die Konvergenz von gesundheitspolitischen Forderungen und medizintechnischen Innovationspotentialen generell. Es fehlt – nahezu unbestritten – an validen Kriterien einer adäquaten Versorgung der Bevölkerung mit medizinischen Leistungen, aber auch an Wissen über die Durchsetzung, Verbreitung und Wirksamkeit medizinischer Technik. Beide Defizienzen werden in der Forderung deutlich, neue Technologien mit „breitem Anwendungsbereich" zu entwickeln, die durch den medizinischen Fortschritt gerechtfertigt und „zum Vorteil breiter Bevölkerungsschichten" in die Praxis umgesetzt werden können.[30] Wie breit der Anwendungsbereich einer neuen Technologie ist, stellt sich zumeist erst im nachhinein heraus – dann nämlich, wenn sie entsprechend breit – und das heißt: unspezifisch genug – appliziert worden ist. Die gleichsam demokratietheoretisch fundierte Forderung nach Breiteneffizienz konterkariert sich selbst – sie läßt sich heute prinzipiell auf jedes neue Gerät anwenden, enthält also kein Selektionskriterium. Abgesehen davon: ließen sich Technologien im Sinne der Maxime „breiter Anwendungsbereich zum Vorteil breiter Bevölkerungsschichten" konstruieren, hätte sie die Industrie schon von ihren Absatzinteressen her gesehen längst angeboten.

---

[29] Insofern fragt sich, woher die Ortskrankenkassen ihre Hoffnung nehmen, daß „die Neugestaltung des Bewertungsmaßstabes einen wesentlichen Beitrag zur Verbesserung der medizinischen Versorgung" darstelle (Pressedienst der Ortskrankenkasse, 2. 10. 87).
[30] Informationen des BMJFG 1978, S. 78.

Damit ist die Notwendigkeit einer gesundheitspolitischen – insoweit kanalisierenden – Reflexion medizintechnischer Innovationspotentiale nicht überhaupt in Frage gestellt. Ich wollte verdeutlichen, wie schnell ohne eine genauere Kenntnis von Sachzusammenhängen gesundheitspolitische Maximen Diffusionseffekte legitimieren, ja befördern können, die den verfolgten Intentionen genau zuwiderlaufen. Das gilt nicht nur für Maximen, die direkt auf das Problemfeld Medizintechnik zielen, sondern – häufiger noch – für solche, die indirekt technologiepolitisch wirken, weil sie eine intensivere Verbreitung und Nutzung von Medizintechnik als "unintended consequences" zur Folge haben. Im Falle der Verbreitung des Nierenlithotripters wirkte das Kostenargument als diffusionsbefördernder Promotor einer kontraproduktiven Entwicklung – wenngleich das ebenso verfolgte Ziel einer Verbesserung der Versorgungsqualität zumindest teilweise erreicht wurde. In einem anderen Fall jedoch hat das Ziel der Kostensenkung Versorgungsqualität zerstört:

Die Krankenhausverweildauer wurde in den letzten Jahren aus Kostengründen erheblich gesenkt. Dem Ziel liegt ein primär somatischer Krankheitsbegriff zugrunde. Mit der Senkung der Verweildauer ging die Klage über eine zunehmend technisierte, enthumanisierte Medizin einher. Ursächlich dafür ist aber nicht die Technik. Was hier als Humanität zu bezeichnen wäre, wird wesentlich definiert durch den Faktor Zeit. Bei einer Verweildauer von 8–10 Tagen haben Ärzte und Pflegepersonal vielleicht Gelegenheit, den Patienten so kennenzulernen, daß sie beginnen könnten, mit ihm zu reden, ihn über den „Fall" hinaus wahrzunehmen. Wieviel Zeit allerdings wird benötigt, bis sich eine solche Wahrnehmung derart verdichtet hat, daß sie sich dem Patienten vermittelt, und wieviel Zeit, bis sie kommunikativ-therapeutisch fruchtbar gemacht werden könnte? Mit der Reduktion der Verweildauer und insofern von Zeit wurde Versorgungsqualität definiert: Krankenhausversorgung ist Technikanwendung und nur in diesem Zusammenhang erforderliche Pflege, ist Auslotung, ggf. Reparatur primär somatischer Ereignisse. Gesundheitspolitik wurde zur Technologiepolitik – in einem freilich fatalen Sinn.

Andererseits läßt sich genausowenig postulieren, neue Technologien mit hochspezifizierten Anwendungsbereichen zu entwickeln, sei das – Planungen erleichternde – Gebot der Stunde,

– gesundheitspolitisch nicht, weil wir nur selten prima facie zwischen Bagatellfällen und schweren Erkrankungen einerseits, zwischen unspezifisch zu behandelnden und methodenspezifisch zu versorgenden Fällen andererseits unterscheiden können,
– medizintechnisch nicht, weil entsprechende Neuerungen vielfach auf der Ausdifferenzierung eines Funktionsprinzips beruhen, auf einer Basistechnologie und ihrer Übertragung auf verschiedene Anwendungsbereiche einerseits, auf bereits seit längerem in Anwendung befindliche, aber technisch noch limitierte Methoden andererseits.

Die Neuerungen sind tendenziell iterativ, sie erschließen sich ihren Anwendungsbereich gleichsam von selbst. Ihre Diffusion verläuft induktiv. Mit dem *Nierenlithotripter* beispielsweise wird z. Z. in einer von Dornier finanzierten multizentrischen Studie die Zertrümmerung von Gallengangsteinen erprobt.[31] Umgekehrt ist der *Gallensteinlithotripter* geeignet, diejenigen Nierensteine zu zertrümmern, die sonographisch erfaßbar sind.

Solche Studien wie die von Dornier in Auftrag gegebene zeigen jedoch: Wie jeder Betrieb sich vor der Beschaffung einer neuen Produktionsanlage Gedanken über deren Nutzung – sei es im Sinne der Rationalisierung, sei es hinsichtlich der Produktionsverbesserung – macht, sollte mit jeder Verbreitung einer neuen medizinischen Technologie deren Evaluation erfolgen,[32] d. h. sowohl die Bewertung ihres medizinischen Nutzens im Sinne eines Zuwachses an diagnostischer Sicherheit oder von Therapiequalität, als auch die Einschätzung der sozioökonomischen Folgen wie Arbeits- und Kompetenzverlagerung, Einsparungen oder Mehrausgaben, Umstrukturierungen des Handlungsbereiches. Nur ergibt sich hier folgendes Dilemma:

– Einerseits existieren weder in der Bundesrepublik Deutschland noch in den anderen westlichen Ländern diesbezügliche Standards.[33] Soweit das Evaluationsproblem in der Bundesrepublik überhaupt bearbeitet wird, geschieht dies meist ex post, zu einem Zeitpunkt also, in dem durch eine Evaluation sich wenig oder nichts mehr ändern läßt.

– Andererseits können Evaluationsstudien die Potentiale und Grenzen neuer Technologien nur unzulänglich ausloten, wenn sie vor der Praxisphase erstellt werden. Sie müssen dann in notwendigerweise lokal und situativ begrenzten Erfahrungsbereichen veranstaltet werden – der Schluß auf die Invalidität der Ergebnisse liegt nicht fern.

Die Konsequenz daraus kann freilich nicht die Fortschreibung des gegenwärtigen Status quo, der Evaluationsverzicht, sondern nur die Verpflichtung zu kontrollierten Ex-ante-, v. a. aber kontinuierlich fortgesetzten Begleitstudien sein. Ist es doch immer wieder erstaunlich, auf welch bedürftigem Informationshintergrund ein Gerät sich durchzusetzen vermochte.

So kann heute kein Zweifel mehr daran bestehen, daß die Computertomographie des Schädels einen beachtlichen diagnostischen Fortschritt darstellt. Angesichts der – für damalige Verhältnisse – ungewöhnlich hohen Kosten des Gerätes sollte man allerdings meinen, daß die Investitionsbereitschaft zumindest auf einer

---

[31] Vgl. Sauerbruch et al. 1986, S. 818ff.; ähnliche Untersuchungen werden mit dem Nierenlithotripter von Siemens durchgeführt (Terpstra et al. 1987).

[32] Die Chance einer Vormarktkontrolle, wie sie die FDA in den USA verlangt, wurde bei der MedGV verschenkt. Unter dem Gesichtspunkt, daß eine Vermarktung ohne vorherige Erprobung am Menschen kaum möglich ist, wird in § 5(10) geregelt, daß im Anschluß an den Nachweis der technischen Unbedenklichkeit des Gerätes vor der Benutzungszulassung die klinische Erprobung am Menschen erfolgen darf. Dabei heißt es ausdrücklich; „diese Ausnahme ist auf einen vom Antragsteller" – sprich: Hersteller – „vorgeschlagenen Anwenderkreis zu beschränken". Hier hätte eine Regelung mit klaren Evaluationskriterien und -bedingungen weitergeführt.

[33] Im Gegensatz zur Bundesrepublik gibt es jedoch in anderen Ländern systematische Ansätze in diese Richtung, wie z. B. das "National Health Technology Advisory Panel" in Australien oder das "Office of Technology Assessment" in den USA. Ein interessanter Versuch sind auch die sogenannten Konsensus-Konferenzen in den Niederlanden und Großbritannien. Zum Themenbereich vgl. Donabedian 1980.

klaren Vorstellung von der diagnostischen Leistungsfähigkeit des neuen Gerätes und damit einer eindeutigen Kenntnis von dessen medizinischem Nutzen beruhte. Sieht man sich aber die diesbezügliche Literatur genauer an, war genau das Gegenteil der Fall.

Nach etwa 2jährigen Versuchen mit einem Prototyp kam der Schädelscanner im Sommer 1973 auf den Markt. Nach etwas mehr als 2 Jahren, Ende 1975, gab es weltweit bereits ca. 250 Geräte, ca. 180 davon in den USA. Geht man davon aus, daß zwischen dem Datum der Investitionsentscheidung und dem der Inbetriebnahme eines Gerätes mindestens ein Zeitraum von 6 Monaten liegt, so bildeten – sieht man von der Firmenreklame ab – die bis Mitte 1975 vorgelegten Kenntnisse und Erfahrungen aus der Klinik die Grundlage, auf der die Leistungsfähigkeit des Gerätes eingeschätzt werden mußte.

In einer 1977 vorgelegten Untersuchung versuchen Creditor u. Garrett,[34] diese Informationsbasis genauer zu analysieren. Von 141 veröffentlichten Untersuchungen waren 66 Publikationen rein technischen Inhalts, 75 berichteten über klinische Erfahrungen. Letztere Berichte stammten aus insgesamt 27 Instituten, durchweg an Universitätskliniken, was wiederum heißt, daß die nicht-universitären Erfahrungen – vor allem die im ambulanten Bereich – gar nicht an die Öffentlichkeit getreten, gar nicht systematisiert und bekannt geworden waren. Die Mehrzahl der 75 klinischen Berichte besaß anekdotischen, d. h. einzelfallorientierten Charakter, ein kleinerer Teil enthielt immerhin Angaben, welche Arten von Läsionen in welcher Zahl ermittelt werden konnten, ohne allerdings Vergleiche der Leistungsfähigkeit gegenüber konventionellen Untersuchungsverfahren zu erlauben. Nur 13 (!) Berichte gestatteten eine Quantifizierung der diagnostischen Genauigkeit, derjenigen Qualität also, deretwegen der CT als eine revolutionäre diagnostische Errungenschaft bezeichnet worden war.

Bei diesen 13 Berichten wiederum war die Zahl der Fälle durchweg klein. Auch blieb aufgrund der unterschiedlichen Fragestellungen (Tumor, intercerebrale Blutungen, Atrophie usw.) die Differenzierung nach falsch-positiven bzw. falsch-negativen Befunden quantitativ zu gering, um brauchbare verallgemeinerbare Aussagen über Spezifität und Sensitivität des Schädel-CT zu gestatten. Die Literatur überzeugt hinsichtlich der Möglichkeit, die Zahl invasiver Verfahren zu reduzieren, insbesondere die Pneumenzephalographie wird als überholt bezeichnet – nur handelt es sich bei ihr um eine wegen ihrer Risiken ohnehin äußerst selten angewandte Methode. Demgegenüber wurde schon damals deutlich, daß sich die Zahl der durchaus risikobehafteten Angiographien im Gefolge der weiteren diagnostischen Abklärung von CT-Befunden nicht unerheblich vermehren würde. (Hierzu sei angemerkt, daß die Frage der Risikominderung bzw. -mehrung im Zuge der Verbreitung der Computertomographie bis heute nicht untersucht worden ist.)

Absicht von Creditor und Garrett war es, den Informationshintergrund derartiger Investitionsentscheidungen aufzudecken. Das Ergebnis war mager. Fraglos bieten – neben den analysierten Publikationen – Seminare, informelle Treffen und Kongresse erhebliche Informationspotentiale, und die Mitteilung dort präsentierter Informationen erfolgt durchweg Monate vor ihrer Veröffentlichung.

---

[34] Vgl. Creditor u. Garrett 1977; Banta 1984.

Es dürfte jedoch unwahrscheinlich sein, daß sie – gerade im Hinblick auf die Wertigkeit des neuen Verfahrens – detaillierter gewesen wären als die publizierte Version. Offensichtlich sind andere Argumente entscheidend für die Investitionsbereitschaft.

Die Lücke zwischen Theorie und Praxis

Erschließen sich also medizintechnische Neuerungen ihren Anwendungsbereich gleichsam von selbst, ist gerade dies – der Quasiautomatismus – problematisch. Seine Funktionsbedingungen sind ungeklärt. Fest steht aber, daß die Produktions-, Rezeptions- und Legitimationsmuster der medizinischen Versorgung ein Diffusionsklima erzeugen, das der induktiven Verbreitung und Nutzung medizinischer Technik ideal entgegenkommt und an dessen Genese diese Technik intensiv beteiligt ist.

Jede „Geldhahn"theorie – sei es die der Umbewertung von Leistungspositionen, der Budgetierung oder der Selbstbeteiligung – unterstellt, daß medizinische Versorgung ein Rechenexempel, ein Kalkulationsproblem sei. Was der Markt im Gesundheitswesen nicht leistet – die Selektion des Wesentlichen und Angemessenen, des Fortschrittsträchtigen und Preisgünstigen –, soll die Mittelverknappung bewirken. Das setzt voraus, daß Qualitätsstandards die Mittelverwendung anleiten. Ohne progredierende Qualitätsstandards keine Selektivität des je Erforderlichen, Wirksamen, Wirtschaftlichen – getreu der Maxime: „Ärztliche Tätigkeit im Gegensatz zu Medizin als einer klinischen oder Grundlagenforschung ... findet ihre Legitimation ausschließlich dort, wo sie in einer Entscheidung mündet, zum Nutzen des Heilung suchenden Individuums zu handeln."[35]

An dieser – individualisierenden – Maxime gemessen erscheint Medizintechnik ökonomisch par excellence und darum einem Konzept der Mittelverknappung besonders förderlich. Zehrt sie doch vom Ideal ubiquitärer Anwendungsbedingungen, Genauigkeit der Messungen, Wiederholbarkeit vergleichbarer Erfahrungen – kurz: von der Standardisierung und Generalisierung ihres Einsatzes und seiner Ergebnisse, letztlich: von der Austauschbarkeit des Arztes, aber auch des Patienten.[36] In der Eliminierung aller Imponderabilien scheint Medizintechnik Mittel und Zweck zugleich. Als solchermaßen „Objektivität" verbürgende trug sie zur Verwissenschaftlichung der Medizin seit der zweiten Hälfte des 19. Jahrhunderts entscheidend bei. Die Entdeckung der Röntgenstrahlen und ihre technische Umsetzung für diagnostisches und therapeutisches Handeln, die Anwendung von physikalisch-chemischen Methoden, von in klinischer Forschung entwickelten, apparativen Meß- und Beobachtungsverfahren markieren die Leitlinien einer Medizin als Naturwissenschaft.[37]

Problem ist nur, daß dieses „iatrotechnische Konzept der Medizin", wie Rotschuh es genannt hat,[38] höchst eingeschränkt praktizierbar ist. Den Zielgrößen

---

[35] Pellegrino 1979, S. 171.
[36] Vgl. Sadegh-Zadeh 1977, S. 77; vgl. Maxmem 1976.
[37] Vgl. Kirchberger 1986a, S. 99ff.
[38] Vgl. Rothschuh 1978, S. 417.

diagnostischer Transparenz und therapeutischer Reparierbarkeit widersprechen durch individuell unterschiedliche Erfahrungshorizonte und unterschiedliche Informationsverarbeitung auf dem Hintergrund unterschiedlicher Lehrmeinungen bedingte ‚Umwege' des ärztlichen Handelns, widerspricht ein Problemlösungsverhalten, das sich als personen- und fallspezifisch einer übergreifenden, theoretischen Formulierung, einer „klinischen Praxistheorie" weitgehend entzieht. Zugleich ist dieser Widerspruch ein für Versorgungspraxis als medizintechnisches Experimentierfeld treibendes Moment. Der vielfach bestehenden Inkompatibilität von Wissenschaftssystemen, Methodenanwendung, Urteilsbildungsprozessen entspricht die Disparität des medizintechnischen Instrumentariums und des Umgangs mit ihm. So kommt es, daß – wie es in einer *Prognos*-Studie aus den 70er Jahren heißt – „der ‚Wert' oder auch die ‚Effizienz' einzelner Methoden bisher nicht in statistisch relevanter Weise ermittelt, objektiviert und in Vergleich zu anderen Verfahren relativiert worden, teilweise … eine Vergleichbarkeit überhaupt nicht gegeben oder nur bedingt möglich" ist.[39]

Daß wiederum Medizintechnik auch strukturierend, nämlich Methoden verdrängend und Sichtweisen prägend, mithin standardisierend wirkt, ist die Kehrseite dieses Prozesses. Das betrifft insbesondere die Frage, ob der technologische Wandel in der medizintechnischen Diagnostik therapeutische Entscheidungsstrukturen dadurch verändert, daß bestimmte Untersuchungen aus pragmatischen Gründen entfallen und damit therapeutische Alternativen aus dem Blick geraten.

Seit Jahrzehnten gibt es in der Gallensteintherapie einen Schulstreit um die Frage, wann eine Cholezystektomie (operative Entfernung der Gallenblase) erforderlich ist, d. h.

- ob jeder zufällig entdeckte, symptomlose Gallenstein operiert werden soll,
- ob für eine Indikation zur Operation leichte Symptome bereits hinreichen, oder
- ob man erst bei einer akuten Cholezystitis, einer biliär bedingten Pankreatitis oder einem Verschlußikterus operieren soll.

Der Streit verläuft im wesentlichen zwischen Chirurgen und Internisten, wobei letztere überwiegend für den Erhalt der Gallenblase votieren, soweit sie funktionstüchtig ist. Immerhin entfällt bei einer Entfernung der Gallenblase deren Speicher- und Dosierungsfunktion, mit der Folge, daß sich die Galle kontinuierlich und nicht mehr in Abhängigkeit von der Nahrungsaufnahme in den Darm entleert, was wiederum Verdauungsstörungen, möglicherweise aber auch ein erhöhtes Krebsrisiko zur Folge haben kann.

Dieser Streit war bislang eine weitgehend akademische Auseinandersetzung. Einerseits war das Operationsrisiko mit einer Letalität von 0,5 % bei Patienten unter 60 Jahren zu erheblich, um bei zufällig entdeckten bzw. gering symptomatischen Steinen bedenkenlos eine Operation empfehlen zu können.[40] Andererseits

---

[39] Prognos AG, Basel 1977/78, S. 33.

[40] Andererseits wird gerade die steigende Letalität bei zunehmendem Alter als Argument für eine frühzeitige Operation auch symptomarmer Patienten angeführt, vgl. z. B. Rinecker 1981, S. 2360.

war die Zahl der zufällig entdeckten, beschwerdefreien Steine minimal bzw. erfolgte der Steinnachweis über eine Röntgenkontrastmitteluntersuchung, die – selbst nicht risikolos – einer klaren Indikation bedurfte. Schließlich spielte sich die Auseinandersetzung fast ausschließlich unter Krankenhausärzten ab, wohingegen die Entscheidung für oder gegen eine Cholezystektomie vorwiegend von den niedergelassenen Ärzten getroffen wurde. Sie praktizierten Therapieverzicht oder griffen zu einer symptomatischen Therapie, überwiesen in die chirurgische Abteilung zur Cholezystektomie oder in die innere – soweit es sich um inoperable Patienten handelte, aber auch, insoweit sie es als zweckmäßig ansahen, die Entscheidung für oder gegen eine Operation an das Krankenhaus zu delegieren. Die Entscheidungsstruktur der niedergelassenen Ärzte ist höchst differenziert, so daß sich bei gleichen oder ähnlichen Krankheitsbildern ein breites Spektrum unterschiedlicher Behandlungsverläufe ergibt.

Mit der raschen Verbreitung der Sonographie bei Internisten und Allgemeinpraktikern verändert sich die Diagnostik des Gallensteinleidens in zwei wesentlichen Punkten. Risikolosigkeit und hohe Treffsicherheit haben die Ultraschalldiagnostik der Gallensteine in kürzester Zeit zu einem Routineverfahren werden lassen und die Zahl der ambulant durchgeführten Cholangiographien um mehr als die Hälfte reduziert.

– Während jedoch die Kontrastmitteluntersuchung zugleich Aussagen über die Funktionsfähigkeit des Gallensystems gestattete, ist dies mit dem Ultraschallverfahren nur bedingt möglich.
– Während die Kontrastmitteluntersuchung einer klaren Indikation bedurfte und stumme Steine daher nur in seltenen Fällen (bei Übersichtsaufnahmen) entdeckt wurden, werden durch die Sonographie aufgrund deren risikoloser Routine zunehmend mehr symptomlose Gallensteine entdeckt.

Hieraus könnte sich folgende Konsequenz ergeben bzw. als Tendenz schon ergeben haben:
Der Nachweis der Funktionstüchtigkeit der Gallenblase – bei labordiagnostischem Ausschluß der Cholezystitis oder anderer Komplikationen war für viele Internisten ein nicht unerhebliches Argument gegen die Cholezystektomie. Wird nun der überwiegende Teil der Cholangiographien durch Sonographie ersetzt, so entfällt diese Information. Andererseits schafft die – wenngleich unsystematische – sonographische „Früherkennung" einen zunehmenden Behandlungsdruck. Da das Operationsrisiko um so geringer ist, je jünger der Patient, steigt die Tendenz zur Cholezystektomie – zumindest solange keine anderen brauchbaren Therapieformen verfügbar sind.

Diese Überlegung ist empirisch nicht gesichert. Sie macht aber deutlich, wie sich diagnostische Informationsstrukturen durch die Verfügbarkeit neuer Technologien verändern und wie hieraus veränderte Therapiebedürfnisse erwachsen können.

Forschungsstrategische Konsequenzen

Psychologisierende Konzepte und pauschalisierende gesundheitspolitische Richtlinien führen also genausowenig weit wie einseitig ökonomisch intendierte Steuerungsversuche. Die Diffusion medizinischer Technik läßt sich aus institutionellen und organisatorischen Rahmenbedingungen des Gesundheitswesens nur bedingt erklären und nur sehr eingeschränkt mit deren Mitteln steuern. Genauso bedeutsam, vielleicht noch wesentlicher ist die praxeologische Erforschung der Generierung und Anwendung medizinischen Wissens mit den sich daraus ergebenden, diagnostischen und therapeutischen Konsequenzen. Hier erzeugt die Innovation und Diffusion neuer Technologien permanente Umstrukturierungseffekte. Sie stellen die eigentlichen Kostenpotentiale dar.[41]

Dabei spielen strukturelle Persistenzen eine wesentliche Rolle. So darf jeder Arzt grundsätzlich diejenigen Verfahren anwenden, die er nachgewiesenermaßen beherrscht. Das Endoskop mit seinen Varianten Bronchoskop, Gastroskop, Rektoskop usw. ist traditionellerweise ein Instrument der internistischen Diagnostik. Seine Weiterentwicklung in den vergangenen 20 Jahren zu einem hochflexiblen Instrument von wenigen Millimetern Durchmesser hat seinen Anwendungsbereich erheblich vergrößert. Sowohl über Körperöffnungen als auch durch perkutane Anwendung erschließen sich selbst Räume wie 8 mm breite Gallengänge. Hohlnadeln zur Punktion, kleine Messer, Instrumente zur Laserchirurgie lassen sich endoskopisch vor Ort bringen, Ligaturen, ja selbst Nähte durchführen. Es lag nahe, daß die internistischen Fachärzte, die seit Jahrzehnten Erfahrungen mit diesem Instrumentarium gesammelt haben, auch die neu erschlossenen therapeutischen Möglichkeiten nutzten. Die erforderlichen Eingriffe waren weniger invasiv und zugleich besser abgrenzbar als in der konventionellen Chirurgie. Damit allerdings eigneten sie sich Arbeitsfelder an, die bislang von Chirurgen wahrgenommen worden waren. Das hätte längerfristig bedeutet, daß den Chirurgen ein Teil ihrer Aufgaben aus der Hand genommen worden wäre. Deshalb ist es kein Zufall, daß seit neuestem die endoskopischen Techniken zum Weiterbildungskatalog der Chirurgie gehören. Wie jede Fachdisziplin versucht auch sie, sich ihr Arbeitsfeld zu erhalten.

Das Beispiel macht – wie alle anderen genannten – deutlich, daß das Problemfeld „Medizintechnik", wie auch immer man es schneiden mag, schon angesichts der Geräte- und ihrer Verwendungsvielfalt einerseits, angesichts der differenzierten Wirkungsketten andererseits nur sukzessive, über Einzelfallstudien erschlossen werden kann. Diffusion und Kosten eines Gerätes können nur adäquat beschrieben werden, wenn dessen Folgen für den jeweiligen Diagnose- und auch Therapiezusammenhang, die Funktionsänderungen anderer Geräte oder auch Diagnose- und Therapieformen, aber auch Qualitätsänderungen und innerprofessionelle Umstrukturierungen mit berücksichtigt werden. Dabei sollte die Verbreitung und Nutzung eines Gerätes bzw. einer Gerätegruppe als Antwort auf eine in der Sache, d. h. in der medizinischen Versorgung latent oder manifest vorhandene Fragestellung begriffen werden, weil anderenfalls spezifische Handlungsrationalitäten nicht rekonstruiert werden können. Erst auf diesem Hintergrund könnte es gelingen, Modelle zu entwickeln, die es gestatten, auf der Grundlage bestimmter Basishypothesen – wie solchen zur strukturellen Persistenz, zur Divergenz von medizinischer Wissenschaft und ärztlicher Kunst, zur Risikoak-

---

[41] Vgl. Kirchberger 1986a, S. 286.

zeptanz, zu Qualifikationsverläufen, zur innerprofessionellen Spezialisierung, zur Medikalisierung von Lebensformen – Diffusionsprozesse abzuschätzen und in ihren Folgewirkungen zu beurteilen.

Literatur

Abholz H-H (1986) Das Dilemma medizinisch-technischer Entwicklungen. Argument [Sonderband] 141:29ff.
Abholz H-H, Borgers D et al. (Hrsg) (1982) Risikofaktorenmedizin – Konzept und Kontroverse. Berlin New York
Altman S, Blendon R (1979) Medical Technology: the culprit behind health care costs? Proceedings of the 1977 Sun Valley Forum on National Health. DHEW, Washington
Altman S, Wallack S (1979) Is medical technology the culprit behind rising health costs? The case for and against. Medical Technology: the Culprit behind Health Care Costs? Proceedings of the 1977 Sun Valley Forum on National Health. DHEW, Washington, S 24ff.
Anderson JG, Hay JS (1985) The diffusion of medical technology: social network analysis and policy research. Soc Q 26:49ff.
Banta D (1984) Embracing or rejecting innovations: clinical diffusion of health care technology. In: Reiser SJ, Anbar M (eds) The machine at the bedside. – Strategies for using technology in patient care. Cambridge
Borgers D (1986) Für eine ganzheitliche Perspektive in der Anwendung medizinischer Technologien. Argument [Sonderband] 141:49ff
Bruckenberger E (1987) Medizinische und wirtschaftliche Konsequenzen des Einsatzes der Extrakorporalen Stoßwellen Lithotripsie in der Bundesrepublik Deutschland. Hyg Med 7/8:285ff.
Burch G, Pasquale NP de (1964) A history of electrocardiography. Chicago
Chaussy C (1985) Wie wirtschaftlich sind Nierentransplantation und extrakorporale Stoßwellenlithotripsie von Nierensteinen? Arzt Krankenh, S 60ff.
Clade H (1980) Medizintechnik in Praxis und Klinik: Zwischen Verlockung und Verantwortung. Prakt Arzt 18:2261
Creditor MC, Garrett JB (1977) The information base for diffusion of technology: computed tomography scanning. N Engl J Med 291:49ff.
Donabedian A (1980) Explorations in quality assessment and monitoring. Michigan
Fagnani F et al. (1987) La planification des équipements médicaux au niveau régional: le cas du scanographe la région P. A. C. A., INSERM Unité 240/40
Gordon G, Fisher GL (1975) The diffusion of medical technology. Cambridge/MA
Graf H (1968) Endoskopie, ihre Entwicklung vom einfachen Einblick durch ein Rohr bis zum Farbfernsehen aus dem Körperinneren. Elektromedizin, S 50ff.
Häussler S (Hrsg) (1985) Diagnose ohne technische Hilfsmittel. Stuttgart
Hartung C (1980) Die Risiken der Medizintechnik verringern. Ärztl Prax
Jonas H (1984) Warum wir heute eine Ethik der Selbstbeschränkung brauchen. In: Ströker E (Hrsg) Ethik der Wissenschaften? Philosophische Fragen. München, S 75ff.
Kirchberger S (1986 a) Medizinisch technische Assistenz in der Gesundheitsversorgung – Zur Berufsgeschichte der MTA. Frankfurt New York
Kirchberger S (1986 b) Technischer Fortschritt in der Medizin: Strukturen der Kostenentwicklung – Strukturen der Leistungserbringung. (Vortrag vor der Gesellschaft für Versicherungswissenschaft und -gestaltung e. V. Köln, Juni 1986). Schweiz Krankenkassenz, S 265ff., 285ff.
Kirchberger S (1988) Unkalkulierte Folgen mangelhafter Planung im Gesundheitswesen – Das Beispiel Nierenlithotripsie. Arbeit und Sozialpolitik 42:320 ff.
Kirchberger S (1991) The Diffusion of Two Technologies for Renal Stone Treatment: Lithotripsy and Percutaneous Nephrolithotomy. (EC Study on the Diffusion of Medical Technology in Europe), London
Lux G, Demling L (1983) 100 Jahre Gastroskopie. Fortschr Med 4:107ff.

Maxmen JS (1976) The postphysician era. Medicine in the twenty-first century. New York London
Mc Neil BJ, Cravalho E (1982) Critical issues in medical technology. Boston/MA
Pellegrino ED (1979) The anatomy of clinical judgements. Some notes on right reason and right action. In: Engelhaardt HT, Spicker S, Towers B (eds) Clinical judgement. A critical appraisal. Dordrecht, pp 169ff.
Prognos AG, (1977/78) Basel, Medizintechnik. – Vorarbeiten für ein Förderungsprogramm des BMFT, Bd I–IV. München
Rassweiler J, Miller K et al. (1985) Kosten und Nutzen der berührungsfreien Nierenstein-Lithotripsie. Lebensversicherungsmedizin 3:80ff.
Reiff G (1986) Gewinnt die Technik ein Übergewicht in der kurativen Medizin (Radiologie, Labormedizin, physikalische Medizin etc.)? Soz Sicherh Landwirtsch 2/3:129ff.
Reiser SJ (1978) Medicine and the reign of technology. Univ Press, Cambridge
Rettig RA (1981) Lessons learned from the end-stage renal disease experience. In: Egdahl R, Gertman P (eds) Technology and the quality of health care. Germantown, S 153ff.
Rinecker H (1981) Gallensteinleiden. Z Allg Med 57:2358ff.
Rosenbrock R (1986) AIDS kann schneller besiegt werden – Gesundheitspolitik am Beispiel einer Infektionskrankheit. Hamburg
Rothschuh KE (1978) Konzepte der Medizin in Vergangenheit und Gegenwart. Stuttgart
Sadegh-Zadeh K (1977) Grundlagenprobleme einer Theorie der klinischen Praxis – Teil 1: Explikation des medizinischen Diagnosebegriffs. Metamed 1:76ff.
Sauerbruch T, Delius M et al. (1986) Fragmentation of gallstones by extracorporeal shock waves. N Engl J Med 314/13:818ff.
Terpestra OT et al. (1987) An experimental study on shock-wave treatment of gallbladder stones. Rotterdam 15. 8. 87. unveröffentlichtes Manuskript
Vilmar K (1980) Medizinische Geräte – Prothesen ärztlichen Handelns? Dtsch Ärztebl 77/19:1249ff.

Weiterführende Literatur zum Thema
"Evaluationsforschung, Qualitätssicherung und Technologiebewertung"

Evaluationsforschung

Bengel J, Koch U (1988) Evaluationsforschung im Gesundheitswesen. In: Koch U, Lucius-Hoene G, Stegie R (Hrsg) Handbuch der Rehabilitationspsychologie. Springer, Berlin Heidelberg New York Tokyo, S 321–347

Kaluzny AD, Veney JE (1988) Evaluating health care programs and services. In: Williams SJ, Torrens PR (eds) Introduction to health services. Wiley, New York, pp 438–453

Schwartz FW (1990) Aufgaben und Schwerpunkte einer zeitgemäßen Evaluation im Gesundheitswesen. Öffentl. Gesundh.-Wes. 52, S 559–566

Wittmann WW (1985) Evaluationsforschung: Aufgabe, Probleme und Anwendungen. Springer, Berlin Heidelberg New York (Lehr- und Forschungstexte Psychologie; 13)

Qualitätssicherung

Sachverständigenrat für die Konzertierte Aktion im Gesundheitswesen (1989) Qualität, Wirtschaftlichkeit und Perspektiven der Gesundheitsversorgung: Vorschläge für die Konzertierte Aktion im Gesundheitswesen, Jahresgutachten 1989. Nomos, Baden-Baden

Schwartz FW, Selbmann H (Hrsg) Qualitätssicherung ärztlicher Leistungen. Deutscher Ärzte-Verlag, Köln (Wissenschaftliche Reihe des ZI; 20)

Selbmann H, Überla KK (Hrsg) (1982) Quality assessment of medical care. Bleicher, Gerlingen (Beiträge zur Gesundheitsökonomie; 15)

Selbmann H (Hrsg) (1984) Qualitätssicherung ärztlichen Handelns. Bleicher, Gerlingen (Beiträge zur Gesundheitsökonomie; 16)

Technologiebewertung

Int J Tech Ass Health Care (1989) 5/1

US Department of Health and Human Services (1989) National Center for Health Services Research and Health Care Technology Assessment (NCHSR) program note

7 Selbsthilfe- und Netzwerkforschung

Staat, intermediäre Instanzen und Selbsthilfe *

F.-X. Kaufmann

Als um die Mitte des 19. Jahrhunderts das Wort „Social-Politik" aufkam, stand es bereits begrifflich im Spannungsfeld der Unterscheidung von „Staat" und „Gesellschaft". Ebenso vielfältig wie die politischen Strömungen waren in der Folge auch die Ausdeutungen des Begriffs, doch blieb zumindest unterschwellig bei Praktikern wie Wissenschaftlern der Sozialpolitik ein Vorverständnis erhalten, das Sozialpolitik nicht ausschließlich in den Bereich des Staatlichen, sondern gerade in das umstrittene Spannungsfeld von Staat und Gesellschaft verweist. Dies gilt zumindest für die deutsche Tradition, die ja sowohl in begrifflicher wie politischer Hinsicht den historischen Primat beanspruchen kann.

Im Vergleich zu anderen Politikbereichen zeichnet sich die Struktur der Sozialpolitik durch das Vorherrschen von Akteuren aus, die weder dem Staat im engeren Sinne noch dem Bereich privater Organisationen wie Wirtschaftsunternehmungen oder Vereinen zuzurechnen sind. Sie haben teils einen öffentlich-rechtlichen Status, wie die Sozialversicherungen oder Kammern, und sind teils privatrechtlich organisiert, wie die Gewerkschaften, Unternehmerverbände und Wohlfahrtsverbände. Wir bezeichnen sie daher in Anlehnung an den älteren Begriff „corps intermédiaires" (Montesquieu) als intermediäre Instanzen. Viele von ihnen haben Vorläufer, die die sozialpolitische Theorie des 19. Jahrhunderts unter dem Begriff der Selbsthilfe faßte, welche neben der Staatshilfe zum akzeptierten Bestand der „socialen Politik" gezählt wurde. [1]

In den letzten Jahren hat der Begriff Selbsthilfe erneut an sozialpolitischem Gewicht gewonnen, und zwar in einem durchaus verwandten, aber nicht identischen Sinn. Selbsthilfe ist für viele zu einem Programm alternativer Sozialpolitik geworden, einem Programm, das die Nachteile und Defizite staatlicher Sozialpolitik zu kompensieren oder diese in Teilen gar zu ersetzen beansprucht. Ohne an dieser Stelle auf die Vielfalt der Wortverwendung und die Dimensionen der Be-

---

* Erstmals veröffentlicht in: Kaufmann FX (Hrsg) (1987) Staat, intermediäre Instanzen und Selbsthilfe: Bedingungsanalysen sozialpolitischer Intervention (Soziologie und Sozialpolitik Bd. 7). Oldenbourg, München, S. 9–38 (Auszug).

[1] Vgl. Pankoke E (1970) Sociale Bewegung – sociale Frage – sociale Politik. Grundfragen der deutschen Socialwissenschaft im 19. Jahrhundert. Stuttgart; Pankoke E (1983) Geschichtliche Grundlagen und gesellschaftliche Entwicklung moderner Sozialpolitik. In: Schäfers B (Hrsg) Sozialpolitik in der Bundesrepublik. Gegenwartskunde, Sonderheft 4. Opladen, S 23–40

grifflichkeit einzugehen[2], können wir die Grundgedanken der mit Worten wie „Selbsthilfe", „Selbstorganisation", „soziale Aktion", „sozialaktive Felder", „Bürgerinitiativen im sozialen Raum", „informeller Sektor" oder „nichtprofessionelle Sozialsysteme" angesprochenen Phänomene dahingehend zusammenfassen, daß zwischen den Phänomenen individueller „Eigenhilfe" und staatlich oder intermediär organisierter „Fremdhilfe" ein breites Feld interaktiv gesteuerter Formen des Beistands, der Wohlfahrtsproduktion und der Interessenvertretung, kurzum: von sozialpolitisch relevanten Aktivitäten aufzuweisen ist, die im Rahmen der überwiegend staatsorientierten theoretischen Reflexionen der jüngeren Sozialpolitiklehre und auch des auf den intermediären Bereich zentrierten praktischen Sozialpolitikverständnisses zu Unrecht vernachlässigt worden sind.

Diese theoretische Rethematisierung von Selbsthilfe als Ressource oder Medium sozialpolitischer Aktivität erfolgte selbst im Horizont der Entstehung einer sich verbreiternden Selbsthilfebewegung, deren Entstehungsbedingungen noch wenig geklärt sind, aber mit Stichworten wie Scheitern einer Politik der inneren Reform, zunehmende Arbeitslosigkeit, Staats- und Fortschrittsverdruß sowie alternative Lebensstile in etwa angedeutet werden können. Wie so häufig, läuft auch hier die Karriere eines sozialwissenschaftlichen Themas mit Bewegungen des Zeitgeistes parallel, was allerdings keinen stichhaltigen Einwand gegen die wissenschaftliche Fruchtbarkeit des Themas bedeutet. Vielmehr haben v. a. Badura et al. in der Einleitung zum 1. Band dieser Schriftenreihe (Soziologie und Sozialpolitik) die Relevanz der Thematik zur Fortentwicklung sozialpolitischer Theorie überzeugend dargestellt.[3]

---

[2] Vgl. hierzu insbesondere Badelt C (1980) Sozioökonomie der Selbstorganisation. Frankfurt New York, S 29–47; Hegner F (1981) Zur Systematisierung nicht-professioneller Sozialsysteme. In: Badura B, Ferber C von (Hrsg) Selbsthilfe und Selbstorganisation im Gesundheitswesen. München Wien, S 219–253, Hegner F (1985) Öffentliche Förderung von Selbsthilfe und Selbstorganisation. In: Keim KD, Vaskovics LA (Hrsg) Wege zur Sozialplanung. Opladen, S 156–181; Behrendt JU et al. (1983) Arbeitsweise von Gesundheitsselbsthilfegruppen und Anregung zu ihrer sozialpolitischen Unterstützung. In: Ferber C von, Badura B (Hrsg) Laienpotential, Patientenaktivierung und Gesundheitsselbsthilfe München Wien, S 9–33; Vilmar F, Runge B (1986) Auf dem Weg zur Selbsthilfegesellschaft? Fulda, S 11–26.

[3] Vgl. Badura B, Ferber C von, Krüger J, Riedmüller B, Thiemeyer T, Trojan A (1981) Einleitung: Sozialpolitische Perspektiven. In: Badura B, Ferber C von (Hrsg) Selbsthilfe und Selbstorganisation im Gesundheitswesen. München S 1–38.

Ergebnisse und Erfahrungen aus dem Forschungsverbund „Laienpotential, Patientenaktivierung und Gesundheitsselbsthilfe"*

C. von Ferber

Zur Überraschung vieler Gesundheits- und Sozialpolitiker hat die Gesundheitsselbsthilfe an praktischer Bedeutung für die Krankenhilfe gewonnen und – denken wir an die Selbsthilfegruppen – politische Aufmerksamkeit zu einem Zeitpunkt gefunden, zu dem in der Bundesrepublik Deutschland wie in vergleichbaren Ländern ein hoher Stand der medizinischen Versorgung erreicht ist. Die ausreichende Abdeckung der Hilfen, deren kranke und behinderte Menschen bedürfen, um in akuten Krankheitsphasen zurechtzukommen, aber auch um mit chronischer Krankheit und mit bleibenden Behinderungen so normal wie möglich leben zu können, wurde offenbar mit dem sozialstaatlichen Ausbau eines medizinischen und sozialen Dienstleistungssystems nicht erreicht. Ja, es werden zunehmend Zweifel angemeldet, ob das angestrebte Ziel auf dem eingeschlagenen Wege über beruflich-entgeltliche Dienstleistungen selbst unter sozialstaatlicher Organisation und Finanzierung überhaupt erreichbar ist.

Um Fragen dieser Art, die für die Sozial- und Gesundheitspolitik von wegweisender Bedeutung sind, auf der Grundlage von Forschungsergebnissen beantworten zu können, ist zweierlei geboten:

1) Es müssen theoretische Konzepte erarbeitet werden, unter denen der Hilfebedarf infolge Krankheit oder Behinderung auch *unabhängig* von der Inanspruchnahme professioneller Krankenhilfen dargestellt und – auf diesen angebotsunabhängigen Bedarf bezogen – unter denen das System der Krankenhilfe, der professionellen wie der Selbsthilfe, in seinen funktionalen Bezügen entwickelt werden kann.
2) Es ist erforderlich, in enger Beziehung zur Entwicklung theoretischer Konzepte die empirische Forschung voranzutreiben, um die Theorieentwicklung ständig an der Wirklichkeit von Krankheit, Krankheitsfolgen und Krankenhilfe zu kontrollieren.

Ein solches Programm, eine „Epidemiologie" der benötigten Hilfen in Verbindung mit einer funktionalen Analyse der Hilfesysteme, kann im ersten Zugriff nur in der Zusammenarbeit mehrerer Forschergruppen, in einem Forschungsverbund also, und auch dann nur *exemplarisch* geleistet werden. Die folgenden Vorhabendarstellungen gründen sich auf eine mehrjährige Zusammenarbeit im Forschungsverbund „Laienpotential, Patientenaktivierung und Gesundheitsselbst-

---

* Erstmals veröffentlicht in: Ferber C von (Hrsg) (1988) Gesundheitsselbsthilfe – Stand der Forschung: Perspektiven der Forschungsförderung: sozialpolitische Implikationen (BPT-Bericht 12). Gesellschaft für Strahlen- und Umweltforschung, München, S. 23–27.

hilfe". Eine ausführliche Darstellung der Verbundprojekte wird im Anhang zum integrierten Abschlußbericht gegeben (Forschungsverbund Laienpotential 1987).

Problemlage

Gemeinhin wird der Bürger, der sog. Laie, als Teilnehmer am Gesundheitswesen nur in seinen Rollen als „Beitragszahler", als einer, der Ansprüche an die Professionellen stellt, sowie in den Phasen akuter Behandlung als „Patient" oder „Fall" gesehen und geht mit diesen stereotypen Rollen in Analysen/Modellrechnungen und Bedarfspläne ein. Gesundheitsbezogene Selbsthilfe wurde erst im Zuge der Diskussion um „Selbstbeteiligungsformen" einerseits und der Formulierung von Zielen einer „Gegenmedizin" andererseits zum Gegenstand politischen und wissenschaftlichen Interesses. Obwohl die nichtprofessionellen Hilfen und Krankheitsbewältigungsstrategien erst in neuester Zeit durch zunehmende Professionalisierung ihre ehedem überragende Versorgungsfunktion verloren haben, leisten sie vermutlich noch immer einen sehr hohen, „unsichtbaren" Beitrag zur Gesundheitsversorgung. Damit wird Selbstverantwortung und Bürgersinn deutlich, die staatlicher oder komunaler Planung und Reglementierung weitgehend entzogen zu sein scheinen.

Der Forschungsverbund „Laienpotential, Patientenaktivierung und Gesundheitsselbsthilfe" wurde aus gesundheits- und sozialpolitischen Überlegungen heraus gegründet, um den Wandel von einer anbieter- zu einer stärker am Konsumenten gesundheitlicher Leistungen orientierten Gesundheits- und Sozialpolitik zu untersuchen. Hierzu mußten die selbsterbrachten Leistungen der Bürger in Situationen schwerer Krankheit oder für einen besseren Schutz ihrer Gesundheit bestimmt werden, und es mußte begründet werden, warum und wie die Bürger zu der Bereitstellung gesundheitsrelevanter Leistungen in einem bisher unterschätzten Umfang beitragen.

Damit stand also grundlagenforschungsorientiertes Arbeiten im Vordergrund, da über das Laienpotential sowohl theoretisch wie empirisch kaum Wissen vorlag und damit jede Voraussetzung für Überlegungen etwa über Steuerbarkeit der Gesundheitsselbsthilfe fehlte.

Die Projektziele wurden dahingehend konkretisiert:

- Welcher Art sind die eigenerbrachten Leistungen der Bürger?
- Auf welchen gesellschaftlichen Voraussetzungen beruhen die eigenerbrachten Leistungen der Bürger?
- In welcher Weise beeinflußt ein hohes Niveau an professionellen Dienstleistungen – bei weiterhin expandierendem Angebot – Umfang und Richtung der eigenerbrachten Leistungen?
- Über die bekannten Sog- und Verdrängungseffekte hinaus sollen implizite Unterstellungen im Umgang mit den Eigenleistungen der Bürger aufgedeckt werden. Was wird den Bürgern zugemutet, ihnen nicht zugetraut, ihnen vorenthalten?
- Woher bezieht Laienhandeln seine Motivation?

Lösungsweg

Die Umsetzung anwendungsbezogener Fragestellungen auf einem so allgemein formulierten Erwartungshorizont und gleichzeitig in einem Verbund von Vorhaben machte eine Differenzierung in konkrete Einzelaufgaben und eine Auswahl von Themen mit Modellcharakter notwendig.

Die Aufgabenstellung des Forschungsverbundes im einzelnen geschah im Hinblick auf Zusammenhänge, innerhalb derer das gesundheitsbezogene Laienhandeln gegenwärtig als wichtig, weil gesundheitspolitisch beispielhaft, oder als problematisch, weil gefährdet, oder aus gesundheitspolitischen Erwägungen heraus positiv eingeschätzt wird. Jedes Vorhaben sollte ein praktisch relevantes Thema bearbeiten. Die Spannweite der im Verbund bearbeiteten Themen umfaßte:

- Selbsthilfe im Gesundheitswesen,
- Gesundheitsselbsthilfegruppen (Arbeitsweise und Anregungen zu ihrer sozialpolitischen Unterstützung),
- Longitudinalstudie zur Herzinfarktrehabilitation (soziale Unterstützung bei chronischer Krankheit),
- patientenorientierte Intensivtherapie und medizinische Technologie,
- Gesundheitsvorsorge am Arbeitsplatz (gesundheitsgerechte Arbeitsgestaltung),
- gemeindebezogene Gesundheitsvorsorge (Förderung des Gesundheitsverhaltens).

Ungeachtet der Originalität ihrer Fragestellungen und der damit verbundenen Eigenständigkeit der Verbundvorhaben waren diese in wesentlichen Fragen miteinander verknüpft. Dieser Zusammenhang ergibt sich unter soziologischer Perspektive aus der Struktur des „Gesundheitsbezogenen Laienhandelns".

Ergebnisse

Die Ergebnisse der empirischen Forschung verschiedener „Kontexte" des gesundheitsbezogenen Laienhandelns erzwingen als Ergebnis des Projekts teilweise eine theoretische Neuorientierung der soziologischen Erklärungsansätze. So hat sich gezeigt, daß der herkömmliche Selbsthilfebegriff zu eng ist, um der Bedeutung der eigenerbrachten Leistungen für das Niveau der Gesundheitsversorgung gerecht zu werden. Der Selbsthilfebegriff ist durch kontroverse ordnungspolitische Diskussionen mit Unklarheiten befrachtet und verführt zu einem falschen dichotomen Vorverständnis: hier Selbsthilfe, da professionelle Dienstleistungen. So zeigt beispielsweise die Analyse der Situation in der Intensivpflege, daß selbst unter maximalem Einsatz professioneller Dienstleistungen von den Angehörigen wesentliche Hilfen für den Kranken erbracht werden, die außerhalb der Reichweite professioneller Hilfemöglichkeiten liegen.

Das Projektergebnis bestätigt, daß die eigenerbrachten Leistungen der Bürger zur Erhaltung und Wiederherstellung ihrer Gesundheit im Vorfeld wie in Verbindung mit einer Inanspruchnahme medizinischer und sozialer Dienstleistungen wesentlich zum Niveau der Gesundheitssicherung beitragen.

Gesundheitsbezogenes Laienhandeln organisiert sich anlaß- und situationsbezogen sowie personengebunden; unter versorgungspolitischen Anforderungen gesehen ist es stets mangel- und lückenhaft. Es kann keine flächendeckende Versorgungsaufgabe übernehmen. Es entfaltet sich in Bereichen, die den professionellen Dienstleistungen verschlossen (psychosoziale Unterstützung) oder ihnen schwer zugänglich sind (Pflege). Gesundheitsbezogenes Laienhandeln hat seine Domäne, in der es durch professionelle Dienstleistungen nicht ersetzt werden kann. Es ist die erste Ressource, die die Bürger befähigt, selbst ihre Situation zu meistern, und auch ihre letzte Zuflucht. Beides macht das gesundheitsbezogene Laienhandeln zu einem unersetzlichen Element der gesellschaftlichen Gesundheitssicherung. Es steht jedoch unter dem Risiko unzulänglicher Erfahrung, mangelnden Könnens und der Selbstüberforderung. Zusammengefaßt zeichnen sich folgende wesentliche Ergebnisse ab:

a) Die empirischen Befunde widersprechen individualistischen Ausdeutungen von „gesundheitlichem Fehlverhalten" und Vorschlägen, die das Individuum mit einem Bonus-Malus-System zu einer gesundheitsgerechten Lebensweise hin sanktionieren wollen.

b) Gesundheitsbezogenes Laienhandeln ist versorgungspolitisch bedeutsam. Das Niveau der Behandlung von Krankheiten ebenso wie der Schutz vor Gesundheitsgefahren und -risiken, die persönliche und soziale Verarbeitung von chronischer Krankheit und bleibender Behinderung hängt auch von den Erfahrungen, der Kompetenz und der Hilfsbereitschaft der Bürger ab.

c) Gesundheitsbezogenes Laienhandeln läßt sich versorgungspolitisch nicht „dienstverpflichten", es organisiert sich nach anderen gesellschaftlichen Prinzipien als professionelles Handeln.

d) Gesundheitsbezogenes Laienhandeln läßt sich, wenn überhaupt, nur in Grenzen durch professionelle Dienstleistungen ersetzen. Es gehört versorgungspolitisch zu den gesellschaftlichen Ressourcen, die nicht „machbar" sind, sondern mit politischen Mitteln erhalten, geschützt, gefördert werden sollten.

e) Gesundheitsbezogenes Laienhandeln wird diskussions-, verhandlungs- und konfliktfähig in den Zusammenschlüssen der Bürger in Selbsthilfegruppen. Die Gesundheitsselbsthilfegruppen stehen für das gesundheitsbezogene Laienhandeln in der Gesellschaft allgemein, wobei diese gesundheitspolitisch mehr vertreten, als an ihren eingeschriebenen Mitgliedern abzulesen ist.

f) Die Perspektive der Betroffenheit und des Mithandelns in der Prävention, in der Akutbehandlung und in der Rehabilitation werden exemplarisch dargestellt 1) in der Situation der Patienten auf Intensivstationen, 2) in der Situation der Herzinfarktpatienten während der programmierten Herzinfarktrehabilitation, 3) in der Situation des Arbeiters, der am Arbeitsplatz nicht nur seine Leistung erbringt, sondern auch seine Gesundheit riskiert, 4) in der Situation des Bürgers, der sich von den in seiner Gemeinde tätigen Einrichtungen eine Förderung gesundheitsgerechter Lebensweise erwartet. Im Argumentationszusammenhang bürgerorientierter Gesundheitspolitik verdeutlichen die 4 Untersuchungen, gerade weil sie ganz verschiedene Situationen im Angebot medizinischer und sozialer Dienstleistungen vorstellen, die Mängel, aber auch die Chancen in der Aktivierung der Patienten, Rehabilitanden, Beschäftigten bzw. Bürger.

In allen 4 untersuchten Bereichen des Versorgungssystems sind wesentliche Verbesserungen in der Qualität der gesundheitlichen Versorgung zu erwarten, wenn Selbsthilfepotentiale besser zum Einsatz kommen können.

Umsetzung

Für eine bürgerorientierte Gesundheitspolitik werden 3 Aktionsrichtungen vorgeschlagen:

- Förderung der Ressourcen der Gesundheitsselbsthilfe im Familienhaushalt: Vermittlung von Kompetenz in Krankheitssituationen und in Gesundheitsfragen, entlastende Hilfe in andauernden und schweren Pflegesituationen,
- Förderung der Gesundheitsselbsthilfegruppen, der Selbsthilfebewegung sowie
- Förderung der Patienten- und Bürgerorientierung in der Organisation medizinischer und sozialer Dienstleistungen sowie unter den Gesundheits- und Sozialberufen.

Hierzu werden jeweils spezifische Vorschläge gemacht. Wenn richtig ist, daß der erreichbare Standard der Vorsorge gegen Gesundheitsgefahren, daß die Bewältigung von Krankheiten und Krankheitsfolgen sowie die Teilhabe von Kranken und Behinderten an einem „normalen" Lebensalltag (die von der Rehabilitation geforderte Integration in Arbeit, Beruf und Gesellschaft) auch von den Eigenleistungen der Bürger abhängt, sollte Gesundheitspolitik nicht nur Gesundheitsgefahren verringern, sondern sie muß bestrebt sein, die Ressourcen der Selbsthilfe in gleichem Maße zu fördern wie das Angebot an professionellen Gesundheitsleistungen. Hierzu gehören:

- Gesundheitserziehung in Schulen, Weiterbildungsangebote in der Erwachsenenbildung, Patientenorientierung in der Ausbildung der Gesundheitsberufe sowie
- die Entwicklung einer gemeindenahen Infrastruktur für beratende, entlastende und unterstützende Gesundheitshilfen, für den Erfahrungsaustausch und für die Förderung von Selbsthilfezusammenschlüssen.

Im Ergebnis wird gefordert, daß die Gesundheitspolitik durch gesetzliche Rahmenbestimmungen der Gesundheitsselbsthilfe mehr öffentlichen Handlungsspielraum, z.B. in der kommunalen Gesundheits- und Sozialpolitik, einräumt, wie es eine sozialleistungs- und anbieterorientierte Gesundheits- und Sozialpolitik seit jeher für die Sozialleistungsträger getan hat.

Eine bürgerorientierte Gesundheitspolitik bedeutet keine ausschließende Alternative zu einer anbieterorientierten Sozialleistungspolitik, kann aber das Qualitätsniveau gesundheitlicher Versorgung heben. Sie kann aber kaum das Kostenniveau der professionellen Versorgung verringern oder die Kostenentwicklung dämpfen.

Daher kann sie es der anbieterorientierten Sozialleistungspolitik nicht abnehmen, Prioritäten zu setzen, die Effektivität der beruflich-entgeltlichen Dienstleistungen zu verbessern, deren Effizienz zu erhöhen sowie die Qualität der erbrachten Leistungen sicherzustellen. Sie ist kein Ersatz für Strukturreformen des Gesundheitswesens, wohl aber kann sie solche Strukturreformen legitimieren und durchsetzen helfen.

In teilweiser Fortführung des oben beschriebenen Projekts wird derzeit die Aktivierung von Laien durch Mediatoren in einer gemeindebezogenen Netzwerkförderung durchgeführt und dieses Bemühen begleitend evaluiert.

Weiterhin wird für eine Gruppe von Rehabilitanden und ihre Familienangehörigen der Ansatz des oben genannten Projektes fortgeführt, um für diese Langzeiterkrankten den Bewältigungsprozeß und seine Anforderungen und Unterstützungsmöglichkeiten auch langzeitlich zu untersuchen.

Gesundheitsförderung durch Selbsthilfegruppen, freie Einrichtungen, Vereine und Initiativen *

A. Trojan, C. Deneke, M. Faltis, H. Hildebrandt

An welchen Elementen der *sozialen Struktur* läßt sich anknüpfen, wenn man Gesundheitsförderung betreiben will? Wer tut schon etwas? Wer ist geeignet, solche Inhalte aufzugreifen und in Aktivitäten umzusetzen?

So wie bei der Versorgung im Krankheitsfall verschiedene „Systeme" helfen, gibt es auch für die Förderung von Gesundheit unterschiedliche Strukturen und soziale Ebenen, die hier eingreifen können. Unsere Studie konzentriert sich auf die Untersuchung einer vermittelnden („intermediären") Ebene, deren Kern im Amerikanischen als "community organizations" oder auch als "social networks" bezeichnet wird (z. B. Keupp u. Röhrle 1987). Damit sind v. a. eigenständige und im weitesten Sinn freigemeinnützige Selbsthilfegruppen, Vereine, Initiativen und Organisationen gemeint. Außerdem rechnen wir auch die aus ihnen entstandenen Einrichtungen, etwa Beratungsstellen, Bildungs- und Kultureinrichtungen hinzu, soweit sie nicht kommerziell oder staatlich betrieben werden.

Soziale Unterstützung, soziale Aktionen, Stärkung von Selbsthilfe- und Durchsetzungsfähigkeit

Unter zwei Gesichtspunkten ist dieser Bereich sozialer Netzwerke und ihrer Einrichtungen (in der Ökonomie auch als Teil des „3. Sektors" bezeichnet) von Bedeutung für die Gesundheit:

1. Soziale Unterstützung. Vereine, Selbsthilfegruppen und ähnliche Organisationen gerieten in den letzten Jahren zunehmend in das Blickfeld der Forschung, weil sie eine mögliche Quelle „sozialer Unterstützung für den einzelnen" darstellen können. Sie können zur Bewältigung von Alltagskrisen, Konflikten oder chronischen Belastungen beitragen. In solchen sozialen Netzwerken kann Erfahrungsaustausch stattfinden, können Tips gegeben werden, wo kompetente fachliche Hilfe zu finden ist, hier kann man sich evtl. aussprechen, Zuwendung, Mitgefühl und Geborgenheit finden. Die steigende Zahl an Einpersonenhaushalten in den bundesrepublikanischen Großstädten gibt für die Vermutung Anlaß, daß ein wachsender Bedarf an solchen Unterstützungen besteht.

Verschiedene großangelegte Untersuchungen konnten nachweisen, daß Personen mit geringen sozialen Beziehungen ein 2- bis 3mal so hohes Sterberisiko haben wie Personen mit intensiven sozialen Kontakten (z. B. Berkman u. Syme

---

* Erstmals veröffentlicht in: Bundesvereinigung für Gesundheitserziehung e. V. (1988) Gesundheit für alle – alles für die Gesundheit. Bonn, S. 189–198 (Auszug).

1979). Aus den Ergebnissen dieser Studien resultiert die Forderung nach „Netzwerkförderung" als Ergänzung anderer präventiver Strategien.

2. Soziale Aktionen und Stärkung von Selbsthilfe- und Durchsetzungsfähigkeit. Das leider weitgehend festzustellende Versagen staatlicher Prävention bzw. Gesundheitsförderung („von oben") lenkt jedoch noch auf einen weiteren positiven Aspekt bei organisierten Netzwerken auf lokaler Ebene sowie ihren Einrichtungen: Die Beseitigung von krankmachenden Faktoren in der Arbeitswelt und im Umweltbereich wird ganz offensichtlich von den bisherigen Instanzen allein nicht geschafft, Anstöße von außen sind dazu immer wieder nötig. Damit tatsächlich etwas gegen die mächtigen, dem Gesundheitsschutz entgegengesetzten Interessen unternommen wird, bedarf es meist erst einer breiten Mobilisierung der Bevölkerung. Träger einer solchen Mobilisierung und Aktivierung, z. B. für Umweltschutz und gegen krankmachende Arbeits- und Lebensbedingungen, sind vielfältige informelle oder (in den Gewerkschaften) auch formellere lokale Gruppen.

Solche organisierten Netzwerke, die sich einer bestimmten Aufgabe oder bestimmten Zielen verschrieben haben, können in zweierlei Hinsicht gesundheitsfördernd wirksam werden. Zum einen durch erfolgreiche Aktionen selber, z. B. durch erreichte Verkehrsberuhigung oder das aufgrund ihrer Aktivitäten erreichte Verbot bestimmter Schadstoffe.

Beispiel:

Tempo 30 in der Stadt senkt die Zahl von Unfällen mit Verletzten erheblich, teilweise um mehr als 50%.

Dieses Forschungsergebnis gibt all den Initiativen recht, die sich aktiv für Verkehrsberuhigung einsetzen. Die Prognose von Tempo-30-Gegnern, Lärm und Auspuffgase würden in den betreffenden Vierteln zunehmen, hat sich als „Schall und Rauch" erwiesen, „eher im Gegenteil" (zit. nach *Spiegel* 1985, 40:98).

Zum anderen können Menschen in organisierten Netzwerken positive Erfahrungen machen und sich dadurch verändern: Das Gefühl, ohnmächtig den Ergebnissen der Entscheidungen anderer ausgesetzt zu sein, sich nicht mehr wehren zu können und seine Lebens- und Arbeitsbedingungen nicht verändern zu können, erzeugt Resignation, „erlernte Hilflosigkeit" und ist ein wichtiger Faktor in der Entstehung von Krankheiten, insbesondere psychosomatischer Natur. Die Stärkung von Selbsthilfe- und Handlungsfähigkeit, die soziale Aktivierung und die evtl. gemachte Erfahrung, vielleicht doch nicht „denen da oben" ausgeliefert zu sein, könnte eine ganz entscheidende Gesundheitsbedeutung für die Aktiven in solchen Gruppen, aber auch für das Umfeld haben.

Bürgerinitiativen, Vereine, alternative Projekte, Stadtteilzentren und andere Einrichtungen sind insofern eine *Infrastruktur für gesundheitsrelevante soziale Reformen und Innovation* und können dem einzelnen Möglichkeiten des Engagements und der Verbesserung der eigenen Lebens- und Arbeitsbedingungen bieten.

Zwischen „oben" und „unten" vermittelnde Ebenen („intermediäre Instanzen", wie sie gelegentlich genannt werden) entfalten zwar offensichtlich viele Möglichkeiten, sind aber selber auch einem ganz schönen Streß ausgesetzt. Es stellen sich die Fragen: Sind sie überhaupt den Anforderungen gewachsen, oder würden sie bei einer Übernahme von weiteren Aufgaben zusammenbrechen? Kann man davon ausgehen, daß Vereine, Initiativen u. ä. sich weitgehend selber

„reproduzieren", daß sie die Gründung von eigenständigen Gruppen fördern? Wo brauchen sie selber Unterstützung, welche Formen der Kooperation wünschen sie sich?

Hamburger Befragung von freien Einrichtungen, Vereinen und Initiativen

Nachdem wir früher speziell den Bereich der Selbsthilfegruppen untersucht hatten (Dobler et al. 1984; Trojan 1986), haben wir in einer Studie mit dem Titel „Gemeindebezogene Netzwerkförderung" (aus Mitteln des BMFT) freie Einrichtungen, Vereine und Initiativen hinsichtlich ihrer gesundheitsförderlichen Aktivitäten befragt. Bei der Suche nach Adressen wurde uns sehr schnell deutlich, daß wir nicht alle an und für sich in Frage kommenden Gruppen und Einrichtungen „jenseits von Markt und Staat" anschreiben konnten, dazu hätten weder die Zeit noch die Arbeitskraft gereicht. Einige Bereiche sind daher nicht in unserer Studie repräsentiert: Sport und Betriebssport, Stiftungen, Kleingartenvereine, private Schulen, Wohnheime und Einrichtungen der therapeutischen Versorgung sowie Berufsorganisationen wurden – aus unterschiedlichen Gründen – nicht in der Befragung berücksichtigt.

Mit einem schriftlichen Fragebogen wandten wir uns zwischen Mai und August 1986 an ca. 1 700 Adressen von Hamburger Vereinen, Initiativen und Einrichtungen. Die Adressen hatten wir in einer mühsamen Suche aus Tageszeitungen, Telefonbüchern und anderen öffentlich zugänglichen Adressenkarteien zusammengestellt. Die Kriterien, nichtstaatlich, nichtkommerziell, für jeden zugänglich und auf Dauer angelegt zu sein, erfüllten 1 163 der Gruppen. Von diesen haben 473 den umfangreichen Fragebogen ausgefüllt (entspricht 40 %).

Aus einem Vergleich der angeschriebenen und der antwortenden Vereine/Initiativen/Einrichtungen geht hervor, daß die Antworter das Spektrum der Angeschriebenen in etwa repräsentieren; nur der soziale Bereich ist leicht überrepräsentiert.

Wer hat geantwortet?

- $^2/_3$ der Einrichtungen und Initiativen wurden nach 1970 gegründet, 18 % zwischen 1945 und 1969;
- 4 von 10 arbeiten stadtteil- oder bezirksbezogen,
  2 von 10 nennen das Stadtgebiet als Wirkungsbereich,
  3 von 10 beziehen auch das Hamburger Umland mit ein;
- 2 von 10 richten ihre Arbeit hauptsächlich auf Kinder und Jugendliche,
  1 von 10 auf Behinderte, Kranke oder Abhängige,
  jeweils 3–7 % nennen alte Menschen, Ausländer, Familien, Erwerbslose oder Frauen;
- 4 von 10 Einrichtungen nennen keine spezifischen Hauptzielgruppen, sondern wollen entweder die Öffentlichkeit allgemein oder eine Vielzahl von Zielgruppen erreichen;

- in $^3/_4$ der Einrichtungen haben die Nutzer bzw. Teilnehmer Einflußmöglichkeiten bei Planung und/oder Durchführung der Arbeit,
- $^2/_3$ stehen einer oder mehreren sozialen Bewegungen nahe, wie Selbsthilfebewegung (24 %), Bürgerinitiativ-, Gesundheits-, Friedens- und Ökologiebewe-
  gung (je 15–17 %), Frauen-, Alternativ-, Jugend- und Menschenrechtsbewe-
  gung (je 11–13 %);
- 4 von 10 verstehen sich als Einrichtung zur Hilfe für andere (Beratung, Bildung, Betreuung, Versorgung), $^1/_4$ als Interessenvertretung;
  $^1/_5$ als Selbsthilfezusammenschluß;
- 3 von 10 verstehen sich als Kultur- oder Freizeiteinrichtung, nur 7% spezifisch als Gesundheitsinitiative oder -einrichtung;
- fast alle (97 %) wenden Arbeitsformen der sozialen Unterstützung an (am
  häufigsten Beratung oder Aufklärung von Einzelpersonen);
- 8 von 10 nennen auch Arbeitsformen der Sozialen Aktion (am häufigsten Öffentlichkeitsarbeit).

Soziale Unterstützung, die den einzelnen hilft, gesundheitsgefährdende Belastungen zu verringern oder abzupuffern

Soziale Unterstützung wird von fast allen befragten Einrichtungen und Initiativen angestrebt, knapp 9 von 10 Antworten streben mindestens ein Ziel sozialer
Unterstützung (von 10 möglichen, die von uns vorgegeben waren) an. Die meisten geben gleich mehrere unterschiedliche Aspekte sozialer Unterstützung an,
die sie mit ihrer Arbeit anstreben. Um einen Eindruck zu erhalten, inwiefern sie
dies auch tatsächlich umsetzen, haben wir sie zusätzlich gefragt, wie gut sie diese
Ziele jeweils erreichen. Zwischen einem Drittel und der Hälfte der Gruppen erreichen diese Ziele – nach ihrer eigenen Einschätzung – gut bzw. sehr gut, ein deutlicher Hinweis auf die geleistete Unterstützung durch diesen Bereich.

Soziale Aktionen für „mehr Gesundheit" und Aktivierung zu Selbsthilfe und Durchsetzungsfähigkeit

Bestimmte gesundheitsbezogene Ziele werden von vielen Einrichtungen gleichzeitig angestrebt. So geben 30 % an, daß sie mit ihrer Arbeit gesündere Umweltbedingungen schaffen wollen (und dies sind nur diejenigen, bei denen diese Arbeit
einen mittleren bis sehr großen Anteil an ihren Gesamtaktivitäten einnimmt). Die
Arbeit für eine gesündere Umwelt reicht also weit über den Bereich derer hinaus,
die sich als Initiativen oder Organisationen in dem Handlungsbereich Umwelt-/
Naturschutz eingeordnet haben (5 %).
     Ähnlich, wenn auch in geringerem Maße, bei der Schaffung gesünderer Ar-
beitsbedingungen: 20 % geben dies als Ziel mit einem mittleren bis hohen Anteil
ihrer Arbeit an, als Haupttätigkeitsfeld hatten dies ebenfalls nur 5 % notiert.
     Allgemein für die Entwicklung gesünderer Lebens- und Arbeitsbedingungen
engagieren sich sogar 4 von 10 mit einem mittleren bis hohen Anteil an ihren Gesamtaktivitäten. Hier können Überlegungen anknüpfen, inwiefern sich mit vielen

Tabelle 1. Zielsetzungen im Bereich sozialer Unterstützung (n = 473)

Wir wollen mit unserer Arbeit:	Ja [%]	Davon: wir erreichen dies gut/sehr gut [%]
– Entlastung durch Gespräche ermöglichen	68	57
– Menschen in Not Zuwendung, Verständnis und Mitgefühl entgegenbringen	63	56
– beim Umgang mit persönlichen Krisen, Krankheiten oder Problemen durch Informationen bzw. Ratschläge helfen	60	49
– über gesellschaftliche Bedingungen von Krankheit oder Gesundheitsbedrohungen und was man dagegen tun kann, informieren	52	35
– durch Kurse und Beratung lebenspraktische Fähigkeiten vermitteln	51	50
– zur Selbstfindung von Menschen beitragen, die „aus der Bahn geworfen sind"	51	38
– anderen Menschen bei für sie schwierigen Aufgaben helfen (z. B. beim Ausfüllen von Formularen)	43	48
– anderen Menschen zu Geld oder Sachleistungen verhelfen (z. B. Kleidung, Unterkunft, Einrichtungsgegenstände)	33	41

dieser Gruppen zu bestimmten einzelnen Themen „Bündnisse" oder „Reformkoalitionen" schließen ließen. Die Bereitschaft dazu und ein gemeinsames Interesse scheinen jedenfalls durchaus vorhanden zu sein.

Die Aktivierung von Betroffenen oder der Bevölkerung allgemein ist ebenfalls ein weite Teile der Befragten bestimmendes Leitmotiv.

– Jeweils fast $^2/_3$ versuchen, das Selbstwertgefühl sowie die Handlungs- und Durchsetzungsfähigkeit Betroffener zu stärken.

- 50 % versuchen, den Zusammenschluß Betroffener zur besseren Interessenvertretung zu fördern.
- Etwa $^1/_3$ versucht, die Bürger zu mehr Mitwirkung in Politik und Gesellschaft zu aktivieren.

Für uns sind diese Angaben ein wichtiges Anzeichen, daß in dem von uns befragten Bereich auf das Selbständigwerden, die Eigenaktivität und Handlungsfähigkeit der Rat- oder Hilfesuchenden bzw. Mitbetroffenen großer Wert gelegt wird.

Gesundheitsziele und -verständnis

Interessante Antworten erhielten wir zu der Frage nach der Bedeutung von Gesundheitszielen in ihrer jeweiligen Arbeit. Insgesamt $^2/_3$ sagen, daß Gesundheit für sie ein Haupt- oder Nebenziel ihrer Arbeit ist, und sogar $^2/_3$ sehen gesundheitliche Auswirkungen ihrer Aktivitäten für die Nutzer ihrer Einrichtung. In den letzten Jahren ist diese Bedeutung bei 3 von 10 Antwortern gestiegen, möglicherweise war die Atomkatastrophe in Tschernobyl daran nicht ganz unbeteiligt (die Befragung erfolgte gerade kurz nach dem Unglück).
Die bisherige Auswertung der Fragen zum Gesundheitsverständnis ergab:

- 4 von 10 wollen „zu mehr gesundheitsgerechtem Verhalten erziehen".
- Mehr als 3 von 10 wollen ein „gesünderes Verständnis von Körper und Sinnlichkeit vermitteln", die gleiche Zahl will auch „ein ganzheitlicheres Gesundheitsverständnis entwickeln".
- 3 von 10 wollen „die gesundheitliche und soziale Versorgung verbessern".
- 5 von 10 würden gern zusätzliche gesundheitsfördernde Aktivitäten durchführen, sofern ihnen genügend Zeit und Mittel zur Verfügung stünden.

Aufhebung von Anonymität und Vereinzelung, Unterstützung und Gründung neuer Beziehungsgeflechte

Fast $^2/_3$ der Einrichtungen beabsichtigen mit ihrer Arbeit die Stärkung bzw. Förderung persönlicher Netzwerke, etwa, indem sie durch die Organisation von Festen zu mehr Kontaktmöglichkeiten in der Nachbarschaft beitragen oder indem sie durch das Zusammenbringen von Menschen Freundschaften und gegenseitige Hilfen ermöglichen.
Die Anregung und Unterstützung neuer Netzwerke/Gruppen haben sich $^3/_4$ aller Einrichtungen zum Ziel gesetzt. Tatsächlich entstanden sind verständlicherweise weniger Gruppen, immerhin aber trotzdem in einem bemerkenswert hohen Ausmaß, nämlich bei 6 von 10 Befragten.
Für den Außenstehenden besonders interessant ist die deutliche Unterstützung, die die befragten Gruppen anderen, von ihnen unabhängig bestehenden, gewähren. Fast $^2/_3$ geben dies in der Befragung an, am häufigsten gewähren sie Unterstützung in Form von inhaltlicher Beratung, dicht gefolgt von der Überlassung von Räumen.

Weil die Abwehr sozialer Vereinsamung wegen steigender Anzahl von Einpersonenhaushalten, der Auflösung der Großfamilie, erhöhter beruflicher und sozialer Mobilität und ähnlichen Entwicklungen immer wichtiger wird, kann man die gesellschaftspolitische Bedeutung der „Netzwerkförderung" durch die von uns befragten Gruppen gar nicht hoch genug einschätzen. Wenn man überdies davon ausgeht, daß neu entstehende Gruppen bzw. „Netzwerke" ebenfalls soziale Unterstützung leisten und gesundheitsrelevante soziale Aktionen durchführen, dann läßt sich schließen, daß Gesundheitsförderung in dem befragten Bereich ein sich selbst verstärkender Prozeß ist. Unsere bisherigen Ergebnisse sprechen für diese Annahme.

Schlußfolgerungen und Ausblicke

Bei aller Vorsicht, die wir angesichts der Vorläufigkeit dieser ersten Auswertung für angebracht halten, läßt sich doch schon in der Tendenz festhalten, daß dem von uns befragten Bereich von Vereinen, Initiativen und freien Einrichtungen in Sachen Gesundheitsförderung ein zentraler Stellenwert zukommt. Aus den Antworten zu einigen Fragen, die wir gestellt haben, geht hervor, daß insgesamt etwa bei zwei Drittel der Einrichtungen und Initiativen Interesse besteht, Aktivitäten im Bereich Gesundheit auszuweiten und zu intensivieren.

Zur Ausweitung oder Intensivierung ihrer Aktivitäten wünschen sich:
- 69 % die Vermittlung von neuem „Gesundheitswissen" aus Forschung und Modellprojekten in den Initiativenbereich,
- 66 % die Einrichtung eines Forums für Erfahrungsaustausch bezüglich Gesundheit und sozialer Unterstützung,
- 63 % inhaltliche Anregungen für gesundheitsbezogene Aktivitäten.

Insgesamt wird aus den Ergebnissen deutlich, daß in den Vereinigungen des von uns angeschriebenen Bereichs schon jetzt vielfältige gesundheitsfördernde Aktivitäten stattfinden. Dennoch ist dies in starkem Maße weiter entwicklungs- und ausbaufähig, falls ausreichend Ressourcen bereitgestellt würden (vgl. Trojan et al. 1987). Die Ergebnisse der Befragung haben wir Ende 1986 auf einer Tagung mit den befragten Einrichtungen und Initiativen diskutiert und auf mögliche praktische Konsequenzen hin untersucht (vgl. Enkerts u. Schweigert 1988).

Nach Ende des Forschungsprojektes wollen wir Gesundheitsförderung durch freie Einrichtungen, Vereine und Initiativen stärken und unterstützen helfen (vgl. ausführlicher Hildebrandt u. Trojan 1987, S. 82 ff.). Dieses Projekt hat den Titel „Werkstatt Gesundheit" und ist inzwischen verwirklicht worden.

Literatur

Anderson R (1983) Health promotion: an overview. Paper prepared for the WHO, Copenhagen (dt. 1984 in: Europäische Monographien zur Forschung in Gesundheitserziehung, S 1–60 „Bundesministerium für Gesundheit und Umweltschutz, Wien)
Berkman L, Syme L (1979) Social networks, host resistance and mortality: a nine-year-follow up study of Alameda County Residents. Am J Epidem 109:186–104

Dobler M, Enkerts V, Kranich C, Trojan A (1984) Wünsche – Wissen – Widerstand. Selbsthilfegruppen diskutieren mit Politikern und Experten. Sozialwissenschaften und Gesundheit e. V., Hamburg. Zu beziehen über: Kontakt- und Informationsstelle für Selbsthilfegruppen, Gaußstr. 21, 2000 Hamburg 50

Enkerts V, Schweigert I (1989) Gesundheit ist mehr! Soziale Netzwerke für eine lebenswerte Zukunft. Ergebnisse, Hamburg

Hildebrandt H, Trojan A (Hrsg) (1987) Gesündere Städte – kommunale Gesundheitsförderung. Materialien und Ideen zum „Healthy Cities"-Projekt der Weltgesundheitsorganisation. Selbstverlag. Bestelladresse: H Neuland, Adenauerallee 45, 2 Hamburg 1

Keupp H, Röhrle B (Hrsg) (1987) Soziale Netzwerke. Campus, Frankfurt am Main

Ottawa-Charta (1987) In: Hildebrandt H, Trojan A (Hrsg) Gesündere Städte – kommunale Gesundheitsförderung. Materialien und Ideen zum "Healthy Cities"-Projekt der Weltgesundheitsorganisation. Selbstverlag

Trojan A (1986) Wissen ist Macht – Eigenständig durch Selbsthilfe in Gruppen. Fischer alternativ, Frankfurt

Trojan A, Hildebrandt H, Faltis M, Deneke C (1987) Selbsthilfe, Netzwerkforschung und Gesundheitsförderung. Grundlagen „gemeindebezogener Netzwerkförderung" als Präventionsstrategie. In: Keupp H, Röhrle B (Hrsg) Soziale Netzwerke. Campus, Frankfurt

Trojan A, Deneke C, Faltis M, Hildebrandt H (1987) Gesundheitsförderung im informellen Bereich. Gutachten für die Gesundheitsbehörde der Freien und Hansestadt Hamburg

Wenzel E (1984) Entwicklung eines Hessischen Programms zur Gesundheitsförderung Bericht. Klausurtagung des Hess. Ministers für Arbeit, Umwelt und Soziales. Schlangenbad, Frankfurt am Main

Weiterführende Literatur zum Thema
„Selbsthilfe- und Netzwerkforschung"

Badura B, Ferber C von (Hrsg) (1981) Selbsthilfe und Selbstorganisation im Gesundheitswesen. Oldenbourg, München

Deutsche Arbeitsgemeinschaft Selbsthilfegruppen e.V. (Hrsg) (1988) Selbsthilfegruppen-Förderung. Eigenverlag, Gießen

Ferber C von, Badura B (Hrsg) (1983) Laienpotential, Patientenaktivierung und Gesundheitsselbsthilfe. Oldenbourg, München

Ferber C von (Hrsg) (1987) Gesundheitsselbsthilfe und professionelle Dienstleistungen: soziologische Grundlagen einer bürgerorientierten Gesundheitspolitik. Springer, Berlin Heidelberg New York Tokyo

Hatch S, Kickbusch I (eds) Self-help and health in Europe. New approaches in health care. World Health Organization Regional Office for Europe, Copenhagen

Levin LS, Idler EL (1981) The hidden health care system: mediating structures and medicine. Ballinger, Cambridge/MA

Soc Sci Med (1989) Special issue "Health Self-Care", vol 29/2

Trojan A et al. (in press) Community groups and voluntary organizations as a setting for health promotion. In: Badura B, Kickbusch I (eds) Issues in health promotion

8 Versorgungsforschung

8.1 Primäre Gesundheitsversorgung

Internationaler Vergleich der ambulanten medizinischen Versorgung in Frankreich, der Bundesrepublik Deutschland und den USA*

E. Schach, H. E. Kerek-Bodden

Im folgenden werden die Ergebnisse eines Vergleichs von Datensätzen aus der ambulanten medizinischen Versorgung der Bundesrepublik Deutschland, Frankreichs und der USA beschrieben, zu dem der EVaS-Datensatz beigetragen hat. Bei der Untersuchung, die sich auf vergleichbare Daten aus den 3 Ländern stützte, ging es v. a. darum, zu überprüfen, welche Ähnlichkeiten und welche Unterschiede sich bei Kontakten in der ambulanten medizinischen Versorgung in den Versorgungssystemen der 3 Länder beobachten lassen (DeLozier et al. 1989).

Daten

Die Daten für diesen Vergleich stammen aus Untermengen von Stichprobenerhebungen in der ambulanten medizinischen Versorgung der 3 Länder (DeLozier et al. 1989). Die Erhebung in Frankreich (LeFur et al. 1981) stützte sich auf eine sich über ein ganzes Jahr (Mai 1982–April 1983) hinstreckende Erhebung bei einer Stichprobe von Ärzten, die in einem ihnen zugewiesenen Dreitageszeitraum über alle Patienten-Arzt-Kontakte berichteten. Die Erhebung in den USA (Tenney et al. 1974) basierte auf Berichten über eine systematische Stichprobe von Kontakten bei einer Zufallsstichprobe von Ärzten in der ambulanten medizinischen Versorgung, die im ganzen Jahr 1981 stattfand. Die EVaS-Daten (EVaS-Studie 1981/82) stammen aus Stichproben von Ärzten, die an 2 aufeinanderfolgenden Wochentagen Stichproben von Kontakten dokumentierten (s. Schach, Schwartz u. Kerek-Bodden 1989, Kap. E. 3). Die Berichtsperiode für die Ärzte war eine Woche. In Frankreich wurde der Sonntag und in der EVaS-Studie wurden Sonnabend und Sonntag aus der Erhebung ausgeschlossen, weil an diesen Tagen eine regelmäßige, ambulante medizinische Versorgung in der Praxis nicht stattfand. Während sich die Erhebungen in Frankreich und in den USA auf die gesamte Ärzteschaft in der ambulanten medizinischen Versorgung der jeweiligen Länder beziehen, stellt die EVaS-Erhebung eine Zufallsstichprobe von 5 Kassenärztlichen Vereinigungen dar, die gemeinsam Strukturgleichheit in bezug auf demographische Merkmale der Bevölkerung und Eigenschaften der niedergelassenen Ärzte mit der Bundesrepublik Deutschland aufwiesen. Die Grundgesamtheiten der Ärzte und der dokumentierten Kontakte unterschieden sich entsprechend den Gegebenheiten der 3 ambulanten Versorgungssysteme und den daraus resultierenden Unterschieden in den Erhebungen. Die Datenerfassung ähnelte sich in

---

* Erstmals veröffentlicht in: Schach, Schwartz u. Kerek-Bodden 1989, S. 204–212.

den 3 Studien, denn in Frankreich und der Bundesrepublik Deutschland wurden die Kontakterhebungen nach einem Einführungs- und Informationsbrief (Bundesrepublik Deutschland) oder Eingangstelefonat (Frankreich) postalisch und in den USA nach anfänglichem telefonischem Kontakt und einem persönlichen Besuch eines Interviewers auch postalisch ermittelt.

Für den internationalen Vergleich wurden vergleichbare Arztgruppen (Allgemeinmediziner, Kinder-, Frauenärzte, Internisten, Psychiater/Neurologen, Dermatologen, Augen- und HNO-Ärzte) und Kontakte (persönliche Arzt-Patienten-Kontakte in der Praxis oder als Hausbesuch) herangezogen.

Unter den erhobenen Variablen gingen folgende in diese Untersuchung ein: Alter, Geschlecht, Bekanntheit des Patienten in der Praxis, Diagnose(n), ausgewählte therapeutische und diagnostische Maßnahmen sowie der Behandlungsplan. Nur ausgewählte Ergebnisse auf der Basis dieser Daten werden hier berichtet.

Methodik

Raten für den internationalen Vergleich stammen aus Jahresschätzungen von persönlichen Patienten-Arzt-Kontakten in der ambulanten medizinischen Versorgung entweder in der Praxis niedergelassener Ärzte oder in Form von Hausbesuchen bezogen auf die jeweiligen Bevölkerungen. Als Bezugsbevölkerungen dienten in Frankreich und den USA die entsprechenden Gesamtwohnbevölkerungen des Bezugsjahres und für die Bundesrepublik Deutschland die Wohnbevölkerung der 5 an der Studie beteiligten Kassenärztlichen Vereinigungen. Schätzungen von Raten wurden entsprechend den Stichprobenplänen der 3 Länder vorgenommen.

Anliegen des Patienten und die dazugehörigen diagnostischen Eintragungen des Arztes wurden in den 3 Ländern unterschiedlich kodiert. In Frankreich wurde dafür der ICD-9, in der Bundesrepublik Deutschland die deutsche Fassung des RVC (Wagner et al. 1989) und in den USA der Reason for Visit (Schneider et al. 1979) Schlüssel für Anliegen und der ICD-9 für Diagnosen verwendet (WHO 1978). Um die Daten der EVaS-Studie mit denen der anderen Länder vergleichen zu können, wurden die diagnostischen Eintragungen nach den Regeln des ICD-9 umgeschlüsselt.[1]

Die hier berichteten Resultate stammen aus den von einer Drei-Länder-Arbeitsgruppe erarbeiteten Ergebnissen des internationalen Vergleichs von Daten der ambulanten medizinischen Versorgung von Frankreich, der Bundesrepublik Deutschland und den USA.[2]

---

[1] Für wichtige Hilfen bei der Umkodierung der diagnostischen Angaben aufgrund der deutschen Fassung des RVC (Wagner et al. 1989) in eine Form auf der Basis der ICD-9 danken wir Herrn Professor Dr. F. W. Schwartz, Hannover, und Frau P. Wagner, Köln.

[2] Alle hier berichteten Ergebnisse wurden von einer international besetzten Arbeitsgruppe erarbeitet, die es sich zum Ziel gesetzt hatte, Daten aus dem Bereich der ambulanten medizinischen Versorgung aus Frankreich, der Bundesrepublik Deutschland und den USA zu vergleichen. Der Arbeitsgruppe gehörten die folgenden Personen an: James DeLozier, H. Elisabeth Kerek-Bodden, Thérèse Lecomte, Andrée und Arié Mizrahi, Simone Sandier, Elisabeth Schach und Kerr L. White.

Ausgewählte Eigenschaften der Gesundheitssysteme

Bevor inhaltliche Ergebnisse des internationalen Vergleichs gezeigt werden, sind zunächst einige Charakteristika der drei Gesundheitsversorgungssysteme zu nennen.

Alle 3 Länder gehören zu den westlichen Industrienationen mit einem hohen Bruttosozialprodukt pro Kopf der Bevölkerung (über 10000 US$ pro Jahr), einem Wirtschaftswachstum von 2–4% und Arbeitslosenquoten zwischen 4,4% (Bundesrepublik Deutschland) und 7,5% (USA), jeweils für 1981.

In allen 3 Ländern ist die Säuglingssterblichkeit im Studienjahr relativ niedrig [zwischen 9,7 (Frankreich) und 11,9 (USA) pro 1000 Lebendgeborene (1981)].

Bezüglich der Charakteristika des Gesundheitssystems zeigt sich:

- eine höhere Arztdichte pro Bevölkerung bei den europäischen Ländern im Vergleich zu den USA. Bei diesen ist hier wiederum die Facharztdichte höher als in Frankreich und in der Bundesrepublik Deutschland.
- daß die Anteile von Ärzten in der ambulanten medizinischen Versorgung an allen Ärzten in der Patientenversorgung in den USA und Frankreich größer sind als in der Bundesrepublik Deutschland.
- daß die Anzahl der Krankenhausbetten pro 1000 Einwohner in der Bundesrepublik Deutschland unter den 3 Ländern am höchsten ist, gefolgt von Frankreich und den USA. Während in Akutkrankenhäusern die Anzahl der Krankenhauseinweisungen in den 3 Ländern sehr ähnlich ist (156 für die Bundesrepublik Deutschland und 169 für die USA pro 1000 Einwohner, 1981), findet man längere Krankenhausverweildauern für Frankreich und die Bundesrepublik Deutschland im Vergleich zu den USA.

Auch bezüglich des Grads der Ausgabenabdeckung für Gesundheitsausgaben bestehen (z. Z. der jeweiligen Studien) Unterschiede zwischen den 3 Ländern. Während in den USA nur Teile der Bevölkerung durch spezifische Programme erfaßt werden, ist in der Bundesrepublik Deutschland und in Frankreich die Mehrheit der Bevölkerung krankenversichert. Weiterhin trägt in den USA der Patient einen erheblichen Teil der Kosten aus eigener Tasche, in Frankreich sind dies etwa 25% der Kosten für ambulante Versorgung und in der Bundesrepublik ein nur geringer Prozentsatz (z. B. etwa 10%[3], nur bezogen auf ambulante Ausgaben für Arznei-, Heil- und Hilfsmittel).

In allen 3 Ländern herrscht freie Arztwahl im ambulanten Sektor. Krankenhauspatienten werden in allen 3 Ländern nur in begrenztem Umfang von ebenfalls in der ambulanten Versorgung tätigen Ärzten betreut. In allen 3 Ländern werden Ärzte in der ambulanten Versorgung nach dem System der Einzelleistungsvergütung bezahlt. Während in Frankreich und in den USA die Bezahlung für ärztliche Leistungen in der Regel direkt vom Patienten an den Arzt erfolgt (wobei die Patienten anschließend den ihnen von Versicherungen zustehenden Teil der Rechnung zurückfordern), gilt dieses Verfahren in der Bundesrepublik Deutschland nur für Privatversicherte.

---

[3] Persönliche Mitteilung von F. W. Schwartz an E. Schach.

Spezifische Studienergebnisse

Da die oben beschriebenen Charakteristiken des Gesundheitswesens einen Einfluß auf die Ergebnisse des internationalen Vergleichs haben, sollten sie bei deren Interpretation im Auge behalten werden. Die folgenden Ausschnitte werden dargestellt:

- Raten von persönlichen Patienten-Arzt-Kontakten in der ambulanten medizinischen Versorgung pro 1000 Einwohner,
- Struktur der diagnostischen Angaben bei persönlichen Patienten-Arzt-Kontakten im ambulanten Versorgungsbereich,
- die Verteilung von Angaben zu ausgewählten Krankheiten oder Symptomen bei persönlichen Patienten-Arzt-Kontakten in der ambulanten Versorgung bei Allgemeinmedizinern und Fachärzten.

Im Vergleich der 3 Länder beobachten wir eine Rate von 6,2 persönlichen Patienten-Arzt-Kontakten pro Person in der Bevölkerung im Jahr 1981 für Frankreich, eine Rate von 10,6 für die Bundesrepublik Deutschland und eine von 2,6 für die USA für die einbezogenen Arztgruppen in der ambulanten medizinischen Versorgung. Die auf die Bevölkerung von Frankreich standardisierten Raten betrugen 10,4 Kontakte pro Person in der Bevölkerung und Jahr für die Bundesrepublik Deutschland und 2,7 für die USA. Bei der Suche nach möglichen Erklärungsfaktoren für diese Differenzen sind die Raten der Arztdichte in der ambulanten Versorgung in den 3 Ländern nicht allein ausschlaggebend, denn sie betragen 1,307 pro 1000 Bevölkerung für Frankreich, 0,86 für die Bundesrepublik Deutschland und 0,775 für die USA (1981) für die 8 Gebietsgruppen, die verglichen wurden. Die Arztdichten pro Bevölkerung der 3 Länder entsprechen also weder der Reihung der Kontaktraten pro Bevölkerung noch deren Relationen zueinander.

Auf die dem internationalen Vergleich unterliegenden 8 Arztgruppen entfallen in allen 3 Ländern hohe Prozentsätze der Gesamtkontakte in der ambulanten medizinischen Versorgung (88,5 % für Frankreich, 91,6 % für die Bundesrepublik Deutschland und 80,9 % für die USA). Teilt man nun die 8 Arztgruppen in 3 Gruppen nach Patientennähe ein, nämlich in Allgemeinmediziner, Primärspezialisten (Internisten, Frauen-, und Kinderärzte) und andere Gebietsärzte in der ambulanten medizinischen Versorgung (Nerven-, Haut-, Augen- und HNO-Ärzte), dann stellt man fest, daß beinahe zwei Drittel in Frankreich, etwas mehr als die Hälfte in der Bundesrepublik Deutschland und weniger als ein Drittel der persönlichen Patienten-Arzt-Kontakte der USA in der ambulanten medizinischen Versorgung in den Praxen von Allgemeinmedizinern registriert werden. Auf die Primärspezialisten entfallen in Frankreich 11,6 %, in der Bundesrepublik Deutschland 26,3 % und in den USA 34,7 % aller persönlichen Patienten-Arzt-Kontakte in der ambulanten medizinischen Versorgung. Damit zeigt sich eine sehr starke Verantwortung der Allgemeinmediziner für die ambulante medizinische Versorgung in Frankreich, eine geringere in der Bundesrepublik Deutschland und eine noch geringere in den USA. Diese Verantwortung wird in den letzten beiden Ländern von den Gebietsärzten der Primärversorgung geteilt.

Ausgewählte Ergebnisse zum Behandlungsplan verhelfen dazu, diese Ergebnisse weiter zu erläutern. Untersucht man zunächst die Anteile der persönlichen

Tabelle 1. Diagnostische Eintragungen nach ICD-Hauptgruppen in der ambulanten Versorgung: Angaben in Prozent aller Eintragungen bei persönlichen Patienten-Arzt-Kontakten nach Ländern.

ICD-Hauptgruppen	Diagnostische Eintragungen in %		
	Frankreich[a] [%]	Bundesrepublik Deutschland[b] [%]	USA[c] [%]
Infektiöse und parasitäre Krankheiten	2,45	2,54	3,10
Neubildungen	1,30	2,03	1,86
Endokrinopathien, Ernährungs- und Stoffwechselkrankheiten, Störungen im Immunitätssystem	3,58	6,18	4,60
Krankheiten des Blutes und der blutbildenden Organe	0,37	0,94	0,59
Psychiatrische Krankheiten	6,89	4,47	4,62
Krankheiten des Nervensystems und der Sinnesorgane	7,72	8,54	10,99
Krankheiten des Kreislaufsystems	16,22	24,21	13,58
Krankheiten der Atmungsorgane	11,84	11,34	13,76
Krankheiten der Verdauungsorgane	6,94	6,40	4,69
Krankheiten der Harn- und Geschlechtsorgane	3,80	5,56	5,10
Komplikationen der Schwangerschaft, Entbindung und im Wochenbett	0,42	0,23	0,30
Krankheiten der Haut und des Unterhautzellgewebes	3,47	3,57	5,44
Krankheiten des Skeletts, der Muskeln, des Bindegewebes	8,47	10,88	6,11
Kongenitale Anomalien	0,24	0,27	0,25
Affektionen mit Ursprung in der Perinatalzeit	0,09	0,02	0,04
Symptome und ungenau bezeichnete Affektionen	14,18	3,33	3,77
Verletzungen und Vergiftungen	2,70	2,78	5,38
Gesamt	90,68	93,29	84,17
Besondere Bedingungen, andere unbekannte Eintragung	9,32	6,71	15,83
Angaben Gesamt	100,00	100,00	100,00

[a] ETM 1982/83.
[b] EVaS-Studie 1981/82.
[c] NAMCS 1981.

Kontakte der 8 einzelnen Arztgruppen, die mit einer Empfehlung für einen Wiederbesuch verbunden sind, so ähneln sich die Bundesrepublik Deutschland und die USA diesbezüglich, denn sie weisen für alle Arztgruppen relativ hohe Anteile solcher Kontakte an allen Kontakten auf (50–60 %). In Frankreich weisen nur die Nervenärzte eine ähnlich hohe Rate auf (65,1 %). Alle anderen Arztgruppen liegen in Frankreich bei der Arztempfehlung für einen Wiederbesuch bei 20 % und darunter. Die persönlichen Patienten-Arzt-Kontakte der untersuchten Arztgruppen, die mit einer Überweisung an einen anderen Arzt verbunden sind, sind in der Bundesrepublik Deutschland am höchsten (7,9 %), gefolgt von Frankreich (4,7 %) und den USA (2,6 %). Ein höheres Kontaktvolumen in der Bundesrepublik Deutschland wird z. T. durch die im Vergleich zu den anderen beiden Ländern erhöhten Wiederbesuchsempfehlungen, denen die Patienten offenbar folgen, und erhöhte Überweisungsraten erklärt.

Von Interesse ist nun zu überprüfen, ob die Erhöhung der Kontaktraten pro Bevölkerung im ambulanten Sektor in der Bundesrepublik Deutschland im Vergleich zu entsprechenden Statistiken in Frankreich und den USA Auswirkungen auf die Kontaktfrequenzen für Krankheitsgruppen[4] oder Einzelkrankheiten hat. Dieser Untersuchung dienen die Tabellen 1–3.

Tabelle 1 zeigt die Verteilung der diagnostischen Gesamtangaben der persönlichen Patienten-Arzt-Kontakte nach ICD-Hauptgruppen in Prozent. Verteilt über 17 spezifische Gruppen weisen sie einen hohen Grad der Übereinstimmung über die Länder hinweg auf, wie im folgenden gezeigt wird:

Pearson-Produktmoment-Korrelationskoeffizienten der relativen Häufigkeiten für die ersten 17 Diagnosegruppen der Tabelle 1:

	Bundesrepublik Deutschland	USA
Frankreich	0,80	0,78
Bundesrepublik Deutschland		0,86

Alle Koeffizienten sind von Null verschieden ($\alpha = 0,01$). Da wir es hier mit relativen Häufigkeiten zu tun haben, ist das Ergebnis so zu interpretieren, daß trotz unterschiedlicher Gesundheitssysteme in den 3 Ländern die Verteilung der persönlichen Patienten-Arzt-Kontakte über die ICD-Gruppen hinweg gut übereinstimmt. Diese Aussage gilt weitgehend auch für alle einzelnen Gruppen der Tabelle 1, mit Ausnahme von „Herz-Kreislauf-Erkrankungen" und „Symptomen und ungenau bezeichneten Affektionen".

---

[4] In den 3 Ländern wurden diagnostische Angaben wie folgt verschlüsselt: In Frankreich wurden beim Patienten-Arzt-Kontakt zwar alle Haupt- und Nebendiagnosen, die für den Kontakt Bedeutung hatten, notiert, aber nicht in diese beiden Kategorien sortiert. In den USA und der Bundesrepublik wurden die dem Anliegen des Patienten entsprechenden Haupt- und Nebendiagnosen unterschieden. Für die Tabellen 1–3 wurden, nach Prüfung der diagnostischen Eintragungen auf Vergleichbarkeit zwischen den 3 Ländern, alle Angaben von Haupt- und Begleitdiagnosen für die Analysen verwendet.

Tabelle 2. Spezifische Krankheiten oder Symptome: Angaben in Prozent aller diagnostischen Eintragungen bei persönlichen Patienten-Arzt-Kontakten nach Ländern.

Krankheit/Symptom	Prozent diagnostischer Eintragungen an allen Eintragungen der Krankheits-/Symptomgruppe		
	Frankreich[a]	Bundesrepublik Deutschland[b]	USA[c]
Essentielle Hypertonie	5,29	6,32	6,35
Rückenschmerzen	3,33	3,99	1,38
Neurose	2,79	0,63	2,48
Ischämische Herzkrankheit	2,15	3,73	2,77
Arthritis	3,40	2,22	2,76
Krankheiten der oberen Luftwege	6,33	3,31	7,49
Diabetes mellitus	1,26	3,15	2,67
Bronchitis	1,65	3,71	1,97
Refraktionsanomalien	1,08	1,67	1,61
Depression	2,11	0,90	0,54
Otitis media	0,99	0,20	3,00
Schlaflosigkeit	2,19	0,24	0,02
Krankheiten der Talgdrüsen	0,37	0,78	1,48
Kontaktdermatitis	0,65	1,34	0,96
Asthma	1,01	0,91	0,75
Gesamt	34,69	33,34	36,22

[a] ETM 1982–83.
[b] EVaS-Studie 1981/82.
[c] NAMCS 1981.

Tabelle 2 zeigt die Verteilung ausgewählter Krankheiten und Symptome aus der Gesamtheit der diagnostischen Eintragungen. Die Auswahl erfolgte im Hinblick auf eine Repräsentanz eng definierter (z. B. Refraktionsanomalien) und häufiger, für bestimmte Krankheitsbilder eher unspezifischer, Beschwerden (z. B. Rückenschmerzen). Dabei zeigt sich das bereits für Tabelle 1 beobachtete Ergebnis. Zunächst repräsentieren die ausgewählten Krankheitsbilder über die Länder hinweg etwa ein Drittel der sich bei Kontakten in der ambulanten medizinischen Versorgung zeigenden Krankheitsbilder in den 3 Ländern (33, 34–36, 22 %). Den Grad der Übereinstimmung der relativen Anteile der diagnostischen Kategorien zeigen die folgenden Korrelationskoeffizienten:

Pearson-Produktmoment-Korrelationskoeffizienten der relativen Häufigkeiten für 15 ausgewählte Krankheitsbilder der Tabelle 2:

	Bundesrepublik Deutschland	USA
Frankreich	0,60	0,79
Bundesrepublik Deutschland		0,61

Tabelle 3. Spezifische Krankheiten oder Symptome: Prozentsatz diagnostischer Eintragungen bei persönlichen Patienten-Arzt-Kontakten an allen Eintragungen der Krankheits-/Symptomgruppen bei Allgemein- und Fachärzten.

Krankheit/Symptom	Prozent diagnostischer Eintragungen an allen Eintragungen der Krankheits-/Symptomgruppe		
	Frankreich[a]	Bundesrepublik Deutschland[b]	USA[c]
Allgemeinmediziner			
Essentielle Hypertonie	93,6	75,1	52,4
Rückenschmerzen	84,2	76,7	48,6
Neurose	65,7	63,6	20,6
Ischämische Herzkrankheit	86,8	66,0	32,4
Arthritis	88,6	81,0	56,6
Krankheiten der oberen Luftwege	84,6	50,5	51,4
Diabetes mellitus	91,3	74,2	47,9
Bronchitis	91,9	69,3	61,3
Refraktionsanomalien	2,1	1,9	2,9
Depression	83,7	66,4	41,6
Otitis media	59,1	10,4	27,2
Schlaflosigkeit	94,5	74,9	25,3
Krankheiten der Talgdrüsen	36,9	48,9	12,6
Kontaktdermatitis	73,8	56,0	38,7
Asthma	83,2	67,7	33,8
Gesamt	[d]	65,4	42,0
Fachärzte			
Essentielle Hypertonie	6,4	24,9	47,6
Rückenschmerzen	15,8	23,3	51,4
Neurose	34,3	36,4	79,4
Ischämische Herzkrankheit	13,3	34,0	67,6
Arthritis	11,4	19,0	43,4
Krankheiten der oberen Luftwege	15,4	49,5	48,6
Diabetes mellitus	8,7	25,8	52,1
Bronchitis	8,1	30,7	38,7
Refraktionsanomalien	97,9	98,1	97,1
Depression	16,3	33,6	58,4
Otitis media	40,9	89,6	72,8
Schlaflosigkeit	5,5	25,1	74,7
Krankheiten der Talgdrüsen	63,1	51,1	87,4
Kontaktdermatitis	26,2	44,0	61,3
Asthma	16,8	32,3	66,2
Gesamt	17,9	34,6	58,1

[a] ETM 1982–83.
[b] EVaS-Studie 1981/82.
[c] NAMCS 1981.
[d] Nicht bekannt.

Auch hier handelt es sich um den Vergleich relativer Häufigkeiten von Krankheitsbildern in unterschiedlichen Gesundheitssystemen. Bei den spezifischeren Krankheitsbezeichnungen der Tabelle 2 erwarten wir aber, wegen geringerer Besetzungszahlen und daher größerer Variabilität der Anteilsschätzungen, eine geringere Übereinstimmung. Alle Korrelationskoeffizienten sind aber auch für die Tabelle 2 von Null verschieden ($\alpha = 0{,}02$). Diese Ergebnisse lassen sich dahingehend interpretieren, daß auch bei ausgewählten, enger oder weiter definierten Krankheitsbildern eine hohe Übereinstimmung der Verteilungen der persönlichen Patienten-Arzt-Kontakte nach Krankheitsbildern über die 3 Länder hinweg zu beobachten ist.

Bemerkenswert ist, daß eher psychische Krankheitsbilder, wie Depressionen, Neurosen und Schlaflosigkeit, unter den betrachteten Krankheitsbildern in Frankreich eine größere Rolle spielen als in der Bundesrepublik Deutschland oder in den USA; in der Bundesrepublik Deutschland beobachten wir erhöhte Anteile von Nennungen für „ischämische Herzkrankheiten" und „Diabetes mellitus" und in den USA für „Krankheiten der oberen Luftwege" und „Otitis media".

Tabelle 3 zeigt die Symptom- und Krankheitsnennungen, die auf Allgemeinmediziner und Fachärzte entfallen, jeweils in Prozent aller Nennungen für eine spezifische Krankheit. Während die in den Tabellen 1 und 2 gezeigten relativen Häufigkeiten von Krankheitsnennungen eher von der Verteilung von Krankheiten beeinflußt sein werden, ist die in Tabelle 3 gezeigte Aufteilung zwischen Allgemeinmedizinern und Fachärzten eher das Ergebnis gesundheitssystemspezifischer Einflüsse. Für die genannten Symptome/Krankheiten sind die von Allgemeinmedizinern versorgten Anteile daran in Frankreich am höchsten, gefolgt von denen der Bundesrepublik Deutschland, und für die USA am niedrigsten. Da insgesamt das Niveau der von Allgemeinmedizinern versorgten Krankheiten bei Kontakten in der ambulanten medizinischen Versorgung in Frankreich am höchsten ist und von der Bundesrepublik und den USA gefolgt wird, ist es auch hier von Interesse zu überprüfen, ob die einzelnen Versorgungsanteile für Allgemeinmediziner (und als Folge davon auch für Fachärzte) sich über die genannten Krankheiten hinweg ähneln. Dies wird durch eine Überprüfung der folgenden Korrelationskoeffizienten bestätigt:

Pearson-Produktmoment-Korrelationskoeffizienten der Versorgungsprozentsätze von Allgemeinmedizinern für 15 ausgewählte Krankheitsbilder der Tabelle 3:

	Bundesrepublik Deutschland	USA
Frankreich	0,83	0,81
Bundesrepublik Deutschland		0,64

Die Korrelationskoeffizienten sind relativ hoch und von Null verschieden ($\alpha = 0{,}01$). Das bedeutet, daß trotz erheblicher Unterschiede in den Rollen von Allgemeinmedizinern in den 3 Gesundheitsversorgungssystemen die von ihnen versorgten Anteile von Kontakten der ausgewählten Krankheitsbilder sich nicht so sehr in der Struktur, sondern vielmehr im Niveau (Menge) unterscheiden.

Zusammenfassung

Die mengenmäßigen Beziehungen der persönlichen Patienten-Arzt-Kontakte in der ambulanten medizinischen Versorgung der USA, Frankreichs und der Bundesrepublik Deutschland verhalten sich wie $1:2{,}4:4{,}1$. Außerdem unterscheiden sich die Gesundheitsysteme der 3 Länder in wesentlichen Punkten. Trotz dieser Unterschiede ist die Übereinstimmung der Verteilungen diagnostischer Angaben nach ICD-Hauptgruppen und für ausgewählte Krankheitsbilder bei persönlichen Patienten-Arzt-Kontakten über die 3 Länder hinweg recht gut. Dieses Ergebnis wird dahingehend interpretiert, daß möglicherweise gleiche Morbiditätsstrukturen der jeweiligen Bevölkerungen etwa gleichartige Morbiditätsstrukturen in der ambulanten Versorgung verursachen. Bemerkenswert ist daran, daß sich dieses Ergebnis trotz deutlicher Niveauunterschiede in den Kontaktraten ergibt.

Literatur

DeLozier J, Kerek-Bodden HE, Lecomte T, Mizrahi A, Mizrahi A, Sandier S, Schach E, White KL (1989) Ambulatory Care: France, Federal Republic of Germany, and United States, 1981–83. National Center for Health Statistics, Series 5, No. 5 Department of Health and Human Services, Public Health Service, US Government Printing Office, Washington DC

LeFur O, Mizrahi A, Mizrahi A (1981) Méthode d'Enquête Morbidité et Thérapeutique Médical. Centre de Recherche pour l'Etude et l'Observation de Vie. Paris

Schach E, Schwartz FW, Kerek-Bodden HE (1989) Die EVaS-Studie. Eine Erhebung über die ambulante medizinische Versorgung in der Bundesrepublik Deutschland Deutscher Ärzte-Verlag, Köln

Schneider A, Appleton L, McLemore T (1979) A reason for visit classification for ambulatory care. National Center for Health Statistics, Vital and Health Statistics Series 2: Data Evaluation and Methods Research No. 78. US Government Printing Office, Washington DC

Tenney JB, White KL, Williamson JW (1974) National Ambulatory Medical Care Survey: Background and Methodology In. National Center for Health Statistics (ed) Vital and Health Statistics Series 2: Data Evaluation and Methods Research No. 61. US Government Printing Office, Washington DC

Wagner P, Schach E, Schwartz FW (1989) A reason for visit classification for ambulatory care. Ein Klassifikationsschema für Kontaktanlässe in der ambulanten Versorgung. Erweiterte deutsche Fassung. Wissenschaftliche Reihe des Zentralinstituts für die kassenärztliche Versorgung in der Bundesrepublik Deutschland, Band 39.2. Deutscher Ärzte-Verlag, Köln

World Health Organization (WHO) (1978) Manual of the International Statistical Classification of Diseases, Injuries, and Causes of Death Genf

Weiterführende Literatur zum Thema „Primäre Gesundheitsversorgung"

Basler HD (Hrsg) (1989) Gruppenarbeit in der Allgemeinpraxis. Springer, Berlin Heidelberg New York Tokyo (Neue Allgemeinmedizin: Angewandte Heilkunde Praxisforschung)
Bengel J, Koch U (1988) Gesundheitsberatung durch Ärzte. Deutscher Ärzte-Verlag, Köln (Wissenschaftliche Reihe des Zentralinstituts für die kassenärztliche Versorgung; 32)
Doherty WJ, Baird MA (eds) (1987) Family-centered medical care: a clinical case book. Guilford, New York
Int J Tech Ass Health Care (1989) vol 5/1
Pendelton D, Schofield T, Marinker M (eds) (1986) In pursuit of quality· approaches to performance review in general practice. The Royal College of General Practitioners, London
Pauli HG (1985) Argumente für eine Forschungsstrategie in der Allgemeinpraxis. Allgemeinmedizin 14, S. 51–54
Sachverständigenrat für die Konzertierte Aktion im Gesundheitswesen (1987) Medizinische und ökonomische Orientierung: Vorschläge für die Konzertierte Aktion im Gesundheitswesen, Jahresgutachten 1987. Nomos, Baden-Baden
Sachverständigenrat für die Konzertierte Aktion im Gesundheitswesen (1989) Qualität, Wirtschaftlichkeit und Perspektiven der Gesundheitsversorgung: Vorschläge für die Konzertierte Aktion im Gesundheitswesen, Jahresgutachten 1989. Nomos, Baden-Baden
Sachverständigenrat für die Konzertierte Aktion im Gesundheitswesen (1990) Herausforderungen und Perspektiven der Gesundheitsversorgung: Vorschläge für die Konzertierte Aktion im Gesundheitswesen, Jahresgutachten 1990 Nomos, Baden-Baden
White KL (1979) Allgemeinmedizinische Forschung und neue Epidemiologie. Arzt 7:906–910
Zentralinstitut für die Kassenärztliche Versorgung (1989) Die EVaS-Studie: eine Erhebung über die ambulante medizinische Versorgung in der Bundesrepublik Deutschland. Band 39.2 Deutscher Ärzte-Verlag Köln

8.2 Geriatrie

Ausdifferenzierung und Vernetzung von medizinischen, pflegerischen und sozialbetreuerischen Leistungen als regional- und strukturpolitische Aufgaben*

H. Radebold

Der über 60jährige kranke und hilfebedürftige Mensch in seiner Umwelt: Unser derzeitiger Wissensstand

Der über 60jährige Kranke ist charakterisiert durch seine Multimorbidität, die Chronifizierung und die schnellere Dekompensationsneigung. Er leidet gleichzeitig an mehreren Erkrankungen (Multimorbidität), die in der Regel unterschiedliche Organ- und Funktionssysteme betreffen; dabei nimmt die Zahl seiner Diagnosen mit weiterem ansteigendem Lebensalter zu.[1] So lassen sich Funktionseinschränkungen der Sinnesorgane (Hören und Sehen), der Beweglichkeit (von dem Wegfall längerer Wegstrecken bis hin zur Bettlägerigkeit), der körperlichen Leistungsfähigkeit wie auch der Stuhl- und Urinkontrolle beobachten. Diese Funktionseinbußen können nur teilweise durch Rehabilitation und/oder Hilfsmittel ausgeglichen werden.

Als Ausdruck der hohen gerontopsychiatrischen Morbiditätsrate (bei den über 65jährigen in 23–24 %) zeigen sich zusätzlich affektive Störungen (depressive Verstimmungszustände, Veränderungen der Kontrolle und des Antriebs) und insbesondere kognitive Einschränkungen (Merkfähigkeit, Erinnerungsvermögen, Orientierung etc.)[2].

Zahlreiche, aus früheren Lebensabschnitten stammende organische, psychosomatische oder psychische Erkrankungen dauern selbstverständlich jenseits des 60. Lebensjahres als chronische Erkrankungen weiter an; der Kranke und seine Umwelt haben sich zwar mit der chronischen Erkrankung arrangiert, er benötigt jedoch in gewissem Umfang weiterhin ständige ärztliche und sonstige Hilfestellung.

Die erstmals im Alter auftretenden (akuten) Erkrankungen sind aufgrund der erheblichen Fortschritte der geriatrischen Medizin (falls entsprechende klinische

---

* Erstmals veröffentlicht in: Ferber C von (Hrsg) (1989) Die demographische Herausforderung: das Gesundheitssystem angesichts einer veränderten Bevölkerungsstruktur (Beiträge zur Gesundheitsökonomie, 23). Bleicher, Gerlingen, S. 189–210 (gekürzt).

[1] Z. B. fanden sich bei 64jährigen Männern im Durchschnitt 4,1 und bei 64jährigen Frauen im Durchschnitt 4,4 Diagnosen, dagegen bei 74jährigen Männern bereits 4,8 und bei 74jährigen Frauen 5,3 Diagnosen (Lindner 1974); s. außerdem Schubert u. Störmer 1973.

[2] Die psychischen Alterserkrankungen in 23–24 % der über 65jährigen umfassen in knapp einem Drittel psychotische, ebenfalls in knapp einem Drittel hirnorganische/dementielle und in einem reichlichen Drittel neurotische, reaktive, psychosomatische Erkrankungen. Bei den im Alter erstmals auftretenden Erkrankungen handelt es sich in der Regel um Demenzen mit deutlicher Zunahme bei den Höchstaltrigen, s. außerdem Cooper u. Sosna 1983, S. 239–249.

geriatrische rehabilitative Einrichtungen und diesbezügliche Fachkompetenz zur Verfügung stehen) teilweise gut und folgenlos behandelbar. Teilweise verbleiben jedoch erhebliche, ebenfalls einer ständigen Behandlung bedürfende Funktionseinbußen im physischen und psychischen Bereich, die eine weitere Gruppe chronisch Kranker verursachen.

Als entscheidendes Merkmal des alternden Organismus (und damit seiner unterschiedlichen Funktionssysteme) gilt die zunehmende Neigung zu schnellerer Dekompensation, d. h. es stehen weniger Reserven zum Ausgleich von zusätzlichen Belastungen zur Verfügung. Die Schädigung eines Funktions- oder Organsystems führt dann entsprechend zur Dekompensation weiterer und schließlich zum völligen Zusammenbruch mit häufiger Todesfolge. Daher bildet die Gruppe der über 80jährigen als die Gruppe der Höchstaltrigen eine weitere geriatrische Risikogruppe, die im Erkrankungsfalle einer umfassenden fachgerechten klinischen Behandlung und im Überlebensfalle einer langfristigen Rehabilitation und/oder weiterer stationärer Versorgung (Heim) bedarf. Die Behandlung dieser Risikogruppe wird noch dadurch erschwert, daß sich mit zunehmendem Lebensalter eine Zunahme dementieller Erkrankungen zeigt (so von 0,2 % bei den 60jährigen auf über 20 % bei den 80jährigen).

Der sich zunehmend abzeichnende nahezu rechtwinklige Abfall der Überlebenskurve weist darauf hin, daß schwere, klinisch kaum noch beherrschbare Krankheitssyndrome im Sinne der Dekompensation bestehender Multimorbidität erst in den letzten 2–3 Lebensjahren der Höchstaltrigen auftreten.

Die Lebenssituation des über 60jährigen ist weiterhin charakterisiert durch ungünstige Lebensbedingungen und soziale Einschränkungen, die ebenfalls (teilweise in Kombination mit der beschriebenen Multimorbidität und ihren Folgen) zur Hilfsbedürftigkeit führt. Der 1982 vorgelegte Fachbericht und auch die späteren Familienberichte der Bundesregierung belegen unverändert, daß ein relativ großer Anteil dieser Altersgruppe, in der Regel die Frauen, unter schlechten sozialen Bedingungen lebt. Dazu zählen insbesondere niedriges Einkommen und schlechte Wohnverhältnisse (Ausstattung mit sanitären Einrichtungen, Heizung und Licht, Erreichbarkeit etc.). Aufgrund ihres in früheren Lebensjahrzehnten erreichten relativ niedrigen Bildungs- und Einkommensniveaus bilden sie jetzt in ihrem Alter erneut die Benachteiligten. Wenn auch inzwischen die Annahme einer großen Gruppe völlig isolierter oder vereinsamt lebender über 60jähriger widerlegt wurde, so ist nicht zu übersehen, daß ein größerer Teil der über 60jährigen Frauen aufgrund frühzeitiger Verwitwung alleinstehend ist und im Einpersonenhaushalt lebt.[3]

Die beschriebenen physischen, psychischen und sozialen Veränderungen und Einschränkungen erweisen sich im Einzelfall als spezifische Problemsyndrome, die häufig in Form mehrerer gleichzeitiger Probleme auftreten. Innerpsychisch werden diese Veränderungen, unterstützt durch den Wegfall bisheriger Funktionen und den Wegfall des Status als im Arbeitsprozeß Stehender, bei gleichzeitig näherrückendem Lebensende, als Verluste, Bedrohungen, Attacken und Kränkungen erlebt, die insgesamt die innerpsychische Stabilität bedrohen und/oder

---

[3] Siehe außerdem Memorandum der Bundesarbeitsgemeinschaft der Freien Wohlfahrtspflege 1984.

die Autonomie schwächen. Verluste gelten dabei, psychosomatisch gesehen, als schwerste psychische Stressoren.

Drei strukturelle Veränderungen der Alternssituation in der Bundesrepublik müssen für eine zukünftige Versorgungsplanung mitberücksichtigt werden: a) das Überwiegen der Frauen, b) die sich reduzierende familiäre Hilfestellung und c) die sich verschlechternde Relation von Jüngeren zu Älteren.

Die deutlich größere Lebenserwartung der Frauen (ab Geburt und insbesondere bei den über 50jährigen) bedingt, daß gerade in den versorgungsrelevanten Gruppen der über 75jährigen die (alleinstehenden) Frauen weitgehend überwiegen. Dazu werden die noch lebenden (wenigen) Männer in der Regel durch ihre Partnerinnen versorgt.

Die sich seit dem 2. Weltkrieg abzeichnenden dramatischen familiären Veränderungen (Rückzug in die Einkindkernfamilie mit ihrer teilweisen Auflösung bei zunehmender Zahl von Alleinstehenden) führt dazu, daß bisher pflegende Töchter und Schwiegertöchter in zunehmenden Ausmaß mehrere hilfs- und pflegebedürftige Elternteile versorgen müssen. Sie sind dazu in immer geringerem Umfang bereit und stehen aufgrund ihres höheren Lebensalters, eigener Krankheit und Hilfsbedürftigkeit weniger dazu zur Verfügung. Die Möglichkeiten, auf familiäre Unterstützung/Pflege zurückzugreifen, nehmen ab.

Gleichzeitig veränderte sich die Relation der unter 75jährigen zu den über 75jährigen dramatisch und wird sich bis zur Jahrtausendwende noch weiter verschieben. Damit stehen zukünftig ebenso weniger potentiell professionell Tätige zur Pflege/Versorgung zur Verfügung.[4]

Aufgabenstellung für eine adäquate Versorgung

Diese Analyse, die sich summarisch auf wichtige sozialgerontologische und geriatrische Forschungsergebnisse aus dem letzten Jahrzehnt für die Bundesrepublik Deutschland stützt, erlaubt, folgende Aufgabenschwerpunkte derzeitiger und zukünftiger Hilfestellung für die Gruppe der über 60jährigen zu benennen:

- Die Komplexität der Alternssituation (Problemkumulation) verlangt eine im engeren Sinne psychosomatische (d.h. neben körperlichen gleichberechtigt auch psychische und soziale Einflußfaktoren berücksichtigende) Gesamtsicht. Diese muß den über 60jährigen als Mitglied seiner Familie und seiner näheren Umwelt begreifen.
- Als primäres Ziel einer Hilfestellung gilt, die Autonomie des über 60jährigen im vertrauten bzw. gewünschten sozialen Milieu zu erhalten oder (erneut, u.U. auf einem niedrigerem als bisherigem) Niveau zu stabilisieren. Diese Zielsetzung erfordert eine die Selbständigkeit fördernde stimulierende, aktivierende und rehabilitative Hilfestellung statt der betreuenden, pflegenden, bewahrenden oder kontrollierenden Hilfe.
- Die Hilfe hat systematisch, (wohn)quartierzentriert und aufsuchend zu erfolgen und muß gleichzeitig (noch) bestehende familiäre und nachbarschaftliche Unterstützungssysteme langfristig stabilisieren.

---

[4] Siehe Rückert 1989, S. 111.

- Als Ergebnis einer (psychosomatischen) Gesamtsicht sind Maßnahmen in unterschiedlichen Teilbereichen (in der Regel unter Einschluß der Medizin) erforderlich, die sich am ablaufenden (Krankheits)prozeß (Akut-, Rehabilitations-, Chronizitäts- und Terminalphase) orientieren müssen. Neben einer im Bedarfsfall zu leistenden Basisversorgung bedarf es aufgrund der Spezifität der Problemsyndrome zusätzlicher differenzierender Maßnahmen.
- Das geriatrische/rehabilitative Angebot muß auf die langfristige Versorgung chronisch Kranker, Behandlung akuter Krankheitssituationen und die umfassende medizinische Versorgung in der Terminalphase vorbereitet sein. Dabei stehen aktivierende/rehabilitative Maßnahmen im Vordergrund; gleichzeitig müssen die erforderlichen Übergangsmaßnahmen und -institutionen für Alleinstehende oder nicht mehr ausreichend familiär Versorgbare bereitgestellt werden.
- Die sich zunehmend einschränkende familiäre Hilfe- und Unterstützungsmöglichkeit erfordert es mehr und mehr, Aufgaben der Versorgung/Pflege von professionell Tätigen mit quartierbezogener, institutioneller Verankerung ausführen zu lassen.
- Diese auf den über 60jährigen und seine familiäre/soziale Umwelt zentrierte (und damit nicht durch den Träger oder das System definierte) Aufgabenstellung erfordert ein systemübergreifendes Finanzierungskonzept mit finanzieller Absicherung der Basisversorgung und der differenzierenden Maßnahmen. Daneben müssen lokale und regionale Planungs- und Entscheidungskompetenz stehen, um einerseits Konkurrenz und Selektivität von Diensten/Trägern zu vermeiden und andererseits die für Gesamtsicht und -behandlung erforderliche Vernetzung und Kooperation von Angeboten zu ermöglichen.
- Eine grundlegende Voraussetzung dafür ist eine bessere Professionalisierung durch entsprechende Aus-, Weiter- und Fortbildung aller in den unterschiedlichen Versorgungssystemen tätigen Berufsgruppen in den Bereichen (Sozial)gerontologie, Geriatrie und Gerontopsychiatrie.

Zur derzeitigen lokalen und regionalen Versorgung über 60jähriger

Wie Untersuchungen über die Inanspruchnahme zeigen, wird die medizinische Versorgung der über 60jährigen in deutlich größerem Umfang als bei anderen Altersgruppen von der allgemeinmedizinischen bzw. internistischen Praxis und dem Allgemeinkrankenhaus getragen. Der über 60jährige Patient stützt sich auf seinen „Haus"arzt, den er langfristig (von einem bis zu mehreren Jahrzehnten) konsultiert und dem er gleichzeitig eine hohe Beratungskompetenz, auch in psychosozialen Fragestellungen, zutraut.[5] Vor Ort relativ leicht erreichbar (mit deutli-

---

[5] In der Mannheimer Untersuchung von Allgemeinarztpraxen bestand ein langfristiges Arzt-Patient-Verhältnis für alle Altersgruppen (1–5 Jahre bei 17,0 %; 5–10 Jahre bei 16,5 % und mehr als 10 Jahre bei 49,6 % aller Patienten). Rund zwei Drittel der Patienten aller Altersgruppen beantworten die Frage, ob sie sich bei allgemeinen Sorgen, sei es familiärer oder beruflich-finanzieller Art oder bei sehr persönlichen eigenen Problemen an ihren Hausarzt wenden würden, mit „ja" oder „möglich". Vgl. Zintl-Wiegand et al. 1980.

chem Stadt-Land-Gefälle), übernimmt der Arzt für Allgemeinmedizin bzw. der Internist die langfristige, sich weitgehend auf Pharmakotherapie stützende Behandlung, bei fast völligem Verzicht auf aktivierende und rehabilitative Maßnahmen. Selten wird an das ambulante psychiatrische/psychotherapeutische/psychosomatische System weiterverwiesen (bzw. verweigert sich dieses seinem Behandlungsauftrag). Eine Kooperation mit anderen Diensten (mit der teilweisen Ausnahme der Sozialstationen) erfolgt ebenfalls kaum.

Die klinische Versorgung stützt sich weitgehend auf Allgemeinkrankenhäuser, welche in den letzten Jahren zunehmend unter dem Druck der Aufenthaltsreduzierung bei Zentralisierung und Spezialisierung stehen. Teilstationäre bzw. Übergangseinrichtungen sowie rehabilitative und/oder psychiatrische/psychotherapeutische/psychosomatische Behandlungsmöglichkeiten stehen für über 60jährige in der Regel vor Ort kaum und auch in weiterer Entfernung (z. B. Abteilungen für Gerontopsychiatrie oder Rehabilitationskliniken) nur in geringem Umfang zur Verfügung. Die sich an der Kosteneffizienz ausrichtenden derzeitigen strukturellen klinischen Veränderungen erlauben lediglich eine Akutbehandlung Älterer ohne weitergehende Möglichkeiten. Es fehlt ein integriertes abgestuftes System der Gesundheitsversorgung Älterer in definierten Versorgungsregionen, welches unterschiedliche Intensitätsgrade ambulanter medizinischer Versorgung über teilstationäre Hilfestellung (Tageskliniken, Tageskrankenheime) bis hin zu einer differenzierten klinischen Behandlung einschl. Rehabilitation ermöglicht. Zusammengefaßt läßt sich feststellen, daß das derzeitige System der Gesundheitsversorgung weder auf die besonderen Bedürfnisse über 60jähriger ausgerichtet ist noch sie mindestens mitberücksichtigt, sondern ein auffallendes Desinteresse gegenüber dieser Altersgruppe zeigt. Es orientiert sich weitgehend an den Versorgungsbedürfnissen 20- bis 60jähriger. Diese einseitige Orientierung wird noch durch das bisher unverändert in der Medizin vorherrschende Defizitmodell des Alterns unterstützt, welches Altern als unabänderlichen (und damit auch unveränderbaren) fortschreitenden organischen bzw. hirnorganischen Abbau versteht, der in Konsequenz nur eine betreuende, pflegende, bewahrende oder kontrollierende Hilfestellung erlaubt. Zusätzlich wirkt sich erschwerend aus, daß Ärzte bisher in der Bundesrepublik Deutschland sowohl während ihrer Ausbildung als auch später während ihrer Weiterbildung zum Facharzt keine systematischen, curricular verankerten Kenntnisse in Geriatrie, Gerontopsychiatrie und Sozialgerontologie erhalten. Ihr Desinteresse belegen auch die nur in geringem Umfang besuchten Fortbildungsveranstaltungen.

Die pflegerische Versorgung stützt sich ambulant zunächst auf die familiäre Hilfestellung (durch Töchter und Schwiegertöchter) und weiterhin auf die inzwischen weitgehend überall eingerichteten Sozialstationen (organisatorische Bündelung der bisherigen Gemeindekrankenpflege) und stationär auf die (Alten-, Pflege-)Heime. Die Sozialstationen gewährleisten inzwischen (bei einem deutlichen Stadt-Land-Gefälle) die verordnete (und finanzierbare) häusliche Krankenpflege. Auch hier mangelt es an unterschiedlichen Intensitätsgraden der Hauskrankenpflege (Tag/Nacht, Wochenende) und an Übergangsmöglichkeiten zwischen Klinik und Zuhause, wie durch Übergangspflegeheime/Tagespflegeheime/ Tagesheime. Stationäre Versorgungs- und Pflegeaufgaben werden durch Heime (bei noch weiterbestehendem Mangel an Pflegeplätzen) abgedeckt.

Die professionelle ambulante und stationäre Pflege ist weiterhin dadurch charakterisiert, daß sie nur in gewissem Umfang mit anderen Berufsgruppen und anderen Diensten kooperiert und kaum systematische Hilfsangebote (z. B. Pflegetraining, vorübergehende Intensivpflege, vorübergehende Aufnahme zur Entlastung) zur familiären Unterstützung zur Verfügung stellt.

Gleichzeitig mangelt es an der Kooperation von medizinischer und pflegerischer Versorgung, die der über 60jährige Kranke meist in Kombination benötigt. Ärzte für Allgemeinmedizin arbeiten nur teilweise mit Sozialstationen zusammen, geschweige denn, daß sie diese beraten oder an der Konzeptentwicklung beteiligt sind; ebenso fehlt es an einer Zusammenarbeit im stationären Bereich (z. B. für Fortbildung, Praxisanleitung, Konzeptentwicklung, psychiatrische Versorgung). Weitere allgemeine und spezifische Dienstleistungsangebote unterschiedlicher Träger (Allgemeine Soziale Dienste, allgemeine und spezifische Beratungsstellen, Sozialpsychiatrische Dienste, Bildungs- und Freizeitangebote etc.) sind ebenfalls auf die Altersgruppe der 20- bis 60jährigen ausgerichtet und berücksichtigen die spezifischen Versorgungsbedürfnisse über 60jähriger kaum, zeigen ebenso deutliches Desinteresse oder verweigern sich sogar ihrem Versorgungsauftrag. Ihre Angebote erfolgen darüber hinaus zentralisiert und müssen aufgesucht werden. Ihre Organisationsform ist hochgradig spezialisiert und selektiv.

Die durch einzelne Institutionen, Wohlfahrtsverbände oder Versorgungssysteme speziell für die Gruppe der über 60jährigen geschaffenen Angebote (Mahlzeitendienste, Wäsche-, Putz- und weitere Versorgungsdienste, Altenberatungsstellen, Altenbildungs- und Freizeitangebote etc.) erfolgen meist in Form von Einzelleistungen und haben noch keine flächendeckende Bedeutung (ebenfalls ausgeprägtes Stadt-Land-Gefälle); dazu sind sie nur teilweise quartierbezogen und aufsuchend; sie kooperieren – eher in Konkurrenz stehend – kaum. Die angebotenen Leistungen sind bisher nicht anhand von „Standardleistungskatalogen" überprüfbar. Außerdem werden selbst von den für Ältere geschaffenen medizinischen/pflegerischen/sozialen Diensten bestimmte Patientengruppen, wie z. B. Demente, ausgespart.

Von den Versorgungsbedürfnissen über 60jähriger (und ihrer Familie/sozialen Umwelt) aus gesehen, sind diese aufgezählten Angebote nur teilweise aufsuchend/quartierbezogen, hochgradig selektiv (und damit unüberschaubar) und berücksichtigen nicht die erforderliche Gesamtsicht und nicht die aufgrund vorhandener Problemsyndrome erforderliche kombinierte Hilfestellung. Sie orientieren sich bisher weitgehend an einem pflegenden, betreuenden, verwahrenden oder kontrollierenden Versorgungsmodell und stützen sich auf eine nicht ausreichende professionelle Fachkompetenz. Insbesondere leisten diese Dienste bislang keine systematische, umfassende Hilfestellung für eine brauchbare Stabilisierung der häuslichen/familiären Versorgungssituation, die dazu noch präventiv auch eine notwendige Stabilisierung der pflegenden Töchter und Schwiegertöchter ermöglicht.

Wie bekannt, mangelt es weiterhin an einem umfassenden Finanzierungskonzept für das notwendige Angebot medizinischer, pflegerischer und sozialer Dienste und für die dafür notwendigen Aufgaben von Kooperation und Vernetzung.

Verbesserungsmöglichkeiten derzeitiger lokaler und regionaler Versorgung

Um die im vorigen Abschnitt genannten Aufgaben der (psychosomatischen) Gesamtsicht und einer spezifischen Gesamtversorgung mit dem Ziel der Erhaltung der Autonomie des Älteren und seiner Umwelt wohnorientiert umzusetzen, müssen professionelle Dienstleistungen ausgebaut, vernetzt und gleichzeitig stärker ausdifferenziert werden.

Das derzeitige Dienstleistungsangebot für über 60jährige ist insbesondere auf dem Lande ebenso wie in kleinen und mittelgroßen Städten quantitativ und qualitativ nicht ausreichend; nur in den Großstädten entspricht es eher den sich aufgrund der bereits eingetretenen demographischen Veränderungen ergebenden Versorgungsaufgaben. Mit Ausnahme der Sozialstationen werden die vorhandenen Dienstleistungen nicht quartierbezogen angeboten, sondern eher zentralisiert.

Für Planungen sollte entsprechend den Modellvorstellungen der Psychiatrie-Enquete[6] von einem gerontologischen Versorgungsgebiet (mit einer Gesamtbewohnerzahl von 150000–250000) ausgegangen werden, bei eindeutig stärkerer Berücksichtigung der quartierbezogenen Versorgung.

Um eine zusätzliche Ghettoisierung der über 60jährigen zu vermeiden, sind vorhandene Dienstleistungsangebote/Institutionen daraufhin zu untersuchen, ob sie zusätzlich definierte Aufgaben (bei Umstrukturierung und/oder zusätzlicher Ausstattung mit Personal- und Sachmitteln) für die Zielgruppe der über 60jährigen übernehmen können. Angesichts der bereits eingetretenen demographischen Veränderungen und der bestehenden Versorgungsbedürfnisse kann ein „spontaner" Umstrukturierungsprozeß nicht mehr abgewartet werden.

Die Vernetzung muß auf mehreren Ebenen erfolgen: a) Jede Versorgungsinstitution bedarf der notwendigen Gesamtsicht, d. h. der Hereinnahme medizinischer, psychosozialer und pflegerischer Aspekte unter einem funktionalrehabilitativen Ansatz; b) vor Ort (im Haushalt, im Wohnquartier) muß die Hilfestellung der unterschiedlichen Dienstleistungen unterschiedlicher Träger für die zu leistende Basisversorgung, einschließlich weiterer differenzierender Maßnahmen koordiniert werden und c) bedarf es der zentralen Abstimmung aller Gesamtmaßnahmen aufgrund fortzuschreibender Planung. Die Einlösung der Gesamtsicht und der notwendigen Basisversorgung kann nicht dem beeinträchtigten Älteren und/oder seiner familiären Umwelt abgefordert werden.

Die Ausdifferenzierung muß sich an der erforderlichen Intensität, dem vorliegenden (Krankheits)prozeß und dem lokal und regional notwendigen Dienstleistungsspektrum orientieren. Die Intensität umfaßt die Zeitperspektive (Wochen-/Feiertag, Sonntag/Nacht, täglich bis wöchentlich, Akut-/Krisenintervention).

---

[6] Die Psychiatrie-Enquete schlug vor, für die psychiatrische Versorgung sog. Standardversorgungsgebiete mit 150000–250000 Einwohnern zu schaffen und diese mit allen notwendigen psychiatrischen Einrichtungen auszustatten. Dabei wurde allerdings von weitgehend zentral einzurichtenden Angeboten ausgegangen, während über 60jährige aufgrund ihrer Funktionseinschränkungen in sehr viel größerem Umfang wohnortorientiert, leicht erreichbare Angebote benötigen. S. den Bericht zur Lage der Psychiatrie in der Bundesrepublik Deutschland. Deutscher Bundestag 1975.

Die Versorgungsspezifität erfordert ambulante/offene, teilstationäre/übergangs-orientierte, stationäre/geschlossene Angebote. Die Orientierung am (Krank-heits)prozeß verlangt Hilfestellung in der Akutphase/Krisensituation, in der Aktivierungs-/Rehabilitationsphase und für die Rückkehr in das häusliche Mi-lieu (unterstützt durch entsprechende Hilfsmittel) als zukünftig erneut Gesunder oder langfristig Kranker. Das auszudifferenzierende Angebotsspektrum umfaßt die quartier-/wohnortbezogene Basisversorgung (medizinische, pflegerische, so-zialbetreuerische einschließlich informierender/beratender Hilfestellung sowie Hilfsmittelverleih, Bildungsangebote etc.) und zentralisiert angebotene Dienste (spezifische Information/Beratung, spezifische ambulante medizinische Versor-gung einschließlich psychiatrischer/psychotherapeutischer Hilfestellung, spezifi-sche Versorgungsdienste wie Essen auf Rädern etc., spezifische klinische Ange-bote einschließlich stationärer Rehabilitation und Gerontopsychiatrie).

Wie erfolgreich werden sich vorhandene Dienste/Institutionen für die skiz-zierten Aufgabenstellungen verändern lassen? Diese Frage soll am Beispiel der allgemeinärztlichen Praxis und am Beispiel der Bündelung sozialer und pflegeri-scher Dienste in einem Dienstleistungszentrum untersucht werden.

Praktisch alle körperlichen Kranken und ebenso die pflegebedürftigen über 60jährigen sind in der Regel seit vielen Jahren, bis hin zu mehreren Jahrzehnten, Patienten eines niedergelassenen Arztes für Allgemeinmedizin,[7] der vor Ort rela-tiv leicht erreichbar ist. Folgende Anforderungen[8] an eine zukünftige geriatrische Basisversorgung lassen sich formulieren:

- frühe Identifizierung von körperlicher/psychischer Krankheit oder Beein-trächtigung einschließlich aller physischen, psychischen und auch sozialen Aspekte;
- umfassende Einschätzung aller mit gesundheitlicher Versorgung zusammen-hängenden Probleme (in Kooperation mit Sozialarbeitern und Pflegekräf-ten);
- rechtzeitige Überweisung zu bzw. Einbeziehung von Fachärzten;
- fortgesetzte Vorsorge- und Nachsorgeuntersuchungen (in Kooperation mit Fachärzten, Sozialarbeitern, Pflegekräften und weiteren Mitarbeitern);
- aktive medizinische Behandlung;
- Veranlassung aktiver pflegerischer Betreuung;
- Information und Beratung über medizinische und präventive Fragestellungen des Patienten, seiner Angehörigen und der näheren Umwelt;
- Vermittlung von entlastenden Hilfen und finanzieller Unterstützung;
- Beratung bei der Vermittlung von Heimunterbringung;
- regelmäßiger Kontakt mit den lokalen und regionalen Diensten und Einrich-tungen der an der Versorgung beteiligten (Teil)systeme;
- Mitarbeit bei Öffentlichkeitsarbeit und Fortbildung;

---

[7] Nach Cooper u. Sosna (1983) befanden sich in der Mannheimer Feldstudie 95% aller psy-chisch Alterskranken in allgemeinärztlicher regelmäßiger Behandlung, lediglich 2 von insge-samt 95 waren früher einmal in fachärztlicher psychiatrischer Behandlung gewesen.

[8] In Ableitung der Forderung an den niedergelassenen Arzt für Allgemeinmedizin bezüglich ge-rontopsychiatrischer Versorgung, s. Mann u. Graham 1986.

– Anleitung für häusliche Rehabilitation und für die Gestaltung des häuslichen Milieus (Milieutherapie);
– konzeptionelle Hilfestellung für Institutionen (z. B. Sozialstationen und Heime).

Die beschriebene Inanspruchnahme des Arztes für Allgemeinmedizin verdeutlicht, daß sich kein ambulantes Versorgungsmodell über 60jähriger ohne niedergelassene Ärzte für Allgemeinmedizin verwirklichen läßt und ebenso verdeutlicht dieser Aufgabenkatalog, daß der Arzt für Allgemeinmedizin diese Schlüsselfunktionen zur Zeit (oder überhaupt?) bekanntermaßen nicht wahrnehmen kann. Verbesserungen bzw. Veränderungen in folgenden Bereichen wären dafür Voraussetzung:

– geriatrische, gerontopsychiatrische und (sozial)gerontologische Aus-, Weiter- und Fortbildung;
– Kooperation mit, wenn nicht sogar Einbeziehung von pflegerischen, rehabilitativen und sozialarbeiterischen Fachkräften in die Praxis;
– lokale Kooperation (Gemeinde, Stadtviertel) mit den Diensten/Institutionen und nichtärztlichen Berufsgruppen anderer Versorgungssysteme;
– Erweiterung des kassenärztlichen Leistungskatalogs bezüglich Information/Beratung von Patienten und Umwelt, langfristiger psychosozialer Hilfestellung einschließlich Sterbebegleitung, ebenso wie Abrechenbarkeit rehabilitativer, koordinierender und kooperativer Maßnahmen, für Verlaufskontrollen und für eine Hilfestellung für besondere Risikogruppen.

Möglicherweise werden selbst diese Veränderungen nicht dazu führen, daß ein umfassendes professionelles Dienstleistungsangebot unter Integration allgemeinärztlicher Leistungen vor Ort möglich wird. Ob die „neue Ärztegeneration" unter dem Konkurrenzdruck infolge der sich abzeichnenden „Ärzteschwemme" zur Erprobung von neuen Praxismodellen bereit ist, muß skeptisch beurteilt werden. Möglicherweise werden völlig neue Modelle erforderlich.

In welchem Umfang sind im nichtmedizinischen Bereich organisatorische und inhaltliche Bündelungen von Dienstleistungen möglich, die sowohl der Aufgabe der Vernetzung als auch der Aufgabe der Ausdifferenzierung entsprechen?

Die Sozialstationen als derzeitige organisatorische Zusammenfassung quartierbezogener, auf körperliche Krankheiten ausgerichteter Krankenpflegeleistungen experimentieren z. Z. mit unterschiedlichen Wegen der Erweiterung ihres Leistungsspektrums. Dazu zählen die Hereinnahme der Berufsgruppe der Sozialarbeiter zur Hilfestellung für psychisch Kranke und bei sozialen Problemlagen (z. B. Berlin, Hamburg, Kassel) oder die Einbeziehung von psychiatrischen weitergebildeten Pflegekräften für die Hilfestellung bei chronisch psychisch Kranken und psychisch Alterskranken (z. B. im Bundesland Nordrhein-Westfalen). Der weitere Ausbau der Sozialstationen zu umfassenderen Dienstleistungszentren zur Versorgung körperlich und/oder psychisch Kranker einschließlich weiterer Hilfsbedürftiger (aller Altersgruppen, wenn auch in Realität in 90 % für über 60jährige) erscheint relativ kurzfristig realisierbar. Derartige Dienstleistungszentren werden seit längerer Zeit in verschiedenen Großstädten erprobt; ihre Einrichtung auf Stadtteilebene erfolgt derzeit z. B. in München. Sie leisten Information/Beratung des über 60jährigen und seiner Umwelt, bieten „Standarddienstleistungen" an und vermitteln weitere Dienste, leihen Hilfsmittel aus und regen Selbsthilfeaktivitäten an.

Als weiterer, bisher wenig genutzter Ansatz, bietet sich die Einbeziehung der im Wohnumfeld gelegenen Alten(pflege)heime an. Immer häufiger verfügen sie über Rehabilitations-, Gymnastik-, Aktivierungs- und Freizeitmöglichkeiten: dazu eine Cafeteria und weitere Räume. Über ihre derzeitigen Möglichkeiten hinaus, z. B. für einen mobilen Mittagstisch und/oder Freizeitangebote, zur Information/Beratung, zur aufsuchenden oder vorübergehenden Hilfestellung, zur entlastenden Aufnahme erscheint ihr Angebot weiter z. B. für Tagepflege- und weitere Übergangseinrichtungen ausbaubar.

Als günstige Voraussetzung verfügt das Heim über zahlreiche Kontakte zu den im Haus mitbehandelnden Ärzten.

Die bisher skizzierten möglichen Verbesserungen im lokalen Bereich durch a) Verlagerung der Basisversorgung in das Stadtviertel/Wohnquartier, b) stärkere aufsuchende Hilfestellung für den über 60jährigen und seine Umwelt und c) weitere Bündelung von Angeboten unter differenzierender Sicht und Einbeziehung von Übergangseinrichtungen bei vorhandenen Institutionen werden nur über gewisse Veränderungen erreichbar werden.

Für die dringend notwendig erachtete Vernetzung werden weitere organisatorische, institutionelle und strukturelle Ergänzungen notwendig:

- Die im immer größeren Umfang anfallenden Transferleistungen (zwischen dem über 60jährigen und der professionellen Umwelt, zwischen den Angeboten verschiedener Berufsgruppen und den verschiedenen Institutionen und während des ablaufenden Krankheitsprozesses) bedingen in großem Umfang Information, Beratung, Vermittlung und Koordination. Diese muß institutionalisiert, wohnortbezogen und für den Älteren und seine Umwelt erreichbar angeboten werden. Organisatorisch empfiehlt sich eine Anbindung an eine bereits vor Ort vorhandene Institution.
- Quartierbezogene Hilfestellung für Ältere und ihre Umwelt muß sich dabei auf zentrale Kompetenz (Einzugsgebiet entsprechend dem Standardversorgungsgebiet der Psychiatrie-Enquete in der Größenordnung von 150 000–250 000 Einwohnern) stützen können. Hilfestellung wird insbesondere für die im Feld tätigen Berufsgruppen/Institutionen benötigt für a) Planung und Konzeptentwicklung, b) durch Krisenintervention, c) differenzierte ambulante/offene Versorgung, d) Assessment, e) Fortbildung/Supervision und f) Institutionsberatung. Diese Kompetenz kann in Form eines „Gerontologischen Zentrums" geschaffen werden.
- Solange das Fernziel einer „Gerontologisierung" aller im Altersbereich tätigen Berufsgruppen, d. h. eine entsprechende Aus-, Weiter- und Fortbildung nicht erreicht ist, muß qualifiziertes gerontologisches/geriatrisches und gerontopsychiatrisches Wissen mit entsprechender Beratungs- und Handlungskompetenz für die Unterstützung aller lokalen/regionalen Aktivitäten im Altersbereich bereitgestellt werden. Bisher erhalten alle Berufsgruppen keine curricular verankerte Aus-, Weiterbildung in Gerontologie/Geriatrie und Ge-

rontopsychiatrie,[9] bis auf die status- und bezahlungsmäßig unter der Gruppe der Krankenpflegekräfte angesiedelte Berufsgruppe der Altenpflegekräfte.
– Die Abstimmung der unterschiedlichen Angebote, die Vermeidung einer Über- bzw. Unterversorgung, die Wahrnehmung von Kooperations- und Koordinationsaufgaben etc. verlangt eine kommunale (Stadt-, Landkreis) Planungs- und Entscheidungskompetenz mit Fortschreibung entsprechender Planungsdaten und entsprechenden Gremien auf Stadtteilebene.

Literatur

Abschlußbericht (1985) Modellprogramm Psychiatrie der Bundesregierung in der Modellregion Kassel. Kassel
Allekotte H (1979) Sicherung der Gesundheitsversorgung älterer Menschen. In: Dieck M, Schreiber T (Hrsg) Gerontologie und Gesellschaftspolitik. DZA, Berlin
Arbeitsgruppe Fachbericht über Probleme des Alterns (Hrsg) (1982) Altwerden in der Bundesrepublik Deutschland: Geschichte – Situationen – Perspektiven, Bd I–III. Deutsches Zentrum für Altersfragen, Berlin
Arie T (ed) (1981) Health care of the elderly: essays in old age. Medicine, Psychiatry and Services. Croom Helm, London
Biron F, Eder S et al. (1980) Ergebnisse der Wiener Gesundheitsstudie 1979. Institut für Stadtforschung, Wien
Bracker M, Hackewitz W, Pressel I, Radebold H (1982) Aspekte heutiger Altenberatung. Vincent, Hannover
Braun H (1985) Die Pflege hilfsbedürftiger alter Menschen durch den Ehepartner. MMG 10:201–207
Bruder J (1983) Zur Gruppenarbeit mit Angehörigen von dementen und nichtdementen alten Menschen. In: Radebold H (Hrsg) Gruppenpsychotherapie im Alter. Vandenhoeck & Ruprecht, Göttingen
Bundesarbeitsgemeinschaft der Freien Wohlfahrtspflege (Hrsg) (1984) Memorandum zur Altenhilfe. Bonn
Bundesarbeitsgemeinschaft der freien Wohlfahrtspflege (1987) Hilfebedürftigkeit im Alter. Bonn
Cooper B, Sosna U (1983) Psychische Erkrankungen in der Altenbevölkerung. Nervenarzt 54:239–249
Dieck M (1978) Art und Ausmaß der Gesundheitsversorgung älterer Menschen. In: Dieck M, Naegele G (Hrsg) Sozialpolitik für ältere Menschen. Quelle & Meyer, Heidelberg
Dieck M (1984) Modelle gerontologischer/geriatrischer Ausbildung in der Bundesrepublik Deutschland und im (west-)europäischen Ausland. Z Gerontol 17:157–166
Deutscher Bundestag (Hrsg) (1975) Bericht zur Lage der Psychiatrie in der Bundesrepublik Deutschland – Zur psychiatrischen und psychotherapeutisch-psychosomatischen Versorgung der Bevölkerung. 7. Wahlperiode. Drucksache 7/4200, Bonn
Deutscher Bundestag (Hrsg) (1986) Altersforschung (Gerontologie) und Alterskrankheiten (Geriatrie). Antwort der Bundesregierung auf die Kleine Anfrage. Drucksache 10/6721. 10. Wahlperiode. Bonn
Falck I (1979) Gesundheitsversorgung älterer Menschen in der Bundesrepublik Deutschland. In: Dieck M, Schreiber T (Hrsg) Gerontologie und Gesellschaftspolitik. DZA, Berlin

---

[9] Lediglich für die Berufsgruppe der Sozialarbeiter/Sozialpädagogen besteht seit 1983 die Möglichkeit, sich durch ein Aufbaustudium im Fachbereich Sozialwesen der Gesamthochschule Kassel sozialgerontologisch zu qualifizieren. Aufbaustudiengänge für Psychologen sind an den Universitäten von Heidelberg und Nürnberg/Erlangen ab WS 1987/88 vorgesehen. Die derzeitig gültige Approbationsordnung für Ärzte verlangt bisher keinen curricular verankerten Erwerb geriatrischer Kenntnisse. Die jetzt vorgenommenen diesbezüglichen Veränderungen der Prüfungsordnungen für Krankenpflege- und Rehabilitationskräfte werden sich erst in ferner Zukunft auswirken.

Ferber C von (1986) Ehrenamtliche soziale Dienstleistungen. Soz Fortschr 35:265–269
Groen J (1982) Psychosomatic aspects of aging. In: Groen J (ed) Clinical research in psychosomatic medicine. Van Gorkum, Assen
Grunow D (1977) Problemsyndrome alterer Menschen und die Selektivität organisierter Hilfen. Arch Soz Arb 8:166–194
Grunow D (1977) Rehabilitation und Administration Probleme organisierter Hilfen für alte Menschen. Soz Sozialpol [Sonderheft der KZfSS] Opladen 1977
Grunow D (1978) Problemsyndrome älterer Menschen und die Selektivität organisierter Hilfen der örtlichen Sozialverwaltung. In: Dieck M, Naegele G (Hrsg) Sozialpolitik für ältere Menschen. Quelle & Meyer, Heidelberg
Grunow D (1986) Selbst- und Laienhilfe in der prämedizinischen Phase. Allgemeinmedizin 15:146–151
Illinger H et al. (1985) Rehabilitation bei Schlaganfallpatienten: Alters- und geschlechtsspezifische Verbesserungen von Alltagsfunktionen. Münch Med Wochenschr 127:522–524
Illinger H et al. (1985) Gruppenspezifische Verbesserungen von Alltagsfähigkeiten bei älteren Schlaganfallpatienten während der Rehabilitationsphase. Z Gerontol 18:231–235
Karl F et al. (1985) Epidemiologie des Schlaganfalles. Untersuchungen im Raum Kassel und im internationalen Vergleich Münch Med Wochenschr 127.306–308
Korte W, Radebold H, Karl F (1988) Gerontopsychiatrische Versorgung. In: Österreich K, Platt D (Hrsg) Psychiatrie und Neurologie, Bd III. Handbuch der Gerontologie. Thieme, Stuttgart
Mann A, Graham N (1986) Open and closed health care for the elderly: comparison of family and home care. In: Häfner H, Moschel G, Sartorius N (Hrsg) Mental health in the elderly. Springer, Berlin Heidelberg New York Tokyo
Olbrich E (1985) Gerontologisch-geriatrische Ausbildung in den USA. Z Gerontol 18:95–99
Ostermann K et al. (1985) Schlaganfall. Hilfs- und Pflegebedürftigkeit der Patienten und ihre sozialen Auswirkungen. Münch Med Wochenschr 127:313–315
Ostermann K (1986) Prognose über 60jähriger Schlaganfallpatienten ein- bis zwei Jahre nach dem Insult. Prakt Geriatr 6
Pallenberg C (1983) Dokumentation der universitären gerontologischen Lehrangebote, Bd 45. Deutsches Zentrum für Altersfragen, Berlin
Pfeiffer E (1976) Ausbildungsprogramme in den Vereinigten Staaten für die gerontologische Psychiatrie und die Gerontologie im allgemeinen. Gerontopsychiatrie 4, Janssen Symposien. Düsseldorf
Radebold H (1982) Psychische Erkrankungen und ihre Behandlungsmöglichkeiten. In: Reinmann H (Hrsg) Das Alter. Enke, Stuttgart
Radebold H et al. (1982) Altentreffpunkt Ulm/Neu-Ulm. Beschreibungen und Analyse eines selbstorganisierten und selbstverwalteten Zentrums für Ältere. Hannover
Radebold H et al. (1985) Altentreff Ulm/Neu-Ulm. Dienstleistungszentrum für Ältere. Entwicklung, Struktur, Angebote und Nutzung 1973–1983 Schriftenreihe des BMJFG, Bd 176. Kohlhammer, Stuttgart
Radebold H, Bruder J (1986) Self-help (possibilities and potentials) in Gerontopsychiatry. In: Häfner H, Moschel G, Sartorius N (Hrsg) Mental health in the elderly. A review of the present state of research. Springer, Berlin Heidelberg New York Tokyo
Rosenmayr L (1983) Die späte Freiheit. Severon & Siedler, Berlin
Rückert E (1989) Die demographische Entwicklung und deren Auswirkung auf Pflege-, Hilfs- und Versorgungsbedürftigkeit, S 111–148
Schubert R, Störmer A (Hrsg) (1983) Multimorbidität. München-Gräfelfing
Sichrovsky P (1984) Krankheit auf Rezept. Köln
Taylor RC (1986) Environmental and behavioral factors in psychiatric disorders in the elderly: an approach through risk groups. In: Häfner H, Moschel G, Sartorius N (eds) Mental health in the elderly. A review of the present state of research. Springer, Berlin Heidelberg New York Tokyo
Uexküll T von (1979) Vorwort zur ersten Auflage. In: Uexhüll T von (Hrsg) Lehrbuch der Psychosomatischen Medizin. Urban & Schwarzenberg, München
WHO (Hrsg) (1977) Expert group on mental disorders in the elderly. Copenhagen
Zintl-Wiegand A, Cooper B, Krumm B (180) Psychisch Kranke in der ärztlichen Allgemeinpraxis. Beltz, Weinheim

Weiterführende Literatur zum Thema „Geriatrie"

Barker WH (1987) Adding life to years. Johns Hopkins Univ Press, Baltimore
Fries JF (1983) The compression of morbidity Milbank Mem Fd Q/Health and Society 61:397–419
Garms-Homolova V, Hütter U, Müller R et al. (1987) Versorgung alter Menschen – Bedarf und Barrieren: care delivery systems for the elderly. Zwischenbericht im Verbundprojekt „Vergleichende Untersuchung der Sozial- und Gesundheitsdienste für ältere Menschen". Berlin: Institut für Soziale Medizin der Freien Universität, Berlin
Häfner H, Moschel G, Sartorius N (Hrsg) (1986) Mental health in the elderly: a review of the present state of research. Springer, Berlin Heidelberg New York Tokyo
Lehr U (Hrsg) (1979) Interventionsgerontologie. Steinkopff, Darmstadt (Praxis der Sozialpsychologie; 11)
Lehr U, Thomae H (Hrsg) (1987) Formen seelischen Alterns: Ergebnisse der Bonner Gerontologischen Längsschnittstudie. Enke, Stuttgart
Sachverständigenrat für die Konzertierte Aktion im Gesundheitswesen (1988) Medizinische und ökonomische Orientierung: Vorschläge für die Konzertierte Aktion im Gesundheitswesen, Jahresgutachten 1988. Nomos, Baden-Baden
Svanborg A (1988) Practical and functional consequences of aging. Gerontology 34 [Suppl 1]:11–15
Taylor R, Gilmore A (eds) (1981) Current trends in British gerontology. Gower, Brookfield
Valkenburg HA (1988) Epidemiologic considerations of the geriatric population. Gerontology 34 [Suppl 1]:2–10
Verbrugge LM (1984) Longer life but worsening health? Trends in health and mortality of middle aged and older persons. Milbank Mem Fd Q 62:397–419
Wattis JP, Hindmarch I (1988) Psychological assessment of the elderly. Churchill Livingstone, London
Wilkin D, Williams EI (1986) Patterns of care for the elderly in general practice. JR Coll Gen Pract 36:567–570

8.3 Psychiatrie

Die wissenschaftliche Evaluation psychiatrischer Versorgungssysteme: Prinzipien und Forschungsstrategien *

B. Cooper, H. Dilling, S. Kanowski, R. Remschmidt

Einleitung

Mitte der 60er Jahre wurde ein Dilemma psychiatrischer Versorgung in der Bundesrepublik Deutschland deutlich erkennbar, das noch immer nicht aufgelöst werden konnte. Ein wachsendes öffentliches Bewußtsein der Mißstände in den Großkrankenhäusern führte zu einem Drang nach humanitärer Reform, während gleichzeitig die Entwicklung und Einführung effektiverer Therapien neue Wege der Patientenbehandlung und der sozialen Rehabilitation eröffneten, die in althergebrachten Strukturen psychiatrischer Institutionen nicht realisiert werden konnten und u. a. die Gründung neuer Einrichtungen teilstationärer und ambulanter Versorgung erforderten. Mit der Psychiatrie-Enquête (Deutscher Bundestag 1975) wurde der Versuch unternommen, die Prinzipien, auf denen eine künftige, humanere Psychiatrie basieren sollte, so klar darzulegen, daß die politisch Verantwortlichen darauf ihre Entscheidungen und Handlungen gründen konnten.

In den letzten Jahren wurde auf mehreren Ebenen angestrebt, die im Enquête-Bericht genannten Prinzipien der psychiatrischen Versorgung zu verwirklichen. Von der Bundesregierung wurde zuerst ein Modellverbund „Ambulante psychiatrische und psychotherapeutisch/psychosomatische Versorgung" (Deutscher Bundestag 1979), kurz danach auch das „Modellprogramm zur Reform der Versorgung im psychiatrischen und psychotherapeutisch/psychosomatischen Bereich" (Bundesminister für Jugend, Familie und Gesundheit 1979) konzipiert und gefördert. Gleichzeitig haben auch die Landesregierungen ihre Psychiatriepläne festgelegt und neue Entwicklungen im extramuralen Bereich gefördert.

Gemäß dem herrschenden Zeitverständnis, das auch politische Entscheidungen zunehmend wissenschaftlich abgesichert sehen will, sind neue Programme wissenschaftlich zu begleiten. So ist es Ziel des Bundesmodellprogramms, das sich auf 14 Modellregionen erstreckt und eine Vielzahl von geförderten Einrichtungen bzw. Diensten umfaßt, die Implementation der im Enquête-Bericht niedergelegten Prinzipien zu fördern und gleichzeitig deren Ausführbarkeit und Wirksamkeit empirisch zu prüfen. Damit sind hohe Ansprüche an die Begleitforschung des Modellprogramms gestellt, die grundsätzlich evaluative Aufgaben zu erfüllen hat. Anreiz für die vorliegende Übersicht war die noch fortlaufende Dis-

---

* Erstmals veröffentlicht in: *Nervenarzt* (1985) 56:348–358.

kussion hiermit verknüpfter Probleme innerhalb der Beraterkommission des Modellprogramms[1].

Obgleich die Entwicklung wissenschaftlich zu begleitender Modellprogramme in der Bundesrepublik Deutschland neue, ungewohnte Anforderungen für die Psychiatrie und sogar für das Gesundheitswesen als Ganzes stellt, ist evaluative Forschung in diesem Bereich – zumindest aus internationaler Sicht – keineswegs als *Tabula rasa* zu betrachten. Im Gegenteil, es besteht schon ein erheblicher Fundus des Wissens, der v. a. auf praktischer Erfahrung der letzten 25 Jahre in den anglo-amerikanischen Ländern beruht (Landsberg et al. 1979; Schulberg u. Baker 1979, Windle 1979; Wing u. Hailey 1972), aus dem sich Leitlinien für die Planung und Durchführung evaluativer Forschungsprogramme auch im deutschsprachigen Raum ableiten lassen. Im folgenden wird versucht, den heutigen Stand der Methodik auf diesem Forschungsgebiet kurz zu umreißen und ihre Relevanz für die deutsche Psychiatrie aufzuzeigen.

Grundprinzipien der Evaluation und ihre Anwendung im psychiatrischen Bereich

Evaluation im breiten Sinne bedeutet einfach Bewertung. Die Bewertungsprozesse, die Bestandteile nahezu aller Formen sozialen Handelns bilden, gleichgültig ob Individuen oder komplexe Organisationen daran beteiligt sind, sind in der Regel von subjektiven und gesellschaftlichen Einflüssen stark geprägt. Die besondere Funktion *evaluativer Forschung* besteht darin, bei sozialpolitischen Entscheidungen die Bewertung soweit wie möglich rational zu begründen und auf jeden Fall den Einfluß wissenschaftlich fundierter Erkenntnisse gegenüber vorgefaßten Meinungen, subjektivem Ermessen oder Modeströmungen zu vergrößern. Evaluative Forschung umfaßt alle Prozeduren der Datenerhebung, -verarbeitung und -analyse, die zur genaueren Einschätzung der Wirkungsweise und der Effektivität von gesellschaftsbestimmten Einrichtungen und Maßnahmen beitragen sollen (Suchmann 1967).

Kern der evaluativen Forschung ist immer das Messen oder Einschätzen von Wirkungen und Wirksamkeit. Alle Einrichtungen medizinischer Versorgung müssen nach dem Erfolg beurteilt werden, mit dem sie ihre Aufgaben erfüllen und ihre Ziele erreichen. Diese Beurteilung geschieht anhand einer Darlegung dessen, was der Dienst eigentlich tun sollte, einer Offenlegung dessen, was er tatsächlich leistet und eines Vergleichs mit anderen Diensten, die ähnliche Funktionen wahrnehmen. Die wissenschaftliche Evaluation ist also im wesentlichen ein vergleichendes Vorgehen.

Über evaluative Forschung in der somatischen Medizin liegt schon beträchtliche Literatur vor (Cochrane 1972; Holland 1983). Auch in der Psychiatrie ist in jüngerer Zeit durch die Entwicklung und den Ausbau neuer Versorgungsangebote ein zunehmendes Interesse für wissenschaftliche Evaluation entstanden (Bie-

---

[1] Die Autoren sind Mitglieder der vom Bundesminister für Jugend, Familie und Gesundheit berufenen Beraterkommission des Modellprogramms, vertreten hier jedoch ihren eigenen wissenschaftlichen Standpunkt.

fang 1980; Gruenberg 1966; Kramer u. Taube 1973; Wing 1975). Hier in besonderem stellt sich sofort eine zentrale Frage: Nach welchen Kriterien soll ein Versorgungsangebot beurteilt werden? Was ein psychiatrischer Dienst eigentlich leisten soll, mag zunächst für selbstverständlich gehalten werden, kann aber in der Tat auch zum strittigen Punkt werden, sobald eine Operationalisierung versucht wird. Die Ansichten eines Forschungsteams können sich z. B. von denen des Auftraggebers, der betroffenen Kliniker oder des Kostenträgers erheblich unterscheiden. Deshalb ist es für die evaluative Forschung notwendig, die Leistung eines Dienstes im Hinblick auf vorher klar bestimmte Absichten und Ziele beurteilen zu können.

Mit Wing (1973) kann man davon ausgehen, daß es letztendlich Aufgabe und Ziel psychiatrischer Dienste – ebenso wie in allen anderen Bereichen des Gesundheitswesens – ist, Morbidität und Mortalität in der Gesamtbevölkerung zu reduzieren oder zumindest deren weitere Ausbreitung und Folgen einzudämmen. Daraus folgen sowohl kurative als auch präventive Tätigkeiten. Die unmittelbare Anwendung so rigoroser Erfolgskriterien in Forschungsprogrammen stößt jedoch auf große Schwierigkeiten. Dies gilt insbesondere in der Psychiatrie, wo es trotz einiger, in den letzten Jahren durchgeführter Feldstudien (Cooper u. Sosna 1983; Dilling et al. 1984) immer noch an populationsbezogenen Morbiditätsdaten mangelt und daher die notwendige epidemiologische Ausgangsbasis für eine Evaluation der genannten Art noch lückenhaft ist. Deshalb muß sich die Forschung derzeit meistens auf die Prüfung einer Reihe von sekundären Kriterien, die allerdings in Zusammenhang mit den oben genannten Zielen stehen sollten und die sich von allgemeinen Grundsätzen der psychiatrischen Versorgung (Deutscher Bundestag 1975; WHO 1980) ableiten lassen, beschränken. Als solche allgemeinen Grundsätze können betrachtet werden:

1) Die Dienste und Einrichtungen eines umgrenzten Einzugsgebietes sollen gemeinsam die Verantwortung für die Versorgung psychisch kranker Personen in dieser Region tragen.
2) Jedes Mitglied der Bevölkerung des Einzugsgebietes soll in Abhängigkeit von der jeweiligen Krankheit das gleiche Recht und die gleiche Chance auf medizinisch bzw. psychiatrisch indizierte Behandlung und Versorgung haben. Das heißt im Klartext, daß Fehlentwicklungen in Richtung einer „Klassenpsychiatrie" zu vermeiden sind.
3) Die Dienste sollen, allein oder in Verbindung mit anderen (z. B. überregionale Einrichtungen) eine angemessene Behandlung und Versorgung für alle psychischen Erkrankungsarten, die in der Einzugspopulation vorkommen, anbieten.
4) Die Dienste sollen, allein oder in Verbindung mit anderen, eine fortlaufende Betreuung über aufeinanderfolgende Krankheitsstadien hinweg, unter Einschluß von Rehabilitation und Wiedereingliederung chronisch kranker Patienten, anbieten. Zwischen den einzelnen Facheinrichtungen innerhalb eines Versorgungsgebietes soll hinreichende Zusammenarbeit entstehen, damit eine koordinierte Behandlung der einzelnen Patienten gesichert ist.
5) Die Dienste und Einrichtungen sollen in der Regel innerhalb ihrer Einzugsgebiete angesiedelt werden und der Bevölkerung leicht zugänglich sein.

6) Die Qualität der angebotenen Behandlung bzw. Versorgung soll für alle psy-
    chisch Kranken übliche Kriterien des Gesundheitswesens erfüllen, d.h. sie
    soll der Behandlungs- bzw. Versorgungsqualität für somatisch kranke Patien-
    ten entsprechen.

Gemeinsam bilden diese Forderungen, die im Bericht der Psychiatrie-Enquête
(Deutscher Bundestag 1975) in 4 Prinzipien (gemeindenahe Versorgung, bedarfsgerechte Versorgung aller Patientengruppen, koordinierte Versorgung und
Gleichstellung psychisch Kranker mit körperlich Kranken) zusammengefaßt
sind, eine mögliche Ausgangsbasis für die Evaluation psychiatrischer Versorgungssysteme, expressiv verbis jedoch *insbesondere* für das z. Z. laufende Modellprogramm. Allerdings können sie nicht ohne weiteres als Meßindizes dienen, da
sie für diesen Zweck zu allgemein und zu abstrakt formuliert sind. Es müssen daher für einzelne Forschungsprojekte oder -programme konkrete Zielsetzungen
festgelegt, Teilkriterien ausgewählt und diese in Form von spezifischen Erfolgsin-
dikatoren operationalisiert werden.

Zielsetzung und Forschungsstrategie

Grundsätzlich sollte evaluative Forschung in psychiatrischen wie in anderen Bereichen im Rahmen eines zyklischen Prozesses ablaufen, in dem Planung und
Einführung neuer Dienstangebote auf einer quasiexperimentellen Basis und empirische Überprüfung und Bewertung sowie daraus sich ergebende Modifikation
des Angebots aufeinander folgen (Borach u. Riecken 1975; Lewin 1947; Riecken
1976). Wichtig ist es dabei, vor Beginn schon zu entscheiden, ob es sich um Beurteilungen handelt, die einem spezifischen Dienstträger und dem betroffenen Personal helfen sollen, das Dienstleistungsangebot zu optimieren (*formative Evaluation*) oder ob die Ergebnisse generalisierbar – d.h. nicht nur für den erforschten
Dienst selbst, sondern auch für andere ähnliche Einrichtungen und damit
schließlich für die Planung auf regionaler und nationaler Ebene – relevant und
bedeutsam sein sollen (*summative Evaluation*) (Cook et al. 1977). Während formative Evaluation von der betroffenen Einrichtung selbst durchgeführt werden
kann, setzt summative Evaluation unabhängige Forschung voraus und stellt höhere Ansprüche an die wissenschaftliche Methodik im Hinblick auf die Generalisierbarkeit der Ergebnisse. Ideologisch geladene Polarisierungen zwischen ‚qualitativen‘ und ‚quantitativen‘ Forschungsmethoden (Cook u. Reichhardt 1979)
oder zwischen Aktionsforschung und konventionellen Forschungsansätzen (Moser 1975) stellen falsche Antithesenbildungen dar und sind wissenschaftlich steril.

Ziele und Definition

Die genaue Festlegung der Forschungsziele und -strategien erfordert eine sorgfältige Definition in dreierlei Hinsicht: *Die Untersuchungspopulation ist abzugrenzen, das Versorgungssystem selbst ist klar zu beschreiben und erfaßbare Indikatoren seiner Effektivität sind zu bestimmen.*

a) Die Untersuchungspopulation. Ein Vergleich des Behandlungserfolgs zwischen
2 oder mehreren Einrichtungen ist nur dann sinnvoll, wenn die Art ihrer Patien-

tenauswahl bekannt ist. Ein Vergleich zwischen Versorgungsdiensten in verschiedenen Regionen wird fruchtlos, wenn man nichts über die Strukturen der jeweiligen Risikopopulationen weiß. Deshalb muß die zu versorgende Population definiert werden, wobei die gesamte Bevölkerung eines Gebietes gemeint sein kann oder bestimmte Untergruppen (z. B. alle Kinder und Jugendlichen).

b) Das Versorgungssystem. Ein psychiatrisches Versorgungssystem ist heute – jedenfalls in den hochentwickelten Ländern – als komplexe Organisation zu betrachten (May 1976; WHO 1971). Es umfaßt eine Anzahl verschiedener Einrichtungen, in denen jeweils mehrere Berufsgruppen vertreten sind, die wiederum eine Vielzahl therapeutischer bzw. rehabilitativer Maßnahmen anbieten. Seine Grenzen sind zudem nicht immer leicht bestimmbar, da in den Randzonen Überlappungen mit nichtpsychiatrischen Einrichtungen und Diensten bestehen: ein Punkt, der v. a. das sog. ‚psychiatrische Vorfeld‘ betrifft.

Die systematische Erfassung und Beschreibung einer gesamten Versorgungsstruktur, die sich dementsprechend komplex gestaltet, kann mit Hilfe differenzierter Dokumentationssysteme gelingen (Häfner u. Klug 1980; Wing u. Hailey 1972). Der darauf folgende Schritt der Bewertung dieser Struktur als Ganzes erscheint jedoch nur schwer lösbar, da die verschiedenen Strukturelemente spezifischen Zwecken dienen und deshalb auch nach spezifisch angepaßten Kriterien zu beurteilen sind. Aus diesem Grund muß sich evaluative Forschung meistens auf die Wirkungen einzelner klar abgrenzbarer Entwicklungen innerhalb einer Versorgungsstruktur (z. B. Eröffnung einer neuen Ambulanz oder Tagesklinik) konzentrieren.

c) Indikatoren der Qualität und Effektivität. Jede Therapie oder jede Dienstleistung kann von einer Reihe verschiedener Standpunkte aus bewertet werden. Der Kliniker dient v. a. an den einzelnen Patienten und die Wirkung der Behandlung auf seinen Zustand, gleichzeitig aber beachtet er die Konsequenzen, die daraus für die Familie des Patienten entstehen. Die Verwaltung muß an Implikationen im Hinblick auf die Bettenbelegung, den Bedarf an Pflegepersonal und apparativer Ausstattung sowie Kostendeckung denken. Die Politiker werden v. a. an finanziellen und makroökonomischen Aspekten des Versorgungsangebots interessiert sein. Prinzipiell sollten alle diese Standpunkte in der Gesamtbewertung des Systems vertreten werden.

Die verfügbaren Indikatoren lassen sich in 5 Hauptgruppen wie folgt einordnen:

1) Kosten und Standards in bezug auf Personalschlüssel, Gebäude, Ausrüstung, Pflegesätze etc.

2) Maße für die Aktivität (z. B. Aufnahme und Entlassungszahlen, durchschnittliche Behandlungsdauer, Zahl der ambulanten Behandlungen) und das Qualitätsniveau (z. B. Prozentzahlen von ausgebildetem Fachpersonal) des Dienstes.

3) Effektivität der Behandlung bzw. Betreuung der einzelnen Patienten (z. B. Indizes der klinischen und sozialen Besserung – Häufigkeit von Frühberentung oder Arbeitslosigkeit – bei Patienten, die vom Dienst behandelt und versorgt werden, nach Möglichkeit mit geeigneten Kontrollgruppen verglichen).

4) Wirkungen auf *populationsbezogene Indikatoren* der psychiatrischen Morbidität (z. B. Suizidraten, alkohol- und drogenbedingte Sterblichkeit, Anzahl der psychisch kranken Gewalttäter etc.).

5) Akzeptanz des Dienstes, gemessen an der Zufriedenheit der Nutznießer, an der öffentlichen Meinung, an der Aktivierung des Laienpotentials sowie an der Arbeitsmoral des Dienstpersonals.

Diese Indikatoren lassen sich auf verschiedene Weise kombinieren. Bei der *Kosten-Nutzen-Analyse* z. B. wird versucht, durch eine Verknüpfung zwischen klinisch-medizinischen und ökonomischen Kriterien, die Effizienz des Dienstes zu überprüfen (Glass u. Goldberg 1977; Kanowski 1978; May 1970). Dabei darf nicht vergessen werden, daß nur klinisch-medizinische und epidemiologische Indikatoren – d. h. die Gruppen 3 und 4 oben – direkte Maßstäbe für die Effektivität sind, da sie die einzigen sind, die sich unmittelbar auf Gesundheit und Morbidität beziehen. Die übrigen können mit Effektivität zusammenhängen, tun es aber nicht notwendigerweise (Mac Mahon et al. 1961).

Die Forschungsstrategie

Die einfachste Stufe der evaluativen Forschung besteht in einer Beschreibung der Aufgabenbereiche eines Dienstes und einer Gegenüberstellung von tatsächlichen Leistungen auf rein deskriptiver Ebene: die sogenannte *Programmevaluierung* (Landsberg et al. 1979; Schulberg u. Baker 1979; Windle 1979). Die gleiche Strategie kann bei statistischen Untersuchungen über die Zahlen behandelter Patienten und ihre Verteilung nach Diagnose, klinischem Schweregrad, soziodemographischen Merkmalen usw. angewendet werden sowie bei Untersuchungen von Trends in der Inanspruchnahme von Diensten (Nielsen et al. 1981). Solche Informationen sind in erster Linie für die formative Evaluation erforderlich.

Differenziertere Strategien werden notwendig, wenn die Ergebnisse generalisierbar sein sollen. Das einfachste Forschungsdesign besteht dann darin, daß man vorbestimmte Indizes der Wirksamkeit (z. B. Anteil der Langzeitpatienten) zuerst vor Einführung eines neuen Versorgungsangebots ("baseline measures") und zu einem oder mehreren Zeitpunkten danach wieder mißt und die gemessene Werte miteinander vergleicht (Kessel u. Hassall 1971). Ein derartiges Spiegelbilddesign mag sich als bestmöglicher Kompromiß empfehlen, wenn eine Kontrollstudie nicht durchführbar ist. Dabei kann es sich aber als recht schwierig oder sogar unmöglich erweisen, spezifische Versorgungseffekte von zufälligen Einflüssen oder bei längeren Beobachtungsperioden, von allgemeinen säkularen Trends zu differenzieren. Deshalb sind Kontrollstudien immer dann vorzuziehen, wenn die Möglichkeit eines sinnvollen Vergleichs besteht.

Für evaluative Kontrollstudien in diesem Bereich besteht kein allgemein anerkanntes Paradigma. Bei der Bewertung somatischer Therapien gibt es zwar ein solches Paradigma, nämlich das des kontrollierten Versuches mit Zufallsverteilung ("randomized controlled trial"), dessen Anwendbarkeit in der evaluativen Forschung bleibt jedoch beschränkt. Hierunter versteht man den Vergleich der Veränderungen zwischen 2 oder mehreren Patientengruppen, die sich in jeder Hinsicht gleichen, außer in der jeweiligen spezifischen Therapie bzw. hinsichtlich präventiver Maßnahmen (Lilienfeld u. Lilienfeld 1980). Wenn überhaupt möglich, wird die Therapie ‚doppelblind' durchgeführt, d. h. weder dem Untersucher noch den Patienten wird bekannt, welche Mittel (z. B. Medikament oder Plazebo) der Patient erhalten hat.

Der wissenschaftliche Wert des randomisierten Versuchs bleibt unbestritten, was die Erprobung neuer Medikamente anbelangt. Er vertritt sozusagen ein Ideal an sauberer Methodik nach der auch die evaluative Forschung streben sollte (Cochrane 1972; Light 1976). Bei der Überprüfung psychologischer und sozialer Therapiemaßnahmen sowie von Versorgungsangeboten entstehen jedoch mehrere methodische Probleme. Zunächst einmal wird – anders als in der Pharmakotherapieforschung – ein ‚Blindversuch' nur ausnahmsweise möglich sein. Darüber hinaus kann eine wesentliche Voraussetzung für eine Zufallseinteilung in experimentelle und Kontrollgruppe nicht immer erfüllt werden, daß nämlich beide aus derselben Patientenpopulation gezogen werden sollen. Drittens muß das Forschungsprojekt in der Regel über mehrere Monate oder sogar Jahre hinweg laufen, wobei es, v. a. im ambulanten Bereich, entsprechend schwieriger wird, den Einfluß verschiedener Störvariablen auszuschließen und deshalb sicher zu sein, daß die Gruppen wirklich vergleichbar bleiben. Und schließlich gibt es manchmal ethische Bedenken gegenüber einer Zufallseinteilung der Patienten in experimentelle und Kontrollgruppen, obgleich sich die in Frage gestellte Therapie oder das Versorgungsangebot als unwirksam oder sogar als schädlich erweisen könnte. Aus allen diesen Gründen wurden bisher nur wenige evaluative Studien in der Psychiatrie realisiert, die sich auf Randomisierungsverfahren bezogen: diese betreffen meistens die Effektivität von Nachsorgeprogrammen für entlassene Klinikpatienten (Chowdhury et al. 1973; Hogarty et al. 1974).

Eine alternative Forschungsstrategie besteht darin, zwei oder mehrere Gebiete bzw. Einzugspopulationen mit kontrastierenden Versorgungsangeboten in bezug auf Indikatoren der oben genannten Art zu vergleichen. Eine Variante des Modells liegt vor, wenn eine Population Zugang zu einem neuen, quasiexperimentell eingesetzten Dienst hat, während eine andere Population weiterhin konventionell – d. h. von einem herkömmlichen, mehr oder weniger typischen – Dienst versorgt wird. Dieses Design, das schon mehrmals bei der Evaluation neu entwickelter gemeindenaher Versorgungsangebote verwendet wurde (Grad u. Sainsbury 1966; Kasius 1966), kommt dem wissenschaftlich-experimentellen Paradigma einen Schritt näher, auch wenn die Voraussetzungen für einen streng kontrollierten experimentellen Versuch immer noch nicht gegeben sind. Es kann sich auch unter Umständen die Möglichkeit eines Vergleichs zwischen parallelisierten Stichproben bieten (Cooper et al. 1975).

Eigentlich sollte bei der Evaluation eines Versorgungsdienstes, wie in der Therapieforschung, immer angestrebt werden, zwischen spezifischen Behandlungseffekten, dem „Milieu-Effekt" und der Interaktion zwischen beiden zu differenzieren (Rashkis u. Smarr 1958). In der Tat kann es jedoch sehr schwierig oder sogar unmöglich sein, diese Komponenten im Rahmen eines Versorgungs- oder Rehabilitationsprogramms getrennt voneinander zu messen. Behandlungsmethoden und Milieu können kaum trennbar sein, worauf beispielsweise Ausdrücke wie „therapeutische Gemeinschaft" und „Milieutherapie" (Krüger 1975; Ploeger 1980) hinweisen. Die Generalisierbarkeit von empirischen Forschungsergebnissen auf diesem Gebiet muß deshalb begrenzt bleiben, zumindest bis die therapeutisch wirksamen Komponenten solcher Programme klarer bestimmt und erfaßbar werden.

Ausgangsdaten, Indizes und Meßmethoden

Die in der evaluativen Forschung verwendeten Meßmethoden und Techniken sind keineswegs spezifisch: im Gegenteil, sie lassen sich von den in der klinischen, epidemiologischen oder sozialwissenschaftlichen Forschung gebrauchten Metho-

den ableiten. Es gibt keine evaluativen Allzweckwerkzeuge oder kein gebrauchs-
fertiges Kompendium von Meßinstrumenten, auf das sich der Forscher verlassen
könnte, unabhängig davon, welche Art von Einrichtung oder welche Zielgruppe
von Patienten er untersuchen will. Vielmehr muß bei jedem einzelnen Forschungsprojekt genau überlegt werden, welche Meßmethoden für die vorgesehenen Zielgruppen unter den gegebenen Rahmenbedingungen geeignet wären. Der
Erfolg von Projekten wird teilweise davon abhängen, ob die Forschung in der
Tat flexibel genug vorgehen und diejenigen Methoden auswählen können, die ihrer Zielsetzung am besten gerecht werden. In dieser Übersicht würde es also sehr
wenig nutzen, Listen von in Frage kommenden Meßindizes bzw. -instrumenten
aufzustellen. Stattdessen wird auf allgemeine Orientierungshilfen hingewiesen,
die im Problemfeld wichtig erscheinen.

Sekundärdatenerhebung und -quellen

Eine für die evaluative Forschung grundlegende Frage betrifft den Umfang, die
Qualität und die Verfügbarkeit der Daten, die im alltäglichen Verlauf eines Versorgungsdienstes aufgezeichnet, gesammelt und gespeichert werden (Kreitman
1975). Solche Daten sind – v. a., wenn ein vergleichbares Dokumentationssystem
benutzt wird (Dilling et al. 1982) – für die wissenschaftliche Bewertung des
Dienstangebotes sehr nützlich. Allerdings sind die meisten Dokumentationssysteme definitionsgemäß auf sog. Basisdaten beschränkt, die für evaluative Zwek-
ke allein nicht ausreichen. Sie müssen mit Hilfe gezielter Forschungserhebungen
ergänzt werden, deren Inhalt und Umfang durch die wissenschaftliche Zielsetzung zu bestimmen sind.

In den wenigen Forschungszentren, wo funktionierende psychiatrische Fallregister auf nationaler (Dupont et al. 1974), regionaler (Baldwin 1971) oder Ge-
bietsebene (Böhm u. Wagner 1981) bestehen, sollte es möglich sein, sowohl die
Qualität der erhobenen Daten zu überprüfen, als auch personenbezogene Daten
aus mehreren Einrichtungen in einer zentralen Datei zu verknüpfen (Acheson
1967). Als ein Gerüst für evaluative Forschung hat ein Fallregister erhebliche
Vorteile, da es sich auf eine definierte Einzugspopulation bezieht und da es Informationen über den Krankheitsverlauf und die Behandlungskarriere aller Patienten liefern kann, die mehrmals Kontakt mit den Einrichtungen aufnehmen (Brooke 1974; Häfner u. Klug 1980; Wing u. Hailey 1972). In letzter Zeit sind jedoch
Fallregister sowohl in der Psychiatrie als auch in manchen anderen medizinischen
Fachbereichen wegen der Datenschutzbestimmungen in große Schwierigkeiten
geraten (vgl. Probleme des Datenschutzes, S. 508).

Patientenbezogene Indizes

Während für die Einschätzung und Messung von Versorgungs*aktivitäten* die Erhebung anonymisierter, einrichtungsbezogener Daten ausreichen kann, werden
für Einschätzung und Messung der Versorgungs*effektivität* patientenbezogene
Daten erforderlich, die für einige Zwecke – z. B. die Erfassung von Mehrfachbe-

treuung – auch einrichtungsübergreifend verfügbar sein müssen. Hierfür kommen mehrere mögliche Datenquellen in Betracht.

a) Wichtig ist v. a. eine systematische Beurteilung des psychischen Zustandes des Patienten sowie der damit verbundenen Beeinträchtigungen und Risiken, die von einem Experten – sei es dem behandelnden Arzt oder einem Mitglied des Forschungsteams – vorgenommen werden soll. Diese Einschätzung soll nach Möglichkeit auf den Ergebnissen eines standardisierten Beurteilungsverfahrens – z. B. eines strukturierten oder halbstrukturierten Interviews, eines Fragebogens oder einer Ratingskala – basieren (Möller u. Zerssen 1983; Mombour 1972). Bei der Verwendung solcher Instrumente muß von Anfang an klar sein, welche Fertigkeiten und Fachkenntnisse bzw. welches zusätzliche methodische Training für eine verläßliche Fremdbeurteilung (z. B. Einschätzung von berichteten Symptomen, Krankheitsschweregrad etc.) erforderlich sind. Dies ist v. a. dann notwendig, wenn die Beurteilung nicht von klinisch erfahrenen Mitarbeitern durchgeführt werden kann.

b) Hinzu kommen Einschätzungen durch die Patienten selbst, die sowohl auf Fragebögen niedergelegte Selbstbeurteilungen (Möller u. Zerssen 1983) als auch Beurteilungen des Versorgungsangebots umfassen können ("consumer evaluation").

c) Schließlich sind Einschätzungen durch Angehörige oder andere Beziehungspersonen wichtig, die den psychischen Zustand des Patienten und seine Anpassungsfähigkeit im alltäglichen Leben betreffen.

Für eine ausgewogene Bewertung kann es erforderlich sein, die Einschätzungen von Patienten, Angehörigen und Betreuern bzw. Untersuchern sowohl miteinander als auch mit den administrativen Indizes zu vergleichen.

Längsschnitt- und Kohortenanalysen

Einzelne Querschnittserhebungen sind für evaluative Zwecke von nur begrenztem Wert. Sie gewinnen in diesem Zusammenhang erst dann an Bedeutung, wenn durch Replikation eine Reihe von Querschnittsanalysen bzw. Bestandsaufnahmen miteinander verglichen werden können oder wenn die einzelne Querschnittsanalyse als Basis für eine follow-up- oder Kohortenstudie dient. In der klinischen Forschung wird das Untersuchungskollektiv in der Regel aus neu aufgenommenen bzw. frisch entlassenen Patienten gebildet, deren späterer Krankheitsverlauf analysiert wird (follow-up-Studien). In der epidemiologischen Forschung hingegen handelt es sich eher *um Kohorten von Personen*, die in bezug auf ein gemeinsames punktuelles Ereignis, wie Geburt, Schulanfang, fünfundsechzigster Geburtstag etc. definiert werden und zur Grundlage einer Längsschnittverlaufsuntersuchung (Cooper 1979) werden. Von besonderer Bedeutung für alle Längsschnitt-Untersuchungen ist die eindeutige Festlegung sogenannter "outcome"-Variablen (Schimmelpfennig 1978; Schulberg u. Baker 1979).

Für die evaluative Forschung sind aus mehreren Gründen Längsschnittstudien erforderlich, in denen Patienten systematisch nachbeobachtet werden, und zwar aus 3 Gründen: 1) Sie bieten eine Möglichkeit, die verschiedenen Behandlungsepisoden miteinander zu verknüpfen und so die „Karriere" psychiatrischer Patienten durch die nacheinander folgenden Stufen ihrer Krankheitsverläufe zu verfolgen. 2) Es wird ermöglicht, den psychischen und sozialen Zustand des einzelnen Patienten zu bestimmten Zeitpunkten (z. B. ein Jahr oder zwei Jahre nach der Klinikaufnahme) festzustellen und auf dieser Basis systematische Vergleiche zwischen Patientengruppen unter verschiedenen Behandlungsbedingungen zu machen. 3) Auf diese Weise können auch diejenigen Patienten in die Untersuchung einbezogen werden, die nach einem oder mehreren Kontakten nicht mehr aufgetaucht sind und deren Schicksal den psychiatrischen Einrichtungen somit unbekannt bliebe.

Aus diesen Gründen stellt die Längsschnittstudie eine wesentliche Ergänzung zur einrichtungsbezogenen Dokumentation der Patientengruppen dar. Da sie aber eine relativ kostspielige und arbeitsintensive Forschungsstrategie ist, sollte sie nur für gezielte Fragestellungen eingesetzt werden. Als Zielgruppen kommen in erster Linie Patienten in Frage, die aufgrund des Krankheitsschweregrades, der Chronizität, der assoziierten Behinderungen oder anderer sozialer Konsequenzen unsere Gesellschaft mit dringlichen Gesundheitsproblemen konfrontieren.

Die Durchführung von Längsschnittstudien setzt gewisse Datenschutzvorkehrungen voraus, die im Abschn. „Probleme des Datenschutzes" (S. 508) abgehandelt werden.

Einrichtungsbezogene Indizes

Der Merkmalsraum einer Einrichtungsdokumentation bezieht sich v. a. auf die ersten 2 Gruppen von Indikatoren (vgl. Zielsetzung und Forschungsstrategie, S. 500), nämlich erstens finanzielle Aspekte (Betriebs- und Investitionskosten) und zweitens Aktivitäts- und Qualitätsmaße (Kanowski 1978; Light 1976). Die grundsätzlich deskriptiven Daten, die im Rahmen einzelner Bestandsaufnahmen erhoben werden, gewinnen jedoch erst dann eine evaluative Bedeutung, wenn eine Vergleichsbasis besteht und wenn sich darüber hinaus die Richtung dieser Unterschiede in bezug auf anerkannte Versorgungsprinzipien als erwünscht oder unerwünscht bewerten läßt. Bei der Planung einer Einrichtungsdokumentation sollten folgende Betrachtungsebenen im Mittelpunkt stehen:

- Standort und Kapazität des Versorgungsangebots im stationären, ambulanten und komplementär rehabilitativen Bereich in bezug auf die Einzugspopulation;
- Art und Breite des Angebotspektrums einschließlich patientenbezogener Kooperation zwischen Einrichtungen;
- Kostenträger und Art und Höhe der Kosten der Versorgungseinrichtungen; Verteilung der Angebotskapazität auf die verschiedenen Kosten- und Einrichtungsträger.

Schwierigkeiten kann die Entscheidung bereiten, ob die Effektivität einer Einrichtung grundsätzlich anhand vorgegebener (kosten)gesetzlicher Regelungen und Verwaltungsvereinbarungen oder eher nach einem von der betreffenden Institution selbst vorgegebenen Konzept beurteilt werden soll. Streng genommen sind die Funktionen und Aufgaben der Einrichtung vom Träger in Vereinbarung mit den zuständigen Behörden zu bestimmen. Allerdings müssen manchmal wegen der begrenzten Kapazität Prioritäten festgesetzt werden, die in der Tat zu einer Konzentration auf bestimmte Zielgruppen bzw. Behandlungsmodi und damit zu Abweichungen von den ursprünglichen Vereinbarungen führen. Dies muß bei der Evaluation in Betracht gezogen werden. So wäre es z. B. täuschend, 2 Tageskliniken nach den gleichen Kriterien zu beurteilen, wovon sich die eine auf die Nachsorge entlassener schizophrener Patienten konzentriert, während die andere v.a. eine Alternative zur stationären Aufnahme chronisch neurotischer und depressiver Patienten anbieten (Bosch u. Veltin 1983). Hier müßte jeweils festgestellt werden, erstens inwieweit die dem Konzept entsprechenden Aufgaben erfüllt wurden und zweitens, wie gut dieses Konzept in das Gesamtbild des Versorgungsangebots für die Einzugspopulation paßt.

Gebietsbezogene Indizes

Die Psychiatrie-Enquête ging in ihrem Bericht (Deutscher Bundestag 1975) von der Voraussetzung einer gemeindenahen Versorgung aus. Dabei hatten die Sachverständigen nicht nur eine gute geographische Erreichbarkeit vor Augen, sondern auch die Vorstellung, daß Einrichtungen, die ein und dieselbe Bevölkerung versorgen, miteinander intensiv kooperieren sollen. Die beiden Gesichtspunkte führten zu dem Vorschlag der Kommission, Standardversorgungsgebiete von 150000 bis 350000 Einwohnern abzugrenzen. Sollen Standardversorgungsgebiete evaluativ miteinander verglichen werden, so ist zu berücksichtigen, daß sie sehr unterschiedliche Aspekte je nach Wohnbevölkerung und deren Charakteristika bieten können, die direkte Vergleiche erschweren. Andererseits erscheint es unbedingt notwendig, neben den einzelnen Einrichtungen in einem Standardversorgungsgebiet auch ihre Leistung insgesamt zu betrachten, um z.B. kritisch zu überprüfen, inwieweit und mit welchem Erfolg sich das im Enquête-Bericht vorgestellte Konzept einer sektorisierten Psychiatrie verwirklichen läßt. Dies kann nur anhand von Indikatoren geschehen, die sich auf Daten von mehreren Einrichtungen innerhalb eines Gebietes beziehen: wie z.B. Rückgang der Anzahl von stationären Langzeitpatienten auf der einen Seite und Zunahme der Behandlungen in ambulanten und teilstationären Bereichen auf der anderen (Kessel u. Hassall 1971) oder Qualität und Umfang einer die Grenzen des Versorgungsgebietes „überschreitenden" Versorgung.

In diesem Zusammenhang wird oft von „Versorgungsnetzen" gesprochen. Damit soll die Notwendigkeit zur Kooperation und Koordination der Dienste in einem Standardversorgungsgebiet ausgedrückt werden. Dieser Begriff ist jedoch schwer zu definieren und in operationalisierte Prüfkriterien umzusetzen. Er hat in der Bundesrepublik Deutschland keine rechtsverbindliche Bedeutung und spielt in den Empfehlungen der Psychiatrie-Enquête keine Rolle. Es ist deshalb vorzuziehen, von Trägern der Standardversorgung und deren Koordination und Kooperation zu sprechen.

Neben einer Analyse von derartigen Beziehungen innerhalb eines Standardversorgungsgebietes müssen auch außerhalb des Gebietes die Einrichtungen und Dienste erfaßt werden, mit denen für Patienten aus dem Gebiet Kooperationsprobleme bestehen. Hierbei werden auch kritische Analysen über Vorteile bzw. Nachteile der Versorgung durch überregionale oder weit entfernte Institutionen zutage kommen.

Im allgemeinen setzt diese gebietsbezogene Evaluation nur geringe zusätzliche Datenerhebungen voraus; im wesentlichen sollte sie sich auf gezielte Analysen der Einrichtungs- und Patientendokumentation sowie der Längsschnittstudien beziehen. Grundsätzlich sind dafür 2 Auswertungsstrategien geeignet: 1) ein Vergleich zwischen der Situation zum Ausgangspunkt und einige Jahre später (1. und 2. Bestandsaufnahme), 2) Längsschnittuntersuchungen des Patientenstroms und insbesondere ausgewählter Patientenkohorten in einer Region.

Probleme des Datenschutzes

Besondere Bemerkungen müssen dem Datenschutz gewidmet werden. Grundsätzlich gilt seit jeher, daß persönlich identifizierbare Daten der ärztlichen Schweigepflicht unterliegen. Es dürfen also identifizierbare patientenbezogene Daten aus medizinischen Einrichtungen nur für bestimmte Zwecke, und zwar normalerweise nur mit Einwilligung der Betroffenen, weitergegeben werden. Lediglich, wenn dies zum Zwecke notwendiger Diagnostik und Therapie geschieht, darf das Einverständnis des Patienten stillschweigend vorausgesetzt werden.

Durch die Entwicklung der elektronischen Datenverarbeitung haben sich die Möglichkeiten vervielfacht, Informationen rasch zu speichern und weiterzugeben, so daß die in den letzten Jahren intensivierten und z. T. politisch kontrovers diskutierten Datenschutzbestrebungen grundsätzlich zu begrüßen sind, soweit sie die Belange des Individuums im notwendigen Umfang schützen. Ein Antagonismus wird offenbar, wenn Datenschutzvorkehrungen die medizinische Forschung in wichtigen Bereichen behindern oder sogar unmöglich machen (Baldwin et al. 1976; Böhm u. Wagner 1981).

Die heutzutage in der Bundesrepublik Deutschland geltenden Datenschutzregelungen und ihre Interpretation sind ein besonders gravierendes Beispiel für die Begrenzung der Möglichkeiten epidemiologischer und evaluativer Forschung. Es dürfen nach diesen Regelungen ohne besonderer Einwilligung der Patienten nur solche Daten dokumentiert werden, die in den behandelnden Einrichtungen im therapeutischen Zusammenhang ohnehin routinemäßig erfaßt werden. Forschungsspezifische Daten, die für einrichtungsübergreifende Untersuchungen erforderlich sind, dürfen demnach ohne Einwilligung der betroffenen Patienten nicht erhoben und weitergeleitet werden. Basisdaten über Patienten müssen vom therapeutischen Personal anonymisiert werden, bevor sie nach außen gehen. Datenauswertungen auf personenbezogener Ebene sind daher nur innerhalb der einzelnen Einrichtungen möglich.

Für die evaluative Forschung ist es nun besonders wichtig, das Funktionieren von Versorgungsprogrammen sowohl in bezug auf Patientenpopulationen als auch auf die Laufbahn einzelner Patienten zu untersuchen. Eine sinnvolle Analyse unter dieser Zielsetzung kann aber nur gelingen, wenn eine personenbezogene Dokumentation ermöglicht wird, die es erlaubt, Wiederaufnahmen und Wechsel zwischen Versorgungseinrichtungen zu erkennen und damit individuelle Krankheitsverläufe nachzuvollziehen (Acheson 1967). Für die Forschung müssen deshalb individualisierbare Daten verschiedener Einrichtungen zur Verfügung stehen. Nur so läßt sich die Verknüpfung der Institutionen und ihr Zusammenspiel prüfen. Auch die Zahl der insgesamt Behandelten sollte festzustellen sein, d.h. daß Mehrfachzählungen ausgeschlossen sein müssen. Will man also Funktion und Effizienz des Versorgungssystems prüfen, so kann dies nur mit Hilfe genauer

Kenntnis der behandelten Patienten und ihren Weges durch die Versorgungskette der operierenden Einrichtungen geschehen.

Bei Beachtung der gegenwärtig engen Auslegung der Datenschutzbestimmungen in bezug auf die Forschung, können solche Untersuchungen kaum noch stattfinden, da eine schriftliche Einwilligung des einzelnen Patienten immer erforderlich wird. Die Notwendigkeit, sich nur auf ausgewählte Gruppen von Patienten zu verlassen, die bereit sind, aktiv an Forschungsprojekten teilzunehmen, indem sie schriftlich in die Weitergabe ihrer Daten einwilligen, hat offensichtliche Beschränkungen und Nachteile. Gerade in der Psychiatrie muß man die Repräsentativität solcher Patientenstichproben bezweifeln, da ein Teil der Patienten aus Krankheitsgründen nicht in der Lage sein wird, rechtsgültige Einwilligungen zu geben, während andere, zum Teil auch aus krankheitsbedingten Gründen, ihre Zustimmung verweigern werden. Auch die Motivation derjenigen, die einwilligen, ist nicht ohne weiteres zu erkennen und kann zu einer weiteren Stichprobenverzerrung führen.

Für die Erprobung eines Versorgungssystems ist also die Untersuchung repräsentativer und individualisierbarer Patientenstichproben unabdingbar. Rein technisch wäre es auch möglich, einrichtungsübergreifende Datenanalysen unter Einhaltung eines hohen Sicherheitsgrades durchzuführen. Dieser Standard ließe sich beispielsweise durch Doppelverschlüsselung der Individualdaten erreichen. Ein solcher Kode muß unabhängig von Ort und Zeit die verschlüsselten Personen eindeutig bestimmen, so daß eine Person nicht mehrere Kodes trägt oder mehrere Personen denselben Kode tragen, andererseits aber eine Identifikation für Außenstehende, d. h. nicht mit dem Kode Vertraute, unmöglich ist. Die Verschlüsselung darf nur durch eine oder sehr wenige autorisierte Personen erfolgen, damit die Geheimhaltung gewährleistet ist. Systeme dieser Art konnten jedoch bisher nicht eingeführt werden, da sie entweder vom zuständigen Datenschutzbeauftragten beanstandet oder vom Forschungsträger für zu lästig und kostspielig gehalten wurden.

Auf diesem Hintergrund stellt sich das Datenschutzgesetz in seiner gegenwärtigen Form zu sehr als ein restriktives Verbot der Datenerhebung bzw. -weitergabe dar, anstatt sich stärker mit notwendigen und einzuhaltenden Voraussetzungen für den Schutz des Individuums im Falle der Datenweitergabe auseinanderzusetzen. Bei einer Novellierung des Bundesdatenschutzgesetzes bzw. der entsprechenden Ländergesetze sollte ernsthaft überlegt werden, ob eine so große Begrenzung der Forschungsmöglichkeiten, die nicht nur für die Psychiatrie, sondern für alle medizinischen Versorgungsbereiche zutrifft, im allgemeinen Interesse der Patienten gerechtfertigt ist. Dabei wäre stärker als bisher der Tatsache Rechnung zu tragen, daß der Fortschritt in der medizinischen Forschung schließlich sowohl dem Individuum als auch der Gesamtbevölkerung zu dienen hat.

Schlußfolgerungen

In der modernen technologischen Gesellschaft ist evaluative Forschung zu einem wichtigen Instrument beim Aufbau bzw. Umbau sozialer Strukturen und bei der Entwicklung sozialer Prozesse geworden. Sie bietet Politikern und Planern eine

Möglichkeit, Fehler zu vermeiden oder mindestens zu minimieren, neue Ansätze zu überprüfen und Schritt mit den sich ändernden Sozialbedingungen zu halten. Forschung dieser Art hat eine besondere sozialpolitische Bedeutung: sie stellt eine der selbstregulierenden Tendenzen dar, die nur in einer offenen Gesellschaft effektiv funktionieren kann, die aber auch für das Überleben der offenen Gesellschaft nötig geworden ist (Cooper 1976).

In keinem medizinischen Fachgebiet ist heute wissenschaftliche Evaluation dringlicher als in der Psychiatrie, wo einem notwendigen Reformbedarf ein Mangel an fundierten Kenntnissen über optimale Behandlung und Versorgung gegenübersteht. Bislang beschränkte sich evaluative Forschung der hier vorgestellten Art – d.h. basierend auf klaren Definitionen, standardisierten Meßmethoden und kontrollierten Vergleichsstudien – auf wenige isolierte Projekte in Universitätsabteilungen und Forschungsinstituten. Auf Praxis und Planung im psychiatrischen Versorgungsbereich hat sie kaum Einfluß ausgeübt.

Eine systematische Anwendung evaluativer Forschung in diesem Bereich ist an 5 Voraussetzungen gebunden:

1) Es müssen Forschungsstrategien und -methoden entwickelt werden, die relativ ökonomisch und leicht anwendbar sind. Es erscheint in diesem Zusammenhang sehr wünschenswert, daß in einigen Regionen der Aufbau bzw. die Weiterführung psychiatrischer Fallregister ermöglicht werden sollte, um die methodische Entwicklung voranzutreiben.

2) Zwischen wissenschaftlicher Forschung und klinischer Praxis müssen Brücken geschlagen werden, so daß die in der Praxis tätigen Fachleute in die Lage versetzt werden, an evaluativen Forschungsprojekten aktiv oder beratend teilzunehmen. Nur auf diese Weise kann sichergestellt werden, daß die Forschungsprojekte auf dem Boden der Realität stehen.

3) Die wissenschaftliche Unabhängigkeit und Neutralität der in der Evaluation tätigen Forscher muß gewährleistet sein.

4) Politiker und Planer müssen bereit sein, die Ansprüche der evaluativen Forschung ernst zu nehmen, d.h. dieser nicht nur eine Alibifunktion zuzuteilen, sondern die Rahmenbedingungen für solche Forschung zu schaffen, ihre Ergebnisse – ob als politisch günstig oder ungünstig betrachtet – bekanntzugeben und ihre Implikationen in den Entscheidungsprozeß einzubeziehen.

5) Schließlich müssen bei der Vorbereitung evaluativer Forschungsprograme die Rahmenbedingungen sorgfältig und rechtzeitig bedacht und ihre Konsequenzen bei der Durchführung des Programms berücksichtigt werden.

Was sind nun die erforderlichen Rahmenbedingungen? Sie betreffen in erster Linie die wechselseitige Abhängigkeit von Modellentwicklung und wissenschaftlicher Begleitung. Einerseits läßt sich Forschung nicht im luftleeren Raum planen, sondern ist von konkreten Fragestellungen her zu entwickeln, die im vorliegenden Kontext von der Art der Versorgungseinrichtungen mitbestimmt werden. Andererseits muß bei der Planung neuer Versorgungsstrukturen auf forschungsimmanente Anforderungen Rücksicht genommen werden. Dabei ist auch zu bedenken, ob aus den Modellversuchen resultierende Kostenprobleme im Rahmen traditionell vorgegebener Finanzierungssysteme gelöst oder auch hier innovative Anregungen entwickelt werden sollten. Der Versuch, neue Vorsorgungsmodi innerhalb eines existierenden starren Finanzierungssystems zu entwickeln, kann Faktoren des Scheiterns von vornherein beinhalten.

Soll die Aussagekraft der Forschungsergebnisse nicht gefährlich eingeschränkt werden, sind Probleme mit Datenschutzvorschriften vor der Phase der Modellimplementation zu klären. Eine Lösung auf der Ebene praktischer Kompromisse kann nur nach Abwägung aller Aspekte – ethischer, juristischer, politischer und wissenschaftlicher – in sinnvoller Weise gefunden werden. Die juristische Kompetenz darf nicht als die allein zuständige angesehen werden.

Schließlich muß der Modellentwicklung und -erprobung eine angemessene Planungsphase vorangehen. Je umfangreicher und komplexer das Modellprogramm, um so sorgfältiger muß diese Phase gestaltet werden, obgleich dies unvermeidlich Zeit- und Geldeinsatz bedeutet. Stellt man die beachtliche Höhe der finanziellen Aufwendungen für Modellprogramme in den psychiatrischen und sozialen Versorgungsbereichen in Rechnung, so wäre es wohl unverantwortlich, Mittel für eine fundierte wissenschaftliche Evaluation nicht aufwenden zu wollen, deren Umfang nur einen kleinen Bruchteil des ganzen Finanzierungsvolumens ausmacht, weil sie allein eine Basis für eine rational begründete Verbesserung der Versorgung psychisch Kranker und Behinderter bieten kann.

Literatur

Acheson ED (1967) Medical record linkage. Oxford University Press, London

Baldwin JA (1971) The mental hospital in the psychiatric service. Oxford University Press, London

Baldwin JA, Leff J, Wing JK (1976) Confidentiality of psychiatric data in medical information systems. Br J Psychiatry 128:417–442

Biefang S (1980) Evaluationsforschung in der Psychiatrie. Fragestellungen und Methoden. Enke, Stuttgart

Böhm K, Wagner G (1981) Datenschutz für Krebspatienten. Interessenkonflikt zwischen Patientenrecht und Forschungszwängen. Dtsch Ärztebl 42:1977–1982

Borach RF, Riecken HW (1975) Experimental testing of public policy. Westview, Boulder/CO

Bosch G, Veltin A (1983) Die Tagesklinik als Teil der psychiatrischen Versorgung. Aktion Psychisch Kranke, Tagungsberichte Bd 9. Rheinland, Köln

Brooke EM (1974) The current and future use of registers in health information systems. WHO Genf

Bundesminister für Jugend, Familie und Gesundheit (1979) Konzept für die Umsetzung der Ankündigung der Bundesregierung, zusätzliche Finanzmittel für neue Modelle in der Psychiatrie bereitzustellen. Drucksache 8/2865

Chowdhury N, Hicks RC, Kreitman N (1973) Evaluation of an after-care service for parasuicide (attempted suicide) patients. Soc Psychiatry 8:67–81

Cochrane AL (1972) Effectiveness and efficiency. Random reflections on health services. Nuffield Provincial Hospitals Trust, London

Cook TD, Reichardt CS (1979) Qualitative and quantitative methods in evaluation research. Sage research progress series in evaluation, vol 1. Sage Publications, Beverly Hills/CA

Cook TD, Cook FL, Mark MM (1977) Randomized and quasiexperimental designs in evaluation research. In: Rutman L (ed) Evaluation research methods: a basic guide. Sage Publications, Beverly Hills/CA, pp 101–140

Cooper B (1976) Die Bedeutung von Forschungsergebnissen für Praxis und Planung in der Psychiatrie. In: Kulenkampff C, Picard W (Hrsg) Gemeindenahe Psychiatrie. Rheinland, Köln, S 144–154

512

B. Cooper et al.

Cooper B (1979) Demographic and epidemiological methods in psychiatric research. In: Kisker KP et al. (Hrsg) Psychiatrie der Gegenwart Bd I, 2. Aufl. Berlin S 685–710

Cooper B, Sosna U (1983) Psychische Erkrankung in der Altenbevölkerung: eine epidemiologische Feldstudie in Mannheim. Nervenarzt 54:239–249

Cooper B, Harwin BG, Depla C, Shepherd M (1975) Mental health care in the community: an evaluative study. Psychol Med 5:373–380

Cranach M von, Wittchen H-U (1980) Epidemiologische Aspekte der Evaluationsforschung in der psychiatrischen Versorgung. In. Biefang S (Hrsg) (1980), S 208–249

Deutscher Bundestag (1975) Bericht über die Lage der Psychiatrie in der Bundesrepublik Deutschland. Deutscher Bundestag, 7. Wahlperiode. Drucksache 7/4200. Heger, Bonn

Deutscher Bundestag (1979) Stellungnahme der Bundesregierung zum Bericht der Sachverständigen-Kommission über die Lage der Psychiatrie in der Bundesrepublik Deutschland. Deutscher Bundestag 8. Wahlperiode. Drucksache 8/2565 Heger, Bonn

Dilling H, Balck F, Bosch G et al. (1982) Die psychiatrische Basisdokumentation. Bericht über die Tätigkeit der Arbeitsgruppe und Vorschlag der DGPN sowie der Bundesarbeitsgemeinschaft der Träger psychiatrischer Krankenhäuser zur Vereinheitlichung der Merkmalskataloge. Spektrum 5:147–160

Dilling H, Weyerer S, Castell R (1984) Psychische Erkrankungen in der Bevölkerung. Enke. Stuttgart

Dupont A, Videbeck T, Weeke A (1974) A cumulative national psychiatric register its structure and application. Acta Psychiatr Scand 50:161–173

Glass NJ, Goldberg D (1977) Cost-benefit analysis and the evaluation of psychiatric services. Psychol Med 7:701–707

Grad J, Sainsbury P (1966) Evaluating the community psychiatric service in Chichester: Results. In: Gruenberg EM (ed) (1966), pp 246–278

Gruenberg EM (1966) Evaluating the effectiveness of mental health services. Milbank Mem Fund Q 44:1–402

Häfner H, Klug J (1980) First evaluation of the Mannheim community mental health service. In: Strömgren E, Dupont A, Nielsen JA (eds) Epidemiological research as basis for the organization of extramural psychiatry. Acta Psychiatr Scand [Suppl] 62:67–78

Hogarty GE, Goldberg SC, Schooler NR, Ulrich RF (1974) Drug and sociotherapy in the aftercare of schizophrenic patients. II. Two-year relapse rates. Arch Gen Psychiatry 31:603–608

Holland WW (1983) Evaluation of health care. Oxford University Press, Oxford

Kanowski S (1978) Zur Problematik der Planung von Kosten-Nutzen-Analysen in der Gerontopsychiatrie. In: Lauter H (Hrsg) Gerontopsychiatrie 6. Janssen, Düsseldorf, S 343–360

Kasius RV (1966) The social breakdown syndrome in a cohort of long-stay patients in the Dutchess County Unit, 1960–1963 In: Gruenberg EM (ed) (1966)

Kessel N, Hassall C (1971) Evaluation of the functioning of the Plymouth Nuffield clinic. Br J Psychiatry 118:305–312

Kramer M, Taube CA (1973) The role of a national statistics programme in the planning of community psychiatric services in the United States. In: Wing JK, Häfner H (eds) Roots of evaluation. The epidemiological basis for planning psychiatric services. Oxford Univ Press, London, pp 35–73

Kreitman N (1975) The use of clinical records in retrospective research. In. Sainsbury P, Kreitman N (eds) Methods of psychiatric research, 2nd edn Oxford Univ Press, London, pp 120–132

Krüger H (1975) Therapeutische Gemeinschaften. In: Kisker KP et al. (Hrsg) Psychiatrie der Gegenwart III. Soziale und angewandte Psychiatrie, 2. Aufl. Springer, Berlin Heidelberg New York

Landsberg G, Neigher WD, Hammer RJ, Windle C, Woy JR (1979) Evaluation in practice. A sourcebook of program evaluation studies from mental health care systems in the United States. Dept of Health Education and Welfare, Rockville/MD

Lewin K (1947) Frontiers in group dynamics. part II: social planning and action research. Hum Rel 1:143–153

Light RJ (1976) Research design and policy inferences. In: Abt CC (ed) The evaluation of social programs. Sage Publications, Beverly Hills/CA

Lilienfeld AM, Lilienfeld DE (1980) Foundations of epidemiology 2nd ed. Oxford University Press, New York, pp 256-275

MacMahon B, Pugh TF, Hutchinson GB (1961) Principles in the evaluation of community mental health programs. Am J Public Health 51:963

May AR (1976) Mental health services in Europe. WHO Offset Publication No. 23 WHO, Genf

May PRA (1970) Cost-efficiency of mental health delivery systems. A review of the literature on hospital care. Am J Public Health 60:2060-2067

Möller HJ, Zerssen D v. (1983) Psychopathometrische Verfahren: II. Standardisierte Beurteilungsverfahren. Nervenarzt 54:1-16

Mombour W (1972) Verfahren zur Standardisierung des psychopathologischen Befundes. Psychiatr Clin 5:73-120:137-157

Moser H (1975) Aktionsforschung als kritische Theorie der Sozialwissenschaften. Kösel, München

Nielsen J, Nielsen JA, Kastrup M, Strömgren E (1981) The Samsø Project. A community psychiatric project in a geographically delimited population. Acta Jutlandica 55

Platt S, Weyman A, Hirsch S, Hewett S (1980) The social behaviour assessment schedule (SBAS) Rationale, contents, scoring and reliability of a new interview schedule. Soc Psychiatry 15:43-55

Ploeger A (1980) Milieutherapie und therapeutische Gemeinschaft. In: Peters UH (Hrsg) Die Psychologie des 20. Jahrhunderts. Band X: Ergebnisse für die Medizin (2): Psychiatrie. Kindler, Zürich, S 1011-1025

Rashkis HA, Smarr ER (1958) A method for the control and evaluation of sociopsychological factors in pharmacological research. Psychiatr Res Rep Am Psychiatr Assoc 9:121-129

Riecken HW (1976) Social experimentation. In: Abt CC (ed) The evaluation of social programs. Sage Publications, Beverly Hills/CA

Schimmelpenning GW (1978) Psychiatrische Verlaufsforschung: Methoden und Ergebnisse. Huber, Bern

Schulberg HC, Baker F (1979) Program evaluation in the health fields. Vol II. Human Sciences, New York

Suchmann EA (1967) Evaluative research: Principles and practice. Russell Sage Foundation, New York

Weismann MM (1975) The assessment of social adjustment: a review of techniques. Arch Gen Psychiatry 32:357-365

Windle C (1979) Reporting program evaluations: Two sample community mental health centre annual evaluation reports. Rockville/MD, U.S. Dept. of Health, Education and Welfare, Public Health Service

Wing JK (1973) Principles of evaluation. In: Wing JK, Häfner H (eds) Roots of evaluation. Oxford University Press, London, pp 3-12

Wing JK (1975) Die Evaluation gemeindenaher psychiatrischer Dienste. Arch Psychiatr Nervenkr 220:245—254

Wing JK, Hailey AM (1972) Evaluating a community psychiatric service: the Camberwell register 1964-71. Oxford University Press, London

World Health Organization (1971) Classification and evaluation of mental health service activities. Second interim report of a working group W.H.O. Regional Office for Europe, Copenhagen

World Health Organization (1980) Changing patterns in mental health care. Euro. Reports and Studies, 25. W.H.O. Regional Office for Europe, Copenhagen

Soziale Isolation, psychische Erkrankung und Altersverlauf. Eine epidemiologische Untersuchung *

B. Cooper, J. Jaeger, H. Bickel

Der Begriff „soziale Isolation" und seine Anwendung in der psychiatrischen Forschung

Seit Durkheim (1973) sind die sich überschneidenden Konzepte Anomie, Entfremdung und soziale Isolation immer wieder als Variablen genannt worden, die den Ausbruch einer seelischen Krise oder einer psychischen Krankheit erklären könnten. So wurden beispielsweise für Suizid (Sainsbury 1955) sowie für die Behandlungsinzidenz von Schizophrenie (Faris u. Dunham 1939) Zusammenhänge mit stadtökologischen Indizes für soziale Isolation festgestellt. Auch die gerontopsychiatrische Forschung hat dieser Variablen Aufmerksamkeit gewidmet, da soziale Isolation von Sozialwissenschaftlern als „ein wesentliches Kennzeichen der Lebensbedingungen alter Menschen" (Parsons 1968) bezeichnet wurde.

Die Bedeutung sozialer Isolation oder Integration für die psychische Gesundheit älterer Menschen bleibt allerdings weitgehend ungeklärt. Zwar weisen mehrere Autoren auf einen allgemeinen Zusammenhang zwischen Isolation und psychischen Alterserkrankungen hin, es ist der empirischen Forschung jedoch bis-

Tabelle 1. Soziale Isolation – Analyseebenen und Kriterien. (Nach Sosna u. Cooper 1980)

Ebene der Analyse	Kriterien
Ökologische Ebene	1. Soziale Isolation als Merkmal von Wohngebieten (z. B. Anteil der Einpersonenhaushalte)
Ebene der sozialen Interaktion	2. Alleinleben
	3. Mangel an familiären und außerfamiliären Kontakten
Psychologische Ebene	4. Subjektive Isolation (z. B. Gefühle der Einsamkeit und Verlassenheit)
	5. Isolation von Gruppennormen (Alienation, Anomie)

* Das Forschungsprojekt wurde zuerst als Teil des SFB 116 (Psychiatrische Epidemiologie) an der Universität Heidelberg, später mit Unterstützung des Bundesministeriums für Jugend, Familie und Gesundheit durchgeführt. Wir danken herzlich den ehemaligen Mitarbeitern dieses Projekts, insbesondere Frau Dr. U. Sosna, die das IMSI entwickelte, und Frau Dipl.-Psych. B. Mahnkopf, die für die soziale Untersuchung der Heimbewohner zuständig war.
Dieser Beitrag erschien bereits in: Angermeyer MC, Klusmann D (Hrsg) (1989) Soziales Netzwerk. Springer, Berlin Heidelberg New York Tokyo, S. 231–246.

lang weder gelungen, Probleme der Definition und Operationalisierung zu überwinden, noch Ursache und Wirkung zu differenzieren. Die in den Studien verwendeten Isolationskriterien lassen sich im wesentlichen in 5 Kategorien gruppie-
ren, die 3 unterschiedlichen Analyseebenen entsprechen (s. Tabelle 1).

Ökologische Ebene

Die meisten Hinweise auf Verbindungen zwischen sozialer Isolation und psychischen Störungen im Alter stammen aus ökologisch orientierten Studien, in denen Isolation nicht als individuelles Merkmal, sondern als Kennzeichen um-
schriebener Wohngebiete gemessen wurde (Cooper u. Sosna 1980). Die Ergebnisse zur Verteilung psychischer Alterserkrankungen sind jedoch weniger konsistent
als die entsprechenden Daten zur Schizophrenie und erlauben keine gesicherten
Schlußfolgerungen.

Ebene der sozialen Interaktion

Zahlreiche Untersuchungen haben gezeigt, daß alleinlebende Ältere erhöhte Auf-
nahmeraten aufweisen und in Altenpflegeheimen mit ihrem hohen Anteil an psychisch kranken Bewohnern überrepräsentiert sind; diese Ergebnisse könnten aber
eine Folge selektiver Einweisungsprozesse sein. Definitive Nachweise dafür, daß
die Inzidenz und Prävalenz psychischer Störungen bei alleinlebenden älteren
Menschen höher liegen als in anderen Gruppen der Altenbevölkerung, stehen
noch aus. Die Forschungsergebnisse entsprechender Feldstudien (Nielsen 1962;
Kay et al. 1964; Lowenthal u. Berkman 1967) sind in diesem Zusammenhang un-
schlüssig und z. T. widersprüchlich.

Alleinleben ist nicht notwendigerweise mit Isolation gleichzusetzen. Viele der
betroffenen Älteren sind eingebunden in ein tragfähiges Netz familiärer und sozialer Beziehungen. So liegt nahe, Isolation auch über die Häufigkeit persönlicher
Kontakte in einem bestimmten Zeitraum zu erfassen. Die bekanntesten Beispiele
dieses Ansatzes sind die englischen Arbeiten von Townsend (1957) und Tunstall
(1966), die ein Scoresystem für Sozialkontakte entwickelt und angewendet haben. Von einem ähnlichen Ansatzpunkt aus haben Lowenthal u. Berkman (1967)
versucht, die Zusammenhänge zwischen Kontakthäufigkeit und psychiatrischem
Krankheitsrisiko zu prüfen. Die kleine Gruppe der nach ihren Kriterien ausgesprochen isoliert lebenden Alten war nicht auffällig häufig psychisch gestört, obgleich bei leichteren Formen von Kontaktmangel eine gewisse Häufung gefunden
wurde.

Diese rein quantitativen Indizes lassen wichtige qualitative Aspekte außer
acht, die in der Feldforschung nur schwer erfaßbar sind, bei der Ermittlung des
Morbiditätsrisikos jedoch von entscheidender Bedeutung sein können. Untersuchungen der Qualität sozialer Kontakte wurden in der psychiatrischen Forschung nur selten durchgeführt (Henderson et al. 1981); in der Gerontopsychiatrie hat man einen derartigen Ansatz bislang nicht verfolgt.

Psychologische Ebene

Subjektive Aspekte sozialer Isolation, etwa Einsamkeitsgefühle, sind mit den
eher objektiven Indizes, z. B. Kontakthäufigkeit, nicht eng korreliert (Bungard
1975). Personen mit relativ vielen Kontakten können durchaus unter Einsamkeit
leiden, wenn diese Kontakte ihre psychischen Bedürfnisse nicht erfüllen können;
auf der anderen Seite klagen Ältere, die schon ein Leben lang kontaktarm gewesen sind, meistens nicht über Einsamkeitsgefühle. Nach den Ergebnissen einer
Reihe von psychiatrischen Feldstudien (Sheldon 1948; Kay et al. 1964; Lowenthal 1964) erscheint es notwendig, die Rolle von Einsamkeit und emotionaler Isolation unabhängig von der Häufigkeit sozialer Kontakte zu untersuchen.

Einige Forscher schließlich haben Isolation als Alienation oder Entfremdung
von kulturellen oder Gruppennormen interpretiert: ein Konzept, das sich, eng
verwandt mit Durkheims Anomie, ursprünglich auf Kollektive bezog, dann aber
als „psychologische Anomie" oder „anomia" auch auf Individuen angewandt
wurde (Srole 1956). Auch dieser Ansatz wurde in der gerontopsychiatrischen
Forschung noch nicht aufgegriffen, obgleich man postulieren kann, daß in unserer Gesellschaft alte Menschen davon besonders betroffen sind.

Dieser kurze Überblick macht deutlich, daß sowohl die Operationalisierung
als auch die psychiatrische Relevanz des Konzeptes „soziale Isolation" divergie-
rend und unbestimmt geblieben sind. Eine adäquate Forschungsstrategie sollte
deshalb versuchen, die unterschiedlichen Aspekte sozialer Isolation getrennt voneinander zu erfassen und ihre Korrelationen untereinander und mit psychischer
Erkrankung zu überprüfen.

Forschungsziele und Methodik

Im Rahmen einer epidemiologischen Feldstudie in Mannheim, die auf einer repräsentativen Stichprobe von 350 in Privathaushalten lebenden über 65jährigen
und einer weiteren Stichprobe von 153 in Alten- und Pflegeheimen untergebrachten Älteren basierte, wurden die Zusammenhänge zwischen Isolation in ihren unterschiedlichen Erscheinungsformen und psychiatrischer Morbidität untersucht.
Der ersten querschnittlichen Erhebung folgte nach 7,8 Jahren bei der Gemeindestichprobe bzw. nach 5,6 Jahren bei den in Heimen versorgten Probanden eine
zweite Befragung, um u. a. die prognostische Bedeutung sozialer Isolation für die
Inzidenz psychischer Erkrankungen, Heimeinweisung und Mortalität zu ermitteln.

Über die psychiatrischen Untersuchungsmethoden und die zentralen Ergebnisse der Querschnittstudie ist schon ausführlich berichtet worden (Cooper u.
Sosna 1983; Sosna u. Wahl 1983; Cooper 1984; Cooper et al. 1984). Im Follow-
up wurde der psychische Gesundheitszustand der überlebenden Probanden anhand des bereits im Erstinterview verwendeten Instrumentes beurteilt. Bei Verstorbenen trat an die Stelle der differenzierten psychiatrischen Diagnostik eine
das letzte Lebensjahr betreffende globale Demenzeinschätzung, die auf einer systematischen Befragung naher Angehöriger oder anderer Informanten beruhte.

Zur Erfassung der Häufigkeit und Verteilung sozialer Isolation bei der Erstbefragung entwickelte die Forschungsgruppe ein Meßinstrument, das alle in Tabelle 1 dargestellten Analyseebenen berücksichtigt: das „Interview zur Messung sozialer Isolation" – IMSI (Sosna 1983). Als ökologische Parameter dienen die den städtischen Statistiken entnommenen Daten über die prozentualen Anteile der Einpersonenhaushalte sowie der Ledigen, Verwitweten und Geschiedenen in den Stadtbezirken, denen die Probanden jeweils angehörten. Die beiden anderen Dimensionen werden durch einen detaillierten halbstrukturierten Fragebogen abgedeckt.

Die Ebene der sozialen Interaktion ist in der Meßvariablen Kontakthäufigkeit repräsentiert. Die Operationalisierung orientiert sich an der von Townsend (1957) entwickelten und von Tunstall (1966) modifizierten Technik, systematisch alle in der Woche vor dem Interview stattgefundenen und mindestens 5 min währenden Kontakte sowohl mit Familienangehörigen (mit Ausnahme des Ehepartners: s. unten) als auch außerfamiliärer Art (Freunde, Nachbarn, Arbeitskollegen, Angehörige medizinischer und sozialer Versorgungsdienste einschließlich des Arztes, Mitarbeiter kirchlicher Einrichtungen, Hilfspersonen, Pflegekräfte im Heim, Heimmitbewohner und sonstige Personen) aufzulisten. Die Summe der mit je einem Punkt verrechneten Kontakte, eine konstante Punktzahl für im Zusammenleben mit dem Ehepartner automatisch gegebene Kontaktmöglichkeiten und Scores für gemeinsam mit Dritten eingenommene Hauptmahlzeiten ergeben, ohne weitere Gewichtung aufaddiert, den Gesamtpunktwert der Kontakthäufigkeit.

Als Indikatoren sozialer Isolation auf der psychologischen Ebene erfaßt das Interview das Ausmaß erfahrener und verfügbarer instrumenteller und emotionaler Hilfe und Unterstützung durch die bestehenden familiären und außerfamiliären Beziehungen, den Grad der Alienation und die subjektiv empfundene Einsamkeit.

Im erstgenannten Aspekt sind zentrale Bedürfnisse des alternden Menschen angesprochen, wie sie von Weiss (1974) beschrieben wurden: Beistand und Hilfe zu erlangen sowohl bei alltäglichen Pflichten und Aufgaben als auch in Konflikten und Auseinandersetzungen mit Dritten oder in Notfällen, zu wissen, daß man gebraucht wird, und zu erleben, daß man sich auf vertrauensvolle Beziehungen stützen und eigene Aktivitäten und Interessen mit anderen teilen kann. Die Erfüllung dieser Bedürfnisse wird nach den Auskünften der Probanden auf 5stufigen Skalen quantifiziert und zu einem Gesamtscore (0–24) aufsummiert. Der Meßwert für Alienation (0–36) leitet sich aus der ins Deutsche übertragenen Subskala „soziale Isolation" von Dean (1961) ab, eine 9 Items umfassende Einstellungsskala. Zum Ausmaß erlebter Einsamkeit schließlich werden die Probanden gefragt, ob sie sich einsam fühlen und ob sie sich für einsamer als andere Gleichaltrige halten.

Bei der Datenauswertung wurde der Struktur der Kontaktsituation auf der Variablen- und auf der Personenebene nachgegangen. Es wurde sowohl geprüft, ob die verschiedenartigen Indikatoren für soziale Isolation konvergieren, als auch der Versuch unternommen, die Stichprobe in homogene Subgruppen zu untergliedern, die hinsichtlich ihrer sozialen Beziehungen typisch für die Altenbevölkerung sind. Zu diesem Zweck wurde ein clusteranalytisches Verfahren verwendet, das zu Lösungen mit vollständiger Zuordnung aller Stichprobenmitglieder in einander wechselseitig ausschließende Gruppen führt.

Um die prognostische Bedeutung sozialer Isolation für zentrale Ereignisse im Alter zu ermitteln, wurde ein Verfahren für die multivariate Analyse von Verlaufsdaten eingesetzt, das Proportional-Hazards-Regressionsmodell von Cox (1972), das für eine Auswertung von Longitudinalstudien günstige Eigenschaften besitzt.

Forschungsergebnisse

Zum Zusammenhang zwischen den Isolationsindizes

Anhand der Daten aus der Gemeindestichprobe wurden die Interkorrelationen der zentralen Isolationsmerkmale berechnet. Die Zusammenhänge waren ausnahmslos positiv und statistisch signifikant, lagen numerisch jedoch nur in einer geringen bis mittleren Höhe. Einsamkeitsgefühle und Alienation korrelierten untereinander und mit den restlichen Variablen in einer Größenordnung zwischen $r = 0{,}10$ und $r = 0{,}35$; Alleinleben, Sozialkontakthäufigkeit sowie der Summenwert des Index „Hilfe und Unterstützung durch soziale Beziehungen" erreichten untereinander Korrelationen bis zu $r = 0{,}54$. Dieses Ergebnis unterstreicht, daß die verschiedenartigen Aspekte sozialer Isolation nicht zufriedenstellend in einem übergreifenden Gesamtindex repräsentiert werden können, sondern getrennt voneinander erfaßt und analysiert werden sollten.

Soziale Isolation in der Mannheimer Altenbevölkerung

In der Gemeindestichprobe lag der Anteil der Frauen bei 64,0%: das mittlere Alter betrug 73,8 Jahre $(s = 5{,}9)$; 41,7% wohnten mit ihrem Ehepartner zusammen; weitere 14,8% führten mit anderen Angehörigen einen gemeinsamen Haushalt; 43,5% lebten allein in einer Privatwohnung.

Die Zusammensetzung der Heimstichprobe wich erwartungsgemäß beträchtlich davon ab. Der Anteil der Frauen belief sich hier auf 84,3%, im Durchschnitt waren die Heimbewohner 80,8 Jahre alt $(s = 6{,}3)$; 96,7% waren verwitwet, ledig oder geschieden; 48,4% hatten einen Altenheim- und 51,6% einen Pflegeplatz inne.

Abbildung 1 und 2 zeigen die Häufigkeitsverteilung des Summenwertes der Sozialkontakte in der Gemeinde- und in der Heimstichprobe. Die Kurven weisen auf eine kontinuierliche Verteilung der Kontakthäufigkeit in der Altenbevölkerung hin; es gibt keine ersichtliche Trennung zwischen „isolierten" und „nichtisolierten" Älteren.

Es stellt sich also die Frage, wo man eine Grenze ziehen soll, unterhalb der mit gewisser Berechtigung von sozial isolierten Personen gesprochen werden kann. Mangels begründbarer Normen ist man hier immer noch auf Konventionen angewiesen, die auf der Grundlage empirischer Forschung beruhen. Tunstall (1966) setzt 5 oder weniger Kontakte von mindestens 10minütiger Dauer pro

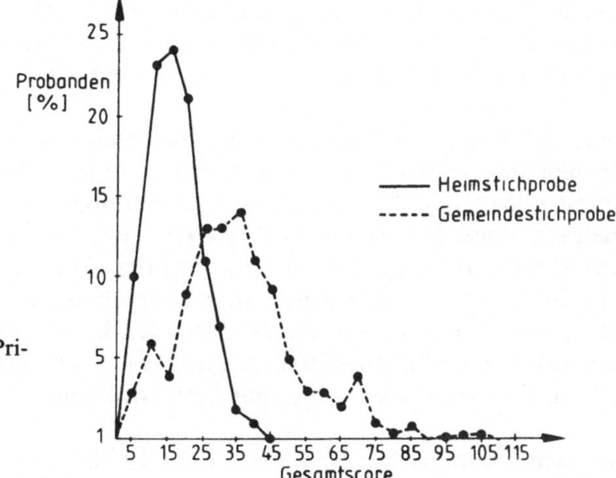

Abb. 1. Verteilung der Sozialkontaktscores bei Heimbewohnern und in Privathaushalten lebenden älteren Menschen. (Aus Cooper et al. 1984)

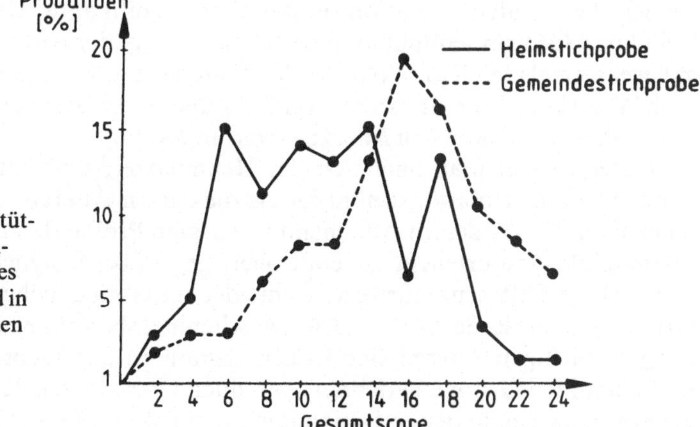

Abb. 2. Hilfe und Unterstützung aus Sozialbeziehungen. Verteilung der Scores bei Heimbewohnern und in Privathaushalten lebenden älteren Menschen. (Aus Cooper et al. 1984)

Woche mit extremer Isolation gleich, bei bis zu 20 Begegnungen in diesem Zeitraum spricht er von Isolation, und Personen, die bis zu 40 Kontakte berichten, bezeichnet er als leicht isoliert oder als Grenzfälle; erst bei darüber hinausgehender Kontakthäufigkeit schätzt er einen Probanden als nicht isoliert ein. Übernimmt man diese Einteilung, so sind 2,4% der Älteren in der Mannheimer Gemeinde extremer Isolation ausgesetzt (gegenüber 4,5% in Tunstalls Stichprobe), isoliert leben weitere 19,4% (gegenüber 16,5%), und knapp die Hälfte (gegenüber 54,0%) der Befragten hat als leicht isoliert zu gelten. Die etwas günstigeren Verhältnisse in der Mannheimer Stichprobe sind teilweise darauf zurückzuführen, daß die Mindestdauer einer Begegnung, die als Kontakt gewertet wurde, mit 5 anstatt mit 10 min angesetzt war.

Die Ergebnisse zum Anteil der in extremer Isolation lebenden alten Menschen korrespondieren recht gut mit den Befunden einer internationalen Studie mit Daten aus den USA, England und Dänemark (Shanas et al. 1968); dort wurde zwar kein vergleichbares Meßinstrument benutzt, aber man fand, daß in diesen Ländern 2–3% der Älteren allein lebten, in der dem Interview vorangegangenen Wochen nicht besucht worden waren und am Tag zuvor keinen Kontakt mit anderen Menschen hatten.

Abbildung 1 macht deutlich, daß die durchschnittliche Kontakthäufigkeit der in Heimen untergebrachten Älteren weit unter der in Privathaushalten lebender Menschen liegt: 10,4% der Mannheimer Heimbewohner müssen als extrem isoliert betrachtet werden, weitere 68,1% als isoliert. Trotz der auf Gemeinschaft angelegten Organisation des Heimlebens und der räumlichen Nähe unterliegen also die in der Institution versorgten alten Menschen einem gegenüber der Gemeindepopulation um das Vierfache erhöhten Risiko, in ausgeprägte soziale Isolation zu geraten. Ein ähnliches Bild vermittelt die Scoreverteilung der aus sozialen Beziehungen verfügbaren Hilfe und Unterstützung, wie aus Abb. 2 hervorgeht.

Selbst nach rechnerischer Elimination der Effekte von Alter und Familienstand, die ohne Zweifel die a priori gegebenen Kontaktmöglichkeiten beeinflussen und in den zwei untersuchten Stichproben ja deutlich voneinander abwichen, bleiben bei beiden Isolationsindizes hochsignifikante Differenzen zwischen Heim- und Gemeindepopulation bestehen. So liegt der Anteil der Heimbewohner mit weniger als 20 Kontakten in der Untersuchungswoche bei 78%, während nach Alterskorrektur ein Anteil von 22% und unter Berücksichtigung des Familienstandes eine Quote von 34% zu erwarten wären.

Unterscheidet man nach Art des Heimplatzes, sind Altenheimbewohner in höherem Maße isolationsgefährdet als diejenigen Älteren, die einen Pflegeplatz innehaben: 17,8% der im Altenheim versorgten Probanden leben, nach der Kontakthäufigkeit zu urteilen, extrem isoliert gegenüber lediglich 1,6% im Pflegebereich. Diese Differenz dürfte v. a. mit der unterschiedlichen Wohnform beider Gruppen zu erklären sein; 97,3% der Altenheimbewohner, aber nur 18,2% der pflegebedürftigen Älteren sind in Einzelzimmern untergebracht. Über 90% der letztgenannten Gruppe berichten denn auch über tägliche Kontakte mit anderen Heimbewohnern, in der erstgenannten knapp 60%. Die auf Pflegestation betreuten Menschen sind auch vermehrt auf Kontakte innerhalb des Heims, sei es mit anderen Bewohnern oder mit dem Pflegepersonal, angewiesen – nur 44% von ihnen erhielten im Verlauf einer Woche einmal oder öfter Besuch von außerhalb der Institution gegenüber 73% der Altenheimbewohner (Mahnkopf 1984). Der durchschnittliche Summenwert von 33 Punkten für Sozialkontakte, der mit dem verwendeten Bewertungsverfahren in der Gemeindestichprobe ermittelt wurde, kommt zu 36% dadurch zustande, daß die Probanden mit ihrem Ehepartner zusammenleben oder mit anderen Angehörigen den Haushalt teilen und die Mahlzeiten gemeinsam einnehmen. Weitere 38% des Gesamtwertes entfallen auf familiäre Kontakte, wobei in erster Linie mit 30% die Kontakte zu Kindern und Enkeln zu nennen sind. Der Anteil außerfamiliärer Kontakte am Summenwert beläuft sich auf 26%.

Bei den Heimbewohnern tragen v. a. Kontakte innerhalb des Heimes zum durchschnittlichen Wert von etwas mehr als 14 Punkten bei. Im Mittel ergeben sich nur 3,2 Kontakte pro Woche zu Personen, die außerhalb des Heimes leben. Dieser Anteil von 22,5% Außenkontakten verteilt sich gleichmäßig auf Kinder, auf andere Angehörige und auf Freunde und Bekannte. Die überwiegende Zahl der Außenkontakte ist auf Besuche im Heim zurückzuführen; Begegnungen außerhalb des Heimes sind selten.

Bei der Frage nach Einsamkeit berichten 35,2% der in Privathaushalten lebenden Älteren, daß sie sich gelegentlich einsam fühlen. Demgegenüber sind aber nur 9,5% der Meinung, einsamer als andere Gleichaltrige zu sein.

Die Heimbewohner antworten in ähnlicher Weise: 47% fühlen sich manchmal einsam, doch nur 6,6% glauben, einsamer als die meisten Gleichaltrigen zu sein.

Typologie der Kontaktstruktur in der Gemeinde

Wie bereits erwähnt, interkorrelieren die verschiedenen Isolationsindizes nicht sehr eng. Darüber hinaus stellt die Sozialkontakthäufigkeit einen Summenwert dar, der sich aus der Zahl der sozialen Begegnungen mit sehr unterschiedlichen Personengruppen zusammensetzt. Das Verteilungsmuster der Sozialkontakte wird in starkem Maße von der Wohnform und von der familiären Situation geprägt, in der die Älteren leben. Es ist deshalb nicht überraschend, daß die Einzelwerte, aus denen sich die Summe der Sozialkontakte ergibt, untereinander nur einen geringen Zusammenhang aufweisen, der von $r = -0,13$ bis $r = 0,56$ reicht. Die Heterogenität auf Variablenebene schließt jedoch keineswegs aus, daß sich Gruppen von älteren Personen unterscheiden lassen, die hinsichtlich der Struktur ihrer sozialen Kontakte und der eher subjektiv gefärbten Isolationsmerkmale homogen zusammengesetzt sind. Zur Überprüfung dieser strukturellen Gemeinsamkeiten wurde eine Clusteranalyse durchgeführt (Dixon et al. 1981), in die sowohl die unterschiedlichen Kontaktquellen als auch die übrigen durch Befragung ermittelten Indikatoren sozialer Isolation eingingen. Aus Gründen der Anschaulichkeit und um die Differenz in den Varianzen auszugleichen, wurden alle Merkmale dichotomisiert. Sofern es sich um Sozialkontakte in der vorausgegangenen Woche handelte, bedeutet eine Null jeweils, daß kein Kontakt, und eine Eins, daß ein oder mehrere Kontakte berichtet wurden. Sofern es sich um kontinuierliche Variablen handelte, wurde eine Unterteilung in unterdurchschnittlich und in überdurchschnittlich vorgenommen. Die Bedeutung der restlichen Merkmale ergibt sich aus Abb. 3.

In Abb. 3 ist eine Lösung mit fünf hinreichend großen und vergleichsweise gut zu interpretierenden Clustern dargestellt. Lediglich fünf Personen ließen sich aufgrund unvollständiger Werte nicht den Clustern zuordnen. Zur Trennung der Cluster tragen mit nur zwei Ausnahmen alle Variablen bei. Die beiden Ausnahmen sind Kontakte durch Berufstätigkeit und Kontakte mit einem Arzt in den letzten sieben Tagen. Alle anderen Merkmale variieren hochsignifikant stärker zwischen den Clustern als innerhalb der Cluster. Am deutlichsten diskriminieren die Variablen „Alleinleben", „verheiratet", „gemeinsame Mahlzeiten", „Hilfe und Unterstützung aus Sozialbeziehungen", „Einsamkeitsgefühle", „Alienation" sowie die Kontakte zu Nachbarn, Kindern und Enkeln.

Cluster 1 umfaßt 22% der Älteren. Es handelt sich dabei größtenteils um Verheiratete in einer insgesamt günstigen Kontaktsituation. Sie verfügen sowohl

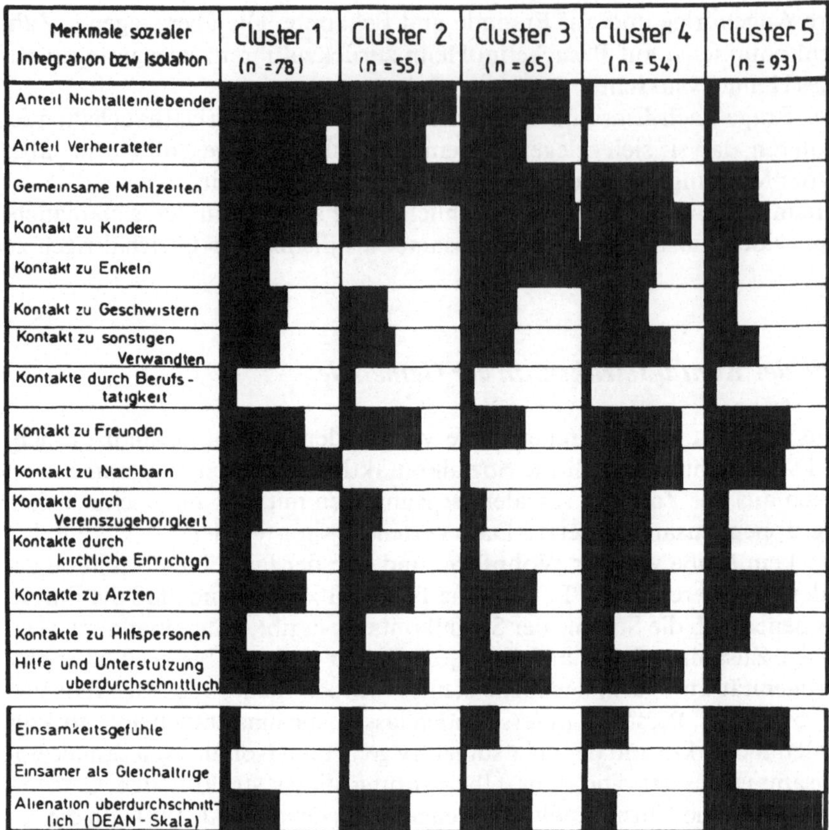

Abb. 3. Profile der Sozialkontakt- und Isolationsmerkmale von 5 per Clusteranalyse ermittelten Personengruppen

über familiäre als auch über außerfamiliäre Kontakte, leiden nicht unter Einsamkeit und erfahren laut eigener Darstellung ausreichende Hilfe und Unterstützung.

Cluster 2 schließt 16% der Stichprobe ein, wobei es sich wiederum überwiegend um Verheiratete, insbesondere um Männer handelt. Einsamkeitsgefühle sind in dieser Gruppe selten; die soziale Stützung erscheint gewährleistet. Die Sozialkontakte verteilen sich nahezu gleichmäßig auf familiäre und auf außerfamiliäre Kontaktpersonen, das Ausmaß der Kontakte ist jedoch leicht vermindert. Im Vergleich mit Cluster 1 fällt besonders auf, daß Kontakte zu den Kindern und zu den Geschwistern seltener sind und keinerlei Kontakte sowohl zu Enkeln als auch zu Nachbarn bestehen.

In Cluster 3 befinden sich 19% der Stichprobe. Diese Gruppe besteht aus Verheirateten und Verwitweten, die selten Einsamkeit empfinden, in hohem Maße soziale Unterstützung erfahren und enge Kontakte zu Kindern, Enkeln und anderen Familienangehörigen haben. Außerfamiliäre Kontakte sind hingegen eher selten.

Cluster 4 wird von weiteren 16% der Älteren gebildet. Charakteristisch für diese Gruppe ist, daß sie fast ausschließlich aus Alleinlebenden besteht, überwiegend aus verwitweten Frauen. Sie zeigen kein erhöhtes Maß an Einsamkeitsgefühlen, halten ihre sozialen Bindungen für sehr tragfähig, nehmen trotz des Alleinlebens ihre Mahlzeiten häufig mit anderen ein und pflegen ein enges Netz familiärer und außerfamiliärer Kontakte.

Diesen sozial integrierten Alleinlebenden stehen die 27% der Stichprobe gegenüber, die Cluster 5 zugeordnet wurden. Es handelt sich zu 85% um Frauen, wovon der größte Teil verwitwet ist; außerdem findet sich hier der höchste Anteil an Ledigen und Geschiedenen. Unschwer läßt sich erkennen, daß die von sozialer Isolation bedrohten Älteren in dieser Gruppe vorherrschen; 90% leben in Einpersonenhaushalten, die Mahlzeiten werden zumeist allein eingenommen, der Kontakt zu Kindern oder zu anderen Angehörigen ist erheblich reduziert. Zwar haben zwei Drittel Kontakt zu Freunden und Nachbarn, doch haben nur wenige im Rahmen von Vereinen oder kirchlichen Einrichtungen weitere Außenkontakte. Die Hilfe und Unterstützung aus Sozialbeziehungen wird fast ausnahmslos als unterdurchschnittlich eingeschätzt, Einsamkeitsgefühle sind häufig, Alienation ist sehr verbreitet. Es scheint demnach, als könne man bei dieser nicht unbeträchtlichen Minderheit der Altenbevölkerung von objektiv geringer Kontakthäufigkeit, verbunden mit dem subjektiven Erleben von Einsamkeit, Isolation und Entfremdung sprechen.

Zusammenhänge zwischen sozialer Isolation und psychischer Erkrankung in der Gemeindestichprobe

Aus der Gemeindeuntersuchung geht hervor, daß objektive und subjektive Indikatoren sozialer Isolation nicht gleichförmig mit der Häufigkeit psychischer Erkrankungen kovariieren. In dieser Stichprobe zeigen sich keine Prävalenzunterschiede in Abhängigkeit vom Haushaltstypus: weder hirnorganische noch funktionelle Störungen treten bei denjenigen, die allein leben, häufiger auf als bei den alten Menschen, die mit ihrem Ehepartner, anderen Angehörigen oder sonstigen Personen in einem gemeinsamen Haushalt leben.

Auch eine geringe Zahl von Sozialkontakten oder mangelnde Hilfs- und Unterstützungsmöglichkeiten sind nicht überzufällig häufig mit psychischer Erkrankung verbunden. Lediglich bei einer Aufgliederung der sozialen Kontakte nach familiären und außerfamiliären Beziehungen läßt sich ein Zusammenhang nachweisen: unter den Älteren, die sehr wenige außerfamiliäre Kontakte haben – rund ein Drittel der Stichprobe – finden sich doppelt so viele psychische Störungen wie unter den Älteren mit größerer Zahl außerfamiliärer Kontakte.

Zwischen dem Ausprägungsgrad der subjektiven Isolation, wie sie als Einsamkeit und als Alienation gemessen wurde, und psychiatrischer Prävalenz besteht hingegen ein hochsignifikanter Zusammenhang. Ältere, die sich als einsam bezeichnen, leiden mit dreifach größerer Wahrscheinlichkeit an einer psychischen Störung als solche, die sich nicht einsam fühlen. Ebenso ist der Anteil psychisch Kranker unter den Älteren mit überdurchschnittlichen Alienationswerten mehr als doppelt so hoch wie unter denen mit unterdurchschnittlichen Alienationswerten.

Bei diesen Zusammenhängen ist jedoch immer eine Kontamination der Variablen zu bedenken. Der Zusammenhang mit subjektiver Isolation kann dadurch zustande kommen, daß die Bewertung der sozialen Situation durch den psychischen Zustand des Probanden gefärbt ist, d. h. weniger mit der sozialen Realität als vielmehr mit der eigenen Bewertung zu tun hat und somit eher als ein Symptom denn als ein Auslöser psychischer Störungen zu verstehen ist.

Ermittelt man die psychiatrische Prävalenz für die aus der Clusteranalyse resultierenden strukturell homogenen Gruppen, so findet man plausible Verteilungsunterschiede, die insgesamt jedoch nicht statistisch bedeutsam sind. In den sozial gut integrierten Clustern 1 und 4 sind psychische Erkrankungen mit einer Häufigkeit von 15% eher selten. In den restlichen 3 Clustern ergeben sich Raten zwischen 25 und 28%, wobei sich unter den nicht allein lebenden Älteren aus Cluster 2 und 3 überwiegend hirnorganische Erkrankungen finden, während die Alleinstehenden aus Cluster 5 v.a. unter funktionellen, psychischen Störungen leiden. In dieser Gruppe sind psychoorganische Störungen selten, da sie nicht mit einer längerdauernden selbständigen Lebensführung vereinbar sind. Damit im Einklang steht, daß die schwerwiegenden, fachärztliche Behandlung erfordernden psychogeriatrischen Erkrankungen nahezu ausschließlich in den Clustern 2 und 3 anzutreffen sind.

Zusammenhänge zwischen sozialer und psychischer Erkrankung in der Heimstichprobe

Die über 65jährigen Bewohner von Alten- und Altenpflegeheimen unterlagen in weitaus höherem Maße dem Risiko sozialer Isolation und waren deutlich häufiger psychisch krank als die Gemeindepopulation. Eine systematische Prüfung der Beziehung zwischen psychiatrischer Morbidität und subjektiver Isolation im Sinne von Einsamkeit und Alienation erwies sich bei dieser Population als nicht durchführbar, da viele Probanden aufgrund ihrer psychischen Beeinträchtigung nicht in der Lage waren, die entsprechenden Fragen vollständig und zuverlässig zu beantworten. Ein allgemeiner Zusammenhang zwischen objektiver Isolation und psychiatrischer Prävalenz ist nicht nachweisbar. Lediglich für eines der erhobenen Isolationskriterien und für eine Untergruppe von Sozialkontakten ergaben sich statistisch gesicherte Zusammenhänge: die auf sozialen Beziehungen basierenden Hilfs- und Unterstützungsmöglichkeiten korrelieren positiv, wenn auch nur gering, mit dem psychischen Gesundheitszustand ($r = 0,26$; $p < 0,01$), und die psychisch beeinträchtigten Probanden haben weniger Kontakte mit Angehörigen oder Freunden, die außerhalb der Institution leben, als psychisch unauffällige Heimbewohner.

Die Vermutung liegt nahe, daß hier die eingeschränkte Mobilität der Pflegeheimbewohner, die auch die höhere psychiatrische Erkrankungsrate aufweisen, eine bedeutsame Rolle spielt. Deshalb wurde in einer weiteren Analyse die Art des Heimplatzes in die Berechnung einbezogen (Cooper et al. 1984). Das Ergebnis bestätigt die Bedeutung sowohl der Unterbringungsart als auch des psychischen Gesundheitszustandes für die Häufigkeit der Außenkontakte. Jeder sechste Heimbewohner – rein rechnerisch eine überzufällig große Gruppe – war pflegebedürftig, psychisch beeinträchtigt und relativ isoliert von Außenkontakten.

Zusammenhänge zwischen sozialer Isolation und dem Altersverlauf

Bei einem im Rahmen einer Querschnittsuntersuchung festgestellten Zusammenhang ist nicht verläßlich zu beurteilen, ob soziale Isolation ein Risikofaktor für psychische Erkrankungen ist oder ob nicht vielmehr eine psychische Erkrankung die soziale Situation verändert, sei es durch Rückzug der Kontaktpersonen vom betroffenen älteren Menschen oder sei es, in umgekehrter Richtung, durch eine vermehrte Zuwendung und durch eine verstärkte Hilfe bei der Bewältigung der alltäglichen Aufgaben. Andererseits kann ein fehlender Zusammenhang zwischen objektiver Kontaktsituation und psychischer Erkrankung dadurch bedingt sein, daß gerade die Älteren mit schweren psychischen Beeinträchtigungen, insbesondere organischen Psychosyndromen, ohne soziale Unterstützung nicht allein leben und in Privathaushalten verbleiben könnten.

Es ist deshalb aufschlußreicher, die Effekte sozialer Isolation im zeitlichen Längsschnitt zu untersuchen. Doch auch hierbei stößt man, insbesondere bei Stichproben aus der Altenbevölkerung, auf erhebliche Probleme. Zum einen ist die soziale Situation nicht unabhängig von anderen Merkmalen wie Geschlecht oder gesundheitlicher Zustand, welche selbst von Bedeutung für den Altersverlauf sind. Zum anderen führt die hohe Mortalität im Alter zu einer starken Reduktion des Stichprobenumfangs und bewirkt eine Auslese der am wenigsten gesundheitlich Gefährdeten. Es scheint aus diesen Gründen erforderlich, multivariate Analysemethoden zu verwenden, die auch andere prognostisch bedeutsame Variablen berücksichtigen, und den Einfluß sozialer Isolation an Verlaufsmerkmalen zu bemessen, die unabhängig von der Mortalität sind, sowie die Überlebenszeit selbst als unabhängige Variable zu betrachten.

Wir beschränken uns deshalb auf objektivierbare Merkmale, deren Auftreten exakt oder zumindest hinlänglich genau datiert werden kann und die zentrale Ereignisse im Altersverlauf darstellen, nämlich die Mortalität, die Inzidenz von progredient und irreversibel verlaufenden Demenzen und die Einweisungen in Alten- und Pflegeheime. Für die Auswertung wird das Proportional-Hazards-Regressionsmodell von Cox (1972) herangezogen, mit dem sowohl der Einfluß mehrerer Kovariaten geprüft werden kann als auch die Fälle einbezogen werden können, bei denen das betreffende Ereignis – Tod, kognitiver Abbau oder Heimeinweisung – im Untersuchungszeitraum nicht eingetreten ist.

Mortalität

Von den Älteren aus der Gemeindestichprobe sind 42% während des Untersuchungszeitraumes gestorben. Obwohl in mehreren Studien ein Zusammenhang zwischen sozialer Unterstützung und Mortalität nachgewiesen werden konnte (Broadhead et al. 1983), ist in der vorliegenden Untersuchung kein Einfluß der Isolationsmerkmale auf die Überlebenszeit nachzuweisen. Weder die Häufigkeit sozialer Kontakte noch die Indikatoren subjektiver Isoliertheit stehen in Beziehung zur Mortalität.

Ein ähnliches Ergebnis findet man auch in der Stichprobe der Heimbewohner, von denen zwischenzeitlich 70% gestorben waren. Sozialkontakthäufigkeit, Kontakte außerhalb des Heimes und Einsamkeitsgefühle kovariieren nicht mit der Überlebenszeit. Der Summenwert für die wahrgenommene „Hilfe und Unterstützung aus Sozialbeziehungen" verfehlt hingegen nur knapp die 5%-Signifikanzgrenze, wenn man Alter, Geschlecht und körperliche Verfassung berücksichtigt.

Andererseits steht die *Besuchshäufigkeit* bei den Heimbewohnern in einer überzufälligen Beziehung zur Mortalität. Auch wenn man die schon genannten Risikofaktoren einbezieht, geht eine größere Besuchshäufigkeit zur Zeit der Erstbefragung mit einer verlängerten Überlebenszeit einher. Die Besuchshäufigkeit wurde auf einer 6stufigen Skala eingeschätzt, die von keinerlei Besuchen im Heim bis zu täglichen Besuchen reichte. Mit jeder Stufe vermindert sich die Mortalitätsrate um 15%, während sie sich pro Altersjahr um 6% erhöht, mit jeder Stufe der Mobilitätsbeeinträchtigung um 49% ansteigt und für Männer um 66% höher als für Frauen ist.

Neuerkrankungen an schweren Demenzen

Ob soziale Isolation einen Risikofaktor für die schwerwiegendsten psychischen Erkrankungen des höheren Lebensalters, die Demenzen, darstellt, wurde bisher noch nicht empirisch geprüft. Durch erneute Untersuchung der Überlebenden und durch eingehende Befragung der Angehörigen oder Pflegepersonen von Verstorbenen gelang es, für 96,5% der Gemeindestichprobe und für alle Mitglieder der Heimstichprobe festzustellen, wer in der Zwischenzeit an einer irreversiblen, wenigstens 6 Monate andauernden, schweren dementiellen Störungen erkrankt war. Es handelt sich dabei um 34 Personen, die zuvor in Privathaushalten gelebt hatten, und um 26 Personen, die in Heimen untergebracht gewesen waren. In der Gemeindestichprobe erkrankten tendenziell die Alleinlebenden häufiger als diejenigen, die einen gemeinsamen Haushalt führten; die jährliche Inzidenzrate pro 1000 Personen betrug für die beiden Gruppen 23,2 bzw. 13,3. In der multivariaten Analyse unter Einbeziehung des Alters, das erwartungsgemäß in signifikantem Zusammenhang mit der Inzidenz stand, ließ sich hingegen weder für die objektiven noch für die subjektiven Isolationsmerkmale ein statistisch bedeutsamer Einfluß nachweisen. Das gleiche Resultat ergab sich auch für die Heimstichprobe. Soziale Isolation scheint demnach kein nennenswerter Risikofaktor für psychoorganische Störungen, die im hohen Alter den überwiegenden Anteil an der psychiatrischen Gesamtmorbidität ausmachen, zu sein.

Einweisungen in Alten- und Pflegeheime

Während des Follow-up-Zeitraums sind 12% der Personen aus der Gemeindestichprobe in ein Heim übergesiedelt. Die Isolationsmerkmale aus der Erstuntersuchung, die in signifikanter Beziehung zur Wahrscheinlichkeit des Heimeintritts stehen, sind „Alleinleben", „Hilfe und Unterstützung aus Sozialbeziehungen" und die Sozialkontakthäufigkeit; Einsamkeitsgefühle haben keine Vorhersagekraft. Die simultane Analyse der Isolationsvariablen zeigt, daß es die gemeinsa-

Tabelle 2. Effekte von Prädiktorvariablen auf die Wahrscheinlichkeit einer Heimeinweisung (Cox-Regression)

Prädiktor	Koeffizient (SE)	Signifikanz	Effekt auf die Einweisungsrate[a]
Alter (Jahre)	0,058 (0,027)	p < 0,05	+ 6%
Geschlecht (Frauen)	0,880 (0,449)	p > 0,05	+141%
Beeinträchtigung der Mobilität (Rating 0–4)	0,429 (0,184)	p < 0,05	+ 54%
Anzahl familiärer Kontakte (Scoreverteilung 0–33)	− 0,047 (0,020)	p < 0,05	− 5%

[a] Die Prozentsätze für die einzelnen Merkmale sind wegen der unterschiedlichen Spannweite der Merkmalsausprägungen nicht direkt miteinander vergleichbar. Der Effekt ist als prozentuale Erhöhung bzw. Verminderung der Einweisungswahrscheinlichkeit pro Anstieg der Merkmalsausprägung um eine Einheit angegeben (z. B. um ein Altersjahr oder um einen Kontaktpunkt).

men Varianzanteile sind, die zur Prognose beitragen, denn der Zusammenhang mit den restlichen Merkmalen wird nullwertig, wenn die Sozialkontakthäufigkeit kontrolliert wird. Bei detaillierter Untersuchung des Einflusses der Sozialkontakte ergibt sich, daß nicht die außerfamiliären sondern ausschließlich die familiären Kontakte mit der Institutionalisierung in Zusammenhang stehen. Dieses Ergebnis bleibt erhalten, auch wenn man die bedeutsamsten demographischen und gesundheitlichen Merkmale in die Vorhersage einbezieht (s. Tabelle 2).

Die in Tabelle 2 dargestellten Resultate zeigen, daß die Wahrscheinlichkeit einer Heimeinweisung mit dem Alter und mit dem Grad körperlicher Beeinträchtigung ansteigt und für Frauen höher als für Männer ist. Darüber hinaus nehmen die familiären Kontakte signifikanten Einfluß auf die Heimeinweisung. Je mehr familiäre Kontakte bei der Erstuntersuchung festgestellt wurden, desto geringer ist die Wahrscheinlichkeit gewesen, im weiteren zeitlichen Verlauf in ein Heim aufgenommen zu werden. Im Durchschnitt reduzierte jeder einzelne Kontaktpunkt das Einweisungsrisiko um 5%. Andere Isolationsmerkmale oder außerfamiliäre Kontakte haben für die Heimaufnahme keine prognostische Bedeutung.

Diskussion

Das für die Mannheimer Feldstudie entwickelte IMSI kann noch nicht als methodisch ausgereiftes Meßinstrument zur Erfassung sozialer Isolation gelten. Insbesondere die Validität von mit Interviewverfahren erhobenen objektiven Isolationsmerkmalen wie Mangel an Sozialkontakten und Mangel an Hilfe und Unterstützung aus sozialen Beziehungen bedarf einer weitergehenden Klärung auf empirischer Basis. Eine sorgfältige Unterscheidung zwischen Isolation als Zustand und Isolierung als Prozeß erscheint ebenfalls notwendig. So haben Lowenthal (1964) und Bennett (1980) beispielsweise darauf hingewiesen, daß geringe Sozialkontakthäufigkeit im Alter nicht in jedem Fall einen unfreiwilligen Verlust an sozialer Integration darstellt, sondern auch ein Charakteristikum eines lebenslang gezeigten Verhaltensmusters sein kann. Es ist anzunehmen, daß unter solchen Bedingungen der qualitative Aspekt sozialer Beziehungen als Quelle emotionaler und instrumenteller Unterstützung und schließlich auch die subjektive Einschätzung erlebter Isolation einen anderen Stellenwert gewinnen.

Dennoch hat sich der mit dem IMSI gewählte methodische Ansatz als nützlich erwiesen. Die Daten der vorliegenden Studie ermöglichen es, die verschiedenen Aspekte von sozialer Isolation im Alter zueinander in Bezug zu setzen, ihre Zusammenhänge untereinander sowie zu anderen personenbezogenen Merkmalen empirisch zu prüfen und ihre Bedeutung sowohl für den psychischen Gesundheitszustand als auch für den weiteren Altersverlauf abzuschätzen.

Die Forschungsergebnisse zeigen, daß nur eine Minderheit der in Privathaushalten lebenden Älteren so weitgehend von sozialen Bindungen abgeschnitten ist bzw. so extrem isoliert lebt, daß von einer Gefährdung gesprochen werden kann. Bei älteren Heimbewohnern kommt (sofern man hier die gleichen Maßstäbe verwenden kann) extreme oder schwere soziale Isolation viel häufiger vor. In der soziologischen Gerontologie sowie in der Gerontopsychiatrie neigt man bisweilen dazu, das Ausmaß und die Wirkung sozialer Isolation im Alter etwas zu überschätzen, v.a. weil man sich verständlicherweise von der schwerwiegenden Isolation der in Alten- und Pflegeheimen untergebrachten alten Menschen beeindrukken ließ (Bennett 1980); z. T. auch weil viele Autoren nicht eindeutig genug zwischen sozialer Isolation als Umweltmerkmal und Einsamkeitsgefühlen als psychologischem Merkmal unterschieden, obgleich die beiden Variablen nicht sonderlich hoch miteinander korrelieren.

Diese relativierende Betrachtungsweise berechtigt jedoch zu keiner Bagatellisierung der sozialen bzw. medizinischen Problematik. Die Daten der vorliegenden Studie weisen darauf hin, daß ungefähr ein Viertel der älteren Stadtbewohner (entsprechend Cluster 5 in Abb. 3) durch mehrere Merkmale von sozialer Isolation – Alleinleben, Kontaktmangel, Mangel an sozialer Unterstützung, Einsamkeit – gekennzeichnet sind und, darüber hinaus, daß diese Merkmale mit einem erhöhten Risiko für Selbständigkeitsverlust und Heimeinweisung verbunden sind. In der Psychiatrie spielt sie bei bestimmten Untergruppen der Altenpopulation, v.a. bei suizidgefährdeten Menschen (Böcker 1975; Bungard 1977), eine wesentliche Rolle. Als ein für die Altenbevölkerung insgesamt gültiges psychiatrisches Morbiditätsrisiko hat soziale Isolation jedoch viel weniger Gewicht als manche andere Belastungsfaktoren, wie z. B. chronische körperliche Erkrankung und Beeinträchtigung, niedriges Einkommen und ungünstige Wohnbedingungen (Sosna u. Wahl 1983; Cooper 1986). Die Interaktion zwischen solchen Belastungsfaktoren und ihre Wirkung auf den Altersverlauf stellt ein wichtiges Forschungsziel für die Zukunft dar.

Literatur

Bennett R (ed) (1980) Aging, isolation and resocialization Nostrand, New York
Böcker F (1975) Suizidhandlungen alter Menschen. MMW 117:201–204
Broadhead WE, Kaplan BH, James SA (1983) The epidemiologic evidence for a relationship between social support and health. Am J Epidemiol 117:521–536

Bungard W (1975) Isolation und Einsamkeit im Alter. Hanstein, Köln

Bungard W (1977) Isolation, Einsamkeit und Selbstmordgedanken im Alter. Aktuel Gerontol 7:81–89

Cooper B (1984) Home and away. The disposition of mentally ill old people in an urban population. Soc Psychiatry 19:187–196

Cooper B (1986) Mental illness, disability and social conditions among old people in Mannheim. In: Häfner H, Moschel G, Sartorius N (eds) Mental health in the elderly. Springer, Berlin Heidelberg New York Tokyo, pp 35–45

Cooper B, Jaeger J (1987) Soziale Isolation als psychiatrischer Risikofaktor im Alter – eine epidemiologische Untersuchung. Nervenheilkunde 6:7–13

Cooper B, Sosna U (1980) Family settings of the psychiatrically disturbed aged. In: Robins LN, Clayton PJ, Wing JK (eds) The social consequences of psychiatric illness. Brunner-Mazel, New York, pp 141–157

Cooper B, Sosna U (1983) Psychische Erkrankung in der Altenbevölkerung. Eine epidemiologische Feldstudie in Mannheim. Nervenarzt 54:239–249

Cooper B, Mahnkopf B, Bickel H (1984) Psychische Erkrankung und soziale Isolation bei älteren Heimbewohnern: eine Vergleichsstudie. Z Gerontol 17:117–125

Cox DR (1972) Regression models and life tables. J R Stat Soc 34:187–220

Dean E (1961) Alienation: Its meaning and measurement. Am Sociol Rev 26:753–8

Dixon WJ, Brown MW, Engelman L, Frane JW, Hill MA, Jennrich RJ, Toporek JD (1981) BMDP statistical software. Univ California Press, Berkeley

Durkheim E (1973) Der Selbstmord. Luchterhand, Neuwied, 65–83. (Soziologische Texte, 32)

Faris REL, Dunham HW (1939) Mental disorders in urban areas. Univ Chicago Press, Chicago

Henderson AS, Duncan-Jones P, Byrne DG (1981) Neurosis and the social environment. Academic Press, Sydney New York

Kay DWK, Beamish P, Roth M (1964) Old-age mental disorders in Newcastle upon Tyne, part I. A study of prevalence. Br J Psychiatry 110:146–158

Lowenthal MF (1964) Social isolation and mental illness in old age Am Sociol Rev 29:70–95

Lowenthal MF, Berkman PL (1967) Aging and mental disorder in San Francisco. Jossey-Bass, San Francisco

Mahnkopf B (1984) Isolation in Institutionen: eine empirische Untersuchung in Mannheimer Alten- und Pflegeheimen. Unveröffentl. Diplomarbeit, Universität Mannheim

Nielsen J (1962) Gerontopsychiatric period prevalence investigation in a geographically delimited population. Acta Psychiatr Scand 38:307–330

Parsons T (1968) Alter und Geschlecht in der Sozialstruktur der Vereinigten Staaten. In: Parsons T, Beiträge zur soziologischen Theorie Luchterhand, Neuwied

Sainsbury P (1955) Suicide in London. Chapman & Hall, London (Maudsley monographs no 1)

Shanas E, Townsend P, Wedderburn D et al. (1968) Old people in three industrial societies. Atherton, New York

Sheldon JH (1948) The social medicine of old age. Report of an inquiry in Wolverhampton. Oxford Univ Press, London

Sosna U (1980) Empirical measurement of social isolation in relation to mental disorders of the elderly. Acta Psychiatr Scand [Suppl] 285:220–229

Sosna U (1983) Soziale Isolation und psychische Erkrankung im Alter. Campus, Frankfurt am Main

Sosna U, Cooper B (1980) Soziale Isolation: begriffliche und praktische Forschungsprobleme. In: Heinrich K, Müller U (Hrsg) Psychiatrische Soziologie. Beltz, Weinheim, S 95–105

Sosna U, Wahl H-W (1983) Soziale Belastung, psychische Erkrankung und körperliche Beeinträchtigung im Alter: Ergebnisse einer Felduntersuchung. Z Gerontol 16:107–114

Srole L (1956) Social integration and certain corollaries. An exploratory study. Am Sociol Rev 21:709–716

Townsend P (1957) The family life of old people. Routledge, London

Tunstall S (1966) Old and alone. Routledge, London

Weiss RS (1974) The provisions of social relationships. In: Rubin Z (ed) Doing onto others. Prentice-Hall, Englewood Cliffs/NJ, pp 17–26

Weiterführende Literatur zum Thema „Psychiatrie"

Bundesminister für Jugend, Familie, Frauen und Gesundheit (1988) Empfehlungen der Expertenkommission der Bundesregierung zur Reform der Versorgung im psychiatrischen und psychotherapeutisch/psychosomatischen Bereich auf der Grundlage des Modellprogramms Psychiatrie der Bundesregierung. Bonn

Cooper B (1987) Mental health care models and their evaluation: the West-German experience. Int J Soc Psych 33/2:99–104

Cooper B, Bickel H (1984) Epidemiologie psychischer Störungen: Folgerungen für die psychotherapeutische Versorgung. In: Baumann U (Hrsg) Psychotherapie: Makro- und Mikroperspektiven. Hogreve, Göttingen

Häfner H, Moschel G, Sartorius H (Hrsg) (1986) Mental health in the elderly: a review of the present state of research. Springer, Berlin Heidelberg New York Tokyo

Häfner H, Pfeifer-Kurda M (1990) Das kumulative psychiatrische Fallregister Mannheim. In: Schmidt MH (Hrsg): Fortschritte der psychiatrischen Epidemiologie. Deutsche Forschungsgemeinschaft, Bonn

Heimann H, Zimmer FT (Hrsg) (1987) Chronisch psychisch Kranke: Problemlage und Stand der Behandlungs- und Forschungssituation in der Bundesrepublik Deutschland. Fischer, Stuttgart

Mechanic D (1989) Mental health and social policy, 3rd edn.. Prentice Hall, Englewood Cliffs

Tress W, Schepank H (1990) Zur Epidemiologie psychogener Erkrankungen in der Stadtbevölkerung. In: Schmidt MH (Hrsg): Fortschritte der psychiatrischen Epidemiologie. Deutsche Forschungsgemeinschaft, Bonn

8.4 Rheuma

Treatment Profiles in Different Groups of Rheumatoid Arthritis Sufferers: Description, Analysis, Evaluation*

H.-H. Raspe, W. Mau, and A. Wasmus

Introduction

Analysis of the incidence and prevalence of certain diseases does not always utilize fully the scientific potential of population-based epidemiological studies. At least in rheumatology, the combination of population-based epidemiology with health services research has rarely been recognized as a source of knowledge. A simple method for accomplishing this combination in the case of rheumatoid arthritis (RA) would be case documentation including both illness variables (e.g., inflammatory activity) and treatment conditions (e.g., remission-inducing drug therapy). In contrast to all registry studies it would then be possible to relate the actual therapy to the concrete situation of patients and to estimate the adequacy of treatment, a basic aspect of the quality of care (Vuori 1982). Additionally, this type of study offers information on the „community effectiveness" (Tugwell et al. 1985) of rheumatological treatment standards that are usually dominated by clinicians. How complete, for example, is the local general practitioner's „compliance" with the recommendations of clinical specialists from their referral centers?

It is remarkable, that this type of study does not appear in the list of seven topics of health services research in rheumatology proposed by Epstein in 1981; these are:

1) Design of clinical research
2) Measurement of functional outcome variables and disability
3) Assembly, storage, retrieval, an analysis of data dealing with populations of persons with rheumatic diseases
4) Epidemiology of the rheumatic diseases
5) Organization of services for persons with rheumatic diseases
6) Costs of care for persons with rheumatic diseases
7) Understanding the patient

It could be included between topics 4 and 5 of this list.

Prior to the introduction of new services or the reorganization of older ones, one should have assessed the current type of care provided to the sick in the community and the factors that determine the expectable variance in care and treatment, and one should try to evaluate the quality of care and the significance of the differences observed. At this point, one becomes aware of a deficit in

---

* First published in a slightly different version in *Scand J Rheumatology* (1989) [Suppl] 79:57–65.

Table 1. Use of RIDs in Rheumatological practice with rheumatoid arthritis

Reference	Country	Type of study	Setting	n	Proportion on RIDs	Drugs
Scott et al. (1983)	United Kingdom	Prospective	Hospital in/outpatients	112	100%[a]	AU > HCQ > DPA > IMSP
Reilly et al. (1988)	United Kingdom	Cross-sectional	Hospital in/outpatients	116	70%	AU = DPA > HCQ
Friesen et al. (1985)	Netherlands	Cross-sectional	University outpatients	153	85%	AU = DPA > AZA > HCQ
			University inpatients	166	79%	AZA > AU > DPA > HCQ
van Saase et al. (1987)	Netherlands	Cross-sectional	Hospital outpatients	397	50%	HCQ > DPA > AU > AZA
Carter et al. (1986)	France	Cross-sectional	Rheumatologists	1153	74%	DPA > AU > HCQ > PYR
Elkeles and Raspe (1988)	West Germany	Cross-sectional	University outpatients	372	56%	AU > HCQ > SASP > AZA

[a] Over 10-year period.
AU, gold salts; HCQ, hydroxychloroguine; DPA, D-penicillamine; AZA, azathioprine; PYR, pyritinole; SASP, sulfasalazine
>, higher prevalence; =, similar prevalence

knowledge and research, which we try to compensate for by this study. We concentrate on three main areas. The first is a description of treatment profiles in four groups of RA sufferers. In this context the therapy with remission-inducing drugs (RIDs) is emphasized. The term remission-inducing is certainly too optimistic. In chronic RA one seldomly succeeds in effecting sustained clinical remission (Wolfe and Hawley 1985). The second area is analysis of the extent of RID use. Two population-based studies have demonstrated frequencies of current RID use of 7% in a California Medicaid population (Jacobs et al. 1988) and 20% in a Tasmanian population (Owen et al. 1986). These prevalence rates are low in comparison with those reported from rheumatological centers (Table 1). These marked differences in the use of RIDs are of interest, and predictors favoring the use of RIDs could be of use. We can assume that disease activity plays a crucial role in patients with active disease receiving RIDs more often than patients with minor disease activity (Raspe 1988). According to a recent cross-sectional Dutch study by van Saase et al. (1987) the disease duration seems to be of some importance; the frequency of RID treatment was found to be higher in patients with a short history of RA. Finally, their use may differ with patient's social and demographic characteristics. The third focus of this study is an evaluation of the adequacy of current RID treatment/nontreatment, based upon an explicitly normative approach.

Studies, Materials, Methods

Our data are based on four independent cross-sectional studies, all of which were carried out in the Hannover region of the Federal Republic of Germany. In the first study, conducted in 1986, we identified a group of 25 RA sufferers out of a total of 246 individuals, all of whom were subscribers of a local health insurance in Hannover (Allgemeine Ortskrankenkasse, AOK, study). All 246 had been on sick leave over the preceding 18 months due to rheumatic disease, coded under ICD 714 (RA). We were surprised to find only 25 individuals actually suffering from RA (Wasmus and Raspe 1988). In the second study, 45 cases of RA were identified in an ongoing population survey of 8044 residents of Hannover, aged 25–74 (EPI study; Wasmus et al. 1988). The third and fourth studies included a total of 262 RA sufferers consecutively referred to the outpatient department of the Hannover Medical School (Medizinische Hochschule Hannover, MHH, study) for a first consultation in 1985 and 1986. Of these, 121 were from Hannover (HA) and 141 from other communities in Lower Saxony (LS).

All patients underwent a complete rheumatological examination. An estimation of current disease activity used an additive activity index. This is a modified version of the remission index for active RA (Pinals et al. 1981), following an early proposal by Sharp (1982). The criteria used in this index are the following:

- Morning stiffness for at least 15 min (yes/no)
- Malaise/weakness within the first 6 h after getting up in the morning (yes/no)
- Arthralgia (yes/no)
- Tenderness on pressure or motion over at least two peripheral joints (yes/no)
- Synovial swelling over at least two peripheral joints (yes/no)
- Erythrocyte sedimentation rate (ESR; Westergren's method) of at least 20 in men or 30 in women after 1 h

Table 2. Four groups of RA-sufferers ($n = 332$)

			MHH	
	AOK ($n = 25$)	EPI ($n = 45$)	HA ($n = 121$)	LS ($n = 141$)
Sex (percentage women)	64	71	83	77
Age (mean, years)	49	59	59	52
Disease duration (mean, years)	8.4	14.0	7.4	5.3
Number of swollen joints (mean)	5	5	9	7
ESR (mean, 1 h)	13	17	43	30
Erosive (percentage yes)	53	51	60	55
Rheumatoid factor (percentage latex positive)	–	24	56	56

The modifications of this additive index include a more detailed definition of fatigue and of the pattern of joint involvement.

All data on the details of treatment are dependent entirely on patients' statements. So far we have not been able to verify their validity. They are probably valid in regard only to the current therapeutic regimen.

Comparison of the four groups of subjects (Table 2) reveals an increased disease activity and severity in the two groups of Hannover patients. The sufferers identified in the surrounding community are remarkable for a long-standing but seldom active disease, as are those from the AOK sample.

Results

Treatment Profiles. Three major areas of care are medical, nonmedical, and inpatient therapy. As regards the first, the group of epidemiologically identified individuals (EPI study) presented with rather low treatment rates, except for that with steroids (Table 3). Evidently, the patients at the university clinic received a

Table 3. Medical treatment in RA sufferers ($n = 332$)

	AOK ($n=25$)	EPI ($n=45$)	MHH HA ($n=121$)	MHH LS ($n=142$)
Nonsteroids, now	56	32	79	82
Steroids, now	20	16	20	16
RiDs				
Now	12	9	19	27
Past 12 months	–	13	–	–
Ever	40	–	43	43

Table 4. Nonmedical treatment in RA sufferers ($n = 307$)

	EPI ($n=45$)	MHH HA ($n=121$)	MHH LS ($n=142$)
Physiotherapy			
Past 3 months	–	31	22
Past 12 months	16	–	–
Local therapy			
Past 3 months	–	31	29
Past 12 months	38	–	–
Ergotherapy, past 3 months	–	3	1
Psychotherapy, past 3 months	–	0	1
Social work, past 3 months	–	0	0

Table 5. Inpatient treatment RA sufferers ($n = 307$)

	MHH		
	EPI ($n = 45$)	HA ($n = 121$)	LS ($n = 142$)
Hospital			
Past 5 years	–	29	28
Ever	24	–	–
Spa treatment			
Past 5 years	–	26	28
Ever	51	–	–
Surgery, ever	–	21	16

rather intensive treatment, which is in accordance with their higher level of disease activity. Among the various nonmedical types of therapy, physical treatments including massage played a dominant role (Table 4). The use of active physiotherapy is rare. Other forms of nonmedical treatment were hardly ever used. No data could be obtained from those in the health insurance study (AOK). And, finally, approximately one-fourth of all patients received inpatient treatment (Table 5). Rheuma-surgical operations were performed on about one-fifth of the two groups of MHH patients with an average disease duration of 7 and 5 years, respectively, in the HA and LS groups.

Evaluation of these data is difficult due to the fact that we could not compare our results with those of other studies, basically because of their virtual nonexistence. However, a cautious assessment does not offer evidence of systematic overtreatment in our four groups. From a clinical point of view there appears to be a significant deficit regarding special forms of treatment, such as active physiotherapy, surgery, and the use of RIDs.

Description and Analysis of RID Treatment. Therapy with RIDs is probably one of the areas offering the greatest likelihood of agreement with respect to efficacy, efficiency and indication . Despite many controversies (see Goddard and Butler 1984), rheumatologists from a large number of countries recognize them to be the cornerstone in antirheumatic treatment (see Table 1). It therefore seems appropriate to analyze the use of these medications. In the four groups of RA sufferers between 9% and 27% were currently on a medical regimen that included remission RIDs (Table 6), and up to 43% had at some time been treated with RIDs.

These figures form the basis for the analysis as to whether present disease activity offers a predictor for the use of these drugs. The influence of disease activity was analyzed (Table 7) in the data from the group (LS) with the highest RID use. Among patients for whom complete data were available ($n = 128$) the frequency of RID use was 24%. In the seven subgroups formed on the basis of activity index scores, the frequency varied between 12% and 67%. Slightly higher values could be found with lower levels of disease activity, possibly as a consequence of the use of second-line drugs. There were no differences among the groups with medium and high levels of disease activity. Those with highly active RA receive

Table 6. Frequency of RID treatment in RA sufferers ($n = 332$)

	AOK ($n=25$)	EPI ($n=45$)	MHH HA ($n=121$)	MHH LS ($n=142$)
RIDs now	12%	9%	19%	27%
RIDs ever	40%	12%[a]	43%	43%

[a] In preceding 12 months.

Table 7. Current disease activity and frequency of RID treatment in RA patients ($n = 128$)

	Activity index points 0 ($n=2$)	1 ($n=3$)	2 ($n=8$)	3 ($n=16$)	4 ($n=41$)	5 ($n=40$)	6 ($n=18$)	Total
Receiving RIDs	1 (50%)	1 (33%)	7 (88%)	12 (75%)	32 (78%)	31 (78%)	13 (72%)	97 (76%)
Not receiving RIDs	1 (50%)	2 (67%)	1 (12%)	4 (25%)	9 (22%)	9 (22%)	5 (28%)	31 (24%)

RIDs just as rarely as those with lower levels. Subjects in the other three studies also did not show a significant relationship between disease activity and RID treatment (data not shown). No systematic association with the use of RIDs was found with disease duration, sex, age, education, or the type of work situation (on/off work). Taken as a whole, these data support the suspicion of a grossly insufficient treatment, especially in patients with more active disease.

Adequacy of Current RID Treatment. We have tried to evaluate the adequacy of present RID treatment in each individual. This evaluation relies on an explicit norm with an empirical criterion and is derived from our clinical standard: An RID is indicated in all cases of active RA with oligo- or polyarticular joint involvement and disease duration of at least 4 months. The cut-off point for active RA was set between scores of 3 and 4 on the activity index; a score of 4 or more points was considered to indicate an active state. Here at least one of the (semi) objective signs is positive, namely pain on motion or pressure over joints, joint swelling, or elevated ESR. In a previous study (Raspe and Wasmus 1988) we had also considered the adequacy of RID therapy; at that time we used the same treatment norm. Patients fulfilling the criteria of an active, at least oligoarticular and chronic RA, and not receiving RID treatment were classified as being „formally" inadequately treated. In the earlier study we had the opportunity to test this formal evaluation in 75 cases of RA against a careful clinical evaluation of each individual case. Subjects included the entire AOK group and 25 each of the EPI and HA groups. Our results showed the cut-off point of 4 to produce a

Table 8. Formal versus clinical evaluation of
adequacy of RID treatment ($n = 75$)

Remission index	Sensi- tivity	Speci- ficity	κ
≥ 2 points	.94	.50	.49
≥ 3 points	.92	.64	.59
≥ 4 points	.70	.80	.44
≥ 5 points	.44	.80	.15

Table 9. Formal adequacy of current RID treatment in RA sufferers ($n = 332$)

	AOK ($n = 25$)	EPI ($n = 45$)	HA ($n = 121$)	LS ($n = 141$)
Disease duration ≤ 3 months	0%	0%	7%	0%
Activity index and disease duration ≥ 4 points > 3 months	60%	67%	79%	77%
On RIDs now	20%	10%	21%	23%
Formally inadequate	80%	90%	79%	77%

sensitivity of 0.70 and a specificity of 0.80 (Table 8). Application of this evaluation scheme in the 332 RA sufferers now examined (Table 9) showed that approximately 60%–80% of those in the four groups should have received RIDs. Of these subjects, between 10% and 23% have received the formally indicated therapy. Thus 77%–90% must be considered as formally inadequately treated.

Discussion

At least four lines of arguments support our normative approach and results. (a) In 1983 Goldman and McDonald had carried out a questionnaire study among 121 rheumatologists in the United States. Of those responding, 99% favored the use of RIDs in a „paper patient" with erosive RA, and more than 75% would prescribe RID therapy for less active or minor cases. (b) Data from various countries indicate that rheumatologists actually behave in accordance with these attitudes. Of all RA sufferers cared for by rheumatologists, 50%–85% are actually receiving RIDs (Table 1). (c) In almost all randomized controlled RID trials in RA, inactive disease is one of the basic exclusion criteria. In a recent study, for example, Suarez-Almanzor et al. (1988) compared parenteral aurothiomalate to methotraxate, including only patients with active disease.

They had to exhibit at least four swollen joints plus two of the following signs or symptoms: morning stiffness for at least 1 h, pain or tenderness in at least six joints, visual analogue pain scale of at least 3.5/10, radiological evidence of progressive erosions during the preceding 18 months, and ESR of at least 20 mm/h. (d) In the 12 months following the first consultation in our outpatient clinic an additional 40% of the 262 MHH patients were placed on RID treatment, mostly upon our recommendation. This is further evidence for a preexisting treatment deficit, and it demonstrates that we behave generally in accordance to our own standards.

Summary

Some 50%–80% of all RA sufferers treated by rheumatologists have received second-line therapy, in contrast to 7%–27% of those treated at the community level (Jacobs et al. 1988; Owens et al. 1986). Disease duration and disease activity do not seem to affect the treatment regimens of primary or other physicians working in or around Hannover. The same holds true for social and demographic characteristics of the patients. RA sufferers are generally undertreated by community-based doctors with regard to RID therapy and disease activity. Approximately 80% of patients with formal indication for the use of RIDs have not received these drugs, despite the fact that a rheumatological department with an outpatient clinic providing more than 3 500 consultations per year has existed 20 years at the medical school for the region. This outpatient clinic is utilized by more than 60% of all general practitioners and internal and orthopedic physicians working in the city of Hannover. We must therefore acknowledge a rather low community effectiveness of our service.

A sensitivity of the formal evaluation scheme of 0.70 and a specificity of 0.80 imply 30% false-negative and 20% false-positive assessments. In view of the larger number of false-negative judgements, one must assume an even greater difference between treatment reality and rheumatological concepts. So far we cannot offer a certain explanation for this unsatisfactory situation. The predictors we have investigated up to now have not proven selective. Nevertheless, practical steps are urgently required to improve rheumatological effectiveness at the community level – at least in the Hannover area.

References

Carter H, Chevallier J, Ghoussoub K, Paolaggi JB (1986) II. Enquête transversale sur le comportement thérapeutique des rhumatologues du RESFR vis-a-vis de 1153 polyarthrites rhumatoïdes: place de la D-penicillamine Rev Rhum 53:335–339

Elkeles B, Raspe HH (1988) Bekommen Patienten mit einer chronischen Polyarthritis die notwendige medikamentose „Basistherapie"? Aktuel Rheumatol 13:108–111

Epstein WV (1981) Health services research in rheumatology. Bull Rheum Dis 31:15–19

Friesen WT, Hekster YA, van de Putte LBA, Gribnau FWJ (1985) Cross-sectional study of rheumatoid arthritis treatment in an university hospital. Ann Rheum Dis 44:372–378

Goddard D, Butler R (eds) (1984) Rheumatoid arthritis. The treatment controversy. MacMillan, London

Goldman AE, Schwartz McDonald S (1983) Practices, strategies, and motivations in treatment of rheumatoid arthritis. Am J Med [Suppl] 30:79–85

Jacobs J, Keyserling JA, Britton M, Morgan GJ, Wilkenfeld J, Hutchings HC (1988) The total cost of care and the use of pharmaceuticals in the management of rheumatoid arthritis: the Medi-Cal program. J Clin Epidemiol 41:215–223

Owen SG, Friesen WT, Roberts MS, Francis H, Flux W (1986) Functional capacity and treatment data from a community based study of patients with rheumatoid arthritis. Ann Rheum Dis 45:293–303

Pinals RS, Masi AT, Larsen RA (1981) Preliminary criteria for clinical remission in rheumatoid arthritis. Arthritis Rheum 24:1308–1315

Raspe HH (1988) Basistherapie bei der chronischen Polyarthritis. Intern Welt 11:13–19

Raspe HH, Wasmus A (1988) Erhalten Kranke mit einer aktiven chronischen Polyarthritis eine "Basistherapie"? Soz Präventivmed 33:197–201

Reilly PA, Feswood J, Calin (1988) Therapeutic intervention in rheumatoid arthritis. Br J Rheumatol 27:102–105

Scott DL, Coulton BL, Chapman JH, Bacon PA, Popert AJ (1983) The long-term effects of treating rheumatoid arthritis. J R Coll Physicians Lond 17:79–85

Sharp JT (1982) Preliminary criteria for remission in rheumatoid arthritis (Letter). Arthritis Rheum 25:1144

Suarez-Almanzor ME, Fitzgerald A, Grace M, Russel AS (1988) A randomized controlled trial of parenteral methotrexate compared with sodium aurothiomalate (Myochrisine) in the treatment of rheumatoid arthritis. J Rheumatol 15:753–756

Tugwell P, Bennett KJ, Sackett DL, Haynes RB (1985) The measurement iterative loop: a framework for the critical appraisal of need, benefits and costs of health interventions. J Chronic Dis 38:339–351

Van Saase J, Vandenbroucke J, Valkenburg H, Boersma J, Cats A, Festen J, Hartman A, Huber-Bruning O, Rasker J, Weber J (1987) Changing pattern of drug use in relation to disease duration of rheumatoid arthritis. J Rheumatol 14.476–478

Vuori H (1988) Quality assurance of health services. World Health Organization, Copenhagen

Wasmus A, Raspe HH (1988) Analyse der Verschlüsselung von Arbeitsunfähigkeitsdiagnosen mit der ICD-Nr. 714 anhand einer rheumatologischen Nachuntersuchung. Öff Gesundheitswes 50:2–8

Wasmus A, Vorbeck A, Kindel P, Raspe HH (1988) Epidemiologie der chronischen Polyarthritis (cP) in Hannover. Z Rheumatol 47:248

Wolfe F, Hawley DJ (1985) Remission in rheumatoid arthritis. J Rheumatol 12:245–252

Weiterführende Literatur zum Thema „Rheuma"

Epstein WV (1981) Health services research in rheumatology. Bull Rheum Dis 31:15–19
Raspe HH, Wasmus A (1988) Erhalten Kranke mit einer aktiven chronischen Polyarthritis eine „Basistherapie"? Soz Präventivmed 33:197–201
Sasse J van, Vandenbroucke J, Valkenburg H et al. (1987) Changing pattern of drug use in relation to disease duration of rheumatoid arthritis. J Rheumatol 14:476–478
Raspe HH (ed.) (1989) Epidemiology of rheumatoid arthritis and of its treatment. Scand J Rheumatology Suppl 79

8.5 Zahnärztliche Versorgung

Epidemiologie von Parodontalerkrankungen

G. Ahrens, J. Bauch, K.-A. Bublitz, I. Neuhaus

Unter Parodont versteht man die Gesamtheit der Stützgewebe, die der Befestigung des Zahnes im Kiefer dienen. Es handelt sich um ein funktionelles System aus Zahnfleisch, Wurzelhaut, Wurzelzement und Alveolarknochen.

Gesunde Parodontalgewebe sind durch Abwesenheit von entzündlichen, atrophischen und traumatischen pathologischen Veränderungen gekennzeichnet. Parodontalerkrankung ist der allgemeine Ausdruck für eine Skala pathologischer Veränderungen an den Stütz- und Weichgeweben der Zähne. Sie verlaufen chronisch und i. allg. ohne Schmerzen. Die lokale mikrobielle Plaque (Zahnbelag) verursacht fast alle Parodontalerkrankungen, die in ihrem Verlauf ihrerseits durch systemische Faktoren ungünstig beeinflußt werden können. Die chronische marginale Gingivitis und Parodontitis sind die am weitesten verbreiteten Parodontalerkrankungen mikrobiologischer Genese (Cutress 1986; Page u. Schroeder 1982).

Während das Ausmaß der Zahnkaries fast in der ganzen Welt durch Statistiken gut dokumentiert ist, sind unsere Kenntnisse über Vorkommen und Verbreitung von Parodontalerkrankungen mangelhaft. Ein Grund dafür ist sicher darin zu suchen, daß das wissenschaftliche Interesse sich vordringlich der Zahnkaries als der Erkrankung zugewandt hat, die in erster Linie zu Schmerzen und bei Nichtbehandlung bereits im jugendlichen Alter zu Zahnverlust führen kann. Die wissenschaftliche und therapeutische Beschäftigung mit den eher schmerzlosen und erst im späteren Alter zu Zahnverlust führenden Parodontalerkrankungen hat die volle Aufmerksamkeit der wissenschaftlichen Zahnheilkunde erst zu einem späteren Zeitpunkt beansprucht.

Ein weiterer Grund liegt in dem Fehlen guter und zuverlässiger Dokumentationsmethoden für Parodontalerkrankungen. Üblicherweise beruhen derartige Methoden auf Indizes. Ein Musterbeispiel hierfür ist der DMF-Index, der für epidemiologische Untersuchungen auf dem Gebiet der Zahnkaries außerordentlich nützlich und gebräuchlich ist und hervorragende Dienste leistet. Bei den Parodontopathien ist es bisher nicht gelungen, einen derartig einfachen und zugleich aussagekräftigen und zuverlässigen Index zu entwickeln. Dies ist auch ungleich viel schwerer, weil man es bei der Karies mit einer einzigen klinischen Ausprägung zu tun hat, während das klinische Bild der Parodontopathien wesentlich vielfältiger ist und infolgedessen differenzierter betrachtet werden muß.

---

* Erstmals veröffentlicht in: Ahrens G, Bauch J, Bublitz K-A et al. (Hrsg) (1988) Parodontalgesundheit der Hamburger Bevölkerung: epidemiologische Ergebnisse einer CPITN-Untersuchung. Deutscher Ärzte-Verlag, Köln, S. 7–13.

Die in epidemiologischen Untersuchungen am häufigsten benutzten Indizes waren bisher der Periodontalindex von Russel (1956) und der Oralhygieneindex von Greene u. Vermillion (1960). Außerdem gibt es eine große Anzahl weiterer Indizes, die unterschiedliche Verbreitung gefunden hat. Neuerdings hat die WHO in Zusammenarbeit mit der FDI den "Community Periodontal-Index of Treatment Needs" (CPITN) entwickelt (Ainamo et al. 1982). Dieser Index erlaubt gleichermaßen das Registrieren verschiedener Erkrankungssymptome und die Berechnung des zu erwartenden Behandlungsbedarfs. (Als vorwiegend epidemiologischer Index ist er aber nicht für die individuelle Befunderhebung und Behandlungsplanung geeignet). Wegen seiner leichten Anwendbarkeit und großen Aussagefähigkeit scheint sich der CPITN-Index international schnell einzubürgern. Er wurde auch in der vorliegenden Untersuchung verwendet, da er sich in vergleichenden und auch in epidemiologischen Studien als brauchbar erwiesen hat (Cutress 1986; Ainamo et al. 1982).

• Die Epidemiologie parodontaler Erkrankungen ist also eine junge Wissenschaft. Die bereits vorliegenden Untersuchungen lassen eine vergleichende Interpretation nur mit allergrößter Vorsicht zu. Die Heranziehung unterschiedlichster Indizes von unterschiedlichen Untersuchern bzw. Untersuchergruppen machen es schwer, zuverlässige Zusammenhänge zu erkennen.

Gleichwohl sind übergeordnete Trends sichtbar, die Allgemeingültigkeit für sich beanspruchen dürften. Einige neuere Untersuchungen sollen hier zitiert werden.

Nach Lange (1980) ergibt sich bezüglich der Parodontalerkrankungen eine Erkrankungsrate von bis zu 90% bei Kindern und Jugendlichen. Nach Curilović (1977) gehen vom 5. Lebensjahrzehnt an mehr Zähne durch Parodontitis als durch Karies verloren (s. Abb. 1).

Gemäß einer Studie des National Center for Health Statistics in den USA gehen in der Altersgruppe von 1–74 Jahren im Schnitt 6,7 Zähne wegen Parodon-

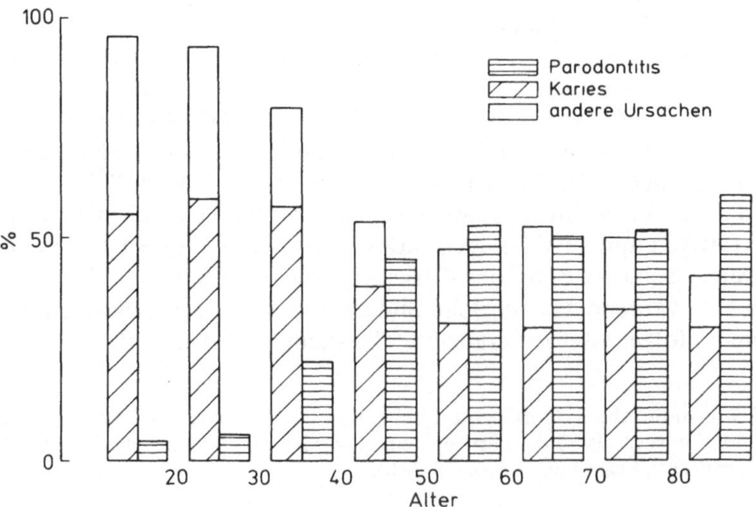

Abb. 1. Ursachen des Zahnverlustes mit steigendem Alter. (Nach Curilović 1977)

talerkrankungen verloren, gegenüber einer Extraktionsbedürftigkeit wegen Karies von nur 0,7 und aus anderen Gründen von 3,2 Zähnen (NCHS 1979; Schicke 1984).

Auch andere Daten zeigen, daß die Prävalenzraten in allen untersuchten Ländern hoch sind. Curilović hat die Ergebnisse einer epidemiologischen Studie von Lange in Münster nach dem PTN-System mit epidemiologischen Studien in Zürich, Oslo, Posen verglichen (Lange 1983): Keine Behandlung nötig hatten in Münster 0,0%, in Zürich 8,8%, in Oslo 1,7% und in Posen 0,0% (s. Tabelle 1).

Motivierung und Mundhygieneinstruktionen waren erforderlich in Münster bei 6,9%, in Zürich bei 7%, in Oslo 7,7% und in Posen bei 0,0%. Überschuß- und Zahnsteinentfernung waren erforderlich in Münster bei 43%, in Zürich bei 37,1%, in Oslo bei 53% und in Posen bei 18%. Chirurgische Taschenelimination war erforderlich in Münster bei 50,1%, in Zürich bei 47,1%, in Oslo bei 37,6% und in Posen bei 82%.

Für die Bundesrepublik Deutschland hat Lange die vorhandenen epidemiologischen Studien zusammengefaßt (Lange 1986):

In einer Untersuchung an Hauptschülern in einer Großstadt im Ruhrgebiet (Bottrop) wurde festgestellt, daß 64,6% der untersuchten Schüler pathologische Zahnfleischtaschen von mehr als 2 mm aufwiesen. In einer internationalen Multi-Center-Studie durch die WHO kamen die Untersuchungsergebnisse von 342 Mädchen und 305 Jungen im Alter zwischen 14 und 16 Jahren im Raum Dortmund zur Auswertung. 7,3% der untersuchten Kinder wiesen pathologische Zahnfleischtaschen auf; 10,4% verfügten über „horizontalen und vertikalen Knochenabbau an den ersten Molaren als Ausdruck einer tiefergehenden Destruktion des knöchernen Zahnhalteapparates" (Wingerath u. Lange 1982).

Tabelle 1. Parodontaler Behandlungsbedarf nach dem PTNI-System. (Lange 1983)

Klasse	notwendige Behandlung	Münster $n=145$ [%]	Zürich $n=159$ (Meier et al. 1979) [%]	Oslo $n=117$ (Hansen u. Johansen 1977) [%]	Posen $n=25$ (Wierzbicka et al. 1977) [%]
0	Keine	0,0	8,8	1,7	0,0
A	Motivierung, Mundhygiene-instruktion	6,9	7,0	7,7	0,0
B	Überschuß- und Zahnstein-entfernung	43,0	37,1	53,0	18,0
C	Chirurgische Taschenelimina-tion (Kürettage, Lappen)	50,1	47,1	37,6	82,0
Gesamt		100,0	100,0	100,0	100,0

Ebenfalls im Rahmen einer Multi-Center-Studie in mehreren europäischen Ländern wurde der Parodontalzustand von 20jährigen deutschen Rekruten erfaßt. Dabei zeigte sich, daß keiner der untersuchten Rekruten gesunde parodontale Verhältnisse aufwies. 75% hatten größere mikrobielle Ablagerungen, 25% hatten eine totale Gebißverschmutzung, 20% wiesen tiefe pathologische Zahnfleischtaschen auf (Lange u. Schwöppe 1981).

Bei einer Untersuchung von 145 35jährigen Münsteranern wurde nach dem PTN-System von Johansen die parodontale Behandlungsnotwendigkeit erfaßt. Es wurde kein Fall festgestellt, in dem keine Behandlung notwendig war, 7% bedurften der Verbesserung der Mundhygiene und professioneller Zahnreinigung, 43% bedurften darüber hinaus intensiver Scalings. Bei 50% waren in mehreren Quadranten operative Maßnahmen angezeigt, bei 6,2% waren diese operativen Maßnahmen in allen Gebißquadranten erforderlich (Lange 1980).

Anhand des CPITN-Indexes (Community Periodontal-Index of Treatment Needs) wurden 353 Münsteraner im Alter zwischen 45 und 55 Jahren untersucht. Bei der Untersuchung in Münster hatten lediglich 0,6 Prozent ausschließlich gesunde Sextanten (Neissen u. Lange 1985).

Code 1 des Indexes (blutet nach vorsichtiger Sondierung) hatten 2,9%. Zahnstein ohne Taschenbildung hatten je nach Altersgruppe zwischen 21 und 34%. Eine Taschentiefe von 3,5–5,5 mm wiesen 32,6% von den 45jährigen und 39,5% von den 50jährigen auf. Taschentiefen von 6 mm und mehr (fortgeschrittene marginale Parodontitis, CPITN-Index Code 4) wiesen 49,9% der 55jährigen auf.

Die Befundungen durch den CPITN-Index geben direkt Aufschluß über den notwendigen Behandlungsbedarf. So waren Mundhygieneinstruktionen bei 1,6% der 45jährigen, bei 3,9% der 50jährigen notwendig. Bei den 45jährigen waren bei 31% komplexe parodontale Behandlungen erforderlich, bei den 50jährigen bei 39,1%, bei den 55jährigen bei 41,9%.

In einer parodontal- und kariesepidemiologischen Untersuchung an 1 075 Rekruten der Bundeswehr (Durchschnittsalter 20,96 Jahre) konnte eine Gingivitismorbidität von 97,2% konstatiert werden. 78,5% der untersuchten Rekruten hatten klinische Sulkustiefen von mehr als 2 mm, somit manifeste Parodontopathien (Rechmann 1984).

In einer von Lieser u. Raetzke 1981 in 4 Kindergärten des Main-Kinzig-Kreises durchgeführten Untersuchung konnte festgestellt werden, daß bereits 56% der Kindergartenkinder an Gingivitis erkrankt waren. In „prophylaxeorientierten" Kindergärten betrug die Gingivitismorbidität dagegen nur 21,7% (Lieser u. Raetzke 1984).

In einer Untersuchung an Kindergartenkindern im Kreis Stormarn konnte ermittelt werden, daß nur 34% der untersuchten Kinder über keine Gingivitiden verfügten, schon bei den 3jährigen waren nur 30,9% entzündungsfrei. Die Zahl der entzündungsfreien Gebisse variierte sozialschichtenspezifisch. In der unteren Sozialschicht waren 24,5% entzündungsfrei, wohingegen in der oberen Sozialschicht 38,9% entzündungsfreie Gebisse aufwiesen (Schiffner et al. 1986).

Aus anderer Sicht wurden diese Ergebnisse der Schichtvariabilität bestätigt. In einer epidemiologischen Studie an Rekruten der Bundeswehr über Gingivarezessionen konnte festgestellt werden, daß Rekruten mit höherer Schulbildung einen höheren Prozentsatz von Gingivarezessionen aufwiesen. Bei 100 Rekruten mit Abitur konnten 67,6% Gingivarezessionen festgestellt werden, bei 100 Rekruten z. B. aus kaufmännischen Berufen waren es nur 27,8% (Mierau u. Fiebig 1986).

In einer nationenweiten Studie in den USA konnte ein Parodontosebefall von 79,1% bei Männern und 69,5% bei Frauen ermittelt werden bei einem PI-Wert von 1,28 für Männer und 0,85 für Frauen (weiße Bevölkerung) (NCHS 1965).

In einer Studie an 500 Kindern in den Altersgruppen 3, 5, 10, 15 und 20 Jahren in Schweden konnte festgestellt werden, daß bereits 50% der 3jährigen einen hohen Plaquebefall hatten, bei den anderen Altersstufen waren es nahezu 100%. 35% der 3jährigen hatten gingivale Entzündungen, bei den anderen Altersstufen wurden Werte von 65–97% gefunden. Pathologisch tiefe Taschen wurden bei 17% der 15jährigen und bei 21% der 20jährigen gefunden (Hugoson et al. 1981).

Bei einer Untersuchung an 1337 erwachsenen Niederländern wurden folgende Werte ermittelt: 19,8% waren zahnlos, 61% hatten Gingivitis, 53% hatten Taschentiefen von 3–6 mm und 10,1% hatten größere Taschentiefen als 6 mm. Die Prävalenz von Gingivitis und pathologischen Taschen wuchs mit zunehmendem Alter und sinkendem Ausbildungsniveau (Plasschaert et al. 1978).

Viele Studien im Ausland befassen sich mit den verschiedenen Einflußsegmenten auf die Zahnfleischgesundheit. So konnte in einer die USA umfassenden Studie nachgewiesen werden, daß der PI-Wert der Erwachsenen mit dem Familieneinkommen in Zusammenhang steht. Bei Personen männlichen Geschlechts mit einem Einkommen unter $ 2000 betrug der PI-Wert 1,99, sank auf 1,66 bei Personen mit $ 2000–3999 Einkommen und auf 1,25 bei einem Einkommen von $ 4000–6999.

In dieser Studie werden auch geschlechtsspezifische Unterschiede (der Parodontalzustand der Frauen ist besser als der der Männer), ethnische Differenzen (Angehörige der schwarzen US-Bevölkerung haben einen schlechteren Parodontalzustand als Weiße) und regionspezifische Unterschiede festgestellt (in ländlichen Gebieten ist der Parodontalzustand schlechter) (NCHS 1965).

In einer argentinischen Studie wurden ethnische Differenzen zwischen der indianischen und caucisischen Bevölkerungsgruppe konstatiert, der Parodontalzustand der indianischen Bevölkerungsgruppe war bei allen Parametern schlechter (De Muniz 1985).

In einer weiteren US-amerikanischen Studie wurde der Einfluß des Rauchens auf die Parodontalgesundheit ermittelt. Die Studie erbrachte den Nachweis eines stringenten Zusammenhanges zwischen Rauchen und schlechterem Parodontalzustand (Ismail et al. 1983).

Die WHO unterhält eine Datenbank, in der die Ergebnisse aller verfügbarer Untersuchungen gespeichert werden. Tabelle 2 gibt einen Überblick über die bisher global verfügbaren CPITN-Daten (Pilot et al. 1986; Barmes 1986). Tabelle 2 kann entnommen werden, daß vollständig gesunde Gebisse weltweit sehr selten waren. Zahnstein und Taschen (CPITN-Code 3) waren die häufigsten Befunde. Überraschend und bisher nicht erklärbar ist der geringe Prozentsatz von Sextanten mit tiefen Taschen (Code 4).

In Tabelle 3 sind Ergebnisse aus einigen Studien zur Behandlungsbedürftigkeit deutscher Bevölkerungsgruppen (unter Einschluß der vorliegenden) zusammengestellt. (Es handelt sich dabei neben dieser Studie, dem Hamburger Paro-

Tabelle 2. Auszug aus der globalen WHO-Datenbank (Stand Juli 1986) 35- bis 44jähriger Probanden. Prozentsatz der Personen mit maximalem CPITN-Index. (Pilot et al. 1986)

Land	Jahr	n	Keine Parodontalerkrankung	Nur Blutung	Zahnstein	Flache Taschen	Tiefe Taschen
Australien	1984	223	11	10	67	8	4
Bangladesch	1982	78	2	0	0	34	65
Elfenbeinküste	1986	355	0	0	1	25	75
ZentralAfrika	1986	108	1	1	14	52	32
Finnland	1984	299	2	7	56	29	6
Griechenland	1985	741	8	13	39	26	14
Hongkong	1982	760	3	4	52	37	5
Hongkong	1984	668	1	0	28	56	16
Ungarn	1985	893	5	8	51	26	8
Indonesien	1984	499	12	3	65	16	4
Indonesien	1985	296	13	10	57	17	2
Indonesien	1986	437	0	0	36	53	10
Italien	1985	21352	3	4	45	36	12
Japan	1984	182	7	4	44	38	7
Kenia	1984	199	1	4	31	49	14
Libyen	1982/83	80	0	0	13	53	34
Marokko	1983	794	4	4	46	28	14
Nepal	1984	131	0	2	45	25	28
Niederlande	1981	85	4	2	18	66	11
Neuseeland	1982	263	7	23	26	36	8
Nigeria	1985	150	4	5	52	35	3
Portugal	1984	616	3	0	47	38	8
Spanien	1985	975	7	7	36	31	18
Sri Lanka	1984	1867	5	1	55	27	10
Tansania	1982	124	1	0	28	63	7
Thailand	1982	128	0	0	50	34	16
Zimbabwe	1986	159	10	0	87	3	1

dontalprojekt, um folgende Studien: MS I, Lange, 1986, MS II, Lange, 1986, Berliner SP, Hohlfeld et al. 1986). Trotz versuchsbedingter Abweichungen sind generelle Übereinstimmungen unverkennbar. Überraschend ist die geringe Zahl gesunder und der hohe Prozentsatz der Gebisse, die einer eingehenden Behandlung bedürfen.

Wenn auch epidemiologische Kenntnisse über Parodontalerkrankungen lükkenhaft sind, läßt sich bereits eine hohe Morbidität und – insbesondere für den europäischen Raum – ein großer Behandlungsbedarf erkennen.

Man kann auch davon ausgehen, daß die Gingivitis

– bereits mit der Kindheit beginnt,
– sich während der Pubertät verstärkt mit dem Gipfel im Lebensalter von etwa 11 Jahren,

Tabelle 3. Zusammenfassung von 4 Studien zur Behandlungsbedürftigkeit deutscher Bevölkerungsgruppen

Behandlungsbedarf	Münster I [%]	Münster II [%]	Hamburger SP [%]	Berliner SP [%]
Keine Parodontalbehandlung	0	0,6	2,8	0
Mundhygieneinstruktion	6,9	2,9	8,6	0
Mundhygieneinstruktion und Entfernen von Zahnstein und Überhängen, Wurzelglätten	42,8	59,7	72,3	46,1
Mundhygieneinstruktion und Entfernen von Zahnstein und Überhängen, Wurzelglätten und chirurgische Behandlung	50,3	36,9	16,3	53,9

Nach PTN- bzw. CPITN-Zuordnungsschlüssel, bei „Münster II" und „Hamburger SP" auf der Basis des höchsten CPITN-Wertes, bei „Berliner SP" auf der Basis von Sextantenmischwerten (zusammengestellt v. W. Micheelis, IDZ, Köln, 1987)

- danach bis zum Alter von 17 Jahren wieder etwas abklingt,
- die Morbidität hoch ist und teilweise bis zu 90 % und darüber beträgt (Stamm 1986).

Daten über den Verlauf von Parodontopathien bei Erwachsenen sind seltener. Als gemeinsame Trends zeichnen sich ein etwas leichterer Verlauf beim weiblichen Geschlecht (Folge besserer Mundhygiene?), ein stärkerer Befall während der Schwangerschaft und eine allgemeine stetige Zunahme mit steigendem Alter ab (Cutress 1986).

Weitere Untersuchungen sind aber erforderlich, um spezielle Details im Verlauf der Erkrankungen besser erkennen und für ätiologisches Verständnis, Prophylaxe und Therapie nutzen zu können.

Literatur

Ainamo J, Barmes D, Beagrie G, Cutress T, Martin J, Sardo-Infirri J (1982) Development of the World Health Organization (WHO) Community Periodontal Index of Treatment Needs (CPITN), Int Dent J 32:281–291

Ainamo J, Parviainen K, Murtomaa H (1984) Reliability of the CPITN in the epidemiological assessment of periodontal treatment needs at 13–15 years of age. Int Dent J 34:214–218

Barmes DE (1986) Epidemiology of periodontal disease acta parodontologica 15/1986. Schw Monatsschr Zahnmed 96:908/88–911/91

Curilović Z (1977) Die Epidemiologie parodontaler Erkrankungen bei Schweizer Jugendlichen und prognostische Konsequenzen, Habilitationsschrift, Universität Zürich

Cutress TW (1986) Periodontal health and periodontal disease in young people: global epidemiology. Int Dent J 36:146–151

Garcia ML, Cutress TW (1986) A national survey of periodontal treatment needs of adults in the Philippines, Comm Dent Oral Epidemiol 14:313–316

Greene JC, Vermillion JR (1960) The oral hygiene index: a method for classifying oral hygiene status. J Am Dent Assoc 61:172–179

Hohlfeld M, Bernimoulin JP (1986) Teilergebnisse einer epidemiologischen Untersuchung des Parodontalzustandes bei 45- bis 54jährigen Berliner Probanden. Dtsch Zahnärztl Z 41:619–622

Hugoson A, Koch G, Rylander H (1981) Prevalence and distribution of gingivitis-periodontitis in children and adolescents. Epidemiological data as a base for risk group selection, Swed Dent J 5·91–103

Ismail AI, Burt BA, Eklund SA (1983) Epidemiologic patterns of smoking and periodontal disease in the United States, J Am Dent Assoc 106:617–621

Johansen JR, Gjermo P, Bellini HT (1973) A system to classify the need for periodontal treatment, Acta Odont Scand 31:297–305

Lange DE (1980) Zur Situation der Parodontologie in der Bundesrepublik Deutschland. Quintessenz 31:91–94

Lange DE (1983) Parodontologie – Daten, Fakten, Entwicklungen und Zielsetzungen. Quintessenz 9:1741–1754

Lange DE (1986) Häufigkeit, Schweregrad und Behandlungsbedurftigkeit von Parodontopathien. ZWR 95:402–406

Lange DE, Schwöppe G (1981) Epidemiologische Untersuchungen an Rekruten der Bundeswehr (Mund- und Gebißbefunde). Dtsch Zahnärztl Z 46·432–434

Lieser H, Raetzke P (1984) Der Effekt regelmäßig durchgeführter Prophylaxe-Maßnahmen auf die Gingivitis- und Kariesmorbidität von Kindern in Kindergärten Dtsch Zahnärztl Z 39:666–668

Mierau H-D, Fiebig A (1986) Zur Epidemiologie der Gingivarezessionen und möglicher klinischer Begleiterscheinungen, Dtsch Zahnärztl Z 41:640–644

Muniz De BR (1985) Epidemiologic oral health survey of Argentine children. Comm Dent Oral Epidemiol 13:328–333

NCHS (National Center for Health Statistics) (ed) (1965) Periodontal disease in adults, United States, 1960–1962, Ser 11, Nr. 12 USDHEW PHS, Washington

NCHS (1979) Basic data on dental examination findings of Persons 1–74, United States, 1971–1974, Ser. 11, Nr 214, USDHEW PHS, Hyattsville/MD

Neissen R, Lange DE (1985) CPITN-Data of 45-to 55-year-old urban residents of Germany. Open Forum, FDI-Congress, Belgrad

Page CR, Schroeder HE (1982) Periodontitis in man and other animals, Karger, Basel

Pilot T, Barmes DE, Leclercq MH, McCombie BJ, Sardo-Infirri J (1986) Periodontal conditions in adults, 35–44 years of age: an overview of CPITN data in the WHO Global Oral Data Bank. Comm Dent Oral Epidemiol 14:310–312

Plasschaert AJM, Folmer T, Heuvel JLM van den, Jansen J, Opijnen L van, Wouters SLJ (1978) An epidemiologic survey of periodontal disease in Dutch adults, Comm Dent Oral Epidemiol 6:65–70

Rechmann P (1984) Parodontal- und kariesepidemiologische Untersuchungen an Rekruten der Bundeswehr. Wehrmed Monatsschr 28:288–296

Russell AL (1956) A system of classification and scoring for prevalence surveys of periodontal disease. J Dent Res 35:350–359

Schicke RK (1984) Sozialmedizinische Aspekte der Zahnheilkunde. Stuttgart New York

Schiffner U, Gülzow H-J, Bauch J (1986) Mundhygiene und Gingivitis bei Kindern aus Stormarner Kindergärten vor und zwei Jahre nach Einführung gruppenprophylaktischer Maßnahmen, Oralprophylaxe 8:22–28

Stamm JW (1986) Epidemiology of gingivitis. J Clin Periodontol 13:360–366

Wingerath H-D, Lange DE (1982) Mundhygieneverhalten von 14- und 15jährigen Schülern unter soziologischen Gesichtspunkten. Dtsch Zahnärztl Z 47:565–568

Weiterführende Literatur zum Thema „Zahnärztliche Versorgung"

Cutress TW (1986) Periodontal health and periodontal disease in young people: global epidemiology. Int Dent J 36:146–151

Micheelis W, Müller PJ (1990) Dringliche Mundgesundheitsprobleme der Bevölkerung in der Bundesrepublik Deutschland: Zahlen – Fakten – Perspektiven. Institut der Deutschen Zahnärzte (IDZ), Köln

Pilot T, Barmes DE, Leclercq MH et al (1986) Periodontal conditions in adults, 35–44 years of age: an overview of CPITN data in the WHO Global Oral Data Bank. Community Dent Oral Epidemiol 14:310–312

US Department of Health and Human Services (1988) Oral health of United States adults – regional findings. NIH publications No. 88–2869, Washington/DC

8.6 Rehabilitationsforschung

Sozialpolitische Rahmenbedingungen, Ziele und Wirkungen von Rehabilitation *

B. Badura, H. Lehmann

Sozialpolitische Rahmenbedingungen

Rehabilitation, verstanden als Prozeß der (Wieder)herstellung körperlichen und seelischen Wohlbefindens und weitestgehender sozialer (Re)integration, wurde in den vergangenen Jahrzehnten zu einem wichtigen Gegenstand moderner Sozialpolitik. Wie die Entwicklung der sozialen Sicherung insgesamt unterliegt auch die Entwicklung von Einrichtungen und Maßnahmen im Bereich der Rehabilitation Einflüssen, die sich nur bedingt an den Problemen und Bedürfnissen der Adressaten dieser Leistungen, der Behinderten, Unfallopfer, Kranken, Pflegebedürftigen, orientieren. Wieviel Mittel für den Rehabilitationssektor insgesamt und für seine Teilsektoren bereitgestellt werden und die Art ihrer Verwendung, d. h. Organisationsstrukturen und Leistungskataloge sozialstaatlicher Rehabilitation, hängen von Rahmenbedingungen und Determinanten ab, die entweder „von außen" auf das System der sozialen Sicherung einwirken (externe Rahmenbedingungen) oder die „von innen" wirken und wegen der Eigendynamik gegebener Institutionen, Regelungsprinzipien und Interessenkonstellationen als gleichsam „hausgemacht" bezeichnet werden müssen (interne Rahmenbedingungen). Wo in diesem Zusammenhang die mittlerweile stattliche Zahl der Behindertenverbände anzusiedeln ist, hängt davon ab, ob sie ihre Aktivitäten schwerpunktmäßig im politischen Bereich (Parlament, Parteien, Ministerialorganisationen etc.) oder direkt über die Träger und Anbieter sozialstaatlicher Leistungen entfalten. Wie authentisch diese Verbände die Bedürfnisse ihrer Mitglieder und der Betroffenen insgesamt vertreten, bedarf einer fallweisen Überprüfung. Behinderte, Kranke, Pflegebedürftige bilden eine sozial höchst heterogene und in der Regel politisch wenig lautstarke Gruppe und sind daher ständig der Gefahr ausgesetzt, daß Politik *für* sie und nicht *mit* ihnen gemacht wird.

Externe Rahmenbedingungen

Solange staatliche Sozialpolitik als Antwort auf die „Arbeiterfrage" primär dem Ziel der Befriedung und politischen Integration des industriellen Proletariats diente und insbesondere in Deutschland dazu bestimmt war, allzu krasse Auswir-

---

* Erstmals veröffentlicht in: Koch U, Lucius-Hoene G, Stegie R (Hrsg) (1988) Handbuch der Rehabilitationspsychologie. Springer, Berlin Heidelberg New York Tokyo, S. 58–73 (gekürzt).

kungen eines sich ungehemmt entfaltenden Industriekapitalismus zu mildern und teilweise auch zu verhindern, solange waren primär externe (ökonomische, politische und soziale) Faktoren ausschlaggebend für die Entstehung und Entwicklung sozialpolitischer Einrichtungen und Maßnahmen. Die für Form und Wirkung Bismarckscher Sozialpolitik charakteristische Dialektik politisch präventiver Absichten auf seiten des Staates und sozialreformerisch bis revolutionärer Absichten auf seiten einer machtvollen und zunehmend wohlorganisierten sozialen Bewegung, ihr „konservativ-revolutionäres Doppelwesen" (Heimann 1980), hat maßgeblich zur Veränderung frühkapitalistischer Machtstrukturen und zur Milderung der sozialen Kosten unseres Wirtschaftssystems beigetragen. Kennzeichnend für die Entwicklung der Bundesrepublik war eine Jahrzehnte und Regierungen wechselnder politischer Couleur überdauernde „Große Koalition" in Sachen Sozialpolitik. „Wachstum und Gedeihen" sozialpolitischer Einrichtungen und Maßnahmen schienen in dieser zweiten Phase deutscher Sozialpolitik „ohne weiteres als begrüßenswert oder auch als tabu" (Achinger 1959, 1971, S. 5). Mit dem „Ölschock" Anfang der 70er Jahre und der sich daran anschließenden wirtschaftlichen Stagnation scheint auch unsere Sozialpolitik an Grenzen ihres, auf Gedeih und Verderb von der gesamtwirtschaftlichen Entwicklung abhängigen, Wachstums gestoßen zu sein. Charakteristisch für die zweite und mehr noch für die dritte Phase staatlicher Sozialpolitik ist, daß es in der einschlägigen Diskussion weniger um Grundlagen und Rahmenbedingungen von Wirtschaft und Gesellschaft insgesamt als vielmehr um die Grundlagen und Rahmenbedingungen sozialpolitischen Handelns geht. In Frage stehen die Einrichtungen unseres Sozialstaates selbst (die „gewachsenen Institute", die „Trägervielfalt", die „dominanten Denksysteme" etc.), ihre Wirksamkeit, Effizienz, Humanität und Bürgernähe (von Ferber, 1967; Badura u. Gross 1976; Kaufmann 1979; Badura 1982).

Insbesondere für den Bereich der Rehabilitation gilt – so die im folgenden vertretene These –, daß ihr gegenwärtiger Zustand und ihre Mängel v. a. „hausgemacht" sind und daher auch auf dem Wege einer auf sich selbst gerichteten Reform staatlicher Sozialpolitik überwunden werden müssen. In einer Gesellschaft, die nahezu ein Drittel ihres Sozialprodukts für das Sozialbudget aufwendet, in der also nicht mehr von „öffentlicher Armut", sondern eher von öffentlichem Reichtum die Rede sein muß, in einer solchen Gesellschaft ist der finanzielle Handlungsspielraum für soziale Maßnahmen eine Sache der Prioritätensetzung, werden die internen Verteilungskämpfe unter den Trägern und Anbietern sozialer Leistungen, die Mitbestimmungsmöglichkeiten der Konsumenten, d. h. die internen Rahmenbedingungen entscheidend für die Entwicklung und die Leistungskraft einzelner Programme und Maßnahmen.

Interne Rahmenbedingungen

Ein erstes bedeutsames Merkmal staatlicher Sozialpolitik insgesamt und damit auch des Rehabilitationssektors ist die *Verrechtlichung* des Leistungsangebots. Verrechtlichung bedeutet in diesem Zusammenhang dreierlei: Zum einen werden Probleme und Leistungen „unter die Kategorie des juristischen Sonderwissens" gestellt (Kaufmann 1984, S. 19), was wiederum in Form von Bürokratisierung und Verberuflichung bestimmte Konsequenzen für die Art der Leistungserbringung und für ihre Wirksamkeit und Angemessenheit hat (vgl. dazu Achinger 1971, S. 87 ff.); zum zweiten hat die Verrechtlichung eines großen komplexen Sozialleistungssystems zur Folge, daß im Falle von Unklarheiten oder einander widerstreitender Interessen Problemlösungen zu einer „immer exklusiveren Angelegenheit von Spezialisten" (Kaufmann 1984, S. 17) werden; zum dritten führt die Verrechtlichung mit ihrer Bindung an die Tätigkeit des Parlaments und der Regierung dazu, daß jede größere Änderung im System sozialer Sicherung – auch die Rücknahme sozialer Leistungen – mit zum Teil erheblichen politischen Kosten verbunden sein kann und somit oft unterbleibt oder an Stellen geschieht, wo der politische Widerstand oder die politischen Kosten als gering eingeschätzt werden. Sind „Einschnitte" nicht mehr zu vermeiden, werden sie daher meist dort vorgenommen, wo sie politisch am leichtesten zu verkraften sind, nicht unbedingt dort, wo sie von der Sache her tatsächlich gerechtfertigt, unter Umständen sogar der Lebensqualität dienlich, oder wo sie am leichtesten zu verschmerzen wären. Nur so läßt sich verstehen, daß in der gegenwärtigen Phase stagnierender Sozialaufwendungen weniger – oder gar nicht – bei den Ausgaben für Arzneimittel oder bei den Einkommen einer mittlerweile recht stattlichen Anzahl von Spitzenverdienern unter den Anbietern sozialstaatlicher Leistungen gespart wird, sondern zu allererst bei den Ausgaben für Schüler, Studenten, Behinderte oder Arbeitslose. Diejenigen, die nach Achinger (1959, S. 44) in den fetten Jahren „in der sozialen Umverteilung am schnellsten zum Zuge" kamen, haben offenbar auch in den weniger fetten Jahren am wenigsten zu befürchten.

Die Verrechtlichung unseres Systems sozialer Sicherung hat insgesamt gesehen sicherlich wesentlich zur Verstetigung und damit zur Berechenbarkeit seiner Leistungen – über gesellschaftliche Umbrüche und tagespolitische Einflüsse hinweg – beigetragen, eine Tatsache, von der gerade bei einem System, das auf „Sicherung" der Bürger abzielt (Kaufmann 1973), eine auch psychologisch nicht zu unterschätzende Wirkung ausgeht. Verrechtlichung hat aber auch zur Starrheit, Innovations- und Anpassungsfeindlichkeit, zur Intransparenz und damit auch zu einer (selbstbewirkten) Bürgerferne und mangelhaften Bedürfnissensibilität beigetragen (Achinger 1971; von Ferber 1967; Kaufmann 1979). Für den Bereich der Rehabilitation wird dies besonders deutlich an der unübersichtlichen *Trägervielfalt*. Bis heute ist es nicht gelungen, die Aufgaben der Rehabilitation einem eigenständigen Zweig der sozialen Sicherung zu übertragen. Rehabilitationsmaßnahmen werden insbesondere von 6 (!) verschiedenen Trägergruppen durchgeführt: von der Rentenversicherung, der Unfallversicherung, der Kriegsopferversorgung, der Bundesanstalt für Arbeit, der Sozialhilfe und der Krankenversicherung. Die Autoren der Sozialenquête hatten bereits 1966, also vor über 20 Jahren, die „Zersplitterung" der Rehabilitationsmaßnahmen und deren negative Folgen für ihre Empfänger bemängelt (Sozialenquête-Kommission 1966, S. 286, 297). Und sie hatten bereits damals eine Reihe von „Organisationsmodellen" zu ihrer Überwindung vorgeschlagen (Sozialenquête-Kommission 1966, S. 297 ff.). An der Trägervielfalt geändert hat selbst diese „hochoffizielle Diagnose" bis heute nichts. Das Rehabilitationsangleichungsgesetz von 1974 hat allerdings einige besonders nachteilige Folgen dieser Situation gemildert.

Eine weitere interne Rahmenbedingung ist die *Selektivität* des Leistungsangebots im Bereich der Rehabilitation und – im Zusammenhang damit – die Bevorzugung bzw. Benachteiligung bestimmter Problembereiche und Personengruppen. Blickt man zurück in die Rehabilitationsdiskussion der 60er und frühen 70er Jahre, so fällt der dort oft als nahezu selbstverständlich erachtete enge Zusammenhang zwischen den *Zwängen des Arbeitsmarktes* und den Zielen der Rehabilitationspraxis auf. In der bereits zitierten Sozialenquête von 1966 heißt es dazu: „Das Brachliegen einiger hunderttausend möglicher Arbeitskräfte sollte angesichts der dauerhaften Neuansprüche des Arbeitsmarktes und der entsprechenden Einsetzung von Gastarbeitern vermieden werden" (Sozialenquête-Kommission 1966, S. 295). Da dieser (externe) Zwang heute entfällt, stellt sich die Frage, ob Rehabilitation damit überhaupt an Bedeutung verlieren oder aber sich einer neuen, nicht mehr primär arbeitsmarktbezogenen Zielsetzung zuwenden sollte. Eine zu enge Verknüpfung von Rehabilitationspraxis und Arbeitsmarktbedürfnissen ist von einigen Rehabilitationsexperten immer schon eher kritisch betrachtet worden. Chronisch Kranke, Unfallopfer, Behinderte und Pflegebedürftige sind zu allererst mit zum Teil schwerwiegenden somatischen, psychischen und materiellen Problemen konfrontiert. Die (Wieder-)Eingliederung ins Erwerbsleben ist für sie der letzte, wenn auch meist hoch bedeutsame Schritt innerhalb einer ganzen Kette zu bewältigender körperlicher, psychischer und sozialer Anpassungsprozesse. (Wieder-)Aufnahme der Erwerbstätigkeit ist in einer „Arbeitsgesellschaft" ein letzter wichtiger Schritt in die „Normalität" (Thimm 1984), ein von gesellschaftlichen Normen und Erwartungen herrührendes Bedürfnis und heute weniger denn je ein Imperativ des Arbeitsmarktes. An diese subjektive Sicht der Betroffenen ist gedacht, wenn an anderer Stelle der Sozialenquête behauptet wird, „daß die berufliche Eingliederung sozusagen das Grundelement der gesellschaftlichen Eingliederung sei" (Sozialenquête-Kommission 1966, S. 283).

Blickt man auf die Statistik der jährlich erbrachten Rehabilitationsleistungen, wird ein weiteres Selektionskriterium deutlich. Weitaus am häufigsten erbracht werden Leistungen im Bereich der *medizinischen Rehabilitation* (Statistik der deutschen gesetzlichen Rentenversicherung 1980, S. 8–13). Auch hier muß die Frage aufgeworfen werden, ob und wie weit diese Schwerpunktsetzung sich mit den tatsächlichen Problemen und Bedürfnissen der Adressaten deckt und welche potentiellen Adressaten dadurch möglicherweise von den Leistungen der Rehabilitationsträger ausgeschlossen bleiben. Wie bereits erwähnt und weiter unten noch im einzelnen auszuführen, sind Unfallopfer, chronisch Kranke, Pflegebedürftige und Behinderte oft mit finanziellen und somatischen Problemen, in jedem Fall aber mit einer ganzen Reihe psychischer und sozialer Probleme konfrontiert, die in einem engen Wechselverhältnis zueinander stehen und daher eine ganzheitliche Betrachtung jedes Einzelfalles mit seiner spezifischen situativen und persönlichen Voraussetzungen notwendig machen. Auch dies ist in der Sozialenquête vor über 20 Jahren bereits erkannt und angesprochen worden. In dem immer noch höchst aktuellen Abschnitt über „Teamwork" wird betont, Rehabilitation sei „in Kenntnis der persönlichen Verhältnisse des Patienten, mit Einschluß der hausärztlichen Kenntnisse und der späteren Mitwirkung am weiteren Lebensverlauf des Patienten ‚zu konzipieren' (Sozialenquête-Kommission

1966, S.296). „Deshalb ist auch die Mitwirkung der freien Medizin, insbesondere also der Hausärzte, die im allgemeinen nach Meinung der ärztlichen Fachkreise weit stärker sozialmedizinisch ausgerichtet werden sollten, mit ins Auge zu fassen" (Sozialenquête-Kommission 1966, S.297). Auch hier ist bis heute recht wenig geschehen. Ähnliches gilt für die Rehabilitation psychisch Kranker (Badura u. Gross 1976, S.230ff.) und die immer noch anstehende Lösung der finanziellen und praktischen Probleme Pflegebedürftiger (Badura 1983).

Eine letzte, für den Stand der Rehabilitation in der Bundesrepublik charakteristische Rahmenbedingung ist die Bevorzugung *stationärer* und überregional *zentralisierter* Rehabilitationseinrichtungen gegenüber Formen ambulanter, ortsnaher Rehabilitation. Auch hierzu finden sich in der Sozialenquête eine Reihe richtungsweisender und bis heute uneingelöster Empfehlungen. So wird etwa den Rentenanstalten als der bedeutendsten Trägergruppe nahegelegt, sie sollten „örtliche Dienststellen schaffen, um auch der Verwaltung die persönliche Kenntnis des Einzelfalles zu ermöglichen und zugleich eine Verbindung zur allgemeinen ärztlichen Praxis herzustellen" (Sozialenquête-Kommission 1966, S.299). An die Infragestellung der völlig tabuisierten Trennung ambulanter und stationärer medizinischer Versorgung haben sich selbst die Autoren der Sozialenquête nicht herangewagt, obwohl es sich auch hier um ein gesetzlich festgeschriebenes und im Ausland völlig unübliches Organisationsdogma bundesrepublikanischer Sozialpolitik handelt, das v.a. den Interessen bestimmter Anbieter und nicht den Bedürfnissen der Konsumenten sozialstaatlicher Leistungen dient.

Auf die bisherigen Ausführungen zurückblickend, drängt sich selbstverständlich die Frage auf, inwieweit die genannten internen Rahmenbedingungen, inwieweit insbesondere die hier feststellbaren massiven Reformwiderstände sich möglicherweise auf einige wenige (mehr oder weniger verdeckte) Interessenkonstellationen und (mehr oder weniger latente) Gestaltungsprinzipien zurückführen lassen. Als erstes wäre das *Eigeninteresse der Träger* von Rehabilitationsmaßnahmen zu nennen und insbesondere deren Furcht, jede Änderung der Organisationspraxis könnte zu einem Verlust an Einfluß oder zum Schaden der eigenen Organisation beitragen. Daß dem so ist, ist offenbar ebenso unbestritten wie unveränderbar: „Viele Sachkenner gehen von der Überzeugung aus, daß zwar eine Vereinheitlichung notwendig sei, daß diese Einheitlichkeit aber die Überwindung der eigenständigen und auf ihren Besitzstand pochenden Verwaltungen voraussetze und daß dieses Hemmnis nicht zu beseitigen sei" (Sozialenquête-Kommission 1966, S.301). Dies zu betonen ist auch und gerade heute von Bedeutung, weil die Tätigkeit dieser Verwaltungen in einem weitgehend von öffentlicher Diskussion abgeschirmten Bereich stattfindet.

Als zweites zu nennen wären der dominante *Einfluß der medizinischen Profession* auf den gesamten Rehabilitationssektor und die geringe Artikulationskraft und Heterogenität der (potentiellen) Adressaten von Rehabilitationsmaßnahmen. Ausbau und Versorgungsniveau unseres Rehabilitationssektors scheinen heute überwiegend daran orientiert, was als medizinisch notwendig und möglich erachtet wird. Alle darüber hinausgehenden psychischen und sozialen Bedürfnisse und Probleme haben versorgungspolitisch einen sehr viel geringeren Rang, obwohl unter Experten seit langem gerade die Bewältigung dieser psychischen und sozialen Probleme als „fast wichtigste Voraussetzung für ein Gelingen der Rehabilitation" angesehen wird (Preller 1970, S. 504). Der tiefere Grund dafür liegt vermutlich nicht allein im professionspolitischen Bestreben nach Kontrolle dieses Sektors, sondern v. a. in einem durch Theorie und Ausbildung bedingten *biomedizinischen Reduktionismus* von Krankheitsbegriff und therapeutischer Praxis moderner Medizin (Engel 1977; McKeown 1982; Badura 1984).

Als weitere Determinante gegenwärtiger Rehabilitationspraxis müssen sozialpolitische Bestrebungen genannt werden, Art und Umfang des Rehabilitationsangebotes den *Zwängen des Arbeitsmarktes* anzupassen. Allerdings, der Slogan „Rehabilitation vor Rente" entstammt noch einer Periode leergefegter Arbeitsmärkte. In Zeiten massenhafter Arbeitslosigkeit hat er seine Bedeutung eingebüßt oder bedürfte einer neuen Begründung. Für die Sozialbeitrags- und Steuerzahler ebenso wie für die Betroffenen wäre dabei eine Lösung am schlechtesten, die sich wie bisher überwiegend an den Interessen der Anbieter (Träger, Professionen) orientiert und die konkreten Lebensverhältnisse und Bedürfnisse der zu Rehabilitierenden als eher nachrangig erachtet. Gegenüber der bisherigen Rehabilitationspraxis plädieren wir:

1) für eine verstärkte Berücksichtigung psychischer und sozialer Probleme der Rehabilitanden und ihrer unmittelbaren Angehörigen;
2) für eine ortsnahe Rehabilitation und eine Förderung der Selbsthilfepotentiale der Betroffenen;
3) für mehr Optionen und verstärkte Mitwirkungsmöglichkeiten der Betroffenen bei der Gestaltung einzelner Rehabilitationsmaßnahmen;
4) für die organisatorische Zusammenfassung der Rehabilitationsträger unter einem Dach.

Die gegenwärtige Situation – Zersplitterung der Träger und Zentralisierung des Leistungsangebots – widerspricht der Logik moderner Dienstleistungsproduktion. Personenbezogene Dienstleistungssysteme erfordern, sollen sie effizient und zugleich wirksam und bedürfnisgerecht produzieren, das Umgekehrte, nämlich eine Vereinheitlichung des Verwaltungsapparates und eine Dezentralisierung der Leistungserbringung (Gross u. Badura 1977; Gartner u. Riessmann 1978).

Thesen zu Wirkungen der Rehabilitation

Die im folgenden diskutierten Thesen zu den alten und neuen Zielen der Rehabilitation basieren auf den Ergebnissen der Oldenburger Longitudinalstudie (Badura et al. 1987), die bei rund 1 000 Erstinfarktpatienten den Rehabilitationsprozeß im ersten Jahr nach dem Infarkt beobachtet hat.

These 1: Biomedizinischer Reduktionismus schmälert den Rehabilitationserfolg

Die ärztliche Tätigkeit erschöpft sich nicht in medizinischer Diagnose und somatischer Intervention. Ein wesentlicher Teil der ärztlichen Arbeit muß sich auch auf Information, Beratung und Zuspruch erstrecken. Ein Vergleich zwischen den Beratungswünschen der Patienten und den Beratungsleistungen der Krankenhaus- und Hausärzte in unserer Untersuchung ergab, daß die Ärzte zu ihren traditionellen, medizinischen Themen Krankheit und Medikamenteneinnahme, Übergewicht und Diät, Rauch- und Trinkgewohnheiten in der Regel die Wünsche der Patienten sogar übererfüllen. Nur die Hausärzte sprechen auch ausführlicher über die Wiederaufnahme der Arbeit. Unzureichend werden in den Augen der Patienten v. a. die Themen Sexualität nach dem Herzinfarkt, Berentung und Pensionierung, nervliche Belastungen in Beruf und Familie behandelt. Auch ist die Informationsleistung zu Heilverfahren und Kuren, zu Sport- und Gesprächsgruppen für Infarktpatienten, zur Inanspruchnahme nichtmedizinischer Leistungen, zu anderen Informationsquellen von den Rehabilitanden stark bemängelt worden.

Am Beispiel dieser Beratungsleistungen ist ersichtlich, daß die Ärzte in der Regel nur zu ihrem Kernbereich, dem biomedizinischen Teil der Krankheit, ausführlich beraten. Sie sind bisher zu wenig bereit oder fähig, die biomedizinischen Fakten im psychischen und sozialen Kontext der Erkrankung zu interpretieren und entsprechend mitzuteilen. Gerade die Beratung aber ist eine ärztliche Leistung, die grundsätzlich diesen biomedizinischen Reduktionismus durchbrechen und sich positiv auf den psychischen Zustand der Rehabilitanden auswirken kann.

Wurde die Beratung vom Patienten als „rundum ausreichend", „klar", „verständlich", und „auf die persönliche Situation zugeschnitten" bezeichnet, so konnten in unserer Studie positive Auswirkungen auf das Wohlbefinden der Patienten nachgewiesen werden. War die Qualität der Beratung dagegen schlecht oder hat die Beratung die Patienten sogar verunsichert, so sind deutliche Verschlechterungen im Wohlbefinden der Patienten zu beobachten. Die nichtmedizinischen Leistungen der Ärzte haben also einen großen Einfluß auf das Befinden der Rehabilitanden. Tritt der Arzt zudem als Vermittler auf, d. h. bezieht er, im Einverständnis mit dem Patienten, den Ehepartner und den Arbeitgeber – als wichtige dritte Personen – in den Behandlungsprozeß mit ein, verbessert dies die sozialen und psychischen Voraussetzungen der Krankheitsbewältigung und erhöht zugleich auch die Patientencompliance. Die Durchbrechung des biomedizinischen Reduktionismus in Behandlung und Therapie durch ausführliche Beratung zu einem weiten Themenspektrum und durch die Einbeziehung wichtiger Bezugspersonen aus dem sozialen Netzwerk der Betroffenen ist ein wesentlicher Beitrag zur Gestaltung einer umfassenden Rehabilitation. Nur durch solche Ausweitungen der Leistungen und durch die Beteiligung weiterer Akteure kann den „neuen" Rehabilitationszielen Rechnung getragen werden.

These 2: Der somatische Gesundheitszustand hat keinen Einfluß auf die Rückkehr zur Arbeit

Legt man, abgeleitet aus dem Ziel der Erhaltung der Arbeitskraft, als Erfolgskriterium für die Rehabilitationsleistungen die Rückkehr zur Arbeit an, so zeigt sich, daß die somatischen Befunde, die durch medizinische Intervention positiv beeinflußt werden können, keine Zusammenhänge aufweisen mit der tatsächlichen Wiederaufnahme der Arbeit (Lehmann 1984). Bei einer Nachbefragung eines stationär behandelten Patientenkollektivs (Kauderer-Hübel u. Buchwalsky 1984) bilden sich sogar inverse Ergebnisse ab, d. h. in ihren körperlichen Funktionen nach einem Myokardinfarkt stark eingeschränkte Personen kehren zur Arbeit zurück, dagegen nehmen Patienten mit geringfügigen Einschränkungen die Arbeit nicht wieder auf. Ähnliche Ergebnisse werden auch von anderen deutschen Studien (Weiß 1984; Krasemann et al. 1984) berichtet. Darüber hinaus zeigt ein Vergleich der Rückkehrquoten und der Zeitdauer bis zur Rückkehr ins Erwerbsleben in ausländischen Studien (Stern et al. 1977; Croog u. Levine 1977) mit den Ergebnissen der Oldenburger Longitudinalstudie, daß in der Bundesrepublik die Anzahl der Rückkehrer niedriger und die Dauer bis zur Rückkehr länger ist als beispielsweise in den USA. Es müssen offenbar andere als medizinische Gründe für die Rückkehr zur Arbeit verantwortlich sein.

Sicherlich hat die jeweilige konjunkturelle Situation auch einen Einfluß auf die Rückkehrerquote, weil von ihr die Arbeitsmarktchancen der Rehabilitanden abhängen. Weitere wesentliche Einflußgrößen auf die Rückkehrerquote konnten in der Oldenburger Longitudinalstudie nachgewiesen werden: das Alter und der Beruf des Patienten, seine eigene Einschätzung der Schädigung des Herzens, seine Beurteilung des Genesungszustandes, sein eigener Rückkehrwunsch sowie das allgemeine Leistungsbild, das sich der behandelnde Arzt, der arbeitsfähig schreibt, vom Patienten macht. Auch kehren Patienten, die im Akutkrankenhaus geringere Ängstlichkeits- und Depressivitätswerte aufzeigen, eher zur Arbeit zurück. Insgesamt gesehen sind also v. a. soziale und psychische Faktoren für die Rückkehr zur Arbeit ausschlaggebend.

Lediglich das Arzturteil hat einen signifikanten Einfluß. Dieses Urteil basiert aber nur zu einem Teil auf somatischen Befunden. Die oben genannten Einflußgrößen wie Alter, Beruf etc. gehen auch hier ein, d. h. auch der Arzt selbst stützt sich auf nichtsomatische Fakten. In dem Maße, in dem „klassische" Leistungen (medizinische Intervention) realistisch beurteilt werden und „klassische" Zielsetzungen (Arbeitsmarktimperative) an Bedeutung verlieren, rückt das Ziel der (Wieder)herstellung bestmöglicher Lebensqualität, rücken Maßnahmen und Leistungen im psychischen und sozialen Bereich ins Zentrum zukünftiger Rehabilitationspolitik. Abhängig von subjektiven Prioritäten, Lebensbedingungen und Optionen im Einzelfall kann aus dieser Sichtweise die Wiederherstellung der Erwerbstätigkeit nach wie vor von hoher Bedeutung sein, wenn es sein muß auch gegen die aktuelle Situation auf dem Arbeitsmarkt.

These 3: Traditionelle Behandlungsphilosophie und überlange stationäre Behandlung wirken iatrogen

Die durchschnittliche Verweildauer im Krankenhaus beträgt für Erstinfarktpatienten 32 Tage. Vergleichbare deutsche Studien (Weiß et al. 1982) kommen zu ähnlichen Ergebnissen. Im internationalen Vergleich gesehen ist dies sehr lang, denn in Großbritannien ist die Verweildauer für Erstinfarktpatienten unter 65 Jahren von 23 (1968) auf 15 Tage (1973) gesunken (DHSS 1977); in den USA werden für unkomplizierte Infarktverläufe 7–14 Tage gerechnet. Wichtigster Bedingungsfaktor für die langen Verweilzeiten ist nicht der körperliche Zustand des Patienten, hierfür von entscheidender Bedeutung erscheinen vielmehr die praktizierte Behandlungsphilosophie, die immer noch Maßnahmen der Frührehabilitation vernachlässigt (Halhuber 1982; Reindell u. Roskamm 1977; Messin u. Demaret 1982) und Imperative der Krankenhausorganisation (Kapazitätsauslastung). Nur ein Viertel der in der Oldenburger Longitudinalstudie beobachteten Patienten konnte als frühmobilisiert bezeichnet werden, obwohl eine entsprechende Behandlungsempfehlung der WHO seit Jahren vorliegt (WHO 1969, 1973). Die im internationalen Vergleich überlange Verweildauer hat – unabhängig vom Alter des Patienten und vom Schweregrad seines Infarktes – einen eigenständigen, negativen Effekt auf die Zukunftsangst. Je länger die Patienten im Krankenhaus sind, desto mehr Angst haben sie vor einem Reinfarkt, vor dem Tod, vor der Wiederkehr der Schmerzen und allgemein vor der Zukunft. Die Patienten werten diesen langen Aufenthalt im Akutkrankenhaus als negatives Signal und glauben, deshalb von dem Infarkt besonders schwer betroffen zu sein.

Eine frühzeitige Rehabilitation verbunden mit kurzen Zeiten stationärer Behandlung scheint also dringend geboten, um iatrogene Schäden im psychischen Bereich mit entsprechenden sozialen Folgen zu vermeiden. Geht man von der arbeitsmarktlichen Zielsetzung der Rehabilitation aus und legt nur medizinische Bewertungskriterien an, so lassen sich die iatrogenen Effekte nicht erfassen. Legt man dagegen Kriterien an, die der neuen umfassenden Zielsetzung entsprechen, und wählt Meßinstrumente, die auch die psychische und soziale Dimension der Rehabilitation erfassen, ist ein Nachweis entsprechender Schäden möglich. Rehabilitation muß also auch unter evaluativen Gesichtspunkten von einem umfassenden Verständnis ausgehen.

These 4: Das Sozialversicherungssystem hat unbeabsichtigte negative Nebenwirkungen

Sozialversicherungsrechtliche Kontrollen, meist Begutachtungen des Gesundheitszustandes der Rehabilitanden zur Beurteilung ihrer Erwerbs- oder Arbeitsfähigkeit, führen zu psychischen Folgekosten bei den Betroffenen. Rund die Hälfte der in unserer Studie erfaßten Rehabilitanden wurde ein- oder mehrmals begutachtet. Unabhängig von der Schwere des Infarktes und unabhängig vom Gesundheitszustand nach der Krankenhausentlassung haben diese Begutachtungen einen negativen Effekt auf Ängstlichkeit, Depressivität und Selbstvertrauen der Betroffenen. Die Begutachtungen, oft durch verschiedene Sozialleistungsträger, verstärken zudem die Rollenunsicherheit und die Zukunftsungewißheit.

Die Trägervielfalt mit den dazugehörigen Auseinandersetzungen über die Zuständigkeiten führt trotz der Bestimmungen in den §§ 5 und 6 des Rehabilitationsangleichungsgesetzes zu hohen psychischen Folgekosten für die Rehabilitanden. Eine Verbesserung der Lebensqualität dieser Personen im Sinne von mehr psychischem und sozialem Wohlbefinden hängt auch davon ab, daß die Begutachtungen erheblich reduziert werden. Umfassende Rehabilitation bedeutet also auch Umgestaltung von Strukturen zur Beseitigung vermeidbarer bürokratischer Streßfaktoren.

Sozialpolitische Perspektiven

Die Diskussion der Rahmenbedingungen, der Ziele und Wirkungen hat gezeigt, daß im Rehabilitationsprozeß bisher im wesentlichen 4 Bereiche sehr unzureichend oder überhaupt nicht berücksichtigt werden. Dies sind einmal die *psychischen Nöte,* in die die Rehabilitanden geraten, sei es durch die Schwere der Erkrankung selbst oder durch unzureichende bzw. falsch angesetzte Behandlungsmaßnahmen oder durch bürokratische Hindernisse. Die psychischen Notlagen erfordern in der Regel keine therapeutischen Interventionen durch einen Spezialisten, sie müssen aber erkannt und durch entsprechende Maßnahmen abgebaut bzw. verhindert werden, beispielsweise durch mehr Beratung und Motivation oder durch Änderung organisatorischer Rahmenbedingungen. Nur zum geringeren Teil werden psychische Notlagen den Einsatz spezialisierter Fachkräfte nötig machen, denn eine Psychologisierung der Probleme erscheint für die Rehabilitation genauso wenig angebracht zu sein, wie die z. Z. noch einseitige somatische Sichtweise. Die Teamarbeit in der Rehabilitation, d. h. die gemeinsame Arbeit verschiedener Fachkräfte und die Mobilisierung der psychischen Ressourcen der Betroffenen erscheint als die beste Lösung zur Berücksichtigung der psychischen Nöte der Rehabilitanden.

Zum zweiten wird das *familiäre Umfeld* des Patienten zu wenig an der Rehabilitation beteiligt. Die Einbeziehung der Familie, in erster Linie des Ehepartners, in den Rehabilitationsprozeß wird noch zu wenig praktiziert. Noch weniger wird auf direkte und indirekte Entlastungsmöglichkeiten gerade dieser familiären Umwelt geachtet, damit diese selbst ihre rehabilitativen und integrierenden Funktionen gegenüber dem Erkrankten erfüllen kann. Die psychischen und sozialen Ressourcen in der Familie werden zwar mehr oder weniger bewußt bei den professionellen Behandlern vorausgesetzt, eine systematische Aktivierung wird aber nicht eingeleitet.

Zum dritten werden die *sozialen Problemlagen* noch zu wenig beachtet. Das Gesetz versteht unter sozialer Rehabilitation in erster Linie Geldleistungen (Einkommenstransfers). Soziale Dienstleistungen sind in der Regel unzureichend und nicht in ein Gesamtkonzept integriert. So fehlt beispielsweise bei der Einleitung von Rehabilitationsmaßnahmen für Herzinfarktpatienten noch eine ausreichende Beratung und Information im Krankenhaus durch Ärzte, Pfleger oder Sozialarbeiter. Beim niedergelassenen Arzt existiert eine Rehabilitation, die auch soziale Dienstleistungen anbietet, nur in Einzelfällen. Allgemein kann festgestellt werden, daß gerade in den Übergangsbereichen aus der eher beschützenden stationären Versorgung in die Alltagswelt eine soziale Hilfestellung nicht angeboten wird. Eine Umstellung auf neu konzipierte, ambulante Versorgungsformen, die näher an dieser Alltagswelt sind, könnte diesen Mangel beseitigen helfen.

Als vierter Punkt bleibt zu erwähnen, daß Rehabilitation vor den Betriebstoren haltmacht. Nur in Fällen persönlichen, ärztlichen Engagements werden zwischen dem medizinischen Bereich und dem *betrieblichen Bereich* Kontakte geknüpft und für die Rehabilitation, insbesondere für die Wiederaufnahme der Arbeit, genutzt. Dieses Defizit wird von Rehabilitationsexperten zwar zunehmend erkannt, aber es gibt einerseits noch zu wenig betriebliche Institutionen (betriebsärztliche Dienste), die sich mit diesen Fragen beschäftigen, und andererseits gehört es im medizinischen Bereich noch nicht zum festen Aufgabenprogramm, solche Kontakte herzustellen. Auch sind betriebliche Rehabilitationsprogramme und Rehabilitationsabteilungen in Großbetrieben (Wagner et al. 1982) bisher kaum vorhanden.

Aus dieser beispielhaften Problemanalyse leiten sich sozialpolitische Forderungen ab, die sich einerseits an die Mediziner und die paramedizinischen Berufe richten, die andererseits die Organisationsstruktur betreffen und die drittens die Stellung des Rehabilitanden tangieren.

Zum einen ist zu fordern, daß die *ärztliche Ausbildung* stärker als bisher sozialmedizinische Grundlagen betont und daß die Ärzte Fähigkeiten auch in Gesprächsführung und Beratung erwerben. Ferner sollte das Fach „Rehabilitation" ein fester Bestandteil medizinischer Curricula werden. Die *paramedizinischen Berufe,* insbesondere Sozialarbeiter und Psychologen, müssen einen eigenverantwortlichen Platz in Rehabilitationsteams erhalten, wie es teilweise schon in Modelleinrichtungen stationärer Art erprobt wird. Diese Rehabilitationsteams müssen aber auch im ambulanten Bereich – vor Ort – gebildet werden.

Organisatorische Veränderungen in den *Trägerstrukturen* müssen diskutiert werden – einschließlich der Idee eines einheitlichen Trägers, denn die diesbezüglichen Lösungsversuche des Rehabilitationsangleichungsgesetzes konnten bisher nicht befriedigen (Silomon 1979). Um eine wirklich bruchlose Rehabilitation zu gewährleisten, ist die starre *Trennung zwischen ambulanter und stationärer Versorgung* aufzuheben. Veränderungen – eher inkrementaler Art – betreffen die Schwerpunktsetzungen innerhalb der bestehenden stationären Rehabilitationseinrichtungen und die Einordnung der Rehabilitationskliniken in die allgemeinen Krankenhausbedarfspläne sowie ihre Öffnung für spezielle Akutversorgungsleistungen in medizinisch schwächer versorgten Regionen. Auch müssen die Chancen zur Praktizierung rein ambulanter Rehabilitation erhalten werden, damit den Rehabilitanden Alternativen angeboten werden können. Diese zuletzt genannte Forderung ist besonders wichtig und auch wohl ohne große politische Kosten realisierbar, um den hochgespielten Gegensatz zwischen ambulanten und stationären Versorgungsformen zu überbrücken.

In der *Rehabilitationsforschung* ist die Aufmerksamkeit verstärkt auf das Zusammenspiel zwischen psychischen, sozialen und somatischen Faktoren im Genesungsprozeß zu richten, insbesondere zum Zwecke der sekundären und tertiären Prävention. Ein weiterer Forschungsschwerpunkt sollte sich mit der Evaluation der Rehabilitationsleistungen beschäftigen. Hier ist in Zusammenarbeit mit den Rehabilitationsträgern noch eine gewisse Distanz zu den Sozialwissenschaften zu überwinden.

Die *Stellung des Rehabilitanden* muß gestärkt werden. Dies gilt in bezug auf seine Mitwirkungs- und Mitentscheidungsrechte bei der Beantragung und Durchführung der Rehabilitationsmaßnahme, dies gilt auch für die Mobilisierung von Selbsthilfe. Diese Mobilisierung kann entscheidend dazu beitragen, aus passiv rehabilitierten Personen echte Partner des Arztes, d. h. den Rehabilitanden zu einem Mitglied des erwähnten Rehabilitationsteams zu machen. Auch die von Patienten gewollte Einbeziehung wichtiger anderer Personen ist geeignet, seine Position im Rehabilitationsprozeß zu stärken, seine aktive Teilnahme zu sichern und die (Wieder-)Gewinnung von Lebensqualität zu erleichtern. Erst in zweiter Linie ist bei der Aufwertung der Stellung des Betroffenen als Kotherapeuten an gesetzliche Maßnahmen gedacht. Diese Aufwertung muß sich auch aus dem professionellen Verständnis der Leistungserbringer, insbesondere auch der Mediziner entwickeln. Zur Stärkung der Stellung des Rehabilitanden gehört daher auch, daß die heilenden Kräfte im Patienten selbst, die Unterstützung aus seinem sozialen Netzwerk und die immer zahlreicher werdenden Selbsthilfegruppen mobilisiert und gefördert werden. Die sozialpolitische Grundmaxime sollte daher lauten: weg vom alten, unterschwelligen Fürsorgegedanken, hin zu einer aktiven und aktivierenden Mitwirkung des Rehabilitanden und seiner sozialen Umwelt.

Literatur

Achinger H (1959) Soziologie und Sozialreform. In: Deutsche Gesellschaft für Soziologie (Hrsg) Verhandlungen des 14. Deutschen Soziologentages. Enke, Stuttgart, S 39–52

Achinger H (1971) Sozialpolitik als Gesellschaftspolitik. Selbstverlag, Frankfurt

Badura B (1982) Soziologie und Sozialpolitik. Alte Themen, neue Aufgaben. In: Beck U (Hrsg) Soziale Welt. Sonderbd 1: Soziologie und Praxis. Göttingen: Schwartz, Göttingen, S 93–106

Badura B (1983) Pflegebedarf und Pflegepolitik im Wandel. Soz Fortschr 32:97–102

Badura B (1984) Thomas McKeown und die ökologische Gesundheitsstrategie. Medizin, Mensch & Gesellschaft 9:151–160

Badura B, Gross P (1976) Sozialpolitische Perspektiven. Eine Einführung in Grundlagen und Probleme sozialer Dienstleistungen. Piper, München

Badura B, Kaufhold G, Lehmann H, Pfaff H, Schott T, Waltz M (1987) Leben mit dem Herzinfarkt. Springer, Berlin Heidelberg New York Tokyo

Bauer J, Lehmann H (1981) Zur Entstehung, Behandlung und Rehabilitation von Herzinfarkt. In: Badura B (Hrsg) Soziale Unterstützung und chronische Krankheit. Zum Stand sozialepidemiologischer Forschung. Suhrkamp, Frankfurt, S 183–257

Beck M, Eissenhauer W, Löffler H (Hrsg) (1984) Rehabilitation heute. Die Reha-Studie Baden. Braun, Karlsruhe

Bundesminister für Arbeit und Sozialordnung (1970) Aktionsprogramm zur Förderung der Rehabilitation. Bundesarbeitsblatt 5.340–342

Bundesminister für Arbeit und Sozialordnung (Hrsg) (1980) Aktionsprogramm Rehabilitation in den 80er Jahren. Eigenverlag des BMAS, Bonn

Croog SH, Levine S (1977) The heart patient recovers. Social and psychological factors. Human Science, New York

DHSS – Department of Health and Social Security (1977) Report on hospital in-patient enquiry for the year 1973, Tables. HMSO, London

Engel GL (1977) The need for a new medical model: A challenge for biomedicine. Science 196:129–136

Ferber C von (1967) Sozialpolitik in der Wohlstandsgesellschaft. Zeit-Buch, Hamburg

Gartner A, Riessmann F (1978) Der aktive Konsument in der Dienstleistungsgesellschaft. Suhrkamp, Frankfurt

Gross P, Badura B (1977) Sozialpolitik und soziale Dienste: Entwurf einer Theorie personenbezogener Dienstleistungen. Köln Z Soziol Sozialpsychol [Sonderheft] 19:361–385

Halhuber MJ (1982) Rehabilitation des Koronarkranken. Perimed, Erlangen

Heimann R (1980/1929) Soziale Theorie des Kapitalismus. Suhrkamp, Frankfurt

Kauderer-Hübel M, Buchwalsky R (1983) Berufsfähigkeit und Sterblichkeit nach Herzinfarkt (Nachbefragung eines AHB-Kollektives). In: Stein G (Hrsg) Probleme um die Wiederaufnahme der Arbeit nach Herzinfarkt. Timmendorfer Strand, Jahrestagung der Deutschen Arbeitsgemeinschaft für kardiologische Prävention und Rehabilitation e. V , 3.–5. Februar 1983 (S. 129–146). Mannheimer Morgen, Mannheim

Kaufmann FX (1973) Sicherheit als soziologisches und sozialpolitisches Problem. Enke, Stuttgart

Kaufmann FX (1979) Bürgernahe Sozialpolitik: Planung, Organisation und Vermittlung sozialer Leistungen auf lokaler Ebene. Campus, Frankfurt

Kaufmann FX (1984) Was heißt Verrechtlichung und wo wird sie zum Problem. In: Kaufmann FX (Hrsg) Ärztliches Handeln zwischen Paragraphen und Vertrauen. Patmos, Düsseldorf, S 9–22

Krasemann EO, Jungmann H, Stein G (1984) Fördert die organisierte Herzinfarkt-Rehabilitation die Arbeitsaufnahme? In: Stein G (Hrsg) Probleme um die Wiederaufnahme der Arbeit nach Herzinfarkt. Timmendorfer Strand, Jahrestagung der Deutschen Arbeitsgemeinschaft für kardiologische Prävention und Rehabilitation e.V., 3.–5. Februar 1983 Mannheimer Morgen, Mannheim, S 147–151

Lehmann H (1984) Erste Ergebnisse der Oldenburger Longitudinalstudie zur Rückkehr zur Arbeit nach Herzinfarkt. In: Stein G (Hrsg) Probleme um die Wiederaufnahme der Arbeit nach Herzinfarkt. Timmendorfer Strand, Jahrestagung der Deutschen Arbeitsgemeinschaft für kardiologische Prävention und Rehabilitation e.V., 3.–5. Februar 1983 Mannheimer Morgen, Mannheim, S 157–164

McKeown T (1982) Die Bedeutung der Medizin. Suhrkamp, Frankfurt

Messin R, Demaret B (1982) Accelerated versus classical early mobilization after myocardial infarction. In: Kellermann JJ (ed) Comprehensive cardiac rehabilitation Karger, Basel, pp 152–155

Preller L (1970) Praxis und Probleme der Sozialpolitik. Mohr, Tübingen

Reindell H, Roskamm H (1977) Herzkrankheiten: Pathophysiologie, Diagnostik, Therapie. Springer, Berlin Heidelberg New York Tokyo

Silomon H (1979) Sechs Beiträge zum Thema: Fünf Jahre Gesetz über die Angleichung der Leistungen zur Rehabilitation – Anspruch und Wirklichkeit. Öffentliches Gesundheitswesen 14:675

Sozialenquête-Kommission (1966) Soziale Sicherung in der Bundesrepublik Deutschland. Kohlhammer, Stuttgart

Statistik der deutschen gesetzlichen Rentenversicherung (1980) Die Leistungen zur Rehabilitation und die zusätzlichen Leistungen in der gesetzlichen Rentenversicherung im Jahre 1980, Bd 57. Verband Deutscher Rentenversicherungsträger, Frankfurt, S 8–13

Stern NJ, Pascale L, Ackermann A (1977) Life adjustment postmyocardial infarction. Arch Internal Med 137:1680–1685

Thimm W (1984) Das Normalisierungsprinzip: Eine Einführung (Bundesvereinigung für geistig Behinderte e.V., Bd. 5, Kleine Schriftenreihe). Marburg

Wagner R, North K, Wampach M, Meyer N, Aniset E (1982) Wiedereingliederung von Behinderten in der Luxemburger Eisen- und Stahlindustrie. Schlußbericht für die europäische Gemeinschaft für Kohle und Stahl. Ergonomische Gemeinschaftsforschung. Differdingen

Weiß B (1984) Rückkehr zur Arbeit nach erstem Herzinfarkt in Hamburg. In: Stein G (Hrsg) Probleme um die Wiederaufnahme der Arbeit nach Herzinfarkt. Timmendorfer Strand, Jahrestagung der Deutschen Arbeitsgemeinschaft für kardiologische Prävention und Rehabilitation e.V. 3.–5. Februar 1983. Mannheimer Morgen, Mannheim, S 73–84

Weiß B, Donat K, Ziegler WJ (1982) Langzeitbeobachtung nach Herzinfarkt. Herz-Kreislauf 14:438–445

WHO (1969) The rehabilitation of patients with cardiovascular diseases. Report on a seminar. Noordwijk ann Zee, 2.–7. October 1967. Copenhagen

WHO (1973) Evaluation of comprehensive rehabilitation and preventive programs for patients after acute myocardial infarction. Report on two working groups. Regional Office for Europe. Copenhagen

WHO (1978) Primary health care. Report of the international conference on primary health care. Alma-Ata, USSR, 6.–12. September 1978. Genf

Weiterführende Literatur zum Thema „Rehabilitationsforschung"

Badura B, Kaufhold G, Lehmann H et al. (1987) Leben mit dem Herzinfarkt: eine sozialepide-
miologische Studie. Springer, Berlin Heidelberg New York Tokyo
Koch U, Lucius-Hoene G, Stegie R (Hrsg) (1988) Handbuch der Rehabilitationspsychologie.
Springer, Berlin Heidelberg New York Tokyo

Anhang

Forschung und Entwicklung im Dienste der Gesundheit *

Bundesminister für Forschung und Technologie

Einführung

Seit 1978 fördert die Bundesregierung das Programm „Forschung und Entwicklung im Dienste der Gesundheit". Seine Aufgabe ist es, die Forschungspolitik in diesem Bereich zu koordinieren und die Förderung des Bundes auf gesundheitspolitisch besonders wichtige Problemfelder zu lenken. Das vorliegende Programm schließt sich an die beiden vorangegangenen Förderprogramme an und führt ihre Zielsetzung mit neuen Akzenten für den Planungszeitraum 1988–1991 fort.

Das Programm „Forschung und Entwicklung im Dienste der Gesundheit" ist als Regierungsprogramm ressortübergreifend angelegt. Dies trägt der Tatsache Rechnung, daß der Forschungsbedarf des Gesundheitswesens die üblichen Grenzen der Forschungsförderung und der Ressortzuständigkeiten übersteigt. Das Gesundheitsforschungsprogramm wird deshalb von den Bundesministern für Forschung und Technologie (BMFT), für Arbeit und Sozialordnung (BMA) sowie für Jugend, Familie, Frauen und Gesundheit (BMJFFG) gemeinsam getragen.

Gesundheitspolitische Zielsetzungen

Ausgangspunkt des Programms sind gesundheitspolitische Leitziele, zu deren Verwirklichung die Forschungspolitik beitragen will. Die Gesundheit ist eines der höchsten Lebensgüter. Es ist das Ziel der Gesundheitspolitik, die Gesundheit der Bürger zu erhalten, zu fördern und im Krankheitsfall wieder herzustellen. Gesünder, länger und aktiver leben zu können, dies für jeden einzelnen Bürger bestmöglich zu gewährleisten und das Gesundheitswesen gleichzeitig finanzierbar zu erhalten, ist die Herausforderung, vor der die Gesundheitspolitik heute und auch in Zukunft steht.

Ziel der Gesundheitspolitik ist damit, eine leistungsfähige und wirtschaftliche Gesundheitssicherung und medizinische Versorgung für alle Gruppen der Bevölkerung zu gewährleisten, wobei auch andere Politikbereiche, z. B. die Umweltpolitik, zu der Erhaltung oder Wiederherstellung von gesundheitsgerechten Lebens- und Arbeitsbedingungen beitragen.

---

* Auszug aus dem Programm der Bundesregierung. Bonn, 1988

Die moderne Medizin hat große Erfolge zu verzeichnen. Sie hat den Bereich der Gesundheitspflege erheblich erweitert. Zur Lösung der Gesundheitsprobleme der Bevölkerung bedarf es dennoch weiterhin großer Anstrengungen aller am Gesundheitswesen Beteiligten, nicht zuletzt der Verantwortung des einzelnen für die eigene Gesundheit. Nicht alle Aufgaben können gleichzeitig und gleichrangig in Angriff genommen werden. Deshalb ist es notwendig, sich über Zielvorstellungen zu verständigen. Ziele und Inhalte einer am Wohl der Bevölkerung orientierten Gesundheitspolitik müssen Gegenstand gesellschaftlicher Diskussion und Konsensbildung sein.

Eine Grundlage für diese Konsensbildung ist die Erarbeitung sog. „prioritärer Gesundheitsziele", eine andere die WHO-(World Health Organization, Weltgesundheitsorganisation)Strategie „Gesundheit 2000", deren Konsequenzen für die Forschung sich in den Vorschlägen *Forschung für Gesundheit im Jahr 2000* der WHO (1985) niedergeschlagen haben. Bei der Bestimmung dieser Prioritäten muß von Kriterien auf der Ebene der individuellen Krankheitsfolgen (Schwere und Dauer der gesundheitlichen Beeinträchtigung, Verfügbarkeit von Behandlungs- und Interventionsmöglichkeiten), wie auch auf der Ebene der gesellschaftlichen Krankheitslasten (Zahl der Betroffenen, Anteil des Problems an den Ursachen der Gesamtsterblichkeit usw.) ausgegangen werden.

Diese gesundheitspolitischen Zielsetzungen und Prioritäten prägen naturgemäß auch die Maßnahmen der Bundesregierung zur Forschungsförderung im Gesundheitsbereich und führen zu Leitkriterien der Forschungsförderung des Bundes, die mit den Stichworten

- Orientierung an den Gesundheits- und Gesundheitsversorgungsbedürfnissen der Bürger und
- Praxisbezug der geförderten Forschungsvorhaben

gekennzeichnet werden können.

Die Erhaltung der Gesundheit und die Heilung und Rehabilitation von Erkrankungen sind für jeden Bürger von höchstem persönlichem Interesse, da der Gesundheit auf dem Hintergrund hohen Lebensstandards und sozialer Sicherheit eine besonders große Rolle für die Lebensqualität des einzelnen zukommt. Die Verantwortung für eine gesunde Lebensweise und die individuelle Krankheitsvorbeugung kann der Staat dem Bürger nicht abnehmen. Es muß aber Aufgabe der Gesundheitspolitik sein, auf gesundheitsgerechte Lebensbedingungen in der natürlichen und der sozialen Umwelt einschließlich der Umwelt am Arbeitsplatz zu achten, Eigeninitiative und Eigenverantwortung zu stärken und eine wirksame und wirtschaftliche Versorgung einschließlich Rehabilitation zu gewährleisten, wobei nicht nur den körperlichen, sondern auch den psychosozialen Gesichtspunkten Rechnung getragen werden muß.

Rolle der Forschungspolitik

In diesem Zusammenhang kommt der Forschung besondere Bedeutung zu. Durch intensive Forschungsbemühungen wird es möglich sein, krankmachende, aber auch gesundheitsfördernde Faktoren, Lebensweisen und Lebensbedingungen zu analysieren, Ursachen von Krankheiten und Möglichkeiten zu ihrer Vermeidung zu erkennen und Verfahren zur frühen Diagnose und zur wirksamen und schonenden Therapie von Erkrankungen sowie geeignete Rehabilitationsmaßnahmen zu entwickeln.

Größere Aufmerksamkeit muß in Zukunft auch im Bereich der Forschung den Möglichkeiten präventiver Maßnahmen geschenkt werden, insbesondere im Hinblick auf ihre wissenschaftliche Untermauerung und ihre ökonomischen Auswirkungen. Hier ist ein deutlicher Paradigmenwechsel zu verzeichnen. Dabei muß jedoch, unabhängig vom Erfolg der Präventivmedizin, die medizinische Versorgung bereits Erkrankter und deren Rehabilitation auf hohem qualitativem Niveau sichergestellt bleiben.

Die Förderorganisationen der deutschen Wissenschaft, die Deutsche Forschungsgemeinschaft (DFG) und die Max-Planck-Gesellschaft (MPG), tragen auf der Basis der Grundfinanzierung der Hochschulen durch die Länder zu einer insgesamt breitgestreuten Förderung der medizinischen Grundlagenforschung unter den prioritären Gesichtspunkten der Originalität und Qualität der Forschung bei. Die Forschungsförderung der medizinischen und pharmazeutischen Industrie konzentriert sich entsprechend der Marktorientierung der Unternehmen auf den Entwicklungs- und Umsetzungsbereich.

In diese Förderlandschaft fügt sich das Programm „Forschung und Entwicklung im Dienste der Gesundheit" ein. Seine Zielsetzungen sind an den gesundheitspolitischen Aufgaben der Bundesregierung ausgerichtet und orientieren sich in erster Linie am Bürger. Es fördert dementsprechend Forschungs- und Entwicklungsvorhaben, die dazu beitragen können, daß

- ein besserer Gesundheitszustand der Bevölkerung erreicht wird;
- einerseits die Möglichkeiten zur Vorbeugung und Verhütung von Krankheiten untersucht und entwickelt, andererseits aber auch die Qualität von Diagnose-, Therapie- und Rehabilitationsmaßnahmen, v. a. bei den stark verbreiteten Krankheiten, verbessert werden;
- die Belastung oder Gefährdung der Patienten durch medizinische Maßnahmen verringert wird;
- die Strukturen von Forschungs- und Versorgungseinrichtungen des Gesundheitswesens den gestiegenen Anforderungen angepaßt werden, auch um die Nutzung neuer Erkenntnisse in den Grundlagenwissenschaften zu verbessern;
- die Kosten von Maßnahmen der Gesundheitsversorgung bzw. die durch Krankheit und Invalidität entstehenden volkswirtschaftlichen Kosten begrenzt werden;
- die Bedarfsgerechtigkeit, Patienten- und Nutzerfreundlichkeit, Leistungsfähigkeit und Wirtschaftlichkeit der Strukturen und Einrichtungen des Gesundheitswesens verbessert werden.

Dabei hat die staatliche Förderung in besonderem Maße die Grenze zu achten zwischen Betreuung im Sinne von Hilfe zur Selbsthilfe und unzulässiger Bevormundung oder vermeidbarer Abhängigkeit von Medikamenten und medizinischer Technik. Die Förderung von Forschung und Entwicklung als Aufgabe der Bundesregierung ist in besonderer Weise verpflichtet, zu mehr Humanität und höherer Qualität im Gesundheitswesen beizutragen, wie es wiederholt vom

Deutschen Bundestag, von der Bundesregierung und von den Gesundheitsministern der Länder nachdrücklich gefordert wurde. Sie wird hierbei die in den letzten Jahren durch neue Entwicklungen in den Grundlagenwissenschaften deutlich gewachsenen Möglichkeiten in vollem Umfang nutzen.

Die ethischen Grundlagen der Medizin werden durch Entwicklungen z. B. in der Medizintechnik oder der Humangenetik mit neuen Fragen konfrontiert. Ihre Beachtung ist Teil der Forschungs- und Gesundheitspolitik, die sich der Menschenwürde verpflichtet weiß.

Nicht zuletzt soll die Gesundheitsforschung Entscheidungshilfen für die Gesundheitspolitik erbringen; dies gilt sowohl für die Qualität und Quantität der im Rahmen der gesetzlichen Krankenversorgung angebotenen Leistungen als auch für Umfang und Struktur der Forschungs- und Versorgungseinrichtungen.

Außer im Regierungsprogramm „Forschung und Entwicklung im Dienste der Gesundheit" fördert die Bundesregierung gesundheitsbezogene Forschung in weiteren Bereichen: sie leistet Zuschüsse zu den großen Institutionen der Forschungsförderung, die von der Wissenschaft selbst verwaltet werden (DFG, MPG, Fraunhofer Gesellschaft) und finanziert überwiegend die Großforschungseinrichtungen wie z. B. das Deutsche Krebsforschungszentrum, die Gesellschaft für Strahlen- und Umweltforschung oder die Kernforschungsanlage Jülich. Darüber hinaus berühren auch andere Regierungsprogramme gesundheitsbezogene Fragestellungen (z. B. die Programme zur Biotechnologieforschung, zur Umweltforschung und zur Humanisierung des Arbeitslebens). Unter diesen Instrumenten der Forschungsförderung im Gesundheitsbereich nimmt das Programm „Forschung und Entwicklung im Dienste der Gesundheit" eine Sonderstellung ein, weil es darauf ausgerichtet ist, die gesundheitspolitische Verantwortung des Bundes durch eine gezielte Politik der Forschungsförderung zu unterstützen.

Programmschwerpunkte

Gesundheit, Lebensweisen und Umwelt

Zwischen den Lebensweisen, die in der Gesellschaft verbreitet sind, und der Gestaltung der biologischen und physikalischen Umwelt gibt es vielfache Wechselbeziehungen. Darüber hinaus gilt für die gesundheitlichen Auswirkungen sowohl der Lebensweisen als auch der Umwelteinflüsse, daß sie zunächst im Vorfeld manifester Erkrankungen liegen und hier durch präventive Maßnahmen beeinflußt werden können.

Der Gesundheitszustand wird neben den Lebensweisen und Umweltfaktoren von genetischen Faktoren und der medizinischen Behandlung beeinflußt. Der Faktor „medizinische Behandlung" kommt erst bei manifesten Erkrankungen zur Geltung und bildet deshalb eine eigenständige Problemstellung. Die genetischen Faktoren nehmen bei dieser Betrachtungsweise eine Sonderstellung ein, weil sie die gesundheitliche Konstitution des Individuums bestimmen sowie die Reaktion des individuellen Organismus auf Umwelteinflüsse, Verhalten und medizinische Behandlung prägen und daher für die Fragen von Gesundheit und Krankheit von ausschlaggebender Bedeutung sind.

Die grundsätzlich wirksamsten Maßnahmen zur Erhaltung der Gesundheit liegen offensichtlich im Bereich der Prävention. Wie das Beispiel vieler Infektionskrankheiten in der Vergangenheit zeigt, waren Änderungen der Lebensweisen (Hygiene, Ernährung, Wohnverhältnisse) und der Umweltbedingungen (Trinkwasserversorgung, Abwässerbeseitigung) mindestens ebenso wichtige Voraussetzungen für die erfolgreiche Bekämpfung der vorherrschenden Infektionskrankheiten wie die Verbesserung der Therapiemöglichkeiten.

In der Folge hat sich die medizinische Forschung v. a. auf den Bereich der medizinischen Behandlung konzentriert: im Mittelpunkt steht dabei die Aufdeckung der Entstehung und des Verlaufs von Krankheiten und die Entwicklung und Erprobung von Verfahren, um Krankheitszustände zu beheben. Es mehren sich jedoch sowohl in Fachkreisen wie in der breiteren Öffentlichkeit die Stimmen, die sich für eine Ausweitung der medizinischen Forschung über den biomedizinischen Bereich hinaus aussprechen, um in einem umfassenderen Sinn auch die anderen Determinanten von Gesundheit systematischer zu erforschen.

Die gesundheitlichen Auswirkungen der Lebensweisen und der Umwelteinflüsse treten als Ansatzpunkte für eine Prävention von Gesundheitsschäden stärker ins Zentrum der Aufmerksamkeit. Die hohe Prävalenz chronischer Krankheiten, die wachsende Lebenserwartung der Bevölkerung, das Auftreten der (vorerst kurativ nicht beherrschbaren) Infektionskrankheit Aids und nicht zuletzt die „Kostenexplosion" im Gesundheitswesen erfordern auch in der Forschung gezielte gesundheitspolitisch ausgerichtete Aktivitäten. Nicht zu übersehen ist allerdings, daß der Wandel zu einer umfassenderen Gesundheitsforschung im erwähnten Sinne gerade erst begonnen hat und sowohl in theoretischer wie in methodischer Hinsicht auf weite Strecken wissenschaftliches Neuland darstellt.

Als vorrangige allgemeine Forschungsaufgaben auf diesem Gebiet sind zu nennen: Erhebungen über Gesundheitsgefahren, die auf Lebensweisen und Umwelteinflüsse zurückzuführen sind, und Untersuchungen zur Entstehung und zum Verlauf lebensweise- und umweltbedingter Erkrankungen. Beide Fragestellungen erfordern neue Formen interdisziplinärer Zusammenarbeit zwischen den medizinischen, naturwissenschaftlichen, sozial- und verhaltenswissenschaftlichen Fächern. Einen wesentlichen Schwerpunkt stellt ferner die Fortführung der Deutschen Herz-Kreislauf-Präventionsstudie (DHP) mit ihrem gemeindeorientierten Präventionsansatz dar.

Wird der Begriff *Lebensweise* im Zusammenhang mit Gesundheit und Krankheit gebraucht, so besteht die Gefahr, daß er ausdrücklich oder unausgesprochen mit individuellem Fehlverhalten gleichgesetzt wird. Der Begriff der Lebensweise ist aber sehr viel weiter zu fassen: er bezeichnet die Muster individuellen Verhaltens, die in einer bestimmten Gesellschaft und ihren verschiedenen sozialen Gruppierungen vorherrschen. Solche Verhaltensmuster dienen der Bewältigung des alltäglichen Lebens in der Arbeits-, Familien- und Freizeitwelt und sind durch eine Vielzahl kultureller, sozialer und wirtschaftlicher Bedingungen geprägt. Gleichzeitig haben die verbreiteten Lebensweisen in vielfältiger Weise direkte und indirekte Auswirkungen auf die Gesundheit.

Dieser Blickwinkel enthält eine grundlegende Konsequenz für die gesundheitsbezogene Forschung: wenn die soziale Umwelt und die individuellen Lebensweisen als Einflußfaktoren für Gesundheit und Krankheit betrachtet werden, dann müssen offensichtlich neben den medizinischen und naturwissenschaftlichen Disziplinen auch, wie es z. B. in den Ernährungswissenschaften geschieht, die Sozial- und Verhaltenswissenschaften einbezogen werden in das wissenschaftliche Bemühen, die Ursachen von Krankheit zu untersuchen und Wege zur Verbesserung der Gesundheit zu finden. Der traditionell vorherrschende biomedizinische Ansatz in der Gesundheitsforschung muß deshalb durch Beiträge aus den Sozial- und Verhaltenswissenschaften erweitert und ergänzt werden.

Die interdisziplinäre Zusammenarbeit zwischen biomedizinischer und verhaltenswissenschaftlicher Forschung ist z. Z. noch nicht ausreichend entwickelt und bedarf besonderer Förderung.

Die vordringlichen Forschungsaufgaben lassen sich in folgenden Themenbereichen zusammenfassen:

Analysen gesundheitsrelevanter Lebensweisen

Eine grundlegende Forschungsaufgabe besteht darin, das verfügbare Wissen über die gesundheitlichen Auswirkungen von Komponenten der Lebensweise zu erweitern, die Verbreitung spezifischer gesundheitsrelevanter Merkmale in den Lebensweisen der verschiedenen Bevölkerungsgruppen zu beschreiben (z. B. in Form einer „Sozialepidemiologie des Ernährungsverhaltens") und ihre Funktionen für das alltägliche Leben zu analysieren. Verstärkter Beachtung bedürfen die gesundheitsfördernden Elemente in allen Bereichen der Lebensweise. Beispielsweise ist es für Bemühungen zur Eindämmung der gesundheitspolitisch bedeutsamen ernährungsbedingten Erkrankungen notwendig, die Kausalzusammenhänge zwischen Fehlernährung und diesen Krankheiten zu erkennen und die zugrundeliegenden Wirkungsmechanismen aufzuklären, um auf dieser Basis sowohl zweckmäßige Wege zur Gesunderhaltung aufzeigen als auch Verfahren der Diagnose und der Therapie entwickeln zu können.

Primärprävention kann in dem Maße gezielter ansetzen, wie Krankheitsursachen besser bekannt sind. Es ist deshalb zu erwarten, daß auch viele Ergebnisse der Krankheitsursachenforschung, z. B. im Bereich der Immunprävention oder der genetischen Konstitutionsforschung, auf längere Sicht die Möglichkeiten für Präventionsmaßnahmen erweitern werden.

Neben den stärker individuell bezogenen Komponenten der Lebensweise bedürfen auch vorwiegend soziostrukturell bedingte Risikofaktoren, denen sich der einzelne kaum entziehen kann, der näheren Untersuchung.

Strategien der Prävention

Maßnahmen zur Prävention von Gesundheitsschäden können ebenfalls auf 2 Ebenen angesiedelt werden:

Bei den Präventionsmaßnahmen, die direkt auf Änderungen des individuellen Verhaltens abzielen, ist der Beitrag der Forschung v. a. in der Evaluation der laufenden oder geplanten Maßnahmenprogramme zu sehen. Die bisherigen Maßnahmen zur Gesundheitserziehung zielen darauf ab, den Informationsstand, die Einstellungen, Überzeugungen und Intentionen in den Zielgruppen zu beeinflussen; über die tatsächlichen Auswirkungen auf das Verhalten und die resultierenden Gesundheitseffekte ist allerdings viel zu wenig bekannt. Besonders vordringlich ist deshalb die Entwicklung von Indikatoren, die sowohl das faktische Verhalten und seine Änderung im Zeitverlauf als auch dessen Wirkungen auf die Gesundheit ausreichend differenziert erfassen können.

Soziostrukturell ansetzende Präventionsmaßnahmen könnten Quellen gesundheitlicher Schädigungen sozusagen „en bloc" ausschalten. Als Beispiel lassen sich die gesundheitlichen Belastungen anführen, die in der Arbeitswelt entstehen: wo Streß und Konflikte strukturell abgebaut werden können, braucht kein spezielles Streßbewältigungsverhalten der betroffenen Individuen eingeübt zu werden; wo durch Einhaltung der Arbeitsstättenverordnung oder der Gefahrstoffverordnung gesundheitsschädliche Einflüsse der Arbeitswelt ausgeschaltet werden, kann insoweit auf das Einüben sicherheitsgerechter Verhaltensweisen verzichtet werden. In diesem Zusammenhang sei auf das Regierungsprogramm „Humanisierung des Arbeitslebens" verwiesen.

Krankheitsverhalten und Krankheitsbewältigung als Bestandteile der Lebensweise

Der weitaus überwiegende Teil der Krankheitsbewältigung, der Pflege und Unterstützung findet nicht in den Einrichtungen des professionellen Versorgungssystems, sondern innerhalb des sog. Laiensystems statt und bildet damit einen Bestandteil der Lebensweise. Gegenwärtig werden in vielen Staaten neue Ansätze zur Strukturierung des Bereichs der Primärversorgung erprobt, die gezielt auf eine enge Kooperation zwischen professionellem und Laiensystem v. a. in den Bereichen der Prävention, der Pflege, der sozialen Unterstützung und der Rehabilitation setzen.

Unabhängig von solchen Strukturfragen ist eine Intensivierung der Forschung über Probleme der Krankheits- und Krisenbewältigung insbesondere innerhalb des Laiensystems erforderlich. Die grundlegenden Konzepte von sozialer Unterstützung, Selbsthilfe und Bewältigungsstrategien bedürfen weiterer theoretischer Klärung und empirischer Studien, die ihre Ausprägungen und Funktionen in den unterschiedlichen gesellschaftlichen Gruppen beschreiben und Ansatzpunkte identifizieren, an denen eine Unterstützung durch die Gesellschaft erforderlich wäre. Die psychosozialen Aspekte der Krankheitsbewältigung in den verschiedenen Lebensaltern müssen allgemein stärker ins Blickfeld der Forschung gerückt werden.

Neben dem Einfluß von Lebensbedingungen und sozialen Umweltfaktoren bedarf auch der Einfluß von physikalischen, chemischen und biologischen *Umweltfaktoren* auf die Gesundheit des Menschen verstärkter Forschungsbemühungen. Die extrem große Zahl solcher stofflicher Umweltfaktoren macht eine auch nur annähernd vollständige Untersuchung denkbarer Wirkungen auf die menschliche Gesundheit unmöglich.

In Ergänzung zur direkt umsetzungs- und maßnahmenbezogenen Ressortforschung beschränkt sich das Regierungsprogramm deshalb darauf, Fragen zum Zusammenhang zwischen stofflichen Umweltfaktoren exemplarisch und in erster Linie im Sinne einer Querschnittsförderung aufzugreifen. Dies bedeutet, daß solche Fragestellungen im wesentlichen dort angegangen werden, wo sie aus anderen Gründen eingerichtete Programmschwerpunkte auf natürliche Weise verlängern und ergänzen.

So sprechen beispielsweise die Förderschwerpunkte zur Lungenforschung und zur Allergologie in erheblichen Teilen Fragen der Wechselwirkung zwischen menschlicher Gesundheit und stofflicher Umwelt an.

Darüber hinaus können in überschaubaren Bereichen einzelne Fragestellungen aufgegriffen werden, für die ein besonderer Forschungsbedarf besteht, die aber gleichzeitig generellen Anliegen des Programms entsprechen, z. B. umweltepidemiologische Untersuchungen, Forschungsansätze zur Klärung von Kausalzusammenhängen durch Untersuchung von Wirkungsmechanismen, oder Arbeiten, die auf Möglichkeiten der Risikoprävention bzw. der Früherkennung abzielen.

Diese Hinweise sind als Rahmen für zukünftige Förderaktivitäten zu verstehen, der in der Diskussion mit Fachwissenschaftlern im Verlauf der Programmdurchführung noch ausgefüllt und inhaltlich präzisiert werden muß.

Leistungsfähigkeit, Qualität und Wirtschaftlichkeit des Gesundheitswesens

Ziel der Gesundheitspolitik und Aufgabe des Gesundheitswesens ist es, die Gesundheit der Bevölkerung unter Beachtung wirtschaftlicher Rahmenbedingungen zu fördern, bestmöglich zu erhalten und wiederherzustellen. Dabei ist Gesundheit nicht nur als individuelles, sondern auch als gesellschaftliches Gut, und ihre Erhaltung und Förderung als öffentliche Aufgabe anzusehen.[1]

Damit umfaßt das Gesundheitswesen sämtliche Personen, Einrichtungen und Institutionen, die an dieser Aufgabe in der gesundheitlichen Versorgung aber auch bei gesundheitlichen Aspekten der sozialen und natürlichen Umwelt tätig sind. Von besonderer Bedeutung ist hierbei die gesetzliche Krankenversicherung. Ihr Gesetzesauftrag ist es, ihren Versicherten und damit rund 90 % der Bevölkerung einen umfassenden Schutz im Krankheitsfall zu gewährleisten. Der Begriff „Gesundheitswesen" geht jedoch weit darüber hinaus.

Die Forschung zum Gesundheitswesen, insbesondere zur Leistungsfähigkeit, Qualität und Wirtschaftlichkeit, bezieht ihre Aufgabenstellung aus den aktuellen und mittelfristigen konkreten Problemen eines zielorientierten Gesundheitswesens. Die zentrale Fragestellung lautet: Wie muß das Gesundheitswesen im einzelnen und insgesamt beschaffen, organisiert und finanziert sein, um auch in Zusammenarbeit mit verschiedenen Politikbereichen einen möglichst guten Gesundheitszustand der Bevölkerung mit wirtschaftlichem Mitteleinsatz und zu gesellschaftlich tragbaren Kosten zu gewährleisten?

---

[1] In dem angelsächsischen Begriff "Public health" kommt diese Orientierung des Gesundheitswesens besonders prägnant zum Ausdruck.

Dabei kann die Forschung insbesondere zu folgenden Bereichen Beiträge leisten:

Der Gesundheitszustand der Bevölkerung und seine Bestimmungsgrößen:
der Beitrag des Gesundheitswesens zur Lebensqualität

Grundvoraussetzung für eine Bewertung der Leistungsfähigkeit, Qualität und Wirtschaftlichkeit des Gesundheitswesens ist es, die Erfüllung seiner oben dargestellten Aufgaben möglichst weitgehend differenzieren und quantifizieren zu können. Dazu gehört insbesondere eine nach Gruppen und Regionen spezifizierte Darstellung des Gesundheitszustands und seiner Entwicklung im Zeitablauf; eine solche Darstellung müßte auf Maßen der Sterblichkeit, Krankheit, Lebenserwartung, Lebensqualität etc. aufbauen.

Solche Daten sind für viele Fragestellungen im Gesundheitswesen von Bedeutung und bilden die Grundlage für Analysen des Versorgungsbedarfs, Organisation des Versorgungssystems, Evaluation und Qualitätssicherung, Prognosen von Entwicklungstrends und gesundheitspolitische Entscheidungen. Von besonderem Interesse ist hier die Entwicklung des Gesundheitszustandes, soweit sie dem Einfluß des Gesundheitswesens zugerechnet werden kann.

Wichtige Forschungsfragen sind:

- Welche Entwicklung der jeweiligen altersspezifischen Lebenserwartung ist welchen Entwicklungen i. allg. und im Gesundheitswesen und welchen damit verbundenen Kosten zuzurechnen, und welche Ergebnisse können von möglichen Entwicklungen im Gesundheitswesen künftig erwartet werden?
- Wie verhält sich diese Entwicklung der Lebenserwartung zur Entwicklung der Lebensqualität, Lebensarbeitszeit, krankheitsbedingten Fehlzeiten, Intensität und Qualität von Arbeit und Freizeit?

Damit kommt der Epidemiologie eine wichtige Aufgabe in diesem Forschungsbereich zu. Gemessen an der Situation in den angelsächsischen und skandinavischen Ländern besteht auf diesem Gebiet in der Bundesrepublik Deutschland ein erheblicher Bedarf an zusätzlicher Forschung und Entwicklung.

Gesundheitszustand und Leistungsfähigkeit/Wirtschaftlichkeit
von Prävention und gesundheitlicher Versorgung

Abgeleitet aus Analysen über den Zustand und die Entwicklung von Gesundheit und Krankheit ergibt sich eine besonders schwierige, zugleich aber auch besonders wichtige Forschungsaufgabe. Sie besteht darin, den Bedarf an Maßnahmen und Versorgungsleistungen sowohl in qualitativer als auch in quantitativer Hinsicht zu analysieren und geeignete „Bedarfsindikatoren" zu entwickeln: In welchen Bevölkerungsgruppen besteht welcher Bedarf an präventiven, kurativen, unterstützenden und rehabilitativen Diensten, und von welchen Bereichen des Gesundheitswesens (professionelles System, soziale Dienste, Laiensystem) können solche Dienste am besten erbracht werden? Wie können neue Wege für die notwendige Zusammenarbeit der unterschiedlichen Bereiche organisiert und gestaltet werden? Im Hinblick auf präventives Handeln ergeben sich dabei Fragen zu den Einflüssen der Organisationsformen. Ohne detailliertere Antworten auf diese Fragen ist es nicht möglich, die Versorgung adäquat zu bewerten und an Wandlungen der Bedarfsstruktur anzupassen (Abbau von Über- und Unterversorgung), die aus Änderungen der Morbidität, des Krankheits- und Bewältigungsverhaltens sowie der demographischen Gegebenheiten resultieren.

Die Zusammenarbeit im Gesundheitssektor, und zwar sowohl in den einzelnen Teilbereichen als auch in ihren wechselseitigen Bezügen innerhalb und außerhalb des Gesamtsystems, stellt eine außerordentlich komplexe Aufgabe dar, bei der u. a. die Forderung nach Zugänglichkeit und Inanspruchnahme bedarfsgerechter Versorgungsleistungen für alle vereinbar sein muß mit der volkswirtschaftlichen Finanzierbarkeit und einem überprüfbar positiven Einfluß auf den Gesundheitszustand der Bevölkerung.

Die Verfügbarkeit zuverlässiger medizinischer und ökonomischer Orientierungsdaten, auf deren Basis Ziele vereinbart werden können, stellt deshalb eine unabdingbare Voraussetzung für eine effektive und effiziente Organisation des Versorgungssystems dar. Die Entwicklung, Bewertung und kontinuierliche Erhebung solcher Orientierungsdaten gehört zu den vorrangigen Forschungsaufgaben: die wichtigsten hier geforderten Einzeldisziplinen sind Epidemiologie, Gesundheitssystem- und Organisationsforschung, Gesundheitsökonomie, Medizinsoziologie und Sozialforschung, medizinische Informatik.

Zu den wichtigsten Anknüpfungspunkten für die Forschung zählen darüber hinaus die Transparenz von Kosten und Leistungen und die Qualitätssicherung. Die Abläufe der Leistungserbringung werden in wachsendem Maße durch Verfahren der Informationsverarbeitung unterstützt; dadurch gewinnt die medizinische Informatik mit den Aufgabenbereichen Kommunikation, Konsultation und Evaluation zunehmend an Bedeutung. Zu den vorrangigen Forschungsbereichen zählt schließlich v. a. die Gesundheitsökonomie: das Versorgungssystem ist offenkundig an der Grenze seiner Finanzierbarkeit angelangt, und die Frage nach der Kosten-Nutzen-Relation durchzieht alle Bereiche, angefangen von der Bedarfsdefinition und -planung bis hin zur Qualitätssicherung.

Präventiven Maßnahmen ist nicht nur im Hinblick auf ihre wissenschaftliche Untermauerung, sondern auch wegen ihrer ökonomischen Auswirkungen größere Aufmerksamkeit zu schenken.

Bei der Organisation des Gesundheitssystems werden zukünftig verstärkt bisher vernachlässigte Bedingungen außerhalb des Versorgungssystems (wie z. B. Selbsthilfezusammenschlüsse, Arbeits- und Wohnverhältnisse, Ernährungsgewohnheiten, Arbeitslosigkeit, Verkehrssicherheit, Beschäftigungswirkung des Gesundheitswesens u. ä.) und die Einflüsse aus anderen gesellschaftlichen Teilbereichen stärker berücksichtigt werden müssen. Zu nennen sind hier v. a. Leistungen zur gesundheitlichen Betreuung und Strategien der Krankheitsbewältigung, die außerhalb der professionellen medizinischen Versorgung stattfinden (Familie, Selbst- und Nachbarschaftshilfe). Hier liegt ein Aufgabengebiet für die Entwicklung und Erprobung neuer Modelle der gesundheitlichen Versorgung, die auch zu erweiterten Aufgabenstellungen des öffentlichen Gesundheitsdienstes und darüber hinaus auf Gemeindeebene führen könnten.

Weitere Forschungsfragen beziehen sich auf die gesamtwirtschaftlichen Auswirkungen von Ausgabenentwicklungen im Gesundheitswesen und insbesondere in der gesetzlichen Krankenversicherung, auf organisatorische Möglichkeiten der Qualitätssicherung, auf Erprobungsmöglichkeiten für präventive Ansätze und auf die volkswirtschaftlichen Kosten von Krankheiten sowie Kriterien und Möglichkeiten zu ihrer Senkung.

Besonderer Aufmerksamkeit bedarf dabei die Ausbildung von qualifiziertem Forschungspersonal im Bereich des Gesundheitswesens. Die in den vorhergehenden Abschnitten genannten Forschungsgebiete sind in der Bundesrepublik Deutschland nicht in ausreichendem Maße entwickelt und erfordern langfristige Anstrengungen zur Ausbildung qualifizierter Forscher. In diesem Zusammenhang ist auch an den Beitrag zu denken, den die bei den angelsächsischen "Schools of Public Health" angesiedelte Forschung leistet.

Entscheidungshilfen für eine zielorientierte Gesundheitspolitik

Eine gesundheitspolitisch bedeutsame Forschungsaufgabe ist daher die Entwicklung einer Gesundheitsberichterstattung, die über die konventionellen Medizinalstatistiken hinausgeht und aggregierte Daten kontinuierlich zur Verfügung stellt und auswertet. Die Aufgabe wird dadurch besonders anspruchsvoll, daß eine Gesundheitsberichterstattung, die Grundlagen für gesundheitspolitische Entscheidungen liefern kann, die Dimension des Gesundheitszustandes der Bevölkerung (u. a. Indikatoren der Morbidität, Mortalität, Risikofaktoren) einerseits und die Dimension des Versorgungssystems (u. a. Leistungserbringung, Inanspruchnahme, Kosten) andererseits zueinander in Beziehung setzen und verknüpft bewerten muß.

Eine mit der Berichterstattung eng verbundene Aufgabe ist die Analyse langfristiger Entwicklungstrends im Hinblick auf den Gesundheitszustand in der Bevölkerung und die Struktur des Versorgungssystems. Beide Komplexe werden von demographischen Entwicklungen, Änderungen des „Krankheitspanoramas", Fortschritten in Diagnose und Therapie, konjunkturellen Entwicklungen und einer Vielzahl anderer Faktoren beeinflußt. Nicht zuletzt sind es die gesundheitspolitischen Entscheidungen selbst, die die Entwicklung des Gesundheitswesens prägen. Die Entscheidungen vorzubereiten und ihre Ergebnisse auszuwerten, ist eine wichtige Aufgabe der Forschung.

Wichtig für die Wirksamkeit dieser Entscheidungshilfe wird daher sein, daß zwischen der Wissenschaft und der Politik eine engere Verbindung hergestellt wird.

In diesem Zusammenhang ist außerdem die Entwicklung und Erprobung neuer Organisationsmodelle für Teilbereiche des Gesundheitswesens zu nennen. In anderen Ländern gibt es beispielsweise Entwicklungen, die auf eine gezielte Erweiterung des Primärversorgungssektors ausgerichtet sind; sie lassen sich charakterisieren durch Stichworte wie: Gemeindezentrierung, Integration der – weniger – spezialisierten kurativen Leistungen mit präventiven, pflegerischen, unterstützenden und rehabilitativen Diensten sowie durch „Laienbeteiligung" bei der Planung und Organisation des Gesundheitswesens auf der Gemeindeebene. Vielversprechend erscheint dabei v. a. die Möglichkeit, langfristige Hospitalisierungen und die damit verbundene soziale Isolierung der Patienten zu vermeiden oder zumindest zu verringern. Möglicherweise liegt in solchen Modellen eine Antwort auf sich abzeichnende Änderungen der Bedarfsstruktur, die aus dem wachsenden Anteil alter Menschen und der hohen Prävalenz chronischer Krankheiten resultieren. Hier wären in der Bundesrepublik Deutschland Modellvorhaben zu erwägen, die eine entsprechende Ausweitung der Primärversorgung erproben und auf Vereinbarkeit mit dem bestehenden System der ambulanten Versorgung prüfen.

Wichtige Forschungsaufgaben sind die Stärkung wettbewerblicher Elemente und Flexibilisierungen in der gesetzlichen Krankenversicherung, die Orientierung von Leistungen und Ausgaben an gesundheitlichen Zielen und die Schaffung wirksamer Anreize für Leistungserbringer, Versicherte und Krankenkassen.